R
RC
731
R468

DO NOT REMOVE FROM LIBRARY

**SOUTH COLLEGE**
709 Mall Blvd.
Savannah, GA 31406

# Respiratory Diseases and Disorders Sourcebook

# Respiratory Diseases and Disorders Sourcebook

Basic Information about Respiratory Diseases and Disorders Including Asthma, Cystic Fibrosis, Pneumonia, the Common Cold, Influenza, and Others, Featuring Facts about the Respiratory System, Statistical and Demographic Data, Treatments, Self-Help Management Suggestions, and Current Research Initiatives.

**Health Reference Series**
**Volume Six**

Edited by
Allan R. Cook and
Peter D. Dresser

Omnigraphics, Inc. • Penobscot Building • Detroit, MI 48226

1995

## BIBLIOGRAPHIC NOTE

This volume contains individual publications issued by the National Institutes of Health (NIH), its sister agencies, and sub-agencies. Numbered publications in this category are: NIH 91-2650; 91-3093; 93-2020; 93-2391; 93-2966; 93-2997; 93-3279; 93-3511; 93-3544 94-1647. Also included are numbered information sheets from the National Sudden Infant Death Syndrome Resource Center (NSIDSRC): #1; 3; and 4, and numbered publications from U.S. Department of Health and Human Services (DHHS): 86-102; 90-8416, and from the U.S. Congress Office of Technology Assessment (OTA): BA-532. The volume also includes unnumbered publications from the Centers for Disease Control (CDC), DHHS, National Cancer Institute (NCI), the NIH, National Institute of Allergies and Infectious Diseases (NIAID), National Heart, Lung, and Blood Institute (NHLBI), unnumbered information sheets from NSIDSRC along with selected articles from National Center for Research Resources *Reporter*, the CDC's *Morbidity and Mortality Weekly Report,* and the FDA's *Consumer*. In addition, the volume includes copyrighted articles from the American Lung Association: 0029; 0139; 0151; 0201; 0204; 0206; 0208; 0213; 0215; 0301; 0426; 0427; 0619; 0694; 1186; 1230; 1551; 1552; and unnumbered, copyrighted articles from the Cystic Fibrosis Foundation and McNeil Pharmaceutical. These are used by permission.

Allan R. Cook
Peter D. Dresser
Editors

Omnigraphics, Inc.

Matthew P. Barbour, *Production Coordinator*
Laurie Lanzen Harris, *Vice President, Editorial*
Peter E. Ruffner, *Vice President, Administration*
James A. Sellgren, *Vice President, Operations and Finance*
Jane J. Steele, *Vice President, Research*

Frederick G. Ruffner, Jr., Publisher
Copyright © 1995 Omnigraphics, Inc.

**Library of Congress Cataloging-in-Publication Data**

Respiratory diseases and disorders Sourcebook : basic information about respiratory diseases and disorders including asthma, cystic fibrosis, pneumonia,the common cold, influenza, and others
. . . / edited byAllan R. Cook and Peter D. Dresser.
    p. cm. — (Health reference series ; v. 6)
Includes bibliographical references and index.
ISBN 0-7808-0037-0 (lib. bdg. : alk. paper)
    1. Respiratory organs—Diseases.  I. Cook, Allan R.  II. Dresser, Peter D.  III. Series.
RC731.R468  1995
616.2—dc20                                                          95-19214
                                                                      CIP

∞

This book is printed on acid-free paper meeting the ANSI Z39.48 Standard. The infinity symbol that appears above indicates that the paper in this book meets that standard.

Printed in the United States of America

# Contents

Preface ............................................................................... xi
Diagram of the Lungs ..................................................... xiii

## Introduction: Understanding the Respiratory System

Chapter 1—The Lungs — Medicine for the Layman ............ 3

## Part I: Common Respiratory Diseases and Disorders

Chapter 2—Asthma ........................................................... 13

       Section 2. 1—Asthma Statistics Data Sheet ......... 14
       Section 2. 2—What You Need to Know About
                   Asthma ............................................ 18
       Section 2. 3—More Than Snuffles:
                   Childhood Asthma .......................... 35
       Section 2. 4—Let's Talk About Asthma:
                   A Guide for Teens .......................... 43
       Section 2. 5—Asthma...At My Age? Facts About
                   Asthma for Older Americans ......... 62
       Section 2. 6—Being a Sport with Exercise-
                   Induced Asthma ............................. 69
       Section 2. 7—Managing Asthma:
                   A Guide for Schools ....................... 73

## Chapter 2—Asthma, continued

Section 2. 8—Management of Asthma During
          Pregnancy ......................................... 85
Section 2. 9—Good News and Great Tips for
          Pregnant Women with Asthma ... 114
Section 2.10—How to Control Asthma Triggers  117
Section 2.11—How to Use a Metered-Dose
          Inhaler ............................................. 123
Section 2.12—How to Use a Peak Flow Meter ... 126
Section 2.13—My Weekly Asthma and
          Peak Flow Diary ........................... 130
Section 2.14—How to Take Your Medicine:
          Adrenegenic Bronchodilators ....... 132
Section 2.15—Asthma Education and Pre-
          vention Materials and Resources  137

## Chapter 3—Chronic Obstructive Pulmonary Disease (COPD) .. 159

Section 3. 1—Chronic Obstructive Pulmonary
          Disease ........................................... 160
Section 3. 2—Facts About Chronic Bronchitis ... 177
Section 3. 3—Facts About Chronic Cough .......... 180
Section 3. 4—Facts About Emphysemia ............. 182
Section 3. 5—Facts about ATT Deficiency-
          Related Emphysema .................... 185
Section 3. 6—Around the Clock with COPD ...... 188

## Chapter 4—Common Cold and Influenza .................................... 211

Section 4. 1—The Common Cold—
          Or Is It the Flu? ........................... 212
Section 4. 2—How to Take Your Medicine:
          Antihistamines ............................. 221
Section 4. 3—Modern Pharmacy's Answer to
          Chicken Soup ................................ 224
Section 4.4—How to Avoid the Flu ..................... 231

## Chapter 5—Cystic Fibrosis ........................................................... 239

Section 5. 1—An Introduction to Cystic Fibrosis
          for Patients and Families ............. 240
Section 5. 2—Living with Cystic Fibrosis: Family
          Guide to Nutrition ........................ 271

## Chapter 5—Cystic Fibrosis, continued

Section 5. 3—Teacher's Guide to CF ............... 291
Section 5. 4—Introduction to Chest Physical
 Therapy ......................................... 294
Section 5. 5—CF Gene: A Fifty-Year Search ...... 315
Section 5. 6—Cystic Fibrosis: Tests, Treatments
 Improve Survival ........................ 320
Section 5. 7—FDA Licenses Cystic Fibrosis
 Treatment ..................................... 330
Section 5. 8—CF and DNA Tests: Implications
 of Carrier Screening .................... 331

## Chapter 6—Histoplasmosis ......................................... 369

## Chapter 7—Pneumonia and Legionnaires' Disease ................... 375

Section 7. 1—Facts About Pneumonia ............... 376
Section 7. 2—Pneumonia Prevention:
 It's Worth a Shot .......................... 382
Section 7. 3—Questions and Answers on
 Legionnaires' Disease ................... 386
Section 7. 4—Legionnaires' and Misters ........... 388
Section 7. 5—Outbreak of Legionnaires' Disease
 Associated with a Cruise Ship ..... 389
Section 7. 6—Legionnaires' Disease Associated
 with Cooling Towers .................... 390

## Chapter 8—Pulmonary Disorders ............................................... 395

Section 8. 1—Pulmonary Embolism: Difficult
 but Crucial Diagnosis ................... 396
Section 8. 2—Primary Pulmonary
 Hypertension ............................... 404
Section 8. 3—Facts about Idiopathic Pulmonary
 Fibrosis ........................................ 414

## Chapter 9—Respiratory Distress Syndrome (RDS)—Infants .... 421

Section 9. 1—Preterm Babies: Get a Double
 Breath of Life ............................... 422
Section 9. 2—Antiviral Drug Benefits Infants
 with Several Respiratory Disease 428

Chapter 9—(RDS)—Infants, continued

    Section 9. 3—Calf Extract Benefits Premature Infants .............................................. 431

Chapter 10—Sarcoidosis ................................................................ 435

Chapter 11—Breathing Disorders During Sleep ......................... 449

Chapter 12—Sudden Infant Death Syndrome (SIDS) and Apparent Life-Threatening Events (ALTE) .......... 469

    Section 12.1—What is SIDS? ............................... 470
    Section 12.2—Facts about Apnea and Other Apparent Life-Threatening Events ............................................. 475
    Section 12.3—Infant Positioning and SIDS ........ 479
    Section 12.4—The Grief of Children ................... 480
    Section 12.5—Infant Apnea Monitors Help Parents Breathe Easy ................... 486

Chapter 13—Tuberculosis .............................................................. 495

    Section 13.1—Questions and Answers About TB ....................................... 496
    Section 13.2—Tuberculosis: Romantic Killer Returns to Challenge Modern Medicine Once More ..................... 508
    Section 13.4—TB Still a Problem ........................ 510
    Section 13.3—Tuberculosis: What Health Care Workers Should Know ................. 531

Chapter 14—Work Related Disorders ........................................... 539

    Section 14.1—Lung Hazards in the Work Place 540
    Section 14.2—Farmers' Lung: Agricultural Lung Hazards ............................. 545
    Section 14.3—Asbestos ......................................... 554
    Section 14.4—Black Lung: Coal Worker's Pneumoconiosis and Exposure to Other Carbonaceous Dusts ....... 559
    Section 14.5—Facts About Fiberglass ................ 567
    Section 14.6—Irritant Gases ............................... 571
    Section 14.7—Silicosis ......................................... 575

## Part II: Controlling Your Breathing Environment

Chapter 15—Biological Agents ....................................................... 581

Chapter 16—Ozone Air Pollution .................................................. 585
Chapter 17—Benefits and Concerns with the Use
  of Humidifiers ........................................................... 589

  Section 17.1—Humidifiers Increase Moisture—
    and Sometimes Bacteria .............. 590
  Section 17.2—Precautions with Certain
    Ventilators, Humidifiers .............. 597

Chapter 18—Environmental Tobacco Smoke ............................... 599

Chapter 19—Health Benefits of Smoking Cessation:
  Report of the Surgeon General, 1990 .................... 607

Chapter 20—Clearing the Air: How to Quit Smoking and
  Quit for Keeps ......................................................... 619

Chapter 21—I Mind Very Much If You Smoke ........................... 641

## Part III: Current Research into Respiratory Illness, Treatment and Prevention

Chapter 22—Respiratory Problems in Minorities ...................... 651

  Section 22.1—Asthma in Minorities ................... 652
  Section 22.2—African Americans and Smoking
    at a Glance ................................... 660
  Section 22.3—Alaska Natives Fight TB ............ 674
  Section 22.4—Minorities Over-Represented in
    Lung Diseases ............................... 676
  Section 22.5—Smoking Education Program
    Sends Out Stop Smoking
    Message ......................................... 678
  Section 22.6—Link Between Respiratory
    Disease and Poverty Needs
    Study ............................................. 680

Chapter 23—Research Highlights ................................................. 683

        Section 23.1—Asthma Allergens: Examining the Role of Eosinophils ................. 684
        Section 23.2—A Trigger for Asthma at the Tip of Your Toes ............................ 688
        Section 23.3—Respiratory Illness Associated with Inhalation of Mushroom Spores ............................................. 689

Chapter 24—New Drugs, Treatments, and Problems ................. 691

        Section 24.1—Specialists Recommend Change in Asthma Treatment ..................... 692
        Section 24.2—FDA Licenses Cystic Fibrosis Treatment ...................................... 693
        Section 24.3—Prevalence of Penicillin-Resistant Streptococcus ................ 694
        Section 24.4—Pneumococcal Polysaccharide Vaccine Recommendations of the Immunization Practices Advisory Committee ......................................... 697
        Section 24.5—Combination TB Drug Approved  705

Chapter 25—Single and Double Lung Transplantation ............. 707

## Part IV: Glossary

Chapter 26—Glossary of Medical Terms ..................................... 717

**Index** ................................................................................................ 757

# Preface

## About This Book

This book contains numerous publications produced by a wide variety of government and private agencies including National Institutes of Health (NIH), the National Sudden Infant Death Syndrome Resource Center (NSIDSRC), the Department of Health and Human Services (DHHS), the U.S. Congress Office of Technology Assessment (OTA), National Institute of Allergies and Infectious Diseases (NIAID), National Heart, Lung, and Blood Institute (NHLBI), the Centers for Disease Control (CDC), National Cancer Institute (NCI), the American Lung Association, the Cystic Fibrosis Foundation and McNeil Pharmaceutical. The documents chosen present basic medical information for the interested layperson and for patients and their families coping with respiratory diseases or disorders.

## How To Use This Book

The introduction describes the operation of the respiratory system, how doctors detect respiratory problems, and some common sources of respiratory diseases and disorders. A diagram of the respiratory system, placed on page xiii provides a convenient visual reference for the entire volume.

# Respiratory Diseases and Disorders Sourcebook

The Parts of this volume are arranged in broad topic areas. Indvidual chapters focus on specific areas of concern. In order to provide complete information, many chapters contain several sections from a variety of reprinted documents from government and private sources. To help you quickly identify areas of interest, a "Chapter Contents" listing appears at the beginning of each chapter containing more than a single document.

Part I: *Common Respiratory Diseases and Disorders* provides detailed information on specific respiratory problems, their detection and treatment, and ways to control symptoms and discomfort. The chapters include statistical data on selected individual conditions and examine some social issues like carrier screening, gene therapy and the effects of peer pressure on effective asthma management. For ease of use, the diseases and disorders are presented in alphabetical order.

Part II: *Controlling Your Breathing Environment* pinpoints common breathing irritants that can be eliminated or minimized in the home and at work. It provides suggestions for identifying and regulating those important sources of respiratory disease.

Part III: *Current Research into Respiratory Illness, Treatment, and Prevention* highlights specific research initiatives and concerns, and presents some topics in the growing field of minority issues.

Part VI: *Glossary* provides a listing and short explanation of some important medical terms used throughout the volume.

## Acknowledgements

The editors wish to thank Margaret Mary Missar for her determined search of medical libraries and government offices which resulted in the documents that make up this volume, Karen Bellenir for her technical assistance and advice, and Bruce the Scanman for his transformational expertise.

## Respiratory Diseases and Disorders Sourcebook

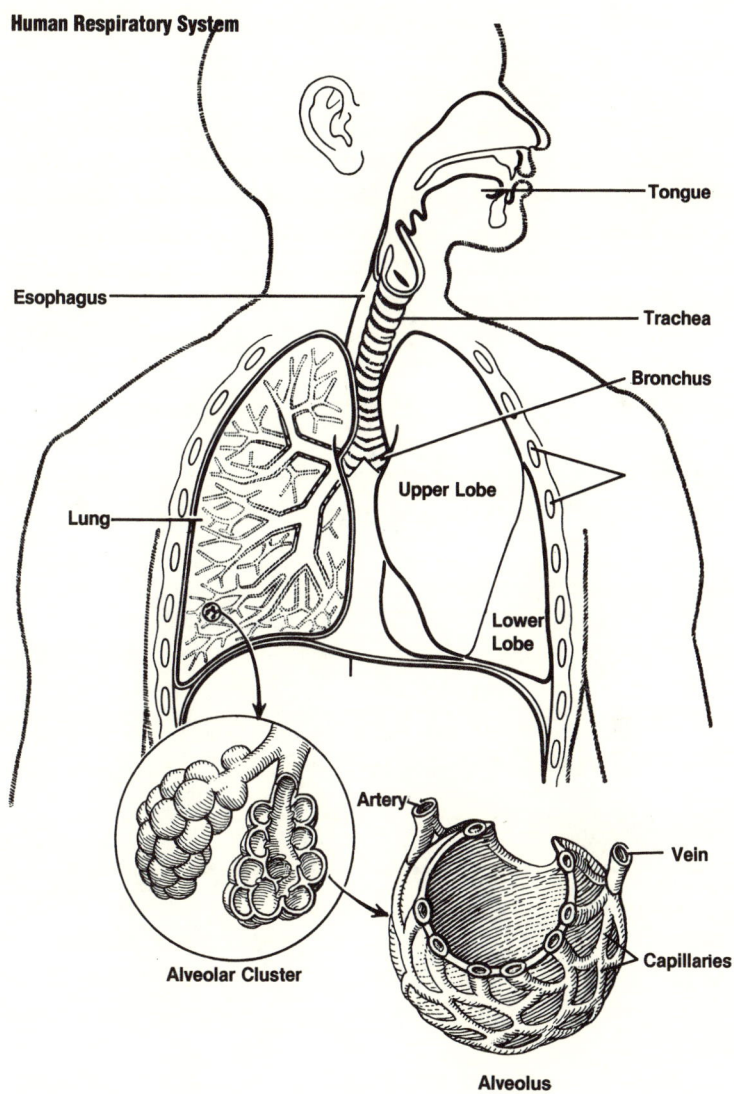

# Introduction

# Understanding the Respiratory System

## Chapter 1

# *The Lungs—*
# *Medicine for the Layman*

The lungs play a critical role in the function of the body. Each time you run up a flight of stairs, sprint to catch a bus, or shovel snow off the walk, you feel the effects of the body's demand on the lungs.

The function of the lungs is to exchange gases between the atmosphere and the body. The lungs must continuously exhale carbon dioxide, a waste product of our cells, and inhale oxygen for those cells. After three to five minutes without oxygen, the cells in the vital organs of our bodies will die.

When you are short of breath, it's your body's signal to exchange more gases with the atmosphere. The more demands you put on your body, the more the lungs need to work.

The lungs occupy most of the body structure of the chest cavity called the thorax. The heart, which is between the lungs, is the only other major organ occupying the thorax. Although fairly large, the lungs weigh only about two pounds and are filled, of course, with air.

The lungs are interdependent with two other systems in the body—the heart and the blood. The heart continuously pumps oxygen carrying red blood cells through the blood vessels (arteries, veins, and capillaries). As the red blood cells reach the cells in the tissues of our body, they deposit oxygen and pick up the waste product, carbon dioxide. Carbon dioxide is picked up by the liquid plasma and by the red blood cells and then transported back to the lungs where the carbon dioxide is unloaded and sent out to the atmosphere.

---

NIH Pub. Medicine for the Layman.

## How the Lungs Function

The air containing oxygen comes in through the main passageway in the throat and travels through the tubular structures of the tracheobronchial tree into the chest to the distal, or far, parts of the lungs.

The main trunk, the trachea or windpipe, divides into two branches, one leading to the right lung and the other into the left lung. From each branch (bronchus) progressively smaller tubes divide into thousands of branch-like tubes, and subdivide into millions of bronchioles, which are the smallest tubes of the tracheobronchial tree. The bronchioles end in tiny air sacs called alveoli. There are about 300 million alveoli in the lungs of the human adult. In the alveoli, oxygen from the atmosphere is exchanged for carbon dioxide from the body cells.

The blood travels through a finely meshed network of capillaries within the walls of the alveoli. When the red blood cells reach the alveoli, they deposit carbon dioxide and pick up oxygen.

Blood carrying waste carbon dioxide from the body cells is pumped from the right side of the heart through the pulmonary artery to the alveoli capillaries. This blood is blue because it carries very little oxygen. As this blood reaches the alveoli, carbon dioxide passes through thin capillary and alveoli walls to the alveoli sacs. At the same time oxygen passes from the alveoli to the oxygen-depleted blood.

The blood, now red because it carries a great deal of oxygen, travels through the pulmonary vein back to the heart, which pumps the oxygenated blood to the cells throughout the body.

The carbon dioxide, discharged by the blood into the alveoli, travels up the tracheobronchial tree and is breathed out into the atmosphere.

There is a partial vacuum in your lungs when you take a breath causing air to rush in. The muscles of the chest pull the chest wall out; and the diaphragm, a muscle separating the chest cavity from the abdominal contents, moves down, which increases the volume of the chest cavity. As a consequence, the air pressure in the chest cavity is lowered; and air rushes in to equalize the pressure.

When you breathe out, the chest muscles relax, causing the ribs to drop and decrease the volume of the chest cavity. The diaphragm muscles also relax, causing the diaphragm to rise to its resting position. The accompanying decrease in the size of the thorax raises the air pressure; and air is forced out of the air sacs of the lungs.

The breathing-in-and-out process takes place about 12-15 times a minute.

## How the Lungs Protect Us

The breathing process is complicated by the fact that the air we breathe is not perfect. In a mechanized urban society automobiles, factories, and many other devices of civilization can pollute the air with substances containing sulfur, particulates (which can be smaller than red blood cells), carbon monoxide, the oxides of nitrogen, hydrocarbons, and material called oxidants.

Two types of cells line the trachea to protect against harmful substances. The goblet cells line the airways like a blanket and produce mucus. The mucus traps harmful substances that might be inhaled, such as pollutants, other particulates, and the more dangerous bacteria and other infectious agents.

The other cell type is called the ciliated cell, containing finger-like projections that sweep the mucus with a wave-like motion. This moves the mucus up toward the throat where it can be cleared out of the airways into the mouth and unconsciously swallowed.

Macrophages, other cells that defend the body, are found in the distal part of the lungs in the alveoli. These scavenger cells have many projections and are able to destroy harmful objects by swallowing them or by releasing enzymes.

## How Physicians Evaluate Your Lungs

Your physician has a number of ways to determine if your lungs are healthy: physical examination; medical history; chest x-rays; pulmonary function tests; and bronchoscopy. If your lungs are not working properly, the doctor can intervene before damage occurs.

**Medical History.** By taking your medical history, the doctor will learn if your lungs have been exposed to harmful substances. The doctor will want to know about the area in which you live, any history of respiratory infection, and any allergies.

**Physical Examination.** After taking your medical history, the doctor will thump your chest, then listen to your lungs with the stethoscope. With the stethoscope placed on the chest, the physician can hear the air rushing into the air sacs and being pushed out while you inhale and exhale. The physician can hear whether or not your lungs are functioning normally. If not, the physician hears sounds that are characteristic of specific disorders and thus can make a differential diagnosis.

**X-Rays.** Another technique for examining the lungs is the x-ray. The chest x-ray provides a picture of the organs of the chest area (the heart, the trachea branching off into the smaller breathing tubes, and the lungs). The x-ray can show lung malfunction or pinpoint the source of a problem.

**Pulmonary Function Test.** The pulmonary function test helps the physician determine how efficiently the lungs work. In one procedure the patient breathes into a machine, and the rate of inhalation and exhalation is recorded. Another more precise test measures the amount of oxygen and carbon dioxide present in the blood during exercise. The patient walks on a treadmill and a fine needle is placed in the artery to draw blood that is analyzed for oxygen and carbon dioxide levels.

**Bronchoscopy.** The technique of putting a tube into the bronchi to see into the breathing apparatus is called bronchoscopy. After the patient inhales an anesthetic to prevent any discomfort, the bronchoscope is guided through the patient's nose into the tracheobronchial tree. The flexible instrument enables light to travel in curved paths, thus permitting the physician to see the breathing structures. The physician can regulate the tip of the bronchoscope to control its direction and illuminate a particular part of the lung.

Several adaptions to the bronchoscope have been developed to enhance the diagnosis and treatment of lung disorders. The bronchoscope can be used to obtain a sample of lung fluid and cells. Fluid is placed in the lung and then suctioned back.

The bronchoscope also can be adapted to take a picture of the tracheobronchial tract. This feature has made the bronchoscope a useful tool for detecting problems before symptoms appear as in the case of asymptomatic tumors. For such problems another adaptation to the flexible fiber-optic bronchoscope can be used to remove small pieces of tissue, which are then biopsied.

Still another attachment to the bronchoscope permits removal of food or objects that have been aspirated into the lungs. This procedure can spare the patient from surgery.

## Industrial Causes of Lung Disease

Sometimes during a medical examination it is fairly obvious that a patient has been inhaling a harmful substance. The risk of lung damage from harmful materials depends on the sensitivity of the individual, the degree of exposure, and the kind of material that is inhaled.

Damage to coal miners' lungs is a serious and costly national health problem. Benefits to coal miners with black lung disease exceed $1 billion a year.

Workers in other industries also risk lung damage. In this country 800,000 people are exposed to cotton dust in mills. More than 1,000,000 workers are exposed to silica in the mining, stonecutting, and construction industries. Twenty thousand workers are exposed to talc, another lung irritant, in the rubber and cosmetic industries; and 250,000 workers are exposed to asbestos.

## Non-Industrial Causes of Lung Disease

Industrial agents are not the only substances capable of causing lung damage. Living matter, which is organic, can cause a number of lung diseases known collectively as hypersensitivity pneumonitis.

Hypersensitivity pneumonitis affects one in 1,000 persons exposed to disease-causing materials from a number of sources.

Organisms that grow in moldy hay can cause a hypersensitivity pneumonitis in farmers; this disorder is known as "farmer's lung." These same organisms can grow in air conditioners and humidifiers. These organisms also are found in sauna baths where they can grow in the wooden water barrel.

## Cigarette Smoking

Smoking cigarettes is the worst thing you can do to your lungs. Lung cancer, emphysema, chronic bronchitis, heart disease, and peripheral vascular disease are all caused by smoking cigarettes. Evidence from research associates cigarette smoking with higher death rates. Deaths among cigarette smokers in this country exceed the expected mortality rate by 60 percent.

Cigarette smoking is associated with the majority of lung cancers. Lung cancer is the major cancer in men and is increasingly prevalent in women. Seventy-five percent of cases of chronic bronchitis and emphysema are associated with cigarette smoking.

## New Diagnostic Techniques

Even with all the methodologies just described, the physician cannot always obtain all of the information needed to determine how well the lungs are working.

Fortunately, some new methods to permit the physician to monitor breathing activity of the lung have been developed at the National Institutes of Health. In these procedures, the patient inhales radioactive gas and is placed in front of a camera that takes picture information of the radioactive gas in the lungs. The picture information is fed into a computer that translates the information into a movie that shows the breathing activity of the lungs.

Using these techniques to observe the movement of gas in and out of the lungs, the physician is able to see if any parts of the lung are not functioning normally.

## How Can You Tell Something Is Wrong?

There are a number of signs and symptoms that indicate problems. Should they appear, call your physician.

- Shortness of breath is a warning signal. Do not worry about the shortness of breath that develops after rapidly running up several flights of stairs, since even the healthiest person will feel short of breath under those conditions. However, be concerned about shortness of breath that happens during routine activities that have not caused breathing difficulty in the past.

- Coughing is a significant symptom of lung disorder. While it is not necessary to worry about a cough accompanying a cold, a chronic cough is not normal and should not be ignored.

- Sputum production, even a small amount, particularly in the early morning, is not normal; it is a sign that you should see a physician.

### The Lungs—Medicine for the Layman

- Blood coughed up is a sign of a serious problem that should receive medical attention immediately.

- Chest pain can have a number of causes, including chronic lung disorders and infection in the lung. Any chest pain should be attended to immediately by a physician.

## How to Protect Your Lungs

First of all, do not smoke.

Work to keep your atmosphere clean; environmental pollutants damage the lung.

Avoid becoming overweight. The heavier a person is, the more the lungs have to work to supply oxygen and to expel carbon dioxide. Extra weight around the waist can push against the diaphragm and make breathing more difficult.

Finally, with any symptoms of lung disease—cough, sputum, shortness of breath, blood coughed up, or chest pain—see your physician immediately. In the early stages, many lung diseases can be treated to prevent serious lung damage. If you wait, it may be too late.

# Part I

# Common Respiratory Diseases and Disorders

# Chapter 2

# *Asthma*

## *Chapter Contents*

Section 2. 1—Asthma Statistics Data Sheet .................................. 14
Section 2. 2—What You Need to Know About Asthma ................. 18
Section 2. 3—More Than Snuffles: Childhood Asthma ................. 35
Section 2. 4—Let's Talk About Asthma: A Guide for Teens ......... 43
Section 2. 5—Asthma...At My Age? Facts About Asthma
　　　　　　　for Older Americans ...................................................... 62
Section 2. 6—Being a Sport with Exercise-Induced Asthma ........ 69
Section 2. 7—Managing Asthma: A Guide for Schools ................. 73
Section 2. 8—Management of Asthma During Pregnancy ............ 85
Section 2. 9—Good News and Great Tips for Pregnant
　　　　　　　Women with Asthma ................................................. 114
Section 2.10—How to Control Asthma Triggers ......................... 117
Section 2.11—How to Use a Metered-Dose Inhaler .................... 123
Section 2.12—How to Use a Peak Flow Meter ............................ 126
Section 2.13—My Weekly Asthma and Peak Flow Diary ........... 130
Section 2.14—How to Take Your Medicine:
　　　　　　　Adrenegenic Bronchodilators ............................... 132
Section 2.15—Asthma Education and Prevention Materials
　　　　　　　and Resources ........................................................ 137

## Section 2.1

# *Asthma Statistics*

Source: U.S. Department of Health and Human Services, May 1992.

Asthma is a serious chronic condition, affecting almost 12 million Americans. People with asthma experience well over 100 million days of restricted activity annually, and costs for asthma care exceed $4.6 billion a year.

The National Heart, Lung, and Blood Institute has initiated the National Asthma Education Program (NAEP) to educate asthma patients, health professionals, and the public about asthma and its treatment. To assist in planning and evaluation of the NAEP, and to encourage program planners, health administrators, and others to become more involved in asthma education, the NAEP has developed this information on Asthma Statistics to indicate the magnitude of the problem.

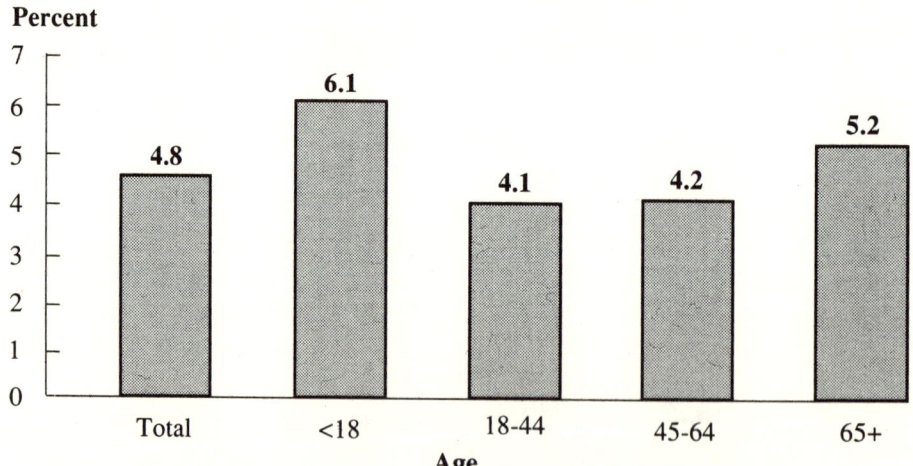

Source: *National Health Interview Survey, National Center for Health Statistics*

**Figure 2.1** Prevalence of Asthma by Age, 1989

## Asthma

### Prevalence

Asthma is much more prevalent among children than adults. Of the 12 million Americans that have asthma, about 4 million of them are under the age of 18. In 1989, the prevalence of asthma among persons under 18 was 6.1 percent compared with 4.8 percent among all other age groups (Figure 2.1). Overall, there is little difference in asthma prevalence by sex (almost 5 percent for both men and women). The percent of blacks with asthma is higher than the percent of whites with the condition (5.3 vs. 4.7 percent, respectively).

The reported prevalence of asthma is increasing. Between 1979 and 1989, the percent of the population with asthma increased by 60 percent (Figure 2.2). This represents an increase in prevalence from 3 percent of the population in 1979 to 4.8 percent in 1989. Increases in the prevalence of asthma have been reported in all age, race, and sex groups.

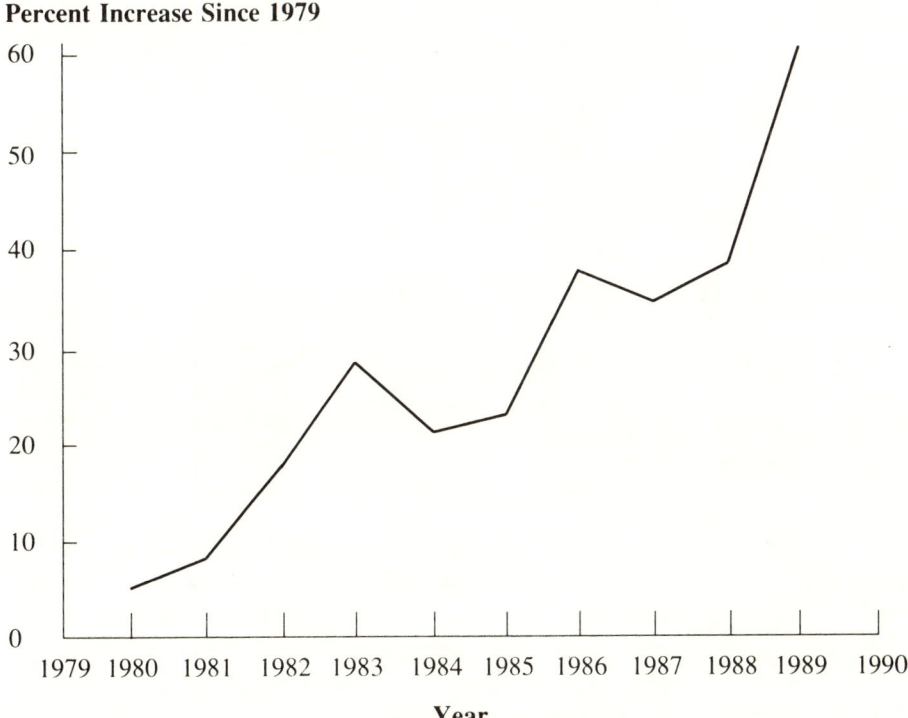

Source: National Health Interview Survey. National Center for Health Statistics

**Figure 2.2** Trends in Asthma Prevalence Percent Increase Since 1979

## Physician Visits

In 1988 there were almost 15 million visits to physicians for asthma. About 35 percent of these visits were made by patients under 20 years of age. Figure 2.3 shows the distribution of physician visits for asthma according to the patients' age.

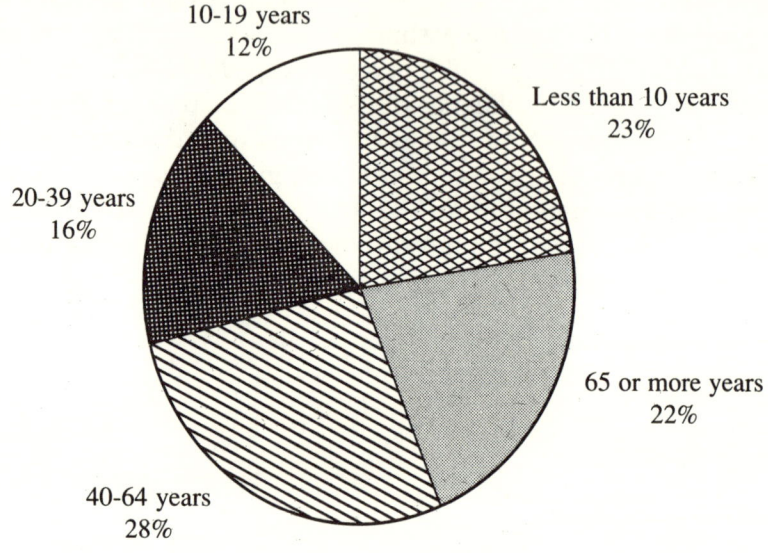

Source: National Disease and Therapeutic Index, IMS America, Ltd.

**Figure 2.3** Distribution of Physician Visits for Asthma by Patient Age, July 1988—June 1989

## Hospitalizations

In 1989, there were over 479,000 hospitalizations in which asthma was the first-listed diagnosis. Hospitalizations for asthma have been increasing among children. For example, from 1979 to 1989, the hospital discharge rate with asthma as the first-listed diagnosis rose 56 percent among children less than 15 years of age, from 19.8 to 30.9 discharges per 10,000 population (Figure 2.4).

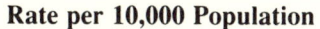

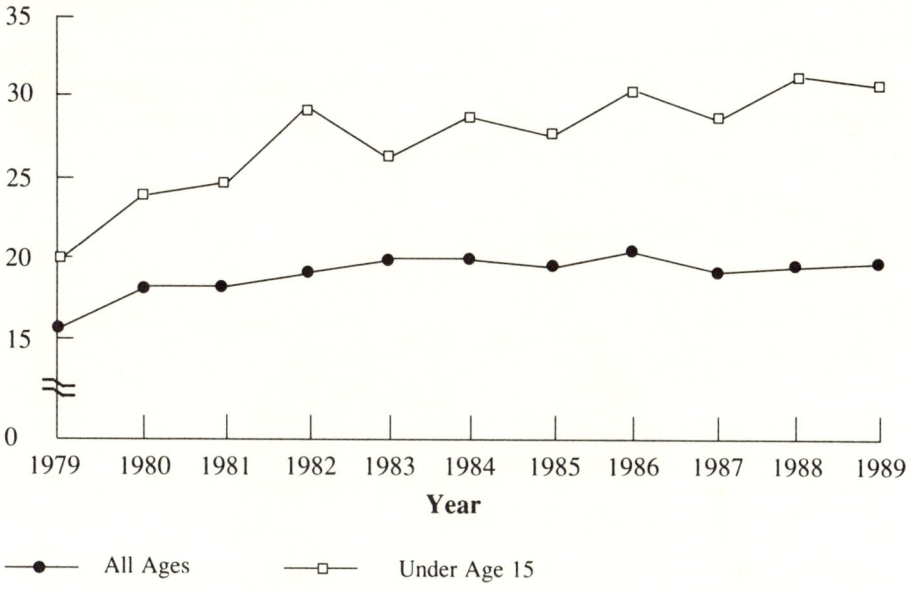

*Source: National Hospital Discharge Survey, National Center for Health Statistics*

**Figure 2.4** *Trends in Hospitalizations for Asthma*

## Mortality

In 1989, 5,150 people died from asthma in the United States. Asthma mortality has increased slightly over the past decade. The greatest increase in the asthma death rate has occurred in those older than 65 years of age.

In 1979, blacks of both sexes were about twice as likely to die from asthma as whites. Over the past decade this ratio has increased, and by 1988 the asthma death rate was almost three times greater among blacks than whites (Figure 2.5).

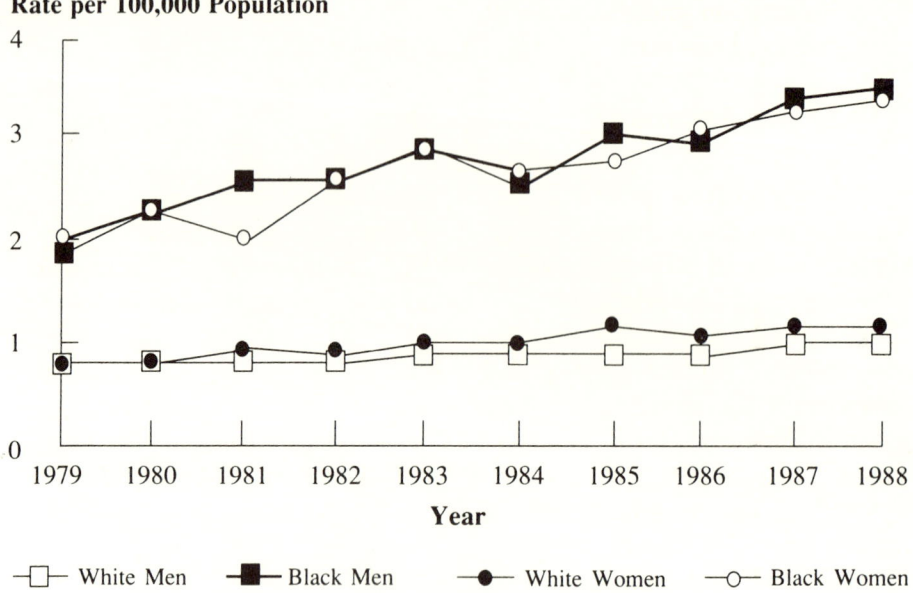

**Figure 2.5** *Trends in Asthma Mortality, U.S. Age-Adjusted Death Rates, 1979-1988*

## Section 2.2

# *What You Need to Know About Asthma*

Source: National Office of Communications, National Institute of Allergy and Infectious Diseases, March 1990, Based on a lecture presented by Michael A. Kaliner, M.D..

### *Bronchial Asthma*

People with asthma suffer from a disease that makes it hard for them to breathe at times. For some people, it is a minor problem, but for others it can be life threatening. Bronchial asthma is characterized by a reversible obstruction-a temporary blockage-of the bronchial airways, the tubes through which you breathe. The obstruction is caused by inflammation and mucus in the airways, contraction of the muscles that surround the airways, and airway swelling.

## *If You Have Asthma, You're Not Alone*

Along with its sister allergic diseases, bronchial asthma is among the most common chronic diseases suffered by Americans. Approximately 15 to 16 million Americans suffer from bronchial asthma; between 30 and 35 million have other allergic diseases. In other words, these are very common diseases.

Asthma is often thought to be a benign disease, but about 4,000 Americans die from asthma each year. The group at greatest risk is older asthmatics, above the age of 50; 10 per 100,000 older Americans die each year from asthma. Among the middle-age groups, 1.5 per 100,000 people die from asthma each year; but below the age of 9, 2 children per 100,000 die per year from asthma.

Asthma is the number one cause of school absenteeism, and the number one cause of pediatric admissions to the hospital. Overall, for adults as well as for children, it is the number six cause of admissions to all hospitals. There are 10 million office visits per year to physicians' offices for asthma. If you take into account office visits for asthma and allergies, the number becomes 30 million. One out of every nine office visits to physicians in the United States is due to asthma or allergic diseases.

Over-the-counter expenses for drugs to treat asthma exceed $2.3 billion dollars. Including prescription drugs, the expense is greater than $3 billion. Including the expense of office visits and hospitalizations, it's a staggering $4 to $5 billion.

## *What's Going On?*

Asthma is not a problem with breathing in but a problem with breathing out. During normal inhalation, air moves smoothly from the mouth, through the trachea, bronchi, and bronchioles into the alveoli. If you're an asthmatic, you can do the same: you lower the diaphragm, you swing the ribs out, and that makes the lungs bigger. If there is an airway obstruction, the airway opens up and air can slide around the obstruction. However, breathing out is passive. Ordinarily, to breathe out all you do is stop breathing in, and you automatically breathe out. But if you're asthmatic, you can't do that. The minute you relax your ribs and let your diaphragm slide up, the obstructed airways block the airflow and air can't get out. You have a lot of dead air trapped in your lungs, and you end up breathing at the top of your lungs.

The four components that cause asthmatics to have trouble in breathing are secretion of excess mucus, swelling in the airway, inflammation in the airway (white blood cells invade the walls of the airways), and muscle spasm.

If you don't have asthma and want to get a sense of how an asthmatic feels, try this: breathe in. Now, don't let the air out. Hold that deep breath and breathe in and out using only the top of your lungs. You're going to find yourself getting tired. It's uncomfortable to breathe up here, and that's what an asthmatic does. You can relax now, but that exercise gives you an idea of what it would be like to have that trapped air.

## Why You Wheeze

Ordinarily, the open airway through which you breathe is empty. The airway itself is lined with ciliated cells, cells topped with little hairs that move mucus. Beneath, there is a very thin basement membrane, an area known as the lamina propria, that is fairly devoid of cells. Next there is a thin muscle layer. Around that are submucous glands that secrete about 10 milliliters of mucus a day, about the amount in a tablespoon.

When an asthmatic's airway is full, it contains not only excessive, very sticky mucus but also a lot of other debris, including two kinds of white blood cells-eosinophils and neutrophils. Also, some of the cells that should be lining the airway lift off and resettle in clumps in the airway. Because the cells lift off, the airway itself becomes denuded; it does not have the normal cells that cover and protect it. The airway becomes hyperirritable; like scraped skin, it's sore. When an asthmatic coughs, or breathes in cigarette smoke or irritating fumes, he or she will begin to wheeze-a whistling sound-because the airways are hyperirritable and have constricted.

The basement membrane becomes very thick because of the deposition of additional materials. The area beneath the basement membrane, which has very few cells in the normal condition, grows full of inflammatory cells such as eosinophils and neutrophils. The blood vessels become dilated and full of white blood cells. The muscle layer thickens and muscle contraction occurs. The mucous glands become enlarged and actively secrete mucus that fills up the airway.

## What Causes Asthma?

The causes of asthma include allergy, infections, industrial chemical exposures, complications from drugs and chemicals, exercise, vasculitis (inflammatory diseases of the blood vessels), and what are called idiopathic causes.

### *Allergy*

Allergy is the number one cause of asthma. About 90 percent of the people under 10 who have asthma have allergies. If you are younger than 30 and have asthma, there is a 70 percent chance that you are allergic. About half the people over 30 who have asthma have allergies.

### *How An Allergic Reaction Works*

Every tissue in the body has "mast" cells, a name derived from the German "mastung," which means well-fed. Mast cells are most heavily concentrated in the mucous membranes (the skin that lines the nose and the airways), where there are about 10,000 mast cells per cubic millimeter. On the surface of mast cells are many IgE antibodies. Antibodies are proteins made by the body, and ordinarily they protect against invaders like bacteria and viruses. In allergy, a special kind of antibody known as IgE is made by plasma cells and is directed against ordinarily harmless materials like pollen, dust, or food. When mast cells that are sensitized by having IgE antibodies on their surface encounter that antigen or foreign substance, they then trigger the release of histamine and other chemicals from inside the mast cells, and this causes the allergic reaction. You don't exhibit an allergic reaction until you have been exposed to the antigen for a period of time. So, for instance, if you think you are safe because you bought a cat last month and you're not sneezing yet, just wait; you still may have an allergic reaction.

Ragweed is a common plant that can illustrate how this works. Ragweed produces about a billion pollen grains per year, per plant. Ragweed pollen is very light and carried far and wide by wind. When inhaled by an allergic person, the pollen will encounter plasma cells that respond to the pollen by making IgE antibodies. The IgE then coats the surface of the mast cells.

After 2 or 3 years (or seasons) of breathing in an allergen like ragweed pollen, the next time that allergic person breathes in that pollen, instead of simply causing IgE to be produced, the mast cells, now sensitized with IgE, release histamine and other chemicals. These substances released from the mast cells interact with the airways and produce the changes that cause asthma. The same allergy mechanism applies to ragweed, grass, dust, mold, animal allergens, and a variety of other allergens that are inhaled. This can also occur in an asthmatic who is allergic to certain foods. In addition, there are mechanisms in the body that trigger the release of these same chemicals from the mast cells not in response to inhaled allergens or to foods, but to exercise. Asthma that is related to exercise is called exercise-induced asthma, and it does not necessarily involve IgE antibodies at all.

Not everybody is allergic and if you're not, your antibody-producing cells won't make IgE antibodies in response to pollen or other allergens. Allergies are hereditary; if you are a parent with allergies, the likelihood is that one in three or one in four of your children will have allergies. If both parents are allergic, all offspring are likely to be allergic, too.

When is allergy likely to be a contributing factor to asthma?

- when a blood relative—mother, father, sister, brother, aunt, uncle, or child has allergies;
- when the asthma begins at a young age;
- when the asthma symptoms occur or worsen seasonally, such as in fall and spring;
- if other allergic symptoms also occur, such as rhinitis (runny nose), hay fever, or eczema;
- if tests show that the blood and sputum contain an increased number of eosinophils.

*Infections*

Infections can also cause asthma. Bronchiolitis is a viral respiratory infection that occurs in children younger than two. It is usually caused by one of two viruses-respiratory syncytial virus or parainfluenza virus. A child may get a fairly bad cold and then develop respiratory distress. The child may cough and wheeze and even have croup. About 50 percent of these children, if they have an allergic parent, will go on to develop asthma. Generally, this asthma is fairly mild and is substantially improved before age ten. Nonetheless, it's a very common cause of childhood asthma. Sporadic asthma can occur when people have an upper respiratory tract infection. Many adults only develop asthma as a consequence of a cold, often a cold that leads to bronchitis.

## *Chemical Causes*

Industrial and occupational exposure can lead to asthma. Inhaled substances can act as allergens or as irritants that do not result in IgE production. The most common cause of occupation-related asthma is the inhalation of substances like toluene diisocyanates, trimellitic anhydrides, and enzymes. Anyone who inhales chemical fumes can develop bronchial irritation or can become allergic to the chemical. It is estimated that as many as 15 percent of asthmatics develop asthma in response to industrial exposure.

A very common cause of asthma is nonsteroidal anti-inflammatory drugs such as aspirin. Aspirin is a very potent drug. The way it takes away pain is to stop the formation of agents known as prostaglandins. There is a whole class of drugs, chemically distinct from aspirin, that acts the same way. About 5 to 10 percent of asthmatics will have asthma triggered by aspirin or other aspirin-like compounds-that includes phenylbutazone, indomethacin, ibuprofen, and other nonsteroidal anti-inflammatory drugs.

Patients with aspirin allergy tend to have chronic sinus infections, and often will have nasal polyposis-growths inside the nose. Aspirin-initiated asthma can be a very severe form of asthma. It can be prevented by avoiding aspirin and, in part, by aggressive treatment of the sinuses.

It was once thought that yellow dyes, the F, D, and C No. 5, known as tartrazine yellow, triggered asthma, and, for a while, physicians discouraged patients with aspirin sensitivity from eating foods containing yellow dye. It turned out not to be a real problem. It was also thought at one time that benzoate preservatives could trigger asthma. There is no convincing evidence that this is true.

One group of chemical additives that has in fact been found to trigger asthma attacks in susceptible people is sulfites.

In ancient times, the Romans began adding sulfites to wines as preservatives, and sulfites have been added to wine ever since. People who have asthma or allergies triggered by wine may be sulfite sensitive.

Most people have heard about asthma attacks occurring after someone eats at a salad bar or restaurant. Sulfiting agents (sulfuric acid derivatives) are added to many perishable foods to keep them from turning color. Generally, any fresh food that would turn brown upon standing could have sulfites added to it to prevent that browning. About 5 percent of asthmatics who ingest high concentrations of sulfites will develop a severe asthma attack.

The Food and Drug Administration requires labeling of sulfite-containing foods and prohibits salad-bar restaurants from adding sulfites to their fresh foods. However, other processed foods that are available at salad bars, for example, still may contain sulfites.

- Foods with the Highest Concentration of Sulfites (ppm)

   Pizza Dough 11-20
   Instant Tea 5-6
   Wine Vinegar 75
   Fresh Shrimp 4-36
   Grapes 15
   Dried Fruits (Apples, Raisins) 275
   Grape Juice 85
   Lemon Juice 800
   Canned Vegetables 5-30
   Instant Potatoes 35-90
   Corn Syrup 30
   Fruit Topping 60
   Molasses 125
   Beer 10
   Wine 150

Beta blockers (beta adrenergic antagonists) have, since their first day of introduction, been recognized to cause asthma. Beta adrenergic antagonists are used for many purposes, including the treatment of migraine headache, glaucoma, rapid heart rate, high blood pressure, tremors, and many other conditions.

If you have asthma and have been advised to take a beta adrenergic blocking agent, tell your doctor that you have asthma and ask if an alternative drug can be prescribed. There is no question that these drugs will make mild asthma more severe and dramatically complicate the treatment of asthma.

## *Exercise*

Exercise is a potent stimulator of asthma. When you exercise, you hyperventilate by taking rapid, shallow breaths. Just as evaporating water cools the skin, hyperventilation cools the airways. A reflex reaction to this cooling of the airways causes asthma.

Exercise is as important for people with asthma as it is for everyone else. Fortunately, there are effective medications that prevent most exercise-induced asthma. Swimming doesn't cause much of a problem in people with asthma, biking causes somewhat more; and running is the worst type of exercise for asthma sufferers. Swimming is best because you are inhaling very moist air, thereby slowing down the cooling of the airway. If you want to exercise without taking medication, you can wear a surgical mask, enabling you to re-breathe humidified air and avoid asthma symptoms. A proper warm-up period also reduces exercise-induced asthma.

## *Vasculitis*

A rare cause of asthma is a type of vasculitis (inflammation of the blood vessels) known as the Churg-Strauss syndrome. In this disease, which occurs equally among males and females, allergic asthma suddenly and for no apparent reason gets much more severe. It is often diagnosed by an abnormal x-ray, which will show a white patch, indicating infiltration of inflammatory cells into the lungs.

## *Idiopathic Causes*

Often physicians can't determine what is triggering someone's asthma, and they call it idiopathic, which is the medical term for "I'm not sure of the cause." This undefined type of asthma occurs most often in older individuals who have some bronchitis, a lot of excess mucus secretion, and perhaps sinus infection. For lack of a better definition, this is called idiopathic asthma, and it accounts for about 25 percent of the individuals above the age of 30.

## **Triggers of Asthma**

Conditions that trigger asthma symptoms include sinusitis, gastroesophageal reflux, pregnancy, intense emotions, and hyperthyroidism.

## Sinusitis

Some asthmatics only have asthma symptoms in relationship to a cold and sinus infection. You'll recognize sinusitis because you will feel mucus dripping down the back of your throat. Often you will have headaches in the sites where the sinuses are, and you may run a fever. Sinusitis commonly causes asthma to worsen. The asthma and the sinusitis should be treated at the same time.

## Gastroesophageal Reflux

Gastroesophageal reflux means the backup of acid from the stomach up into the esophagus, or swallowing tube. In this case, asthma generally occurs at night, because when you are lying in bed, acid can leak out of your stomach and into your esophagus, thereby irritating the lining of the esophagus, setting up a reflex reaction in the chest, and triggering nighttime asthma.

## Pregnancy

Asthma complicates pregnancy about 1 percent of the time; about 1 woman in 100 develops asthma because of her pregnancy. But many asthmatics get pregnant. About half of people with asthma are women. And when those women become pregnant, one-third of them get better, one-third of them get worse, and one-third of them don't change.

In the one-third who get worse, the asthmatic symptoms that occur during the first pregnancy are generally the same in the second, third, and fourth pregnancies.

Fortunately, the asthma medications now in use do not have any bad effects on the unborn baby. Asthmatic patients go on to have normal pregnancies, normal deliveries, and normal children.

## Emotions

Intense emotions can trigger asthma. That doesn't mean that asthma is all in your head, it means that psychological stress can cause an asthmatic attack the same way that sinus inflammation and gastroesophageal reflux can.

## Asthma

*Hyperthyroidism*

Hyperthyroidism, which means over-activity of the thyroid gland, often causes an increase in asthmatic symptoms. It is one of the possibilities doctors consider when an asthmatic who has been stable suddenly gets much worse.

## Diagnosis

When a person with asthma symptoms comes into the doctor's office, the doctor usually gives the patient pulmonary function tests, which, for example, measure tidal volume. That is the amount of air you breathe in and out with a regular breath; it's usually about 500 milliliters. The doctor will then ask the patient to take a maximum inhalation and a maximum exhalation. By measuring the maximum expiratory level and the maximum inspiratory respiratory level, the doctor will calculate total lung capacity.

In a healthy person, about 75 to 85 percent of the air comes out within 1 second of a maximum exhalation (blowing out as hard as possible). By 3 seconds, the lungs have been essentially emptied. Asthmatics can't breathe in as much, because they have all that air trapped in the back of their lungs. Even at 6 and 7 seconds, they are still blowing out air. At that point, the normal person would have already been ready to breathe in again. But a person with asthma can't move air out.

## Treatment

There are two major ways to treat asthma: by avoiding substances or events that trigger asthma, and by using various medications.

*Avoidance*

**Pets.** If an asthma sufferer is allergic, the best treatment is avoidance of the irritating substance. You should avoid cats, for example, if you are allergic to them. The source of allergen from both cats and dogs is saliva. Cats preen themselves, and it's the dried saliva left on their skin that becomes aerosolized and acts as such a potent allergen. Dogs hardly ever clean themselves, so generally a dog turns out to be a much less important source of allergen than is a cat.

People who are allergic to cats should not live with cats. People who are allergic to dogs should not have dogs. But many animal lovers are very attached to their pets. If you must have a dog or cat indoors, at least don't let your pet in the bedroom. Give yourself 8 hours away from inhaling the allergen, if you can. Even birds should be avoided indoors, since feathers are a potent allergen. Feather pillows are another major source of allergy.

**Pollen.** If you have to be outdoors, recognize that airborne pollen levels are highest in the early morning on bright, sunny, windy days. Use air conditioning in your car during pollen season whenever possible.

**Dust.** A major source of allergens in dust is the dust mite. This microscopic bug lives mostly during the summer. During the winter, house dust contains parts of dead dust mites and their feces, which are actually the major source of dust allergens.

Dust mites live in wall-to-wall carpeting, in the springs and mattresses of beds, and any place dust collects. You can cover the springs and mattresses with allergy-proof encasements. You can keep table tops free from knickknacks. Shades are preferable to venetian blinds or curtains. Hardwood floors, or linoleum floors, and washable throw rugs are preferable to wall-to-wall carpeting. Closets are particularly laden with dust, so, if possible, use a clothes closet outside of the bedroom.

**Air-filtering Devices.** Air conditioning is extremely effective at clearing air particles, so during the pollen season, if you have air conditioning throughout the house, you will be less likely to suffer from allergy-induced asthma.

Electrostatic air precipitators are now safe and effective, although expensive. Older models produced ozone, which, even in very low concentrations cause asthmatic symptoms to get worse, since ozone is an irritant to mucosal membranes-the skin that lines the nose and the bronchi. But room air filters (the most effective ones are known as HEPA filters, high-efficiency particulate activating filters) are less expensive and are very efficient in removing air particles and don't produce ozone. Before buying a filter, rent one for your bedroom and see if it makes a difference.

If you have a choice, hot-water heat or radiator heat is better than forced hot-air heat. Forced hot-air heat distributes dust and mold throughout the house every time it circulates the air; radiators don't do that.

## *Medications*

**Cromolyn Sodium.** There is a preventive drug for allergies. It is known as cromolyn sodium. It is used in an inhaled form for asthma, in an eye-drop form for allergic eye diseases, and in a nasal spray for allergic rhinitis. What this drug does is prevent the mast cell from secreting the chemicals that cause allergies.

Unfortunately, cromolyn sodium does not work for everybody, but for those persons in whom it works, it works well. For anyone with allergic asthma, this drug is worth a try. It is also excellent for preventing exercise-induced asthma.

**Bronchodilators.** More commonly used than cromolyn sodium are bronchodilators. Bronchodilators relax the smooth muscles that line the airways, thereby opening those airways, if the muscle is contracted. There are three classes of bronchodilators: anticholinergics, methylxanthines, and beta adrenergic agonists.

- **Anticholinergic Drugs.** Known as atropine or atropine-like drugs, stop the action of acetylcholine, which triggers the muscles to contract. They relax the muscle by blocking its contraction. These are medium-potency drugs, certainly less potent than beta adrenergic agonists. Their duration of action is shorter. They are very important for the treatment of patients who produce excess mucus, and will be very important in the treatment of patients who have chronic pulmonary disease, but they are less important for treating asthma. However, clinical practice, particularly in some children and adults, has shown them to be very effective.

- **Methylxanthines** have been around for quite a long time but have only become popular in the last 15 to 20 years. That's because we now have ways of monitoring methylxanthine blood levels, and we now have pills that can be taken once or twice a day. Therefore, methylxanthines are the major drug used in the United States for the treatment of asthma. The most commonly known methylxanthine is theophylline. People who can't tolerate theophylline can usually take another compound called oxtriphylline. By the way, caffeine, found in coffee and tea, is a derivatve of methylxanthines. Caffeine is a very mild bronchodilator so it wouldn't be effective to treat asthma with coffee or tea.

Theophylline acts by stopping some of the enzymatic actions in smooth muscle cells and thereby relaxing them. This is a very potent, very popular form of therapy, and there are no long-term complications from its use.

- **Beta Adrenergic Agonists.** The last class of bronchodilators is beta adrenergic agonists. These are drugs related to the chemical adrenaline. When you are frightened, your heart starts beating more rapidly, your airways dilate, and the pupils of your eyes dilate, due to adrenaline. Because adrenaline causes the airways to dilate, scientists were abe to modify it into a very specific agent that works only in the lungs, causing them to open without affecting the rest of the body. One of the most impressive things that's happened in the past 15 years in the treatment of asthma has been the creation of inhaled bronchodilators. We can now deposit bronchodilators, like these beta adrenergic drugs, directly into the airways and have the site of action only on the airways. They work very quickly, within minutes, and their effects last up to 6 to 8 hours. So these are the mainstays of therapy. Bronchodilators like methylxanthines and beta adrenergic agonists are the two drugs most prominently used in the treatment of asthma.

**Corticosteroids.** These are clearly the most effective drugs for the treatment of asthma. However it is important to know how to use them, when to use them, who should use them, how long to use them, and when to stop them. They work by reducing swelling, reducing mucus secretions, stopping inflammation, reducing mast cell number and secretion, and even stopping the production of the IgE antibody.

On the other hand, corticosteroids are powerful drugs with serious side effects: they cause osteoporosis, a thinning of the bones; they cause weight gain; they lead to peptic ulcers; they can cause diabetes and increased infections; in children, they can stop growth.

Should we use them? Knowing how to use them properly minimizes the negative effects. Also over the past 5 to 10 years, inhaled steroids have been introduced; these have been pharmacologically engineered to work only in the lungs and have no systemic action. They work on asthma but don't create side effects. That's been the major breakthrough in the treatment of asthma in the past 10 years. While we once hesitated to use corticosteroids because of their side effects, we now use inhaled corticosteroids on many, if not most, asthmatics because of their safety and effectiveness.

**Immunotherapy.** Also known as allergy shots, immunotherapy is appropriate in people whose asthma has clear-cut allergic causes that are not adequately controlled with medication and avoidance of triggers. When immunotherapy works, it reduces not only the need for other treatments but also the disease itself.

*Peak Flow Meters*

In addition to avoidance of triggers and careful use of medications, the use of a peak flow meter can contribute to effective asthma management, particularly in children. This simple device helps patients monitor their own breathing. It measures the peak expiratory flow rate, which means the ability to breathe out quickly. A normal peak flow rate is first determined when an asthmatic child is feeling well, by blowing into the meter as hard and fast as possible several times. This measurement indicates how open the large airways are. The highest reading is recorded.

Peak flow monitoring is usually done several times a day or when the child feels ill. If the rate drops significantly, it may indicate that additional medication is needed to prevent asthma symptoms. Taking medication before severe symptoms are noticeable may prevent a full-blown asthma attack.

## Some Myths About Asthma

Though very common, asthma is not very well understood by most people. Misconceptions about its causes and treatment abound. Here are a few of these misconceptions:

1. "There's no sense treating my child. He's going to outgrow his asthma." This is both true and false. About 50 percent of the asthmatic children whose asthma develops between the

ages of 2 and 10 will not have asthma in their teenage years; they'll have a spontaneous reduction in their asthma. But often the asthma recurs when those people reach their thirties. So it goes away, but it doesn't go away permanently. Lung function tests of former childhood asthmatics show that they still have abnormal airways disease.

Should you wait to treat them? No. Asthma is a serious disease. It impairs the capacity of your child to exercise, it impairs your child's self-image, and it shouldn't be ignored. There are effective ways to treat asthma, and there is no reason to let a child suffer, waiting to get better. Have your child seen by a specialist in asthma and allergies, and have him or her treated adequately.

2. "Asthma is all in your head." Or, "Parents can cause asthma." Asthma is not "all in your head," and parents can't cause it. Psychological stress is one of the things that triggers asthma, but that doesn't mean that asthmatics are crazy or that parents are responsible. Emotional stress can make asthma worse, but you shouldn't feel guilty that your child has asthma. Your child has asthma because of other conditions over which you had no control. Psychological stress can trigger asthma symptoms, but it does not cause the disease.

3. "Asthmatics shouldn't exercise." Asthmatics should go out and exercise just like their friends. Eight percent of the athletes who represented the United States in the 1988 Olympics had exercise-induced asthma. They were able to perform in the Olympics because of proper medications to prevent asthmatic attacks caused by exercise.

4. "Allergic mothers shouldn't breast-feed." In fact, by breast-feeding, you reduce the opportunities for your child to become allergic to foreign proteins. Although breast milk is a distillate of proteins that you've eaten, your breast-fed child has a reduced exposure to non-human proteins. When a baby is born, its gastrointestinal tract is immature and it absorbs proteins that are much larger than proteins absorbed by adults. Adults break those down to very simple

amino acids. By absorbing proteins that are macromolecules, the infant's body recognizes these as foreign antigens and makes antibodies to them. That's one reason children have such a high incidence of food allergy. Mothers who are themselves allergic, and therefore are more likely to have an allergic child, should breast-feed for at least 6 months to a year, if at all possible.

5. "Recurring asthmatic attacks lead to emphysema." Patients can have asthma all their lives and when they die, their lungs don't show any more damage than those of a non-asthmatic. There are two exceptions to this. There is a rare disease known as alpha-1-antitrypsin deficiency, which is a congenital enzyme deficiency that can present as asthma and leads to a very early and very destructive form of emphysema. The second is an unusual condition called allergic bronchopulmonary aspergillosis, which is an infection in the airways that leads to destruction of the airways. Other than those two very unusual causes of asthma, asthma does not lead to emphysema. Asthma is a fully reversible disease in its uncomplicated state. If you have asthma, don't worry about emphysema, but don't ignore the asthma; you still need to be treated.

6. "Smoking does not affect asthma." Asthmatics should not smoke. Inhaling someone else's smoke is also harmful to an asthmatic because smoke further irritates the airways. Parents should be very concerned. Recent studies suggest that children of smoking parents are at greatly increased risk of developing asthma.

7. "Certain foods can cause asthma." Clearly, foods can cause allergies, But they are rarely a cause of asthma. Except in the case of sulfites, foods should not be restricted for asthmatics.

8. "Over-the-counter drugs are all an asthmatic needs." If over-the-counter drugs were as potent as prescription drugs, they would not be sold without a prescription. Over-the-counter drugs are used much more than prescription drugs for asthmatics because they are easier to get to and they don't nec-

essarily involve the expense of an office visit, but you sacrifice potency and specificity in the treatment. The drugs that are available over-the-counter are mild, non-specific agents that are mild bronchodilators, far less potent and far less effective than the drugs you can get by prescription. If you or your child has asthma, you should see a specialist, an allergist, or a pulmonologist who understands asthma and its treatment. As stated earlier, the two major advances in asthma treatment in the past 20 years, inhaled steroids and beta adrenergic agonists, are both prescription-only drugs.

## Research

At many research institutions around the country, including the National Institute of Allergy and Infectious Diseases, scientists are working to better understand the mechanisms involved in asthma, to develop new and improved treatments for asthma, and to find better means of preventing asthma symptoms. We have come a long way in our search to improve the quality of life for people with asthma and certainly hope that we will make even more progress in the decade ahead.

## For Further Information

American Academy of Allergy & Immunology
611 East Wells Street
Milwaukee, WI 53202
1-800-822-ASMA

American College of Allergy & Immunology
800 E. NW Highway, Suite 1080
Palatine, IL 60067
1-800-842-7777

American Lung Association
1740 Broadway
New York, NY 10019

Asthma & Allergy Foundation of America
1717 Massachusetts Avenue, NW, Suite 305
Washington, DC 20036
1-800-7-ASTHMA

Mothers of Asthmatics
10875 Main Street, Suite 210
Fairfax, VA 22030
(703) 385-4403

*Based on a lecture presented by Michael A. Kaliner, M.D. Chief, Allergic Diseases Section Laboratory of Clinical Investigation, National Institute of Allergy and Infectious Diseases, National Institutes of Health*

## Section 2.3

## *More Than Snuffles: Childhood Asthma*

Source: *FDA Consumer.* July/August 1991

  As a child, author John Updike, like many other children, had the snuffles in the winter and hay fever in warm weather. It wasn't until years later as an adult, however, that Updike's asthma was diagnosed during a physical exam. Noting Updike's spread rib cage, or barrel chest—the sign of the chronic asthmatic—and the characteristic wheezing sounds heard through the stethoscope, a doctor correctly identified his condition.

  While some children eventually "outgrow" asthma as the size of their breathing tubes increases, Updike's disease grew worse in maturity. He describes an acute episode that occurred on a visit to his parents' farm in Pennsylvania on a summer day, at the height of the pollen season, in the company of a dog and cats, and surrounded by dust, mold, and plants and trees in full bloom:

*An asthma attack feels like two walls drawn closer and closer, until they are pressed together. Your back begins to hurt, between the shoulder blades, and you hunch. I could not stand up straight and looked down at the flourishing grass between the sandstones. I thought, This is the last thing I'll see. This is death. The breathless blackness within me was overlaying the visual world, this patch of my mother's grass, with a thin gray film, and the space between the two walls I was struggling to pry apart felt hardly wide enough for a razor blade. My children and parents had come out on the back porch to watch me, and a rictus twitched my face as I thought how comic this performance must look, this wrestle with invisible demons. . . . I felt immensely angry at my own body and at everybody. Like a child blind in his tantrum I thought, Serve them right, and waited to die, standing bent over and gasping, of suffocation.* (Copyright 1989 by John Updike. Reprinted with permission of Alfred A. Knopf from *Self-Consciousness*.)

Updike didn't die. After a quick visit to the hospital emergency room and two injections of adrenaline, he experienced that "opening of the bronchial tree which is to asthmatics an interior sunrise, a rebirth into the normal world."

Such scenes are played out in emergency rooms throughout the United States, most of the time with a similar euphoric ending. But sometimes not. In 1988. according to statistics from the National Institutes of Health, 4,580 Americans died from asthma, some of them children. Though asthma can come on with such suddenness and severity that medical help is not available in time, doctors believe that most asthma deaths are preventable.

## Common Childhood Disease

Asthma is the most common chronic childhood disease. It causes more hospital admissions and visits to the emergency room and is responsible for more school absenteeism than any other chronic disease in childhood.

Estimates of the number of children under 17 with asthma vary from 3 million to 8 million, but Nancy Sander, founder of the national organization Mothers of Asthmatics, Inc., believes the incidence is much higher than the statistics show. Says Sander: "Asthma is often

## Asthma

misdiagnosed as acute infectious bronchitis [inflammation of the bronchi] or bronchiolitis [infectious inflammation of the bronchioles]—viral diseases—or recurrent pneumonia."

Though asthma can occur at any age, about 80 percent of the children who will develop asthma do so before starting school. The common "trigger" is a viral upper respiratory infection.

Childhood asthma appears to be increasing worldwide. In American children 3 to 17 years old, asthma's prevalence rose 50 percent in the 1980s, according to the National Center for Health Statistics, and the death rate for children under 14 doubled from 1977 to 1983. Health professionals don't know why asthma is on the rise, but they think that air pollution or other environmental changes may be implicated.

### What Is Asthma?

Asthma is a bronchial disease in which the airways are so sensitive that they sometimes become blocked, making breathing difficult. Of the many factors involved in this airway hypersensitivity problem, the one most experts are sure about is heredity. With the appropriate triggers or stimuli, people who have inherited a susceptibility to asthma may develop the disease. People without this potential don't get asthma. Though many people with asthma have allergies, all allergic people are not asthmatic.

The airways primarily affected are the bronchi, the two main branches of the trachea (or windpipe), and their smaller extensions, the bronchioles. Wrapped around the bronchial tubes are bundles of muscles that control the size of the air channel. When bronchial muscles tighten up, the air channels narrow; when they are relaxed, air channels are of normal size. Contraction and relaxation of these muscles are completely involuntary.

The bronchi are lined with a mucus membrane that is a continuation of the lining of the nose, mouth and throat. Glands embedded in the bronchial wall produce secretions (mucus) that keep the inner surfaces of the bronchial tubes moist.

In asthma, the bronchial tubes, mucus membranes, and mucus glands react abnormally to stimuli. Bronchial muscles clamp down around the bronchial tubes, causing a condition known as bronchospasm. The mucus membranes inside the tubes become inflamed and swollen, further narrowing the air channels. The bronchial glands start producing large amounts of a particularly thick and sticky mucus that is hard to cough up and often forms plugs that further obstruct airflow. As a result of these changes, not enough oxygen can get into the body, and air loaded with carbon dioxide is trapped inside the lungs' air sacs. Asthmatics have to fight to exhale.

Forcing air out through clogged, narrowed airways causes vibrations of the bronchi and the mucus trapped inside the bronchi, resulting in high-pitched whistling sounds, or low- pitched rumbles or rattles, all known as wheezing. Sometimes wheezing is clearly audible; other times it is difficult to hear without a stethoscope.

Coughing is another important symptom, especially in very young children. Scratching the neck or chest or yawning a great deal should alert concerned parents that an attack is on the way. Shortness of breath, spitting up mucus, a pale, sweaty face, and a tight chest are other symptoms. When the attack is severe, wheezing sometimes disappears because the smaller airways are completely blocked, a dangerous stage. Other signs of trouble are fast breathing (hyperventilation), a hyper-inflated chest due to trapped air, and an exhalation time twice as long as the inhalation time.

An asthma episode can last for hours or days, occur once in a lifetime, or every day. It can be mild, or so severe that the child requires hospitalization to treat respiratory failure. Though asthma can strike at any time, attacks often begin during the night. Asthma is an intermittent, reversible illness.

## Medications

Medications for asthma have come a long way since the days of the ancient Egyptians, who treated the disease by administering camel or crocodile dung, or by burning herbs on a hot brick and having the asthma patient inhale the fumes. Or even, for that matter, since the days of the great twelfth century physician and Jewish theologian Moses Maimonides, who prescribed—what else?—hot chicken soup.

Asthma can't be cured, but modern physicians have a powerful array of drugs to help prevent an attack or to relieve one that has already started. For some children, one medication will work; others need a combination of drugs.

Most drugs fall in three major groups: bronchodilators, an anti-allergic mediator agent (cromolyn), and anti-inflammatory agents (corticosteroids)

## Asthma

### *Bronchodilators*

These drugs dilate (open) the narrowed bronchial tubes, allowing oxygen to enter and carbon dioxide to exit the lungs more freely. Bronchodilators can be taken orally or inhaled in the form of an aerosol.

**Theophylline.** Relaxes the muscles surrounding the bronchial tubes, has been used as a bronchodilator in asthma therapy since 1922. The chemical was first isolated from cocoa in 1888, and is related to caffeine, whose bronchodilating effects were noted as early as 1698.

The drug is usually taken orally in immediate-release or slow-release tablets, beads or capsules. It is used to treat occasional episodes and as a preventive medication for long-term use. In emergencies, it may be given intravenously.

Theophylline doses must be carefully adjusted and monitored, based on body weight and how quickly the child eliminates the drug from the body. Too high a dose may result in stomachaches, headaches, high blood pressure, anxiety seizures, and other side effects. But if the dose is too low, the drug is ineffective. Younger children break down theophylline more rapidly than do older children and adults, and thus require a higher dose of theophylline per kilogram (pound) of body weight.

**Epinephrine.** Or adrenaline is another drug that opens up the bronchial tubes. Usually given by injection, epinephrine works fast. It may increase the heart rate and produce other side effects such as headache, jitteriness, anxiety, and sometimes nausea and vomiting.

**Beta-adrenergics or beta-agonists.** These epinephrine-like drugs can be inhaled or taken orally in liquid or tablet form. Although not approved for use in children, epinephrine-like drugs are nevertheless prescribed by some physicians when, in their judgment, the benefit to the child outweighs the risks. Used to treat occasional attacks and as a preventive medication on a long-term basis, they are longer-acting and cause fewer side effects than epinephrine.

These drugs can be used in a device called a metered-dose inhaler, which delivers a specific amount of the drug directly to the bronchial tubes in the form of an aerosol spray. Very young children who can't master the inhaler can use a compressor-driven nebulizer, which sends a fine mist of the drug to the lungs through a mouthpiece or face mask, or they may take oral forms of adrenergic drugs.

To prevent exercise-induced asthma, inhaled adrenergic drugs should be used at least 15 minutes before exercise. Over-use of the inhaler can be dangerous, because it can cause irregular heartbeats, chest pain, and worsening of asthma. Over-use may also mean that the asthma is not under control.

### *Cromolyn*

Unlike bronchodilators, which treat only symptoms, cromolyn treats the specific cause of asthma: airway hyper-reactivity and inflammation. Cromolyn makes airways less sensitive to factors that can trigger asthma episodes and, when an allergic reaction does occur, prevents the release of histamine from certain cells (mast) that cause bronchial tube inflammation.

Cromolyn is inhaled, either as a liquid in a metered-dose inhaler or from a nebulizer, or as a powder using a spinhaler, a propeller device specifically designed for cromolyn use. Cromolyn can be used as long-term preventive treatment. It can also be used to prevent an attack, especially before exercise or exposure to cold air or known allergens, but it is of no use when an asthma attack is under way. The drug has a few mild side effects, such as a bad taste in the mouth, throat irritation, and coughing from the powder.

### *Corticosteroids*

Other drugs used to treat the disease rather than the symptoms are corticosteroids, which are related to cortisone, a hormone produced by the adrenal glands. (These steroids are not to be confused with anabolic steroids used by body builders.)

"Steroids have been, without question, the major advance in the treatment of asthma for the last 20 years," says Michael Kaliner, M.D., head of the Allergic Diseases Section, National Institute of Allergy and Infectious Diseases, National Institutes of Health. "They cause inflammation of the airways to go away, and reduce airway irritability." They also decrease mucus production and swelling, and allow other medicines to work more effectively.

When taken by mouth for more than a week or two, however, they can produce severe side effects, including growth suppression in children, a characteristic "moon" face, bone thinning, acne, cataracts, increased blood pressure, increased blood sugar, and more.

Inhaled steroids may produce the good effects of oral corticosteroids and decrease some of the bad effects, and thus can be used daily as preventive medication.

Sander states: "Parents know about the side effects of oral steroids and are afraid to have their children use inhaled steroids. They shouldn't be.... Inhaled steroids go right where they're supposed to go."

However, the inhaler is difficult for small children to use, and continued use may also irritate the throat. Occasionally, inhaled corticosteroids cause a yeast infection called thrush to settle in the back of the throat. Rinsing the mouth and gargling with warm water after use should help prevent this infection.

Inhaled corticosteroids are not useful in severe or acute attacks of asthma, but they can reduce their frequency. For difficult-to-manage asthma, the more effective oral corticosteroids are probably the most valuable drugs.

Doctors rely on oral corticosteroids when allergy treatment and other medications—including adrenergic drugs, theophylline, inhaled steroids, and cromolyn—have been unable to control asthma symptoms. Occasional short-term use of oral corticosteroids—less than two weeks—may not result in significant side effects.

Finding the right doses of the right medicines that will benefit a child often takes a period of trial and error. The doctor will fine-tune the treatment as much as possible, taking into account the child's symptoms and the medications' adverse effects. With good management, a child with asthma should be able to lead a normal, active life.

## Care of the Asthmatic Child

Many factors can trigger an asthma "flare" in a susceptible child, but the most common are allergens, colds, flu, and other respiratory infections. Exercise is also a common trigger in children, as well as adults.

Irritants such as perfumes, cigarette smoke, wood smoke, hair sprays, paint odors, cotton or wood dust, industrial chemicals and fumes, and outdoor pollution may also bring on an attack. Cold air and changes in the weather, in which winds sweep in from other areas carrying irritants, pollution or different pollens, often cause a flare. A cough, shout or laugh may stimulate the vagus nerve that leads to the lungs, and cause an attack.

Allergies play a part in triggering attacks in a large percentage of children with asthma. Some of the most common offenders are animal dander, pollen, mold, ragweed, house dust, bacteria, dust mites, fungi, and animal and human skin fragments. Certain foods, such as chocolate, shellfish, milk, orange juice, eggs, nuts and peanut butter, along with foods or drugs containing sulfites and other preservatives, can also trigger attacks. Some children may develop severe bronchospasm from aspirin and non-steroidal anti-inflammatory drugs such as ibuprofen, naproxen and piroxicam.

A recent study performed at the National Jewish Center for Immunology and Respiratory Medicine, Denver, Colo., found that children with severe asthma suffer from depression and guilt feelings, often have problems in school, and limit their normal activities because of the disease. Asthma's damage extends to the family, whose lifestyles are often affected. When the cost of medication and devices is added in, it can be seen that severe chronic asthma can be a burden on the family.

Doctors advise parents of asthmatic children whose attacks are allergy-related to help the child avoid the allergen whenever possible, which means that sometimes the family pet must go or more rigorous dust-control measures must be instituted. With unavoidable allergens, allergy shots given year-round are helpful in most cases. Moving to another area to escape allergens is not recommended unless the new area is given a trial in all seasons of the year. It is quite possible that after a "honeymoon" period in the new area, the child may begin to react to local allergens.

Since asthma attacks can happen anytime, anywhere, parents of children with asthma need to communicate with school personnel if their children must take medicine at designated times or use devices such as inhalers. Unfortunately, many teenagers try to ignore asthma symptoms at school because they don't want to be seen using an inhaler, especially before sports activities. The result is often out-of-control asthma.

Parents should see that the child eats a nutritious diet, including plenty of fluids, has adequate rest and exercise, and is knowledgeable about factors that will set off an episode.

To avoid reliance on emergency rooms and hospitals, parents and child need to be alert to the early signs of asthma and have a definite medical regimen to follow when an attack begins. Medications should be taken exactly as prescribed. A supportive and sympathetic doctor, who can provide the parents with an asthma prevention plan as well as care for acute episodes, is a necessity.

Children with well-controlled asthma should be encouraged to take part in exercises or sports-activities. Besides increasing lung capacity, exercise improves breathing and may eliminate or lessen the severity of asthma attacks. An added bonus: Doing what other children can do increases self-esteem. In 1984, 66 of the U.S. Olympic competitors had been diagnosed as having exercise-induced asthma. Forty-one of those athletes won medals in the games.

*—by Evelyn Zamula*

Evelyn Zamula is a freelance writer in Potomac, Md.

## Section 2.4

## *Let's Talk About Asthma: A Guide for Teens*

Source: American Lung Association Pub. No. 1552. 1993. Used by Permission.

The American Lung Association has provided this information to teens with asthma as a public service. The information is general in nature, and the specific needs of individuals may vary widely. It is not a substitute for regular care from a doctor. Do not change your asthma treatment plan or your medication schedule without first speaking with a doctor.

The American Lung Association does not endorse any specific commercial product.

### Introduction

As a teenager with asthma, you probably have many questions about your condition and how it can be treated.

Maybe what interests you most is whether asthma will affect your day-to-day activities, like gym class or work, or how you can control your condition so that a sudden asthma episode doesn't develop. You may be concerned about how friends, classmates, teachers, work supervisors, parents, and other important people in your life will react to your condition. And you may want to know how to talk with those people about your asthma.

This chapter provides you with the facts about asthma and describes how to spot early warning signs of an asthma episode. It explains ways to prevent asthma symptoms from getting out of control and it gives you realistic tips about living life as a normal teenager who happens to have asthma.

By reading this chapter, you are taking an important step toward doing all you can to control your asthma so that you can lead a full and active life. Read on to learn more about asthma and ways you can help yourself.

## *The Facts*

Some people think that asthma is not a physical disease, that it's all in your mind. They're wrong—it's all in your lungs.

Asthma is a chronic or long-term condition that causes the tiny air passageways in your lungs (called bronchioles, pronounced bronk-eeols) to become narrowed or blocked when they react to something in the environment. It is a disease of the respiratory system, the lungs and system of air tubes that lead to them. During an acute asthma episode (or "asthma attack"), several things happen. First, the smooth muscles around the airways tighten, making the airways narrow and making it hard for air to flow in and out of the lungs. Then, the lining of the airways themselves gets thicker so that the airways become even more narrow. Finally, the cells in the airways make more mucus than they should and this extra mucus also blocks the airways. (No wonder it feels like you can't breathe.) Asthma episodes can be mild or moderate or severe. During a mild episode it may be hard to breathe or a cough may begin. Severe episodes may include coughing spasms or chest pain, and you may find yourself gasping for breath.

If you have been diagnosed as having asthma, you are not alone. More than 10 million people in the United States have asthma (including Olympic and professional athletes, actors and actresses, maybe even one of your teachers). And asthma seems to be on the rise, which may be due to increased air pollution or other environmental changes. Asthma is not associated with other lung diseases such as emphysema (em-fe-see-ma), tuberculosis or lung cancer. That is, having asthma won't increase or decrease your chances of developing those conditions. Asthma is not contagious, so no one can "catch" it from being around you.

One-third of all people with asthma are under 18. More than 3.7 million people under 18 have been diagnosed with asthma, and experts think that many other young people have asthma but that symptoms have not been correctly diagnosed. Most teenagers with asthma have a mild form of the condition that often can be controlled through teamwork: you working together with your family and health-care team. With this team, you can figure out a combination of strategies that will be helpful in managing asthma and preventing it from interfering with your day-to-day life.

For teens whose asthma is moderate or severe, asthma episodes may happen more often and they may stay home from school at times. They also may need to visit the emergency room or stay in the hospital. But even if you are one of these teens, you can still work with your family and health-care team to reduce the number and severity of asthma episodes.

You have probably heard your doctor use the term "trigger" to describe those things that cause an acute asthma episode. Just as holding a lighted match to paper can start a fire, being exposed to a trigger can start an asthma episode. Some people have specific, identifiable triggers, others do not. If you have specific triggers, learning what they are is important for managing your asthma. Common triggers are colds and other respiratory infections, allergic reactions, exercise, cold air or sudden temperature changes, and exposure to cigarette smoke, fumes, air pollution, and strong odors.

Although asthma is not a psychological condition (remember, it's "all in your lungs," not all in your head), occasionally, strong emotions, stress or excitement can trigger an asthma episode, especially at a time when there might be other triggers present. Some teens with asthma also have allergy triggers. That means they might be allergic to such things as animal hair, some types of food, mold or pollen. When these people come in contact with their allergy triggers, an asthma episode may result.

Signs of asthma are coughing, wheezing (a high-pitched, whistling sound made when air is forced through narrowed airways), shortness of breath, a gagging or choking sensation, and chest tightness commonly described as "feeling like an elephant is sitting on my chest." You don't need to have all these signs for you to have asthma. Sometimes signs are more subtle, like finding it hard to catch your breath at the top of the stairs. What's important is for you to learn to recognize when your symptoms are under control or appear to be getting worse.

## Take Charge

If you're like most teens, you lead a busy life with family, school, work and social activities, and asthma is an annoyance you wish would disappear.

Many teens do outgrow their asthma. Others may think they've outgrown their asthma because they've slowly decreased their level of activity and thus have fewer symptoms. But even if you are one of those lucky enough to leave asthma behind with adolescence, researchers have found that the people who take responsibility for managing their asthma are better able to avoid asthma episodes When you were younger, your parents probably took control of your health care, making sure you took your medicines and taking you to the doctor. Your parents or guardians are still there to help you, but now that you're older, you are on your own more and want and need to be more independent. As it should be, the responsibility for handling your asthma is ultimately in your hands.

Asthma can be managed if you put your mind to it. Let's take a look at how you can get started with a program that will help you breathe easier.

Your first step is a bit like playing detective. You need to figure out what triggers your asthma symptoms or a full-blown episode. You know your body better than anyone else and you probably already know some of the triggers that start an asthma episode. You may begin to wheeze if you are around cats or dogs or other animals. Walking into a smoke-filled room may set off an asthma episode. Other triggers can include house dust, perfumes, air fresheners, or fumes from cleaning agents or soaps. You might be sensitive to other, more subtle things or changes in the weather. House dust is a major trigger for most people with asthma. House dust contains small amounts of dirt, dust mites, mold spores and other things you may be allergic to. Microscopic dust mites are often the culprits behind chronic asthma symptoms. Of course, it is impossible to get rid of every speck of dust where you live, but there are things you can do that will keep dust to a minimum and make cleaning easier.

A good place to start is with your bedroom. You spend a lot of time there, including when you are asleep, so anything you can do to eliminate triggers there will help. Carpeting, especially wall-to-wall, drapes, curtains and other fabrics hide dust. Your room should be vacuumed and dusted (wiping down surfaces with a damp cloth) at least twice a week, more often if possible. Ideally, someone other than you should vacuum and clean so that you won't breathe in the dust. Try trading household chores so that, for example, you wash the dishes or cook instead of vacuuming. If you must vacuum or dust, wear a dust mask and gloves. (You can buy heavy paper dust masks at hardware stores. Some pharmacies sell washable cotton dust masks.)

Stuffed animals are notorious dust catchers. Banish them from your room or wash them at least once week. (In fact, the more unnecessary things you can get rid of, the less you, or anyone else, will have to dust.) Avoid feather, foam, or down-filled pillows (they can harbor mites and molds). Instead, choose polyester fiberfill. Wash your pillow once a month and get a new one every year. Don't use a blanket that has a fuzzy surface; use a tighter, woven fabric, like a cotton thermal blanket, instead. Cover your mattress with a plastic cover or sheet and use a mattress pad on top of the plastic cover. Wash all bedding, including the mattress pad, weekly. (Water must be at least 130°F.) Keep your closet orderly, too. Airing woolen items or washing clothes after each wearing prevents mildew from forming.

Keeping your bedroom in order is not a one-time job; keep checking for problem areas that you might have missed before. If warm temperatures are a trigger for you, you may also want to keep a fan on hand for warm evenings. Take a look around the rest of your home, too. Are there other areas where you spend lots of time, like a family room or kitchen, that could be organized with fewer asthma triggers? Are pets a problem for you? If they are, you must work out a good solution for you and your family. There really is no such thing as a "non-allergenic pet." Almost all pets can cause allergies, including dogs, cats, birds, hamsters, and guinea pigs. Keeping tropical fish might be a good alternative. Ideally, all pets, except fish, should be removed from the home; at a minimum, they should never be allowed in your bedroom. But this should be something your whole family talks about in order to figure out the best solution for everyone. Maybe your beloved cat can live outside the house only. Perhaps the dog can be cared for (fed, groomed, walked) by other family members and never allowed up on furniture. Ask your parents and other family members to cooperate in helping you limit exposure to triggers.

Tobacco smoke is another common trigger. Smoking cigarettes is a health hazard for anyone; if you smoke and have asthma, you run the risk of sudden and severe asthma episodes. You also should not expose yourself to others' tobacco smoke. If family members smoke, ask them to do so outside the house. If your friends smoke, ask them not to smoke around you, including not smoking in cars.

Air pollution triggers asthma in some people. Many TV and radio stations report the pollen count and pollution index on the news. Tune in to find out this information if you think it will help you prepare for the day.

Sinus or bronchial infections may make your asthma worse. Talk to your doctor if you have such infections frequently.

You're in the best position to know what triggers your asthma episodes. But sometimes it's hard to find the clues since an episode may not start until several hours after you have been exposed to an irritant. The more you can learn about your triggers, the better able you will be to prevent asthma episodes.

You may think that an asthma episode begins suddenly-when you find yourself choking for air—and ends just as suddenly after you use your inhaler and are able to breathe easily again. Actually, changes in your airways take place gradually, both at the beginning and end of an episode. Some experts advise using a peak flow meter, a simple device that measures how much air is flowing from your lungs. Talk to your doctor about whether using a peak flow meter will help you and, if it might, how best to use it. By using a peak flow meter daily, you will learn when changes occur and get an early signal that an episode is developing. There are several different peak flow meters; all are easy to use and may provide you with early warning—perhaps days in advance that an episode is in the works.

If you've ever had an asthma episode, you know that it can be frightening. The fact is, asthma can be a serious disease. It causes more absenteeism from school than any other major illness. But death from asthma is extremely rare and experts say that even the few deaths that do occur might have been prevented if people had followed a good treatment plan and talked to a member of their health-care team when their symptoms became worse. The moral to this story is: Don't try to "tough it out" and ignore asthma's early warning signs, thinking they will go away by themselves. Take your medication as indicated. Using medication at an early stage may prevent an episode from continuing and eliminate the need for additional doses.

## *Partners: You and Your Doctor*

Working together with your doctor is one of the most important ways to fight asthma.

Give your doctor the best information you can about your asthma: when episodes occur, the severity of the episodes, what the triggers might be, how your medication does or doesn't work. If you get side effects from the medication, tell your doctor about that, too; don't just stop using it. Your doctor may be able to prescribe a different medication or give you the medication in another form, such as a pill or inhaler.

Before you visit your doctor, make a list of things you want to talk about. Having a written list to look at will help you remember the things you want to go over. Look back over your journal entries to remind yourself of possible triggers or symptoms to talk about. Don't hesitate to bring up things that are on your mind. Do you want to know more about how a peak flow meter can help you? Are you puzzled about the best way to use an inhaler? Do you want to talk about what sports you can play? Do you want more information about your prescribed medications? These are important questions.

Bring your list and talk these and other questions over with your doctor. Write down the doctor's answers and any new instructions. In fact, it's a good idea to do that right in the office and have your doctor look over what you wrote down to see if you understood what was said.

To work together well, you should feel confident and comfortable with your doctor. Not all doctors are familiar with asthma and not all doctors are comfortable with teenage patients. By law, what you talk about with your doctor must remain confidential. That means she or he cannot tell your parents, school nurse or anyone else what you have talked about. But you should clarify this with your own doctor so that you know how he or she interprets this responsibility. To form the best partnership, your doctor must know about other prescribed drugs, such as birth control pills or antibiotics, and over-the-counter medication, such as diet pills or tranquilizers, you may be taking. Feel free to ask your doctor questions about illegal drugs, too. Some, such as cocaine or uppers, may be particularly dangerous to take along with some asthma medications. Others, such as marijuana or crack, can trigger an asthma episode. If you think you may be pregnant, make sure you tell your doctor that as well. Your asthma medications may affect the developing fetus.

Sometimes people are unable to control an asthma episode and need medical help. Ask for guidance in deciding when to call your doctor or when to go to the hospital emergency room. Your doctor or another doctor who can get your medical records should be available 24 hours a day in case of emergency. Ask your doctor who to call at night if you need to, so that you will not worry about disturbing anyone. Talk about what to do if you do end up in the emergency room and your doctor can't be reached.

Ask for one of your doctor's cards to put in your wallet or carry a completed asthma treatment plan, as described in the next section. This information will be helpful in an emergency. Wearing a medical I.D. bracelet is a good idea so no one will have to rummage through your wallet. (You can buy medical I.D. bracelets at the drugstore and many schools have scholarship funds to help pay for their purchase. Check with your school nurse.)

## Handling Asthma Episodes

With your doctor, you should work out a detailed treatment plan to put into effect if an asthma episode develops. The plan should include what medications to take if you feel like an episode is beginning and how long to wait and what to look for after taking those medications before getting more medical help. The plan should also include your doctor's name and phone number, who to call if your doctor is not available, the name and phone number of the hospital you would choose to go to in an emergency, and a list of all medications you take. If you are in school, share this plan with your school nurse. If you work, share the plan with your supervisor. And keep a copy of this plan and your emergency phone numbers with you in your wallet. It's a lot easier to pull something out of your wallet than to explain all this when you can't breathe.

Be alert to early signs that an episode is coming: persistent cough, mild wheezing, breathing somewhat faster, taking longer to breathe out than to breathe in, shortness of breath. When you first recognize these signs, start the treatment plan you and your doctor have developed.

If you are using a peak flow meter, check your peak flow rates and use medication according to your asthma management plan.

Use an inhaler or other medications your doctor may have prescribed to prevent the episode from getting worse. We've said it before but we'll say it again: Don't try to "tough it out." The right medicine at this point can save you from a full-blown episode later on.

Although it may seem impossible, try to relax. When people get anxious or worried, they usually start to breathe faster. That's not what you want when your asthma symptoms are already making it hard to breathe. See the next section for tips on relaxing.

If your medication and relaxation exercises are not controlling your symptoms after the time limit or dosage set by your doctor, ask someone to help you get emergency medical attention.

## Medications

Taking medication as your doctor tells you helps the medicine to be most effective in lowering your chances of having an acute asthma episode.

For people with mild asthma, this may mean taking medicines as you need them. For most people with moderate or severe asthma, this means taking medicines even when you feel OK.

Here's a description of the most common asthma medicines. There are three major kinds of medicines used to treat asthma:

### *Preventive Medicines*

Preventive medicines keep asthma attacks from starting. The two main kinds are Cromolyn (krow-mow-lin) and inhaled corticosteroids.

Cromolyn (brand name Intal) prevents asthma attacks by blocking swelling in the airways and keeping the surrounding muscles from tightening. It must be taken every day to prevent asthma attacks. It can take two to three weeks for it to start working so, if you have an acute episode in the meantime, **DO NOT STOP** taking this medicine without consulting your doctor. The medication only works if it is taken regularly.

Cromolyn may also be prescribed to prevent symptoms that happen after exercise or contact with an animal. It should be taken five minutes to one hour ahead of time and the preventive effect lasts three to four hours.

Inhaled corticosteroids—brand names Beclovent (bek-lo-vent), Vanceril (van-sir-el), Azmacort (asthma-cort), Aerobid (air-oh-bid)-act in the same way as oral steroids but, since they are targeted directly at the lungs, little of the medication is absorbed by other parts of the body and side effects are minimized. It may take one to four weeks before this medicine is fully effective. Like Cromolyn, if you have a severe asthma episode, **DO NOT STOP** taking the medication without consulting your doctor. It, too, only works if it is taken regularly.

One possible side effect from inhaled steroids is developing thrush, a yeast infection in the mouth. Another side effect may be a sore throat. People with braces, retainers or other mouth appliances are especially susceptible. To avoid this, use a holding chamber on your inhaler or rinse your mouth with water after using the inhaler.

*Oral Corticosteroids*

Oral corticosteroids (kor-ti-co-steer-oidz) reduce the swelling and inflammation in the airways, help relax the surrounding muscles, decrease the amount of mucus being produced, and make the airways more responsive to adrenaline-like medicines. Brand names include Prednisone (pred-ni-zone), Methylprednisone (meth-il-pred-nizone), Cortisone (cor-ti-zone), Decadron, etc. Oral steroids are usually taken for three to seven days. After one day they may cause increased appetite, a feeling of well-being, or sleeping problems. You may feel moody for a few days after you finish your medicine. These medicines can cause long-term side effects and should only be taken as prescribed and under the supervision of your doctor. These are not the body-building steroids taken by some athletes.

*Bronchodilators*

Bronchodilators (bronk-odie-lay-tors) relax the muscles that have tightened around your airways. There are three kinds of bronchodilators: adrenaline (uh-dren-au-lin)-like medicines, theophylline (thee-ahfelin) and ipratropium (e-pra-tro-pee-em).

The adrenaline-type medicines include Ventolin (ven-to-lin), Proventil (pro-vent-il), Alupent (alyou-pent), Metaprel (met-e-prel), Bricanyl (bric-an-il), Brethine (bretheen), etc. If you inhale this medicine, you should feel relief within a few minutes. Pills and liquids can take more than 20 minutes to work. Possible side effects are shakiness, jitteriness or rapid heartbeat. It can take several weeks for these side effects to wear off. If they don't seem to be decreasing, talk to your doctor about changing medications.

Theophyllines include Theo-Dur, Slobid (slow-bid), Slo-Phyllin, Somophyllin, Quibron, Elixophyllin (e-licks-ahf-e-lin), Aminophylline (amin-ahf-e-lin), etc. Other medicines that teenagers might be taking, such as Erythromycin and Tetracyclin (antibiotics), Retin-A, or birth control pills can also increase your levels of theophylline. It's important to let your asthma doctor know if you are taking any of these medicines, too, since the combination may be dangerous. Side effects of theophyllines can include feeling hyperactive, upset stomach and headaches.

Ipratroprium (brand name Atrovent) is sometimes added to adrenaline-like medicines to increase the opening of the airways. It takes effect after several hours. Possible side effects can include dry mouth and cough. Some of these medicines are available in pill or liquid form, others are nose sprays or are inhaled using a nebulizer (neb-you-li-zer) or inhaler (a device that gives a measured amount of medication in mist form. Patients breathe in the mist through their mouths).

Don't decide to skip taking your asthma medicine because you are feeling well and think you won't need it. By taking medication to control a mild asthma episode you might prevent a more serious one. However, taking more medication than is prescribed can be dangerous. Taking other drugs that are not prescribed by your doctor can also be risky. For example, tranquilizers could cause you to miss important signs of breathing trouble; diuretics cause mucus to get drier, which is exactly the opposite of what you want; diet pills and No-Doz can speed up your heart rate, which may already be speeded up as a side effect of your asthma medicine. Some asthma medications may make you less tolerant of alcohol, so that you will feel the effects of alcohol much more quickly.

Finally, illegal drugs can also interact with your asthma medicine or make your asthma worse. Smoking crack cocaine is like inhaling Drano, smoking marijuana is like inhaling woodstove smoke neither of those are any good for your asthma or for the rest of you. If you have an asthma episode while under the influence of a mind-altering drug, it can be hard for you to remember what you are supposed to do. Downers can slow down your breathing, potentially dangerous for people with asthma. And uppers can increase your heart rate, which may already be increased by your prescribed asthma medications.

## Relaxation Techniques

When asthma symptoms worsen, it can be very frightening. Most people's first reaction is to become tense. This tightens muscles all over your body and makes you breathe faster. It's a vicious cycle; the more tension builds up, the more difficult it is for you to breathe normally and the more scared you become.

It would be nice if you could simply tell yourself "relax," and let tension drift out of your body, helping you to breathe freely. It's not that easy, but there are things you can learn that will help you relax. One good exercise is called "progressive muscle relaxation." By practicing this technique before you have an asthma episode, you will find it easier to keep calm when symptoms begin to develop.

Find a quiet, open spot and turn the lights down low. You might play soft background music or just tune into the quiet around you. Lie down (make sure the carpet has been vacuumed), close your eyes, let your body sink slowly into the floor and begin to breathe slowly and deeply.

Begin at the top of your head and imagine each part of your body tightening and tensing and then relaxing. Tighten your scalp and then relax it, then your forehead, your eyebrows, your eyes, your jaws, and so forth. Work down your body, telling each part to tighten and then release.

Take your time and notice small differences as each part tenses and relaxes. Include your arms and legs and don't forget the tops of your feet, the soles, ankles and toes.

The entire process should be done slowly and easily. After each tense/relax stage you should "let go" of the part of your body on which you have focused. After you have finished the head-to-toes relaxation, mentally check through your body to see where pockets of tension remain and tense and relax those areas again. When you have completed this exercise, enjoy the feeling of relaxation in your body. Breathe slowly and easily.

If you are in school or in another public place, you can do a mini version of the relaxation exercise, progressively tensing and then relaxing main parts of your body as you sit in a chair. Concentrate on your breathing, keeping a slow, natural rhythm. Imagine yourself floating on a cloud or drifting through space in a timeless, free way. Another exercise to practice is "pursed-lip breathing." Sitting in a chair, relax, letting your neck and shoulders drop. Breathe in slowly

## Asthma

through your nose. Purse your lips like you are going to whistle, and blow out through your mouth slowly and evenly. Try to take at least twice as long as you did breathing in. Use this technique during an asthma episode to stop gasping for air and gain control of your breathing.

Other relaxation techniques include visualizing a calm, peaceful place or practicing yoga. Your library has books about these and other relaxation techniques Being alert to what makes your asthma symptoms get worse is the key to controlling severe asthma episodes.

### Keep Track

You may know, for example, that being around cats gives you asthma symptoms. But other times you may start wheezing and not know what triggered it. Other early signs of a coming asthma episode may include not sleeping well, coughing (especially at night), chest tightness, rapid breathing, or itchy throat.

A written record may help you identify your triggers and avoid them. A daily journal will give you information you need to recognize patterns about your asthma.

Your journal need not be a fancy one; any notebook will be fine. The important thing is to remember to write in it each day. Take a few minutes to jot down facts about your asthma. Describe whether or not you had any symptoms or an episode, what you think might have triggered it, the weather conditions, types of food you ate, and activities you were involved with, such as exercise or crafts work, and how you felt during and after the activities. Note anything that you think might have contributed to the symptoms or episode. For example, was the grass being cut at school on a day you had asthma symptoms? If the cat is in the house, are your symptoms worse? Were you working with a new kind of model glue or paint?

It's useful to write a journal entry even if symptoms did not develop. What happened or didn't happen on symptom-free days may give you clues about steps to take to control your asthma.

If you enjoy writing, you might like to use your journal to express your thoughts about having asthma. Putting your ideas down on paper is a way to understand and get a handle on your concerns. Remember, your journal is your personal record book. Reading through the entries can help you understand the things in your life that may be contributing to your asthma.

## Talking With Others About Asthma

Having asthma can make you feel different, frustrated, angry and even embarrassed, just as having other conditions, from diabetes to acne, can cause you to feel bad.

At one time or another, everyone has problems. Learning to handle problems is one of the signs of a mature person.

It isn't always easy to talk about a sensitive subject, but you probably will want to talk about your asthma with some of the important people in your life. They will be glad that you opened up the discussion.

Your friends probably already know you have asthma, but they may have questions about it that they have been afraid to ask. They may be interested to know about the steps you take to control asthma and how you can exercise or do other activities. If you use an inhaler, explain how it works and how helpful it is. It can be embarrassing to use an inhaler at school or work but you're less likely to feel embarrassed if you've told your friends why you use it. Your friends may want to know how they can help if your asthma gets out of control. When you are having an asthma episode is another time when you may feel embarrassed and you may tell your friends to go away when you really want them to stay. Talking about how you feel ahead of time will help your friends be able to do what's best for you.

Make friends with other people who have asthma. If you are a student, talk with your school nurse about forming a support group for students with asthma. Maybe you could write an article for the school newspaper about teens with asthma.

If you are in school, let the school nurse know you have asthma and share your asthma plan with her. Your teachers also need to know about your asthma. You may want to talk directly to your teachers about it or you may want the school nurse to tell them. If your asthma causes you to miss school, you'll probably want to talk to your teachers yourself. Then you and your teachers can plan how you can get assignments and keep up with your work. Some teachers may have misunderstandings about asthma. They may think they have to be extra careful not to upset you, or they may think you're trying to get attention or "faking it" to get out of class. If you have a teacher who doesn't seem to understand your condition even after you've talked about it, see if you can set up a meeting with you, the teacher, and the school nurse to try and work out the issues. It's also important for school staff to know about your asthma so they are prepared to help you if you have an asthma emergency. If you work, tell your supervisor about your asthma for the same reasons.

## *Exercise and Asthma*

You may be wondering if asthma will limit your activities.

There is no single answer to that question, but for many people having asthma is only a minor annoyance and they are able to do most things they want to.

One activity that doesn't have to go by the wayside is exercise. Yes, it is true that exercise can trigger asthma. In fact, there is a special name for asthma episodes that are triggered just by exercise: exercise-induced bronchospasm (EIB). But having asthma doesn't mean you shouldn't exercise or play sports. On the contrary: because exercise helps to build up the endurance of your heart and lungs and can keep your weight in check, it can actually decrease your body's need for oxygen, a real plus for those with asthma. Swimming, an excellent exercise for anyone, is especially good if you have asthma because you breathe in warm, humid air as you swim. Sports that have some "down time" (like baseball) might be easier to manage than those that keep you in constant motion (like soccer). But if you love a sport or activity, chances are that, working with your health-care team, you'll be able to figure out a way to play.

If exercise does trigger asthma episodes for you, talk with your doctor about taking a preventive dose of inhaled medication before exercising. To help warm the air you take in, breathe in through your nose instead of your mouth and wear a scarf or mask over your nose and mouth if you are outside in cold weather. Warm-up and cool-down periods also help.

You probably do lots of things that you don't think of as "exercise"—you just think of them as fun. Maybe you go to dances or on walks or play Frisbee in the park. As far as your asthma is concerned, however, you may want to treat these activities as exercise and take the same precautions you would if you were going out to play tennis or for a run.

One final word about exercise and asthma: In the 1984 Olympics, 67 athletes with asthma won 41 medals in sports ranging from basketball to track and field to wrestling. In the 1988 games, 53 athletes with asthma won 16 medals. Exercise and asthma are not incompatible, you just need to have a plan, follow it and learn to read your body's signals.

## Social Life

Let's face it, asthma can be a nuisance. It can pop up at exactly the wrong time.

You probably go out with friends to movies, concerts, dances or parties. You may worry that the excitement of getting ready for a date or party, or the romantic or sexual activities that may follow, could put extra stress on you and trigger an asthma episode. You might want to discuss your asthma with your friends or date so that they will understand it better. If you think it might be a problem, be sure to tell them that cigarette and marijuana smoke can trigger an asthma episode. If perfumes or after-shaves cause you problems, talk about those ahead of time, too. And if you're embarrassed about starting off your date with a list of "asthma do's and don't's," just explain that you are sensitive to certain things.

Remember that you can control asthma. If you have shopping to do to get ready for a party or date, don't wait until the last minute to do it. Plan ahead so that you won't be rushing around trying to meet a deadline. If you expect to be under pressure, it is especially important to take your medication. Don't skip any because you are in a rush and be sure to take medication with you when you go out so that you'll have it handy if you need it. Dancing is exercise so take a preventive dose of medicine before you hit the dance floor if your doctor has prescribed pre-exercise medication. Taking care of yourself can be no big deal, and if that's your attitude, others will feel the same way. But if you forget to look out for yourself, your night out could end in the emergency room—a crummy way to end a date.

## Depression

Having a disease like asthma for which there is treatment but no cure can be depressing, especially when it's difficult to control.

You may feel like you "live on medications" or you may be embarrassed to ask for help especially if you need help because you forgot to take your medications. Talking about your feelings with someone close to you, a parent, school guidance counselor or therapist, can help you feel better. They can also help you think through your options—you may have many more than you can see by yourself.

Even if you get depressed, keep taking your asthma medication. Some researchers think that depression can start a chain of events in your body that may lead to worsening asthma episodes. Although the experts are still studying this possibility, they advise teenagers with asthma to be sure to continue taking medication and not to delay seeking medical help if asthma symptoms get worse.

## Questions and Answers

### Are asthma and allergies related?

Many people with asthma are also allergic to things. Allergies do not cause asthma but they may trigger an asthma episode. Try to avoid things you are sensitive to. Depending on the nature of your allergic responses, your doctor might suggest that you fight allergies with medication or get allergy shots.

### Why do teenagers sometimes "outgrow" asthma?

Perhaps it is misleading to say that teenagers outgrow asthma. More accurately, as you grow, the diameter of your airways expands. Even if they narrow or become filled with mucus and cells during an asthma episode, because they are larger, there is still enough space for air to pass through. But, throughout your life, your airways will be especially sensitive to triggers. Some people may not have asthma episodes as they get older; others will. Even people who think they no longer have asthma may be surprised with an episode if they are exposed to a strong trigger.

### Will cigarette smoking or smoking marijuana affect asthma?

Smoke of any kind, including that from marijuana and tobacco, can be a strong asthma trigger. If you are a smoker, contact your local American Lung Association for help in quitting. Another reason to avoid marijuana smoke is that the marijuana leaf can have a type of mold called Aspergillus, which can cause permanent lung damage.

### When should I call a doctor to treat an asthma episode?

If medications do not reduce wheezing, shortness of breath or rapid breathing, get in touch with your doctor. Fever or vomiting during an acute asthma episode are other signs saying "get medical help." Both of these conditions can cause dehydration (dee-hi-dray-shun: loss of water from your body), which can make your asthma symptoms worse and can be serious. Discuss these and other guidelines with your doctor so you will have a plan and know when you need emergency medical help.

### Can I die from an asthma episode?

Death from asthma is extremely rare. When deaths do occur, experts say that most of them might have been prevented if people had followed a good asthma treatment plan and sought medical help sooner. Having an asthma episode can certainly be frightening and asthma can be a serious disease. Sticking to your asthma treatment plan gives you the best control over your life.

### Is asthma inherited?

The tendency to have asthma can be inherited, but no gene has yet been identified that controls asthma. If a parent has asthma, it does not necessarily mean a child will inherit the disease. Experts are studying other theories to explain why some people seem to develop asthma for the first time when they are adults.

### *Tips for Using an Inhaler*

Ask your doctor to give you a practice inhaler, also called a placebo (ple-see-bow) that has a propellant in it but no medicine so that you can practice using one. Ask for detailed instructions about how to operate it and show your doctor so that you can change what you are doing, if you need to.

Ask your doctor about a spacer or holding chamber to use with your inhaler. A spacer catches the mist from an inhaler and holds it until you are ready to breathe in. That way, you don't have to coordinate releasing the medicine and breathing in. It also lessens the bad taste of the medicine and may feel more gentle.

Here are some other suggestions:

- Be sure your inhaler is clean (keep it capped when it's not in use and wash it with soap and water, or run it through the dishwasher every once in a while).

- You can count the number of puffs you usually use per day. Then calculate how many days an inhaler should last (ask your pharmacist how many puffs are in the inhaler), and mark that day on a calendar. That's the day you should refill your prescription.

- Be sure your inhaler has medicine in it. (To tell if your canister has medicine in it, fill a basin with water and put your canister in it. If it sinks, it's full; if it bobs up with just a bit of the bottom end above the water, it's half full; if it floats like a dead fish, it's empty.

- Stand up while using the inhaler; sit upright if you cannot stand.

- Shake the inhaler a few times before using it.

- Hold your mouth the way your doctor showed you to make sure the medicine gets where it is supposed to.

- First breathe out, then, as you begin to inhale, depress the canister; continue inhaling for 2-3 seconds and then hold your breath for about 10 seconds longer.

- Wait one to two minutes before giving yourself the second dose of a bronchodilator.

- Don't neglect to take a second puff if it has been prescribed; the second dose is needed to get enough medication.

- If your doctor has told you to use a spacer or holding chamber, follow the manufacturer's instructions.

### *Where to Get More Help*

One of the best things you can do for yourself is to keep learning more about asthma and to find resources in your local community. Call your local American Lung Association (ALA) office at 1-800-LUNG-USA.

The ALA has offices in each state that can provide you with information about services in your community. You might even want to volunteer to help offer services to other teens with asthma. Ask your doctor for more information about teens with asthma.

## Section 2.5

## Asthma... At My Age?

Source: American Lung Association. Pub. No. 1551. Used by permission.

Many people who develop asthma as adults remember that they had breathing problems as children. Asthma is a breathing problem that can affect people at any age. Sometimes people have asthma when they are very young and it goes away as they grow up. It may come back later in life. Sometimes people get asthma for the first time when they are older.

Many people have asthma. It can develop at any age. More than 10 million people have asthma and almost 1.1 million of those people are 65 or older.

Asthma is a breathing problem that makes it more difficult for you to get air in and out of your lungs. When you breathe in (inhale), fresh air comes in through your nose. It passes down through tubes (called bronchi) to your lungs. When you breathe out (exhale), stale air from your lungs is breathed out through the same tubes.

When a person has asthma, the breathing tubes are sensitive. They may react to smoke, pollen, dust, air pollution, allergies, or other triggers. In a person with asthma, the breathing tubes may tighten, becoming inflamed and swollen. When the breathing tubes react or when they get inflamed, they become narrow. That makes it harder for you to breathe fresh air in and stale air out. Your difficulty in breathing may change. Sometimes you will feel fine. Other times you may have breathing problems.

## Is Asthma Common in Older People?

Asthma and symptoms like asthma are very common among adults. More than a quarter of the people over 65 included in two studies had some form of wheezing, a common symptom of asthma. They may wheeze with or without colds, or may have attacks of shortness of breath with wheeze. You can have asthma even if you don't wheeze.

In older people, it is sometimes difficult for the doctor to decide whether the problem is asthma or another lung disease. Other lung diseases that cause similar problems are bronchitis and emphysema, particularly in people who smoke. In some adults, bronchitis and emphysema may seem like asthma. Or asthma may seem like bronchitis and emphysema. Heart disease may also cause breathing problems, and a person can have heart and lung disease at the same time.

## The Symptoms of Asthma

The symptoms of asthma can be confusing, but the most common symptoms are:

1. A wheezing sound when you breathe. Sometimes this happens only when you have a cold.

2. Cough. You may cough up mucus. The cough often comes back and it may last more than a week.

3. Shortness of breath. You may have difficulty breathing only now and then, or you may have problems quite often. It feels as if you can't get enough air into your lungs.

4. Chest tightness. Your chest may feel tight in cold weather or during exercise. Chest tightness may be one of the first signs that your asthma is getting worse.

Asthma is a serious health problem. And it is a continuing problem. But the good news is that it can be successfully treated. People with asthma can live normal, productive lives. They need regular medical care from an experienced doctor. However, without proper treatment, asthma can be extremely dangerous, even fatal. Scientists are not sure why some people have asthma and others don't. For some people, a tendency to asthma may be inherited. Other factors may also be involved. Among the things that scientists know are involved are:

- **SMOKING.** Smoking cigarettes, cigars, pipes, or anything else, increases your risk of developing asthma symptoms. If you smoke at home, your child has a greater chance of developing asthma. It's smart to avoid smoke and people who smoke.

- **IN THE FAMILY.** Asthma can "run in the family." It can be inherited. It may be common in Hispanic people, especially those who come from Puerto Rico. If you have a blood relative with asthma or allergies (father, mother, sister, brother, son, daughter), you may be at higher risk of getting asthma.

- **ALLERGIES.** People who are allergic to pollen, pets, or dust are at higher risk of developing asthma.

- **MEDICATIONS.** Some medications may cause asthma symptoms or make asthma worse. Make sure your doctor and your pharmacist know all the medications you are taking. Keep an up-to-date list of all medications you use—both prescription and over-the-counter medicines.

People used to think asthma was a psychological problem. It is not. Asthma is a real medical problem, but too much stress can make asthma worse.

### Treatment of Asthma

Most people with asthma can be treated very successfully. The treatment may mean medication that you inhale (breathe in from an inhaler or puffer) or pills.

Successful treatment of asthma is a partnership. It takes cooperation between the patient and the doctor. You and your doctor will work out an asthma treatment plan. The treatment plan will tell you what to do for your asthma when you're feeling well—and when you're sick.

## Asthma

Your treatment plan will help you know when to take your medications. You will understand what the medications should do. You will know when to call your doctor, especially if your asthma is getting worse.

If you have asthma, you have to know your own body well so you can notice when changes happen. Asthma gives early warning signs of trouble. You also have to work closely with a doctor. You need to know what the best treatments are for you. You need to know the signs of trouble and when to call your doctor. You need a doctor who will talk to you and answer all your questions. You need a pharmacist who can give you information about any medicine you use.

Many good treatments for asthma are available today. The treatments will relax the air tubes in your lungs and help you breathe easier. The treatments reduce the swelling and inflammation in the air tubes.

It's important to follow your doctor's advice about your treatment. Some medicines help prevent asthma. You need to take these medicines all the time, even when you feel well. Other medicines may be needed if your asthma starts to get worse. If your asthma is getting worse, it's important to start treatment early, as soon as your symptoms begin.

Remember that asthma is a problem that does not go away. It is a chronic disease, like diabetes or heart problems. You need a doctor who knows how to treat asthma. Regular care is part of your treatment plan. Don't wait until you have problems to see the doctor.

You have to keep on top of asthma, working with the help of your doctor. Your doctor will teach you how to use medications and tell you the signs of serious problems. Be sure you understand. Don't just smile and say "OK." If you don't understand what your doctor said, ask questions until you do understand. Your doctor will tell you :

- what medications you should take
- when you should take them
- what your medications are supposed to do
- what the signs of problems are
- when to call your doctor for advice
- when to go to an emergency room

**Special Tools for People with Asthma.** There are several different devices that may help you control your asthma and use your asthma medicine better. Ask your doctor about a peak flow meter and a spacer or holding chamber. There's even a special device to help people with arthritis use their medication inhaler more easily.

**Drugstore Remedies.** They may help a little. But everyone is an individual and needs their own asthma treatment plan. If you have asthma, you need an experienced doctor. Good treatment for your asthma means working with your doctor on a regular basis, not buying drugstore remedies that may be expensive and may not treat the problem.

## Medications to Avoid

Some drugs may cause problems for people with asthma. Tell your doctor what medications you are taking for other conditions. Some asthma drugs may cause irregular heartbeats (cardiac arrhythmias). Tell your doctor if this happens to you.

As a reminder, here are some drugs that may interact with asthma medications:

**Blood pressure and heart drugs.** Some people with asthma find that their asthma gets worse when they take certain blood pressure drugs. Some of these drugs are called beta-adrenergic blockers (such as propranolol, nadolol, timolol). Others are called ACE inhibitors.

**Aspirin.** Some people with asthma may have problems if they take aspirin or drugs related to aspirin. Such drugs include many drugstore cold remedies and pain remedies.

**Sleeping pills and tranquilizers.** Sleeping pills, tranquilizers and other sedative drugs may also cause problems for older people with asthma. These drugs make you breathe more slowly and less deeply. That can be dangerous if you have lung problems such as asthma. Remind your doctor about your asthma every time you are given a new prescription.

## What to Do When Having Problems with Asthma

**ACT NOW!** The best control of asthma starts with an asthma treatment plan and early treatment for asthma problems. Serious problems from asthma may result if you delay treatment.

## Asthma

**DON'T WAIT!** If you are having breathing problems or if your medication is not working, **CALL YOUR DOCTOR**. Follow your doctor's advice. If you cannot reach your doctor, go to the nearest hospital emergency room.

Call your doctor right away, even if you are worried about bothering your doctor. Do not wait to see if you feel better. Asthma can be serious! It's better to be safe than sorry.

### Asthma and Older People

Treatment of asthma means recognizing asthma triggers, understanding your asthma treatment, knowing your asthma's early warning signs, and talking with your doctor. Those rules are the same for young people and older people.

Older people are more likely to have other health problems. They have high blood pressure or heart problems. They may take medication for these problems. Sometimes a drug that is good for one health problem is bad for another. Your doctor should know about all your health problems and medications. Your doctor should know all the drugs you are taking.

If you have more than one doctor, remember to tell each doctor what your problems are and what drugs you are taking. If you have a problem, ask the doctor whether one drug might be interacting with another to cause your problem. Keep an up-to-date list of all the medicines you take. Carry the list with you. Many older people still smoke. Smoking makes asthma and other lung problems worse. Tell your doctor if you smoke or if someone in your household smokes. You may be at high risk for lung problems. Other people in your home may also be at high risk for lung problems.

### Good News

You can control your asthma! Good treatment is a partnership between you and your doctor.

- You need an asthma treatment plan.
- You have to talk to your doctor.
- Your doctor has to talk to you.

Young and old people can control asthma. For more information about asthma and asthma programs in your community, call your local American Lung Association. Check the white pages of your telephone book.

*When you can't breathe, nothing else matters.*


## Section 2.6

## *Being a Sport with Exercise-Induced Asthma*

Source: Food and Drug Administration

You wouldn't call Nicholas, 16, a jock. He harbors no dreams of Olympic glory, has no intention of trying out for a school sports team, and has faked more injuries to get out of gym class than even he can count. His hobbies run more to the creative and intellectual—playing bass guitar in a garage band and fooling around on his computer.

But Nicholas (who asked that his last name not be used) didn't always avoid sports. At one time, he was an avid basketball player. But all that changed about four years ago.

"We were supposed to run a mile in gym, and about halfway through, I started coughing, wheezing and felt nauseous. I told the teacher I couldn't go on, but he said that he didn't like quitters. I tried to finish, but I couldn't," he recalls. Nicholas went to the doctor and found out he had exercise-induced asthma.

"My friends stopped inviting me to play B-ball or soccer after school because they were afraid that I would have an attack in the middle of a game. Some of the kids called me 'wheeze boy'," Nicholas says. "After a while, I decided they were right, so even though I loved sports, I gave up on all physical activities."

Asthma is a lung disease that is either inherited or may develop as a severe allergic reaction to pollen, viruses, dust, cigarette smoke, and other "triggers" (but not everyone with allergies develops asthma and not every asthmatic has allergies). Exercise-induced asthma (EIA) is a common form of asthma. It occurs only when a person exercises. People who have chronic asthma, on the other hand, can develop symptoms whenever they are exposed to a trigger.

About 80 to 90 percent of people who have chronic asthma also have EIA. But you can have EIA even if you don't have chronic asthma. Nicholas is among the 35 to 40 percent of people with seasonal allergies who have EIA, and his symptoms are always worse during the spring and fall when gym classes are held outdoors.

## How an EIA Attack Happens

During an asthma attack, the bronchial airways (the large and small tubes that bring air into the lungs) become partly blocked. A trigger, such as pollen, causes immune system cells in the lungs to release histamine and other chemicals. These chemicals cause the lining of the airways to swell, making them narrower. At the same time, tiny rubber-band-like muscles wrapped around the outside of the bronchi (the two large tubes that branch out from the windpipe into the lungs) tighten in what is known as "bronchospasm." Completing the process, mucus cells in the airways produce secretions that plug up the works even more.

In about half of chronic asthmatics, the initial attack (known as "early response") is followed by a delayed reaction ("late response"). This delayed reaction happens because lung inflammation makes the airways and lungs extremely sensitive to irritation. Some asthma specialists believe that EIA differs from chronic asthma because exercise-induced bronchospasm (another name for EIA) does not cause lung inflammation, so there is no late response.

With asthma, the problem isn't getting air into the lungs, but exhaling air out through the obstructed airways. (People who don't have asthma can get an idea of what an asthma attack feels like by taking a breath and holding it for a second, then trying to take another breath without exhaling first.)

Cold, dry air is believed to trigger EIA. So, exercising outdoors in the winter or breathing through your mouth during heavy exertion is likely to set off an attack. (Breathing through your nose warms and moistens the air before it reaches the lungs.) EIA symptoms typically occur after three to eight minutes of strenuous activity, and can last 20 to 30 minutes. They can range from mild to severe, and include coughing, wheezing, tightness or pain in the chest, shortness of breath, and reduced stamina.

## EIA Need Not Bench You

"Many people who have EIA don't know it because they blame their symptoms on being out of shape," notes John Weiler, M.D., a professor in the department of internal medicine at the University of Iowa Hospitals and Clinics in Iowa City. Others may experience symptoms only when they push themselves to the "max" or exercise outdoors when air quality is poor.

But if you're susceptible to it, EIA can affect you, regardless of your fitness level or athletic ability. In fact, according to various studies, 10 to 12 percent of athletes have EIA. At the 1984 summer Olympics in Los Angeles, 67 of the 597 members of the American team had EIA; among them, they won 41 medals.

Obviously, EIA need not limit participation or success in vigorous activities. Today it can be medically managed and its effects minimized.

"In the past, doctors discouraged people with asthma from exerting themselves to avoid triggering an attack. But the current thinking is that it is important for asthmatics to engage in regular exercise to condition and strengthen their lungs," says Stanley Szefler, M.D., director of clinical pharmacology at the National Jewish Center for Immunology and Respiratory Medicine in Denver.

Swimming in an indoor pool may be the ideal exercise for asthmatics because the warm, humid air keeps the airways from drying and cooling. However, "with proper management, virtually no sport is off-limits," says Szefler.

Proper management of EIA, Szefler says, includes monitoring air flow with a peak-flow meter, avoiding allergic triggers, and using medication before exercise.

Asthma symptoms can change a lot. They are often worse at night than during the day. They may be worse in the winter or during "allergy seasons" when pollen counts are high. The new National Heart, Lung, and Blood Institute guidelines recommend that people 5 years or older who have moderate to severe asthma use a peak-flow meter twice a day (morning and evening).

A peak-flow meter measures how fast you blow air out of your lungs. When a person blows into the device—which looks something like a kazoo—a slide indicates the force of the exhaled air. The farther the slide is pushed, the greater the peak flow.

"Peak-flow meters can help asthmatics monitor their symptoms so attacks can be better anticipated," explains Michael Gluck, D.Sc., chief of FDA's anesthesiology and respiratory devices branch.

Once a doctor determines normal peak flow, a treatment approach can be tailored just for you. For instance, your doctor may instruct you to take more medicine than usual if your peak flow drops a certain amount, say 70 percent of normal, or to get medical help right away if it falls to 30 percent of normal.

"In the past, a vague sense of not feeling well was the only indication a person had that an asthma attack was imminent. By that time, it was often too late to head off the attack," says Gluck. "Peak-flow meters give you ... a much earlier indication of an oncoming attack."

"Drugs that relax the muscle spasm in the walls of the bronchial tubes to open them are often the first line of treatment in preventing EIA," says Tunde Otulana, M.D., a medical reviewer in FDA's oncology and pulmonary drugs division. Such drugs are called bronchodilators. They are typically prescribed in aerosol (inhalant) form. They are sprayed into the mouth and breathed directly into the lungs. Doctors recommend using the medication from five minutes to an hour before exercise. If breathing problems develop during exercise, you may need to take another dose. The most common side effect of bronchodilators is feeling jittery, says Otulana.

Cromolyn sodium is often prescribed to treat athletes who have EIA. This drug, which is also an inhalant, prevents the lining of the airways from swelling in response to cold air or allergic triggers, explains Otulana, and must be taken on a regular basis for the treatment of asthma. Cromolyn sodium can be used up to 15 minutes before engaging in physical activity.

Cromolyn has few side effects, according to Otulana. "The most common complaint is that it leaves an unpleasant taste in the mouth for a few seconds. Some people may experience coughing due to dryness and throat irritation and, in rare instances, patients have become nauseated."

In addition to bronchodilators and Cromolyn, which are used primarily to head off an attack of EIA, the National Heart, Lung, and Blood Institute treatment guidelines recommend the use of inhaled corticosteroids for patients with moderate to severe chronic asthma. "Instead of using a 'rescue' approach to treat episodes of breathlessness, doctors are now focusing on the big picture and using a preventive approach to treat airway inflammation, which is the underlying cause of asthma," says Szefler.

"Corticosteroids work by reducing swelling in the bronchial tubes and by enhancing the action of bronchodilators. They are meant to be used as preventive medication, usually on an ongoing basis," says Otulana.

Corticosteroid inhalants can occasionally cause throat irritation and thrush (a fungal infection in the mouth), says Otulana. (He advises gargling with warm water after using the inhaler to help avoid both side effects.) Prolonged use of very high doses may increase the risk of the same type of health problems associated with the drug in pill form: high blood pressure, diabetes, and softening of the bones.

"It is very difficult to recognize EIA, especially when exercise is the only trigger for asthma," says Weiler. "If you can't keep up with the other kids, can't seem to be able to 'get into shape' no matter how much you exercise, or experience problems after exercise that your classmates don't, EIA may be to blame."

Today, Nicholas carries a bronchodilator with him and uses Cromolyn 20 minutes before gym class. Although he still dislikes exercise, he doesn't cut gym now that he can keep up with the other kids. "If I premedicate, I have no problems," he says. "Asthma can be a setback, but it doesn't have to be—if you learn how to deal with it."

## Tips on Coping with EIA

- Start with a 15-minute warm-up to allow the lungs to adjust to the increased demand for oxygen.

- In cold weather, cover your mouth and nose with a scarf to help warm the air before it gets to the lungs.

- Avoid triggers that may cause or worsen EIA (for example, don't exercise outdoors when pollen counts are high).

- End with a 15-minute cool-down rather than stopping abruptly.

- Follow your doctor's instructions about using medication before or after exercise. If you're on a team, let your coach know about your doctor's instructions.

- If you have symptoms, use a bronchodilator right away. Remember, Cromolyn and corticosteroids are not recommended during an asthma attack because they do not immediately open the airways.

*—Ruth Papazian*

## Section 2.7

## *Managing Asthma: A Guide for Schools*

NIH Pub. No. 91-2650. September 1991.

### *Foreword*

The guide that makes up this chapter was developed as the first of a series of collaborative projects between the National Heart, Lung, and Blood Institute (NHLBI), National Asthma Education Program (NAEP), National Institutes of Health, U.S. Department of Health and Human Services, and the Fund for the Improvement and Reform of Schools and Teaching, Office of Educational Research and Improvement (OERI), U.S. Department of Education. These agencies are working together because of the serious and chronic nature of asthma. It affects over 1 in 20 children but, with proper treatment, can be controlled. This material is intended to provide school personnel with practical ways to help students with asthma participate fully in all school activities.

The NHLBI supports comprehensive school asthma education and has as a major objective the development and dissemination of asthma education materials. The focus is to encourage school personnel such as teachers, school nurses, physical education teachers, and coaches to recognize asthma as a disease requiring ongoing care. Giving proper treatment and education will improve the performance of students who suffer from asthma. Thus, the NAEP encourages developing a partnership among physicians, school personnel, patients, and families in managing and controlling asthma.

The OERI is particularly interested in school programs for asthma management because it relates directly to national education goals developed by the President and state governors. Two of the six goals include statements which apply to asthma management. The first states that "all children in America will start school ready to learn." Part of being "ready to learn" means being physically able to take advantage of learning opportunities. Students who are not well enough to attend school, or do not receive school support to control their illness, cannot learn effectively.

The second goal describes the need for "safe, disciplined, and drug-free schools" in America. Safety for asthmatic students is knowing that adults at home and at school can help them properly manage asthma episodes and emergencies. Safety is also knowing that school personnel understand the feelings that accompany asthma and the treatment side effects. Safety, like health, is a basic need that must be satisfied before learning can begin.

AMERICA 2000, the strategy for achieving these national education goals mentioned earlier, emphasizes looking "beyond...classrooms to our communities and families." One community that can contribute to better education is the medical community. Health care professionals can help inform school staff and parents about medical issues that may affect a student's ability to learn.

This chapter outlines how school personnel can help in asthma management. The specific roles and actions that various staff should perform are specified. We hope that schools will take advantage of this important material. For further information please contact the National Asthma Education Program, 4733 Bethesda Avenue, Suite 530, Bethesda, Maryland 20814; (301) 951-3260.

—*Claude Lenfant, M.D.,*

*Director, National Heart, Lung, and Blood Institute,
U.S. Department of Health and Human Services.*

—*Diane Ravitch,*

*Assistant Secretary and Counselor to the Secretary,
Office of Educational Research and Improvement,
U.S. Department of Education.*

## Asthma: A Leading Cause of Absenteeism

Asthma is one of the leading causes of school absence for illness. Approximately 3 million children under the age of 18 have been diagnosed with asthma, and that number may be higher. School staff can play an important role in helping the student with asthma manage the disease at school.

***Effective management of asthma at school can help:***

- promote a supportive learning environment for students with asthma,
- reduce absences,
- reduce disruption in the classroom,
- provide the necessary support in the event of an emergency, and
- achieve full participation in physical activities.

This guide is designed for any member of the school staff, regardless of their medical background. The information in the guide will help you develop and maintain an asthma management program for your school. Included in the guide are:

- a brief definition of asthma,
- a list of common "triggers" or stimuli that cause asthma episodes,
- a description of effective asthma management in schools,
- a description of an asthma management program for schools,
- action plans for school staff, and
- resource information on asthma including an asthma action plan to be used for each student with asthma.

## Asthma Is a Chronic Lung Disease

Asthma is a chronic lung disease characterized by acute episodes or attacks of breathing problems such as coughing, wheezing, chest tightness, and shortness of breath. These symptoms are caused by airway swelling, blocked airways, and increased responsiveness of the airways to a variety of stimuli or "triggers." The triggers that cause an asthma episode vary with individuals, but there are common triggers.

## Asthma Can Be Controlled With Effective Management

Asthma can be controlled with proper diagnosis and management. It cannot be cured. Traditionally asthma care has focused on treating acute episodes. New approaches emphasize preventing episodes by reducing the constant presence of inflammation in the lungs. With long-term therapy, people with asthma need not suffer from symptoms. Consequently when asthma is managed effectively, the student can enjoy unrestricted participation in all school activities.

Effective management of asthma will allow a student to maintain a normal activity level, prevent acute symptoms and episodes, and avoid side effects from medications.

This can be accomplished by:

- Recognizing the early warning signs of asthma. These may include shortness of breath, coughing, increased breathing rate, and wheezing.

- Avoiding or controlling triggers. Refer to the list below.

- Taking medication as directed. A person with asthma often needs two types of medications. One form is used to relax the airways The other is used to decrease the inflammation in the airways and prevent episodes from occurring.

- Monitoring asthma with a peak flow meter, if available. A peak flow meter measures how well air is moving through the lungs. When the airways are narrow, this measurement will be decreased.

Effective management of asthma requires a partnership among the student, parent(s) or guardian(s), the physician, and other adults who work with the child. The school team can play an important role in helping students manage their asthma by providing support through the development of an asthma management program.

### Common Asthma Triggers

- allergens such as pollen, animal dander, dust mites, and molds.

- irritants such as cold air, strong odors, weather changes, and cigarette smoke.

- upper respiratory infections such as a cold or flu.

- physical exercise, especially in cold weather.

## Develop an Asthma Management Program in Your School

Developing an asthma management program shows that your school is responsive to the needs of students with asthma. Such a program will also ease the burden on school staff. By creating procedures that outline responsibilities, an asthma management program will alleviate any anxiety the staff might have about helping a student with asthma. A management program should contain:

- school policies and procedures for administering medications,

- specific actions for staff members to perform in the asthma management program,

- an action plan for asthma episodes.

This action plan should include management guidelines for each student with asthma. The plan should describe the student's medical information and specific steps in asthma management. The asthma action plan should contain:

- a list of medications the student receives, noting which ones need to be taken during school hours,

- a specific plan of action for school personnel in case of an acute episode, and

- emergency procedures and phone numbers.

This action plan should be signed by a parent and the physician and kept on file at school. Because every individual's asthma is different, the action plan must be specific to the student's needs. The sample asthma action plan included in this guide may be adapted to fit the needs of individual students and your school. The following sections of this guide provide two sets of reproducible handouts for use by school staff in their asthma management efforts.

- Managing Asthma in the School-Actions for School Staff
- Resource Information on Asthma.

Each staff member should always remember: the student's action plan should be referred to at the first sign of an acute episode of asthma.

## Managing Asthma in the School: Actions for School Staff

- Principal
- School Nurse or Other Health Personnel
- Classroom Teacher
- Physical Education Instructor and Coach
- Guidance Counselor

## Actions for the Principal

- Involve your staff in the asthma management program. A school asthma management program is a cooperative effort that involves the student, parents, teachers, school staff, and physicians. Many members of the school staff can play a role in maintaining your school's asthma management program, although the principal or the school nurse may be most instrumental in getting a program started. Take the steps listed below to help set up an asthma management program in your school.

- Develop a clear policy on taking medication during school hours. Work with parents, teachers, the school nurse (if available), and others to provide the most supportive policy that your school system allows so that the student can get the medication he/she needs.

- Designate one person on the school staff to be responsible for maintaining each student's asthma action plan.

## Asthma

- Provide opportunities for staff to learn about asthma and allergies by setting up in-service courses. You may get assistance from your school nurse, or a local hospital or medical society. Other sources of information are the American Lung Association, Asthma and Allergy Foundation of America, National Jewish Center for Immunology and Respiratory Medicine, and the Mothers of Asthmatics.

- Establish an asthma resource file of pamphlets, brochures, and other publications for school personnel to provide an opportunity for the staff to get additional information about asthma. Many of the organizations cited above offer materials for this purpose. Make general information available to students as well.

- Schedule any extensive building repairs or cleaning to avoid exposing students to fumes, dust, and other irritants. When possible, try to schedule painting and major repairs during long vacations or the summer months.

- Support and encourage communication with parents to improve school health services.

### Actions for the School Nurse or Other Health Personnel

- Maintain the asthma action plan for every student with asthma. Include information on medications, dosages, triggers, and emergency procedures.

- Alert staff members about students with a history of asthma.

- Use the warning signs presented in the publication, *Managing Asthma: A Guide for Schools*, to help identify students with uncontrolled asthma. Provide this information to parents with the encouragement to see a physician.

- Assist with the administration of medication in accordance with school policy.

- Monitor response to treatment using a peak flow meter. (Refer to resource section on "Use of a Peak Flow Meter" in "Sample Patient Handouts.")

- Communicate with parents about acute episodes, if any, and about the student's general progress in controlling asthma at school.

- Conduct in-services on asthma, and consult with staff to help develop appropriate school activities for students with asthma.

- Collaborate with the PTA to consider offering a family asthma education program in school. Consult organizations on the resource list in the publication, *Managing Asthma: A Guide for Schools*, for assistance.

If there is not a nurse at your school these tasks should be assigned to an appropriate staff member.

### Actions for the Classroom Teacher

- Know the early warning signs of an asthma episode.

- Have a copy of the asthma action plan in the classroom. Review it with the student and parents. Know what steps to take in case of an asthma episode.

- Develop a clear procedure with the student and parent for handling schoolwork missed due to asthma.

- Understand that a student with asthma may feel: drowsy or tired, different from the other kids, anxious about access to medication, embarrassed about the disruption to school activities that an asthma episode causes, and/or withdrawn.

- Help the student feel more comfortable by recognizing these feelings. Try to maintain confidentiality. Educate classmates about asthma so they will be more understanding.

## Asthma

- Know the possible side effects of asthma medications and how they may impact the student's performance in the classroom. Refer any problem to the school nurse and parent(s). Common side effects of medicine that warrant referral are nervousness, nausea, jitteriness, hyperactivity, and drowsiness.

- Reduce known allergens in the classroom to help students who have allergies. Common allergens found in classrooms include chalk dust, animals, and strong odors (perfumes, paints).

- Encourage the student with asthma to participate fully in physical activities.

- Allow a student to engage in quiet activity if recovery from an acute episode precludes full participation.

### Actions for the Physical Education Instructor and Coach

- Encourage exercise and participation in sports for students with asthma. When asthma is under good control, students with the disease are able to play most sports. A number of Olympic medalists have asthma.

- Appreciate that exercise can cause acute episodes for many students with asthma. Exercise in cold dry air and activities that require extended running appear to trigger asthma more readily than other forms of exercise. However, medicines can be taken before exertion to help avoid an episode. This preventive medicine enables most students with exercise-induced asthma to participate in any sport they choose. Warm-up and cool-down activities appropriate for any exercise will also help the student with asthma.

- Support the student's treatment plan if it requires premedication before exercise.

- Understand what to do if an asthma episode occurs during exercise. Have the child's asthma action plan available.

- Encourage students with asthma to participate actively in sports but also recognize and respect their limits. Permit less strenuous activities if a recent illness precludes full participation.

- Refer your questions about a student's ability to fully participate in physical education to the parents and school nurse.

## Actions for the Guidance Counselor

- Help all school personnel understand that asthma is not an emotional or psychological disease—it is not "all in the child's head." Strong emotions such as laughing or crying can trigger an acute episode because this irritates and constricts the sensitive airways of a person with asthma.

- Recognize that learning to cope with asthma, as with any chronic illness, can be difficult. Teachers may notice low self-esteem, withdrawal from activities, discouragement over the steps needed to control asthma, or difficulty making up schoolwork. Special counseling with the student and/or parents may help the student handle problems more effectively.

## Early Signs of an Asthma Episode

Students who have asthma often learn to identify their early warning signs—the physical changes that occur in the early stage of airway obstruction. These early warning signs usually happen long before more serious symptoms occur. Being aware of these early warning signs allows the student to take medication at a time when asthma is easiest to control. Teachers should encourage students to be aware of these early symptoms, and to take the proper action immediately.

Knowing the signs of a beginning episode will help you and other staff take appropriate measures to avoid a more serious medical emergency. There should be no delay once a student has notified the teacher of a possible problem.

*Asthma*

A student may exhibit one or more of these signs during the initial phase of an asthma episode.

1. Changes in breathing may include: coughing, wheezing, breathing through the mouth, shortness of breath, and/or rapid breathing.

2. Verbal Complaints. Often a student who is familiar with asthma will know that an episode is about to happen. The student might tell the teacher that: the chest is tight, the chest hurts, he/she cannot catch a breath, the mouth is dry, the neck feels funny, and/or a more general "I don't feel well."

3. Other signs may be: an itchy chin or neck—some people may rub their chin or neck in response to this feeling, or "clipped" speech—the student may speak in very short, choppy sentences.

**Resources Available to Schools to Help Manage Asthma**

*For more information contact:*

The National Asthma Education Program
(301) 951-3260
Information Center
4733 Bethesda Ave.
Suite 530
Bethesda, MD 20814-4820

The following organizations can provide additional materials and additional information about asthma:

Asthma and Allergy Foundation of America
1-800-727-8462
National Headquarters
1717 Massachusetts Ave., NW
Suite 305
Washington, DC 20036

## Respiratory Diseases and Disorders Sourcebook

American Lung Association
Call your local Lung Association

National Jewish Center for Immunology and Respiratory Medicine
1-800-222-5864
1400 Jackson St.
Denver, CO 80206

American Academy of Allergy and Immunology
1-800-822-2762
611 East Well St.
Milwaukee, WI 53202

National Allergy and Asthma Network,
1-800-878-4403
Mothers of Asthmatics
3554 Chain Bridge Road
Suite 200
Fairfax, VA 22030

American College of Allergy & Immunology
1-800-842-7777
800 East Northwest Hwy.
Suite 1080
Palatine, IL 60067

Section 2.8

# Management of Asthma During Pregnancy

NIH Pub. No. 93-3279. September 1993. Extracted from the Report of the Working Group on Asthma and Pregnancy.

## Introduction

Asthma is one of the most common illnesses that complicate pregnancy. Asthma may occur for the first time during pregnancy, or it may change during pregnancy; about one-third of pregnant women with asthma experience worse asthma during pregnancy, one-third remain the same, and one-third improve. In any case, pregnant women with asthma need treatment to control their asthma and thus protect their health and the health of their fetus. Asthma is a chronic, persistent disease of the airways characterized by coughing, wheezing, chest tightness and difficulty breathing that are usually reversible, but that can be severe and sometimes fatal. Recent studies demonstrated that inflammation is a critical factor in the pathogenesis of asthma, and therefore asthma therapy is predicated on medications to reverse and prevent this abnormality.

Pregnant women with asthma require long-term management to maintain lung function and blood oxygenation to ensure oxygen supply to the fetus. Uncontrolled asthma during pregnancy can produce serious maternal and fetal complications. Maternal complications include preeclampsia, gestational hypertension, hyperemesis gravidarum, vaginal hemorrhage, toxemia, and induced and complicated labors. Fetal complications include increased risk of perinatal mortality, intrauterine growth retardation, preterm birth, low birth weight, and neonatal hypoxia. When asthma is controlled, however, pregnant women with asthma can maintain a normal pregnancy with little or no increased risk to themselves or their fetuses.

The goals of therapy for pregnant women with asthma are to control symptoms, including nocturnal symptoms; maintain normal or near-normal pulmonary function; maintain normal activity levels, including exercise; prevent acute exacerbations of asthma; avoid any adverse effects from asthma medications; and deliver a healthy infant.

To achieve these goals, the Working Group on Asthma and Pregnancy strongly recommends that asthma be as aggressively treated in pregnant women as in non-pregnant women. Underestimation of asthma severity and undertreatment of of exacerbations are two common errors that may lead to adverse maternal and fetal outcomes.

Asthma care should be integrated with obstetric care. Effective management of asthma includes ongoing management to prevent asthma exacerbations and control chronic symptoms, and early intervention to relieve acute exacerbations. There are four integral components of effective asthma management.

*Use Objective Measures for Assessment and Monitoring*

**Maternal Lung Function.** Objective measures of lung volumes or flow rates are essential for assessing and monitoring the severity of asthma in order to make appropriate therapeutic recommendations. Using an office spirometer in the initial assessment of all pregnant patients being evaluated for asthma, and periodically thereafter as appropriate, is recommended. The single best measure of pulmonary function for assessing severity is forced expiratory volume in 1 second ($FEV_1$).

Peak expiratory flow rate (PEFR), which can be measured reliably with inexpensive portable peak flow meters, correlates well with $FEV_1$. Home peak expiratory flow monitoring should be considered for patients who take medications daily. Regular monitoring can help detect early signs of deterioration, indicate when asthma therapy might be changed, and assess response to therapy. Women with asthma may have minimal symptoms but still have abnormal pulmonary function tests and potentially impaired fetal oxygenation. Peak flow measurement will also help differentiate asthma from other causes of dyspnea during pregnancy.

**Fetal Monitoring.** Fetal evaluation is based on objective measurements made by different techniques used according to gestational age and risk factors (12 to 20 weeks) sonography provides a benchmark for progressive fetal growth. Sequential sonographic evaluations of fetal growth are indicated in second and third trimesters if asthma is moderate or severe or if growth retardation is suspected. Electronic fetal heart rate monitoring and ultrasonic determinations of fetal behavior in the third trimester should be used as needed to ensure fetal well-being. For many third trimester patients weekly fetal assessment is sufficient, but frequency should increase if fetal problems are suspected. Daily maternal recording of fetal activity or "kick counts," should be encouraged.

Immediate antepartum fetal assessment is indicated in asthma exacerbations with an incomplete or poor response to therapy or with significant maternal hypoxemia. One reasonable approach to antepartum fetal assessment is continuous electronic fetal heart rate monitoring.

When women with asthma are admitted in labor, careful fetal monitoring is essential. Intensive fetal monitoring (either continuous electronic fetal heart rate monitoring or intermittent auscultation) is recommended for those patients who enter labor with uncontrolled or severe asthma and with a nonreassuring admission test of fetal assessment or other risk factors.

*Avoid or Control Asthma Triggers*

The identification and control of triggers— factors that induce airway inflammation or precipitate asthma exacerbations— are important in controlling asthma during pregnancy. Avoiding exposure to identified allergens and irritants can reduce asthma symptoms, airway hyperresponsiveness, and the need for medication. In addition, eliminating all exposure to tobacco smoke is important for pregnant women with asthma. Although immunotherapy should not be started during pregnancy, ongoing immunotherapy may be continued to reduce the response to a specifically identified allergen.

*Establish Medication Plans for Chronic Management of Asthma and for Managing Exacerbations Using Preferred Medications*

**Chronic Management of Asthma.** Asthma is a disease that varies among patients, and the degree of severity may change for individual patients from 1 month or season to the next or during pregnancy. Therefore specific therapeutic regimens must be tailored to individual needs and circumstances. A step-wise approach to pharmacological therapy, in which the number and frequency of medications are increased with increasing asthma severity, permits this flexibility. Once control of asthma is sustained for several weeks or months, a reduction in therapy— a step down— can be carefully considered because the aim of pharmacological therapy is to use the least medication to maintain control. The step-wise approach presented with detailed recommendations in this chapter emphasizes that anything more than mild occasional asthma requires daily therapy with inhaled anti-inflammatory agents, either cromolyn sodium or beclomethasone. Further, all patients must have inhaled beta$_2$-agonist to relieve symptoms, but it is essential that patients should not rely on frequent use of bronchodilator agents to control their asthma. An increased need for inhaled beta$_2$-agonist is an indication that the asthma is deteriorating and anti-inflammatory therapy should be instituted or increased.

An extensive review of the animal and human studies on the effects of asthma medications found few risks of adverse effects to the fetus. The known risks of uncontrolled asthma are far greater than the known risks to the mother or fetus from asthma medications.

**Managing Exacerbations.** Anticipatory or early intervention is important in treating acute exacerbations. This reduces the likelihood of an episode progressing to severe airway obstruction with impaired maternal/fetal oxygenation. Every patient needs to have a written action plan for recognizing and responding early to signs of worsening asthma. The action plan indicates how to increase medications in response to decreased PEFR or increased symptoms and how to obtain medical advice at any time.

Patients should not delay seeking medical help in the emergency department or hospital if any of the following occur: therapy does not provide rapid improvement, the improvement is not sustained, there is further deterioration, the asthma exacerbation is severe, or fetal kick count decreases.

Treatment in the emergency department or hospital emphasizes intensified administration of inhaled beta$_2$-agonists, oxygen supplementation and the early introduction of systemic corticosteroids.

Monitoring is essential because, in the presence of moderate to severe exacerbation, deterioration can be rapid and a decrease in maternal $P_aO_2$ (especially below 60mmHg) and fetal $P_aO_2$ can result in profoundly decreased fetal oxygen saturation and fetal hypoxia. Furthermore, fetal distress can occur even in the absence if maternal hypotension or hypoxia. Aggressive monitoring of fetal well-being is essential during critical maternal illness.

**Managing the Asthma During Labor and Delivery.** The patient's regularly scheduled asthma medications should be continued during labor and delivery. The patient's PEFR should be taken upon admission to labor and delivery and, subsequently, every 12 hours. Asthma is often quiescent during labor and delivery. However, if asthma symptoms develop, PEFR should be monitored after asthma

## Asthma

treatments. The patients should be kept well hydrated and be provided adequate analgesia to limit the risk of bronchospasm. Patients who have required chronic systemic corticosteroids during pregnancy should be given hydrocortisone to treat for possible adrenal suppression.

Narcotic analgesics that cause histamine release should be avoided; fentanyl is a preferred agent. Lumbar epidural analgesia reduces oxygen consumption and minute ventilation during the first and second stages of labor, which offers the patients with asthma considerable benefit. If a general anesthetic is necessary, preanesthetic use of atropine and glycopyrrolate may provide bronchodilatory effect. For induction of anesthesia, ketamine is the agent of choice. Low concentrations of halogenated anesthetics can provide bronchodilation to the patient with asthma.

For labor induction, oxytocin is the drug of choice. Prior to term, the use of 15 methyl prostaglandin $F_2$-alpha should be avoided because it may cause bronchospasm; use of prostaglandin $E_2$ suppositories or gel has not been reported to cause bronchospasm.

For postpartum hemorrhage, oxytocin is the recommended agent. If additional agents are required, methylergonovine as well as ergonovine should be avoided if possible because they may cause bronchospasm. If their use is unavoidable, pretreatment with methylprednisolone is recommended. If prostaglandin treatment is necessary, the safest analog is $E_2$, which is less likely to cause bronchospasm.

The treatment of preterm labor in a patient already receiving asthma medication creates a risk of dangerous drug interactions. During an asthma exacerbation, uterine contractions are common and usually do not progress to preterm labor. Successful treatment of the exacerbation will usually abate the contractions. If tocolytic therapy is necessary, care should be taken to avoid the use of more than one type of $beta_2$-agonist. Magnesium sulfate is recommended to treat uterine contractions if the patient is already taking a systemic $beta_2$-agonist for her asthma.

### *Educate Pregnant Patients to Develop a Partnership in Asthma Management*

It is of the greatest importance for pregnant women with asthma to understand that they are "breathing for two." These women need information on how to properly control and manage their asthma during pregnancy to reduce the risk to the fetus. Concerns of pregnant women need to be elicited and addressed. Open communication, joint development of a treatment plan by the clinician and patient, and encouragement of the family's efforts to improve prevention and treatment of the patient's symptoms will assist in promoting maternal and fetal safety and well-being. Providing support to pregnant women with asthma during this potentially anxious time is important.

## Maternal Physiology and Interactions with Asthma

### IMPACT ON FETAL OXYGENATION

Changes in maternal respiratory, cardiovascular, and circulatory systems during pregnancy influence fetal oxygenation and acid base status. This section looks at these physiological alterations and their clinical implications.

### Respiratory System Changes

A relative hyperventilation during pregnancy is seen beginning in the first trimester, with minute ventilation increasing up to 48 percent by term. This change is due to an increase in tidal volume; respiratory rate is relatively unchanged during pregnancy, so tachypnea in pregnancy (respirations more than 20 per minute) is an abnormal finding that must be investigated. Increased tidal volume change is due principally to increased placental progesterone production, which also accounts for a sensation of shortness of breath ("dyspnea of pregnancy") that is common in pregnancy. The hyperventilation of pregnancy is associated with significant changes in arterial blood gas with a resting arterial carbon dioxide tension ($PCO_2$) below 35 mmHg. This chronic respiratory alkalosis is partially compensated for by increased renal bicarbonate excretion. Total oxygen consumption and basal metabolic rate also increase by 20 percent and 15 percent, respectively, accounting for increased maternal oxygen tension, which is also common in normal pregnancy. Normal values of $PO_2$ range from 106 to 108 mmHg during the first trimester and decrease slightly in the third trimester (Prowse & Gaensler, 1965; Templeton & Kelman, 1976). Oxygenization is significantly influenced by postural effects. Twenty-five percent of pregnant women experience arterial oxygen tensions of less than 90 mmHg in the supine position, and there is also an increased likelihood of developing increased alveolar-arterial oxygen gradients in the supine, compared to the upright, position.

In terms of pulmonary function, the following are seen by term: a decrease in residual volume, functional residual capacity, expiratory reserve volume, and total lung capacity; an increase in inspiratory capacity; and no change in vital capacity or forced expiratory volume in 1 second ($FEV_1$). All the changes just discussed have the potential for profound impact upon the clinical interpretation of pulmonary function studies and blood gas measurements in the pregnant woman with asthma and must be clearly kept in mind in the clinical interpretation of such data. In general, however, those measurements of pulmonary function in common clinical use (such as respiratory rate or $FEV_1$) do not change with pregnancy, so any changes in these measures should be considered abnormalities and treated as such.

Recent information suggests that during painful labor there is relative hypoventilation between contractions resulting in decreased maternal $PO_2$. With normal pulmonary function, the fetal implications of this phenomenon are negligible. However, this information forms a rationale for the liberal use of oxygen in laboring patients with any degree of respiratory impairment. Maternal oxygen saturation must remain greater than 95 percent to assure adequate fetal oxygenation (Clark, 1990).

## *Cardiovascular System Changes*

During normal pregnancy, resting cardiac output is significantly increased by 6 weeks gestation, peaking at 30 to 50 percent over nonpregnant values by the early part of the third trimester (Clark et al., 1989). This increase is a result of increases in both heart rate and stroke volume and is sustained throughout the pregnancy. In the third trimester, cardiac output is significantly decreased in either the supine or standing positions. Up to 10 percent of women may experience the "supine hypotensive syndrome," a marked drop in blood pressure resulting from venacaval occlusion in the supine position (Holmes, 1960). Supine hypotension can have important maternal hemodynamic consequences and, because of decreased uterine perfusion, may result in fetal hypoxia and bradycardia. Thus recumbent pregnant women should avoid the supine position and favor the lateral decubitus or lateral tilt position.

Further significant increases in cardiac output are seen in the peripartum period. Labor is associated with an additional 1 to 2 liters per minute by the second stage (Ueland & Hansen, 1969). This increase may be minimized by having the patient labor in the lateral recumbent position with epidural anesthesia (Clark et al., 1991). In the immediate postpartum period, cardiac output is increased further, by up to 40 to 50 percent (Ueland et al., 1969), as a result of the "autotransfusion" phenomenon-the release of venacaval obstruction and expulsion of blood from the utero/placental bed into the central circulation. Thus the period of maximum risk for patients with compromised cardiovascular function is during the peripartum period. Cesarean section does not appear to reduce this risk.

*Circulatory System Changes*

**Blood volume.** Blood volume increases markedly in pregnancy, with an increase in plasma volume at term averaging 40 to 50 percent over nonpregnant values (Clark et al., 1989). This increase, due to estrogen stimulation of aldosterone, begins as early as 4 to 6 weeks gestation, plateaus at approximately 32 to 34 weeks gestation, and then remains unchanged until delivery. There is a concomitant increase in red cell mass, erythropoiesis being stimulated by chorionic somatomammotrophin, progesterone, and possibly prolactin. Because red cell mass is increased 20 to 25 percent as opposed to the greater increase in plasma volume, a "physiologic anemia" of pregnancy may be produced. In absolute terms, it is estimated that blood volume in single pregnancies is increased 1,600 cc, with an average 2,000-cc increase observed by 32 weeks in twin gestations.

**Blood pressure.** Systolic and diastolic arterial blood pressure decrease until mid pregnancy and gradually return to nonpregnant values by term (Wilson et al., 1980). These changes appear to be secondary to hormonally mediated decreases in systemic vascular resistance. Thus blood pressures that might be considered frankly hypotensive in the adult male may be normal in the pregnant female, especially during the second trimester of pregnancy. In evaluating blood pressure in the seriously ill pregnant patient with asthma, a comparison of prenatal blood pressure records is important.

**Other Hemodynamic Changes.** Systemic vascular resistance falls by the second trimester, rising toward normal by late third trimester. However, even in the late third trimester, systemic vascular resistance is decreased by 20 percent compared to nonpregnant controls (Clark et al., 1989). Similarly, pulmonary vascular resistance falls 35 percent by late pregnancy compared to nonpregnant values. Left ventricular stroke work index, pulmonary capillary wedge pressure, and central venous pressure all remain unchanged. The pulmonary-capillary-wedge pressure/colloid-oncotic pressure gradient decreases significantly, however, by the third trimester of pregnancy. This predisposes the pregnant woman to pulmonary edema, either because of increased intravascular pressure (i.e., increased fluid overload) or increased pulmonary capillary permeability.

## THE EFFECT OF ASTHMA ON MOTHER AND FETUS

### Epidemiologic Studies

Two large epidemiologic studies published in the early 1970's most clearly define the potential adverse effects of maternal asthma on pregnancy and the infant. One study (Bahna & Bjerkedal, 1972) described pregnancy outcomes in 381 women with asthma compared to a control population of 112,530 pregnant women with no medical illness. There was a statistically significant increase in preterm births and low birth weight infants, decreased mean birth weight, increased neonatal mortality, and increased neonatal hypoxia in the pregnancies of women with asthma compared to control pregnancies. The study also found a statistically significant increase in hyperemesis gravidarum, vaginal hemorrhage, and toxemia as well as a significant increase in induced and complicated labors in pregnant women with asthma versus control pregnant women. The study did not find an increased incidence of congenital malformations.

The second study (Gordon et al., 1970) compared the pregnancy outcome of 277 women with asthma to the pregnancy outcome of the entire cohort population of 30,861 women. This study found a statistically significant increase in perinatal mortality in pregnant women with asthma versus pregnant women without asthma. Neonatal mortality was not specifically reported in this series. Maternal "chronic hypertensive disease" was present in three of the eight cases of fetal death. The data also suggested that pregnant women with severe asthma were at particularly high risk.

Subsequent controlled studies have reported increases in low birth weight infants (Lao & Huengsburg,1990), chronic hypertension (Dombrowski et al., 1986), and preeclampsia (Stenius-Aamiala et al.,1988) in pregnant women with asthma compared to pregnant women without asthma. In addition to fetal morbidity and mortality, severe asthma during pregnancy may be a cause of maternal mortality (Gordon et al., 1970; Schaefer & Silverman, 1961; Williams, 1967). These epidemiological studies have found that pregnant women with asthma have increased risk of perinatal mortality, prematurity, intrauterine growth retardation, gestational hypertension, and other adverse effects. These studies, however, do not define the mechanisms of the increased risk.

## *Mechanisms*

Definition of the mechanisms of asthma's adverse effects on pregnancy would allow institution of optimal intervention strategy. Potential explanations for the adverse effects of maternal asthma on pregnancy and the neonate include: (1) poor asthma control, (2) asthma medications, (3) increased prevalence of cigarette smoking among pregnant women with asthma versus pregnant women without asthma (Dombrowski et al., 1986), (4) extrapulmonary autonomic nervous system abnormalities, such as uterine muscle hyperreactivity (Bertrand et al.,1985), and (5) an increased proportion of African Americans among asthma patients (Centers for Disease Control,1990a) with associated excess perinatal morbidity (Centers for Disease Control, 1990b). The published data do not fully define the mechanism(s) of maternal asthma's potential adverse effects on pregnancy and the infant. However, available information does suggest that poor asthma control may be the most important factor (see table 2.6). The information available also supports the important generalization that adequate asthma control during pregnancy is important in improving maternal/fetal outcome.

## EFFECTS OF PREGNANCY ON ASTHMA

## *Epidemiology*

A number of studies suggest that the course of asthma may change during pregnancy. In a combined series of 1,087 patients from the literature, the course of asthma was reported to improve in 36 percent, worsen in 23 percent, and remain unchanged in 41 percent (Gluck & Gluck, 1976). However, individual studies differed substantially in their results (Gluck & Gluck, 1976). This pattern is maintained in recent studies (Gluck & Gluck, 1976; Juniper et al., 1989; Schatz et al., 1988a; Stenius-Aamiala et al., 1988; White et al., 1989), in which 18 to 69 percent of patients improved while 6 to 42 percent worsened. There are at least two reasons for this variability: (1) the

- Acute asthma may be associated with hypoxia, hypocapnia, and alkalosis.
- Maternal hypocapnia/alkalosis may impair fetal oxygenation.
- Relative maternal hypoxia is associated with lower infant birth weight in high altitude pregnancies.
- Chronic maternal hypoxia is associated with increased prevalences of prematurity and intrauterine growth retardation in women with uncorrected congenital heart disease.
- No increase in perinatal mortality occurred in recent studies in which asthma was managed by specialists (Stenius-Aamiala et al., 1988; Greenberger & Patterson, 1983; Schatz et al., 1975; Greenberger & Patterson, 1988).
- Lower mean birth weight was manifested by infants whose mothers were hospitalized for asthma during pregnancy (2,920 g) compared to infants whose mothers did not require emergency therapy for their gestational asthma (3,354 g) (Greenberger & Patterson, 1988).
- Impaired pulmonary function was associated with lower birth weight and asymmetric intrauterine growth retardation in infants of asthmatic mothers (Schatz et al., 1990).
- Acute asthma is associated with hypertension that improves with amelioration of the asthma.

* Modified from Schatz and Zeiger, 1991.

**Table 2.6.** *Relationship Between Poor Asthma Control and Perinatal Mortality/Morbidity*

method by which the course of asthma was assessed and (2) the asthma severity of the population studied. Review of the data suggests that women with severe asthma prior to pregnancy are more likely to deteriorate during pregnancy (Gluck & Gluck, 1976; White et al., 1989). The variable effect of pregnancy on the course of asthma appears to be more than random fluctuations in the natural history of the disease because the changes generally revert toward the prepregnancy level of severity within 3 months postpartum (Schatz et al., 1988a). It is also of interest that asthma severity is often consistent among successive pregnancies in individual women (Schatz et al., 1988a; Williams, 1967).

## Other Clinical Observations

A study that prospectively evaluated methacholine sensitivity in 16 pregnant women with asthma (Juniper et al., 1989) found a twofold improvement (decrease) in airway responsiveness during pregnancy compared to preconception and postpartum. An associated improvement in clinical asthma severity, as indicated by a reduction in minimum medication requirements, was also observed. Individually, 11 of 16 subjects demonstrated improved airway responsiveness. Change in responsiveness was not closely related to serum concentrations of progesterone or estriol.

Additional observations have identified factors contributing to worsening asthma during pregnancy. Upper respiratory tract infections appear to be the most common precipitants of asthma exacerbations during pregnancy (Williams, 1967). Patient noncompliance with medical regimens may also be associated with poor asthma control during pregnancy, especially among adolescents (Apter et al., 1989). The peak incidence of exacerbations appears to be between the 24th and 36th weeks of gestation (Gluck & Gluck, 1976), particularly in women whose asthma worsens with pregnancy (Schatz et al., 1988a). In contrast, women with asthma, in general, tend to experience fewer symptoms during weeks 37 to 40 of pregnancy than during any prior 4-week gestational period (Schatz et al., 1988a). Finally, asthma generally remains quiescent during labor and delivery. Ninety percent of 360 women with asthma in one study had no symptoms of asthma at all during labor and delivery (Schatz et al., 1988a). Of those who did, approximately half required no acute treatment, some used inhaled bronchodilators, and only two required intravenous aminophylline.

## Mechanisms

The mechanisms responsible for the altered course of asthma during pregnancy are unknown and represent a fertile area for additional research. There are multiple biochemical, physiological, and psychological factors that could potentially ameliorate or exacerbate asthma during pregnancy (see table 2.7 on the next page). It seems probable that the importance of individual factors varies from individual to individual, and presumably a combination of these factors determines what effect, if any, pregnancy will have on the course of asthma.

## Asthma Drugs in Pregnancy and Lactation

When considering the possible effects of drugs and disease on pregnancy, it is important to keep in mind the background incidence of adverse pregnancy outcome in the general population. For example, congenital anomalies are recognized in 3 to 8 percent of live-born infants, miscarriage occurs in 20 to 25 percent of clinically diagnosed pregnancies, and severe mental retardation occurs in 1 to 2 percent of births. In addition, although birth defects are the most dramatic evidence of embryogenesis gone amiss, other endpoints of abnormal development are equally significant. These include spontaneous abortion (miscarriage), fetal death (stillbirth), and functional abnormalities such as impairments in the nervous or immune systems. Growth retardation, preterm labor, and other obstetric complications are also developmental problems of clinical importance. The challenge is to determine whether a drug or disease exposure increases the incidence of adverse outcome over the background incidence.

It is also important to remember that drug-induced birth defects are unusual: Of the 3 to 8 percent of newborns with congenital anomalies, only 1 percent or fewer of these are attributable to drug exposures (Czeizel & Racz, 1990).

### PHYSIOLOGIC CHANGES IN PREGNANCY AFFECTING DRUG DISTRIBUTION

With the profound physiologic changes that occur during pregnancy, it is reasonable to suppose that these changes affect the manner in which drugs are handled by the body. Pharmacokinetics is the

*Table 2.7. Physiologic Changes During Pregnancy That May Affect the Course of Asthma*

**Factors that may improve asthma:**

- Progesterone-mediated bronchodilation
- Estrogen- or progesterone-mediated potentiation of beta-adrenergic bronchodilation
- Decreased plasma-histamine-mediated bronchoconstriction (due to increased circulating histaminase)
- Pulmonary effects of increased serum-free cortisol
- Glucocorticosteroid-mediated increased beta-adrenergic responsiveness
- Prostaglandin-E-mediated bronchodilation
- Prostaglandin-$I_2$-mediated bronchial stabilization
- Atrial-natriuretic-factor-induced bronchodilation
- Increased half-life or decreased protein binding of endogenous or exogenous bronchodilators.

**Factors that may worsen asthma:**

- Pulmonary refractoriness to cortisol effects because of competitive binding to glucocorticosteroid receptors by progesterone, aldosterone, or deoxycorticosterone
- Prostaglandin-$F_2$-alpha-mediated bronchoconstriction
- Decreased functional residual capacity with resultant airway closure during tidal breathing and altered ventilation-perfusion ratios
- Increased placental major basic protein reaching the lung
- Increased viral- or bacterial-respiratory-infection-triggered asthma exacerbations
- Increased gastroesophageal-reflux-induced asthma
- Increased stress
- Increased pulmonary capillary permeability.

\* Modified from Schatz and Zeiger, 1991.

## Asthma

study of drug absorption, distribution, metabolism, and elimination in the body. Although few therapeutic agents have been completely studied as to the effect of pregnancy on the drug's pharmacokinetics, the following changes have been shown to occur during pregnancy and are clinically relevant:

- **Reduction in plasma proteins.** This is largely caused by a decrease in serum albumin concentration (Dean et al.,1980). During pregnancy, drugs bound to serum albumin show a reduction in protein binding and a corresponding increase in the available free fraction of the drug (Connelly et al., 1990; Frederiksen et al.,1986; Gardner et al.,1987). This change in protein binding implies that for certain drugs plasma concentrations should be reduced or kept at the lower end of the therapeutic range during pregnancy (Connelly et al., 1990). For example, the protein binding of theophylline decreases by 10 to 15 percent during pregnancy; therefore, the therapeutic range for theophylline needs to be modified to account for the corresponding increase in the free fraction of theophylline. During pregnancy, theophylline plasma concentrations between 8 and 12 $\mu$g/ml are therapeutically equivalent to concentrations of 10 to 15 $\mu$g/ml in the nonpregnant patient.

- **Increased total body water and plasma volume.** Several studies, however, have shown that this change does not affect the volume of distribution for drugs if the weight of the patient is taken into consideration (Aldridge et al., 1981; Frederiksen et al.,1986; Gardner et al.,1987; Philipson,1977; Philipson & Stiernstedt,1982). Therefore, to achieve the therapeutic drug concentration usually recommended, the mg/kg dose should be calculated using the actual weight of the patient. For example, to calculate a loading dose of aminophylline or theophylline for a pregnant patient not previously receiving a methylxanthine, use the recommended 6-mg/kg regimen and the actual weight of the patient at the time therapy is instituted.

- **Decreased gastrointestinal motility.** This change does not affect the overall absorption of even poorly absorbed drugs, such as ampicillin (Philipson, 1977); however, the time to peak drug concentration is prolonged, and the peak concentration is lower (Philipson, 1977). This may in part explain the observation that an oral dose of 500 mg of ampicillin during pregnancy gives a plasma peak concentration 40 percent lower than in a nonpregnant patient, and the peak concentration occurs approximately 1 hour later.

- **Altered drug elimination.** Pregnancy can alter the manner in which drugs are eliminated from the body, with the greatest effect occurring in the last trimester of pregnancy. Renal elimination of drugs may increase for such drugs as theophylline, ampicillin, and cefuroxime due to the increase in glomerular filtration rate that occurs during pregnancy (Frederiksen et al., 1986; Philipson,1977; Philipson & Stiernstedt, 1982). Metabolic elimination of drugs is less predictable; some drugs, such as methadone, have an increase in metabolic clearance (Pond et al., 1985) and others, including theophylline, have a decrease in metabolic clearance (Frederiksen et al., 1986; Gardner et al., 1987). Therefore, the elimination route and characteristics of each drug must be considered, and frequent use of therapeutic drug monitoring is indicated. Thus, because the overall elimination rate of intravenous methylxanthine decreases by 30 percent in the last trimester of pregnancy, the recommended dose for intravenously administered methylxanthine is a continuous infusion rate of 0.4 mg/kg/hr theophylline (or 0.5 mg/kg/hr aminophylline) in order to maintain serum theophylline concentrations within the range of 8-12$\mu$g/ml.

As a general rule most medications administered to pregnant women will cross the placenta and can be detected in fetal blood. However, extremely large molecular weight drugs, or highly polar compounds, such as heparin, do not effectively cross the placenta in measurable amounts.

*Breast Feeding*

Nearly all medications enter breast milk by diffusion from plasma. Milk concentrations are typically very low, and it is unusual for infants to receive a dose sufficient to produce toxic effects. Recommendations concerning drugs and breast feeding have been made by

## Asthma

the American Academy of Pediatrics Committee on Drugs (1989) and by the World Health Organization (Bennett, 1988).

| Drug or Class | Effect |
| --- | --- |
| Systemic corticosteroids | Impaired fetal growth (about 300 to 400 g decrease in birth weight) |
| Theophylline | Fetal tachycardia with maternal plasma drug levels greater than 20 µg/mL. Neonatal jitteriness, vomiting, tachycardia with neonatal drug levels greater than 10 µg/mL. Neonatal effects are most often seen when maternal plasma drug levels are greater than 12 µg/mL. |
| Systemic beta$_2$-agonists | Fetal tachycardia. Neonatal tachycardia, hypoglycemia, tremor. |
| Topical sympathomimetic decongestants | Fetal heart rate alterations attributed to uterine vasoconstriction. Effect seen at high doses, perhaps only with overdosage. |

*Table 2.8.* Potential Fetal/Neonatal Adverse Effects of Asthma Drugs

- Alpha-adrenergic compounds (other than pseudoephedrine)
- Epinephrine
- Iodides
- Sulfonamides (in late pregnancy)
- Tetracyclines
- Quinalones

*Table 2.9.* Drugs for Asthma and Associated Conditions That Generally Should Be Avoided During Pregnancy

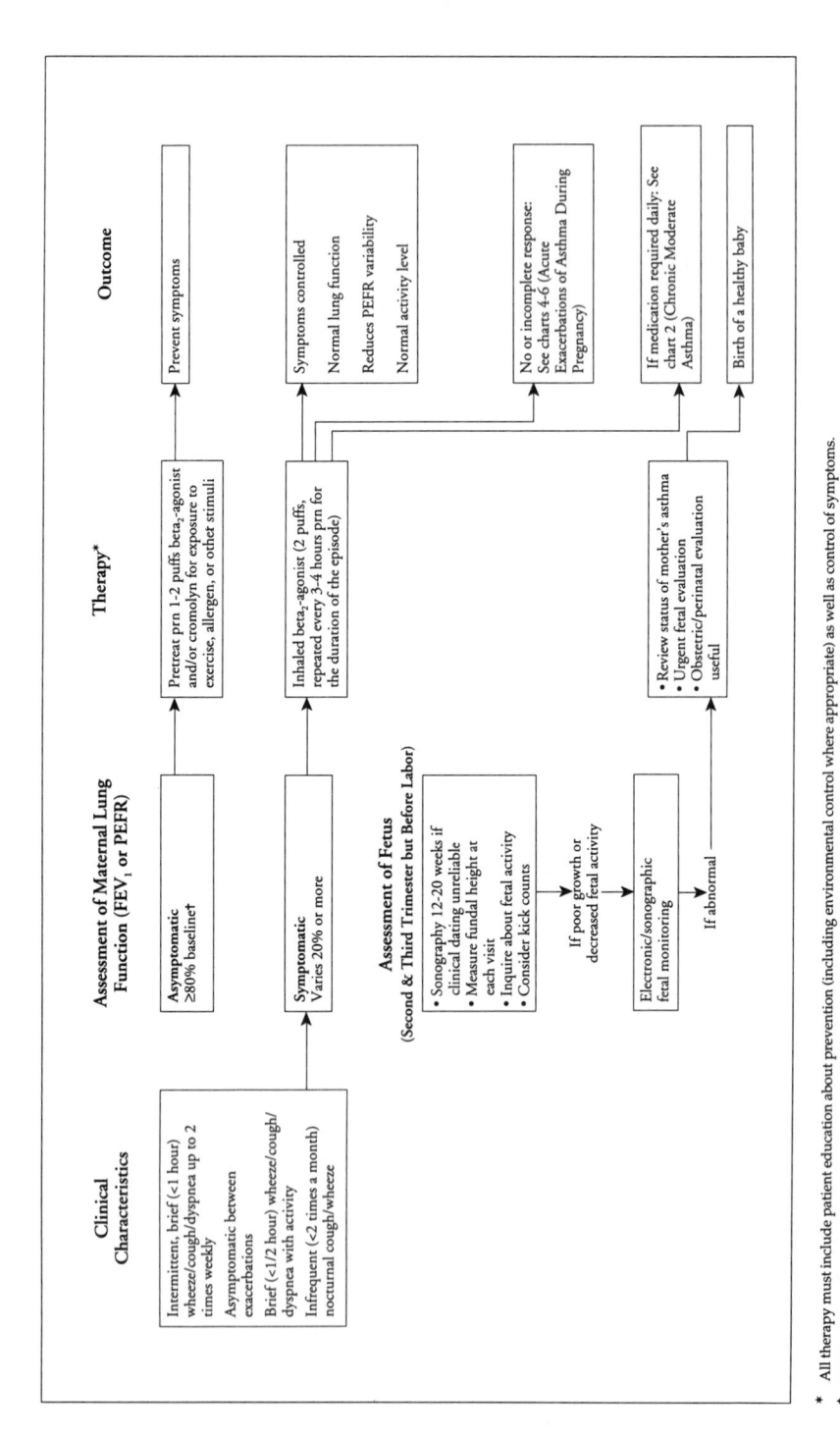

## Respiratory Diseases and Disorders Sourcebook

| Clinical Characteristics | Assessment of Maternal Lung Function (FEV₁ or PEFR) | Therapy* | Outcome |
|---|---|---|---|
| Intermittent, brief (<1 hour) wheeze/cough/dyspnea up to 2 times weekly; Asymptomatic between exacerbations; Brief (<1/2 hour) wheeze/cough/dyspnea with activity; Infrequent (<2 times a month) nocturnal cough/wheeze | Asymptomatic ≥80% baseline† | Pretreat prn 1-2 puffs beta₂-agonist and/or cromolyn for exposure to exercise, allergen, or other stimuli | Prevent symptoms |
| | Symptomatic Varies 20% or more | Inhaled beta₂-agonist (2 puffs, repeated every 3-4 hours prn for the duration of the episode) | Symptoms controlled; Normal lung function; Reduces PEFR variability; Normal activity level |
| | Assessment of Fetus (Second & Third Trimester but Before Labor) | | No or incomplete response: See charts 4-6 (Acute Exacerbations of Asthma During Pregnancy) |
| | • Sonography 12-20 weeks if clinical dating unreliable<br>• Measure fundal height at each visit<br>• Inquire about fetal activity<br>• Consider kick counts | | If medication required daily: See chart 2 (Chronic Moderate Asthma) |
| | If poor growth or decreased fetal activity → Electronic/sonographic fetal monitoring; If abnormal → • Review status of mother's asthma<br>• Urgent fetal evaluation<br>• Obstetric/perinatal evaluation useful | | Birth of a healthy baby |

\* All therapy must include patient education about prevention (including environmental control where appropriate) as well as control of symptoms.
† PEFR percent baseline refers to the norm for the individual, established by the clinician. This may be percent predicted based on standardized norms or percent of patient's personal best.

*Figure 2.10. Management of Chronic Mild Asthma During Pregnancy*

## Asthma

| Clinical Characteristics | Assessment of Maternal Lung Function (FEV₁ or PEFR) | Therapy* | Outcome |
|---|---|---|---|
| Symptoms >1-2 times weekly<br>Exacerbations affect sleep or activity level<br>Exacerbations may last several days<br>Occasional emergency care | 60-80% baseline† (may be normal when asymptomatic)<br>Varies 20-30% when symptomatic | **Anti-inflammatory agents**<br>• Cromolyn (2 puffs qid) *or*<br>• Inhaled corticosteroids (2-4 puffs bid, 168-336 µg/day)<br>*and*<br>**Inhaled beta₂-agonist** prn to tid/qid††<br><br>If symptoms persist<br><br>**Additional therapy**<br>• Increase inhaled corticosteroids *and/or*<br>• Sustained release theophylline *and/or*<br>• Oral beta₂-agonist | Symptoms controlled<br>Pulmonary function values optimal for patient<br>Reduced PEFR variability<br>Normal activity level<br>Rarely awakened at night<br>Infrequent exacerbations<br>Reduced frequency of prn inhaled beta₂-agonist |
| | **Assessment of Fetus**<br>(Second & Third Trimester but Before Labor) | | |
| | • Sonography for dating and growth evaluation<br>• Measure fundal height at each visit<br>• Daily kick counts<br>• Consider serial antepartum fetal assessment beginning at 32 weeks | | |
| | If poor growth or decreased fetal activity | • Review status of mother's asthma<br>• Urgent fetal evaluation<br>• Obstetric/perinatal consultation useful | Birth of a healthy baby |
| | Electronic/sonographic fetal monitoring | | |
| | If abnormal | | |
| Increasingly frequent symptoms | Varies more than 30% during worst exacerbations | **Oral corticosteroids**<br>• Short course of oral prednisone followed by inhaled corticosteroids | Symptoms reduced<br>Peak flow values stabilized<br>Get specialist consultation |
| | | See chart 3: Chronic Severe Asthma<br>Get assessment by specialist | No or intermittent response |

\* All therapy must include patient education about prevention (including environmental control where appropriate) as well as control of symptoms.
† PEFR percent baseline refers to the norm for the individual, established by the clinician. This may be percent predicted based on standardized norms or percent of patient's personal best.
†† If exceed 3-4 doses a day, consider additional therapy other than inhaled beta₂-agonist.

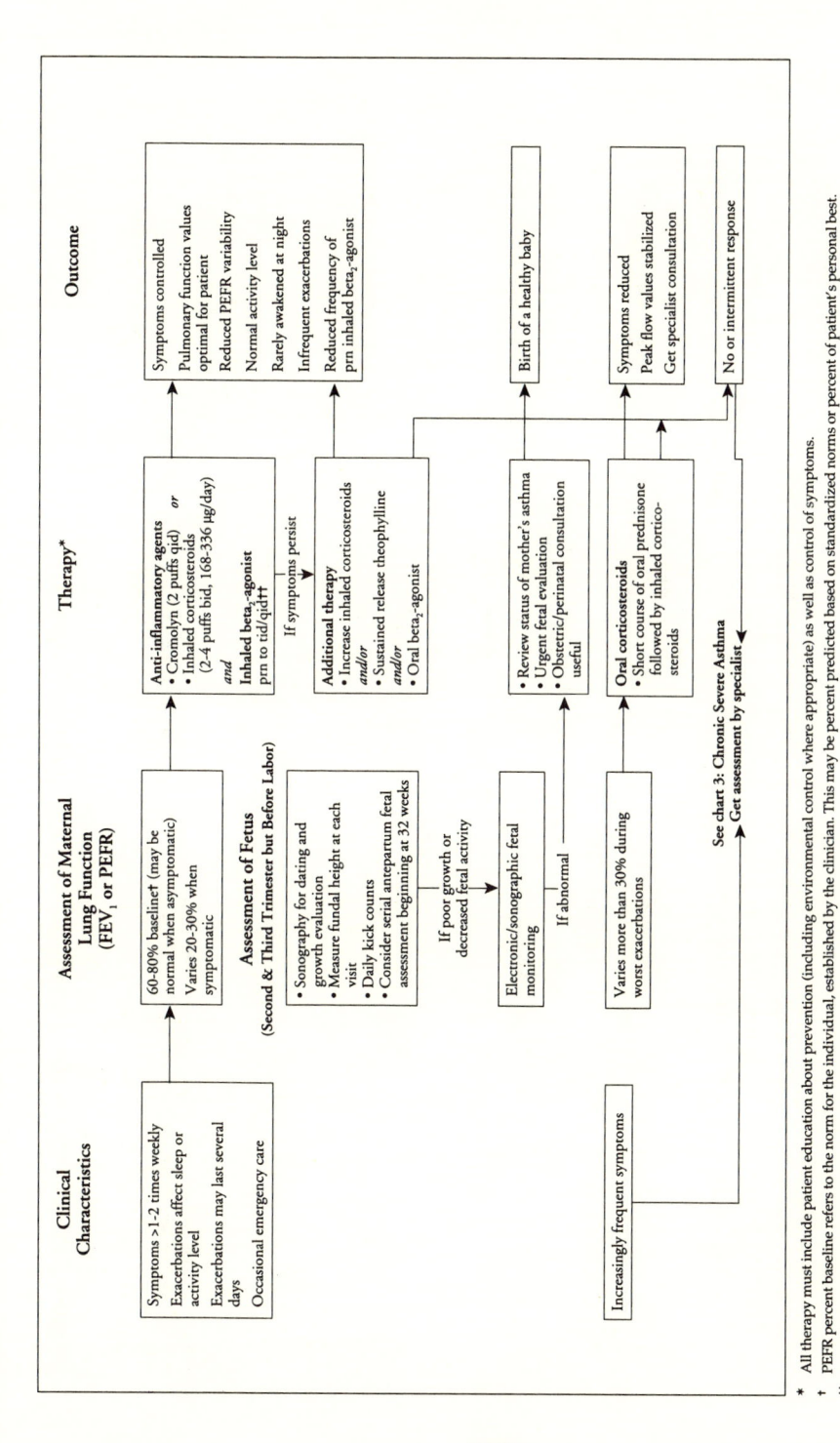

**Figure 2.11. Management of Chronic Moderate Asthma During Pregnancy**

# Respiratory Diseases and Disorders Sourcebook

| Clinical Characteristics | Assessment of Maternal Lung Function (FEV₁ or PEFR) | Therapy* | Outcome |
|---|---|---|---|
| Continuous symptoms<br>Limited activity level<br>Frequent exacerbations<br>Frequent nocturnal symptoms<br>Occasional hospitalization and emergency treatment | <60% baseline†<br>Highly variable: 20-30% changes with routine medicine | **Anti-inflammatory agents**<br>—Inhaled corticosteroid 4-6 puffs bid or 2-5 puffs qid (336-840 μg/day)<br>*with or without*<br>—Cromolyn 2 puffs qid<br>*with or without*<br>(especially for nocturnal symptoms)<br>—Oral sustained-released theophylline, *and/or*<br>—Oral beta₂-agonist<br>*and*<br>• Inhaled beta₂-agonist prn-qid†† | Improved pulmonary function<br>Reduced peak flow variability<br>Almost normal activity<br>Infrequent awakening at night<br>Reduced frequency of exacerbations<br>Reduced frequency of prn inhaled beta₂-agonist<br>Reduced need for corticosteroid burst<br>Reduced need for emergency department treatment |
| | Varies more than 50% during worst exacerbations | *with*<br>• Episodic extra beta₂-agonist (2-4 puffs MDI or nebulized treatment) for exacerbations<br>*and*<br>**Oral corticosteroids**<br>• Burst for active symptoms (40 mg a day, single or divided dose, for 1 week, then tapered for 1 week)<br>*Consider*<br>• Daily or alternate day use (single dose a.m.) | |
| | **Assessment of Fetus**<br>(Second & Third Trimester but Before Labor) | | |
| | • Sonograms for dating and growth evaluation<br>• Measure fundal height at each visit<br>• Daily kick counts<br>• Consider serial antepartum fetal assessment beginning at 32 weeks<br>• Perinatal consultation useful | • Review status of mother's asthma | |
| | If poor growth or decreased fetal activity | | |
| | Electronic/sonographic fetal monitoring | | Birth of a healthy baby |
| | If abnormal | | |
| | • Urgent fetal evaluation<br>• Perinatal consultation useful | | |

**Note:** Individuals with severe asthma should be evaluated by an asthma specialist.
\* All therapy must include patient education about prevention (including environmental control where appropriate) as well as control of symptoms.
† PEFR percent baseline refers to the norm for the individual, established by the clinician. This may be percent predicted based on standardized norms or percent of patient's personal best.
†† If exceed 3-4 doses a day, consider additional therapy other than inhaled beta₂-agonist.

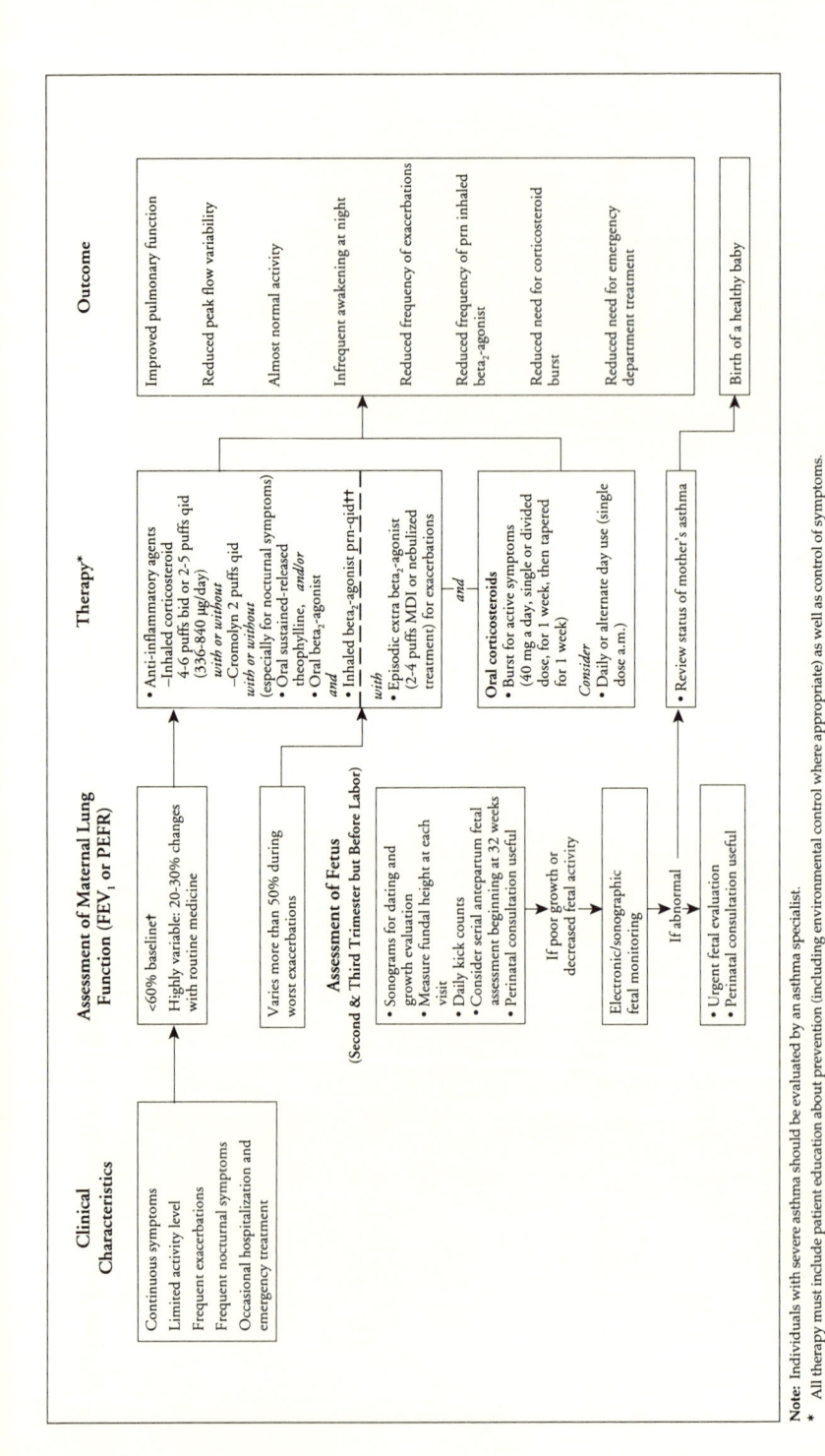

***Figure 2.12. Management of Chronic Severe Asthma During Pregnancy***

## Asthma

**Assess severity**
Measure PEFR, cough, breathlessness, use of accessory muscles, wheeze, chest tightness, presence of fetal activity

- Inhaled beta$_2$-agonist 2-4 puffs every 20 minutes up to 1 hour if needed

**Good response**
- Mild wheeze, cough, breathlessness or chest tightness
- Symptoms occur with activity, but not at rest
- Can climb 1 flight of stairs without stopping to rest
- PEFR >70-90% baseline*
- Appropriate fetal activity

- Continue treatments every 3-4 hours for 6-12 hours as needed
- Continue routine medications
- Contact physician if symptoms recur

**Good response**
PEFR >70-90% and sustained over 4 hours

Continue assessment

- Contact physician if good response is not sustained over 4 hours or symptoms recur
- Contact physician for followup instructions

**Incomplete response**
- Marked wheeze, breathlessness, or chest tightness; repetitive cough
- Symptoms occur while at rest and may interfere with daily activity
- Cannot climb 1 flight of stairs without stopping to rest
- PEFR 50-70% of baseline*
- Decreased fetal activity

Contact physician *or*
Go to emergency department

**Poor response**
- Severe wheeze or breathlessness; speech fragmented by rapid breathing
- Severe symptoms at rest
- Unable to walk 100 feet without stopping to rest
- PEFR <50% of baseline*
- Decreased fetal activity

Go to emergency department

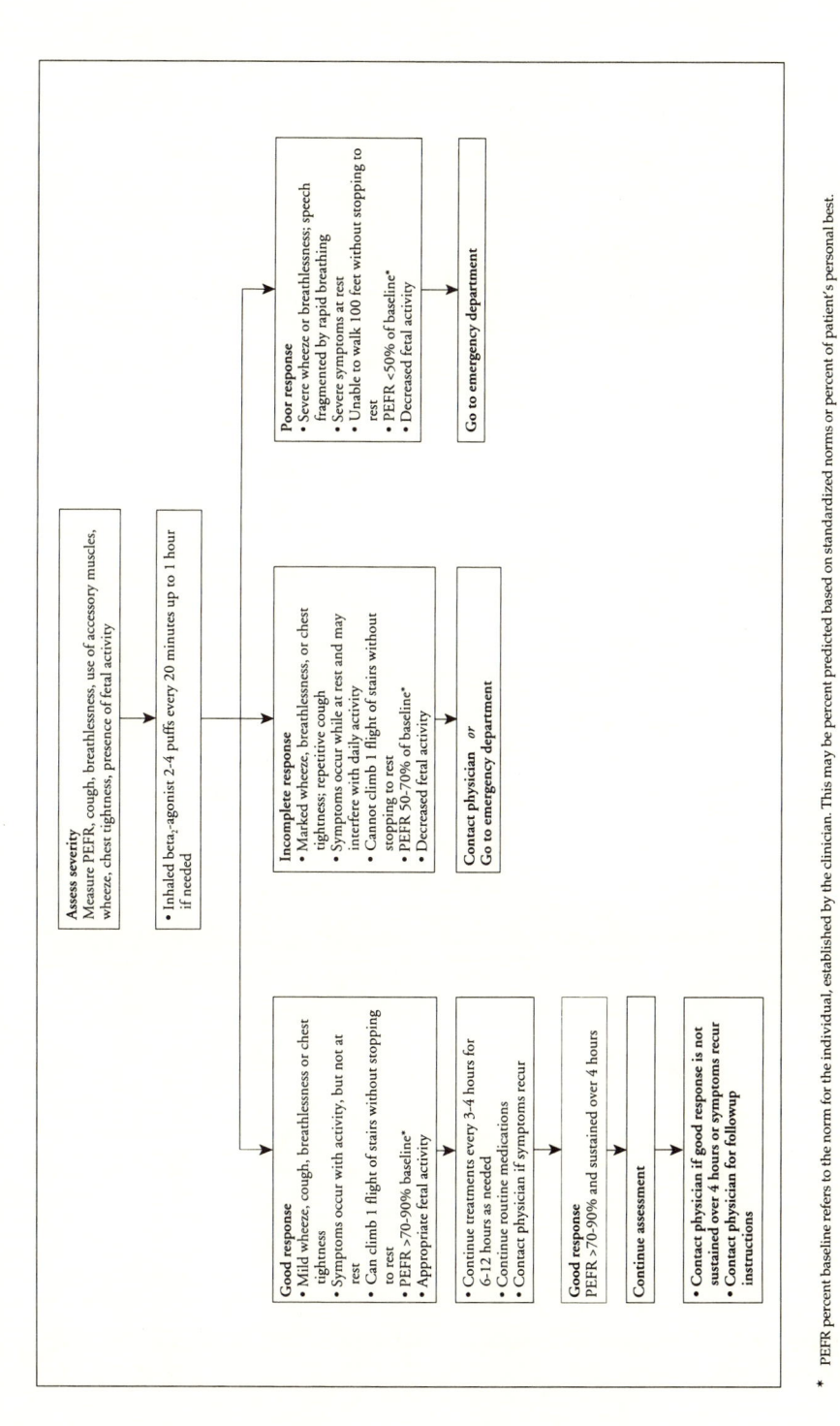

*Figure 2.13. Home Management of Acute Exacerbations of Asthma During Pregnancy*

\* PEFR percent baseline refers to the norm for the individual, established by the clinician. This may be percent predicted based on standardized norms or percent of patient's personal best.

# Respiratory Diseases and Disorders Sourcebook

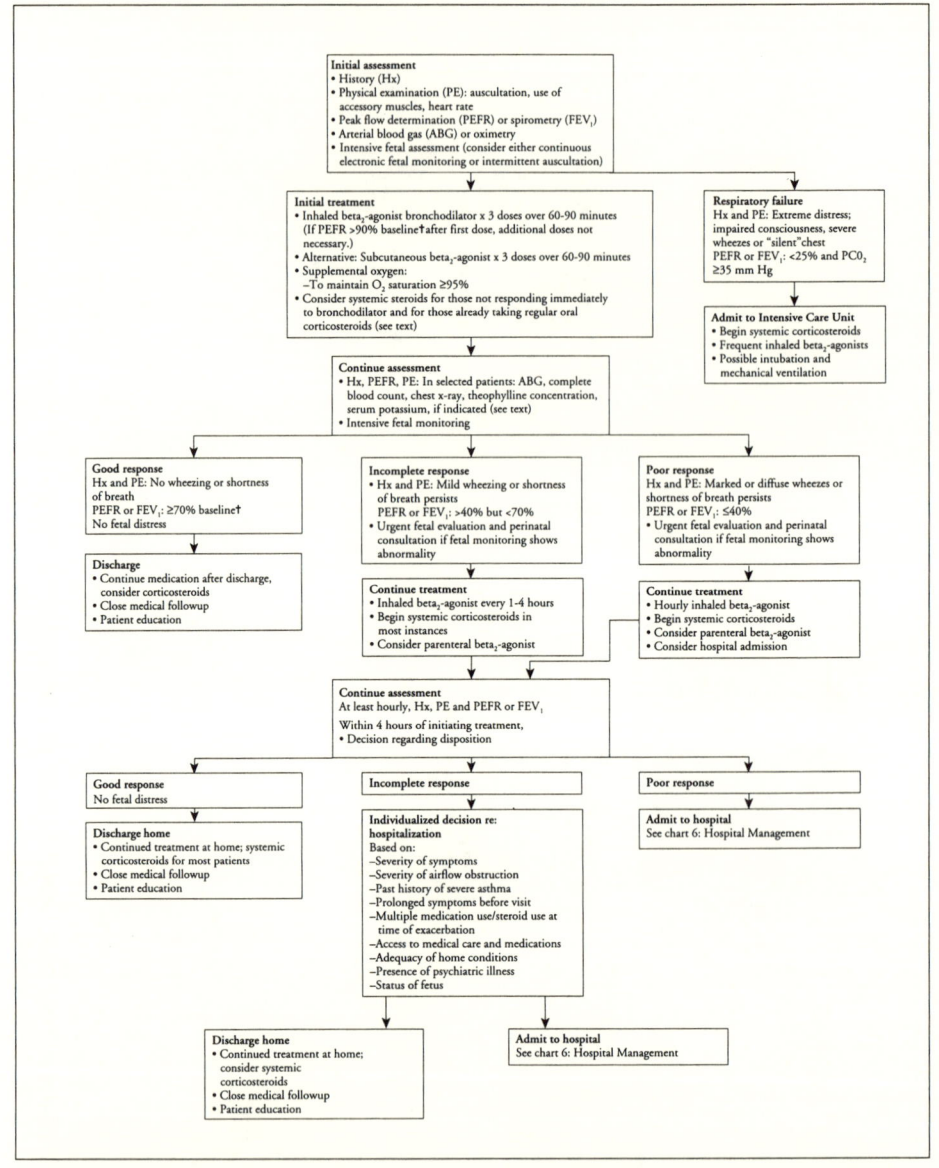

**Initial assessment**
- History (Hx)
- Physical examination (PE): auscultation, use of accessory muscles, heart rate
- Peak flow determination (PEFR) or spirometry (FEV$_1$)
- Arterial blood gas (ABG) or oximetry
- Intensive fetal assessment (consider either continuous electronic fetal monitoring or intermittent auscultation)

**Initial treatment**
- Inhaled beta$_2$-agonist bronchodilator x 3 doses over 60-90 minutes (If PEFR >90% baseline† after first dose, additional doses not necessary.)
- Alternative: Subcutaneous beta$_2$-agonist x 3 doses over 60-90 minutes
- Supplemental oxygen:
  – To maintain O$_2$ saturation ≥95%
- Consider systemic steroids for those not responding immediately to bronchodilator and for those already taking regular oral corticosteroids (see text)

**Respiratory failure**
Hx and PE: Extreme distress; impaired consciousness, severe wheezes or "silent" chest
PEFR or FEV$_1$: <25% and PCO$_2$ ≥35 mm Hg

**Admit to Intensive Care Unit**
- Begin systemic corticosteroids
- Frequent inhaled beta$_2$-agonists
- Possible intubation and mechanical ventilation

**Continue assessment**
- Hx, PEFR, PE: In selected patients: ABG, complete blood count, chest x-ray, theophylline concentration, serum potassium, if indicated (see text)
- Intensive fetal monitoring

**Good response**
Hx and PE: No wheezing or shortness of breath
PEFR or FEV$_1$: ≥70% baseline†
No fetal distress

**Discharge**
- Continue medication after discharge, consider corticosteroids
- Close medical followup
- Patient education

**Incomplete response**
- Hx and PE: Mild wheezing or shortness of breath persists
- PEFR or FEV$_1$: >40% but <70%
- Urgent fetal evaluation and perinatal consultation if fetal monitoring shows abnormality

**Continue treatment**
- Inhaled beta$_2$-agonist every 1-4 hours
- Begin systemic corticosteroids in most instances
- Consider parenteral beta$_2$-agonist

**Poor response**
Hx and PE: Marked or diffuse wheezes or shortness of breath persists
PEFR or FEV$_1$: ≤40%
- Urgent fetal evaluation and perinatal consultation if fetal monitoring shows abnormality

**Continue treatment**
- Hourly inhaled beta$_2$-agonist
- Begin systemic corticosteroids
- Consider parenteral beta$_2$-agonist
- Consider hospital admission

**Continue assessment**
At least hourly, Hx, PE and PEFR or FEV$_1$
Within 4 hours of initiating treatment,
- Decision regarding disposition

**Good response**
No fetal distress

**Discharge home**
- Continued treatment at home; systemic corticosteroids for most patients
- Close medical followup
- Patient education

**Incomplete response**

**Individualized decision re: hospitalization**
Based on:
– Severity of symptoms
– Severity of airflow obstruction
– Past history of severe asthma
– Prolonged symptoms before visit
– Multiple medication use/steroid use at time of exacerbation
– Access to medical care and medications
– Adequacy of home conditions
– Presence of psychiatric illness
– Status of fetus

**Poor response**

**Admit to hospital**
See chart 6: Hospital Management

**Discharge home**
- Continued treatment at home; consider systemic corticosteroids
- Close medical followup
- Patient education

**Admit to hospital**
See chart 6: Hospital Management

\* Therapies are often available in a physician's office. However, most acute severe exacerbations of asthma require a complete course of therapy in an emergency department.

† PEFR percent baseline refers to the norm for the individual, established by the clinician. This may be percent predicted based on standardized norms or percent of patient's personal best.

*Figure 12.14. Emergency Department Management of Acute Exacerbations of Asthma During Pregnancy*

## Asthma

**Initial assessment**
- Detailed medical history (Hx)
- Complete physical examination (PE)
- Expiratory flow measurement: PEFR or $FEV_1$
- Chest radiograph
- Arterial blood gas/oximetry (see text)
- Intensive fetal assessment (consider either continuous electronic fetal monitoring or intermittent auscultation)

Special attention for:
- past history of respiratory failure
- suspicion of intrauterine growth retardation
- uterine irritability
- complicating medical conditions
- history of steroid-induced complications (e.g., psychosis)

**Intensive Care Unit**
- $PCO_2 \geq 35$ mm Hg with PEFR or $FEV_1$ <25%
- Deterioration despite maximal therapy

**ICU treatment**
- Nebulized $beta_2$-agonists every 30-60 minutes; may supplement with parenteral $beta_2$-agonist
- IV corticosteroids
- IV aminophylline
- Oxygen supplementation
- Intubation and mechanical ventilation for hypercapnic respiratory failure

**Not improved**
Deterioration despite maximal therapy
Fetal monitoring indicates abnormality; seek urgent fetal evaluation and perinatal consultation

Transfer ICU

**Treatment**
- Inhaled $beta_2$-agonists up to every 1-2 hours
- Systemic corticosteroids; e.g., IV methylprednisolone 60-80 mg every 6-8 hours
- Supplemental oxygen to maintain $O_2$ saturation ≥95%
- Consider IV aminophylline or oral theophylline

**Continued assessments**
- Hx, PE, PEFR or $FEV_1$ (measured at least twice daily; before and after bronchodilator desirable)
- Intensive fetal monitoring until patient stabilized

**Improved**
Suggested goals prior to discharge:
- Hx and PE: Minimal or no wheezing; ≤1 awakening at night with mild symptoms; good activity tolerance
- PEFR or FEV: ≥70% of baseline*
- No fetal distress

**Preparation for discharge**
- Inhaled $beta_2$-agonist no more than every 3-4 hours
- Oral corticosteroids; role of inhaled corticosteroids discussed in text
- Oral theophylline if indicated
- Adequate oxygen saturation breathing room air
- Provide patient education, especially
  - medication use, including inhaler technique
  - PEFR measurement at home
  - need for followup and chronic care (contact with physician within 7-10 days of discharge recommended)

Home with patient education, medications, and followup plan

* PEFR percent baseline refers to the norm for the individual, established by the clinician. This may be percent predicted based on standardized norms or percent of patient's personal best.

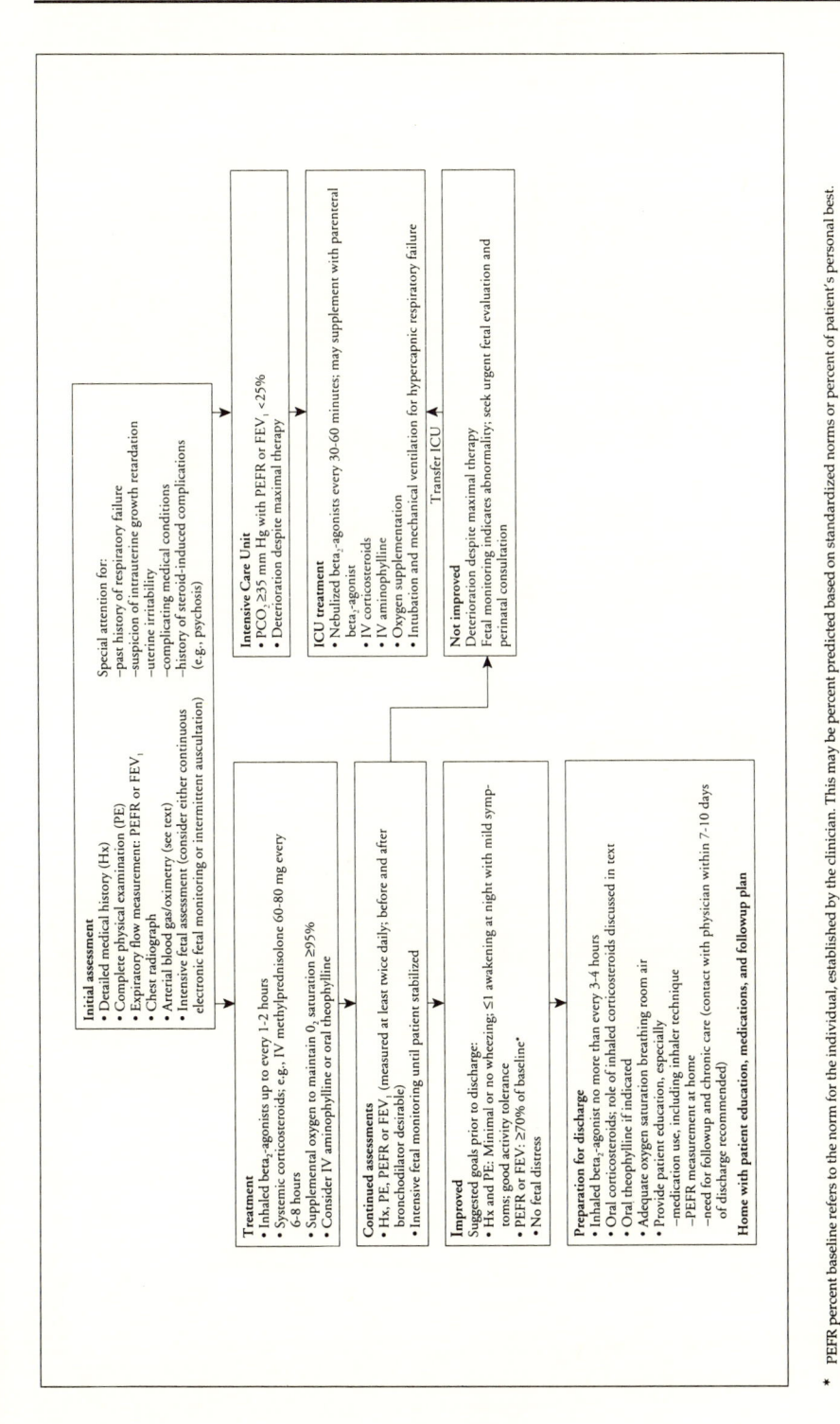

***Figure 12.15. Hospital Management of Acute Exacerbations of Asthma During Pregnancy***

107

# Respiratory Diseases and Disorders Sourcebook

**Assessment at admission**
- Medical history
- Physical examination
- Expiratory flow measurement (PEFR or FEV$_1$)
- Careful fetal monitoring (consider electronic fetal monitoring for at least 20 minutes–admission test)

**Well controlled asthma**
(PEFR/FEV$_1$ ≥80% baseline, no/minimal symptoms)
- Continue routine asthma medications
- Administer hydrocortisone every 8 hours until postpartum if systemic steroids were taken within 4 weeks
- If labor is induced, avoid 15-methyl prostaglandin F$_2$ alpha
- Analgesia
  – Avoid morphine and meperidine
  – Consider fentanyl
  – Consider lumbar epidural

**Exacerbation of asthma**
(PEFR/FEV$_1$ ≤80% baseline)
Symptoms: wheeze, cough, breathlessness, or chest tightness)
- Anesthesia consultation useful
- Treatment (See chart 5 Emergency Department Management)
  – Inhaled beta$_2$-agonist
  – IV corticosteroids
  – Hydrocortisone (100 mg every 8 hours) if systemic steroids taken within 4 weeks
  – Oxygen to maintain O$_2$ saturation ≥95%
- Analgesia
  – Consider fentanyl
  – Consider epidural analgesia

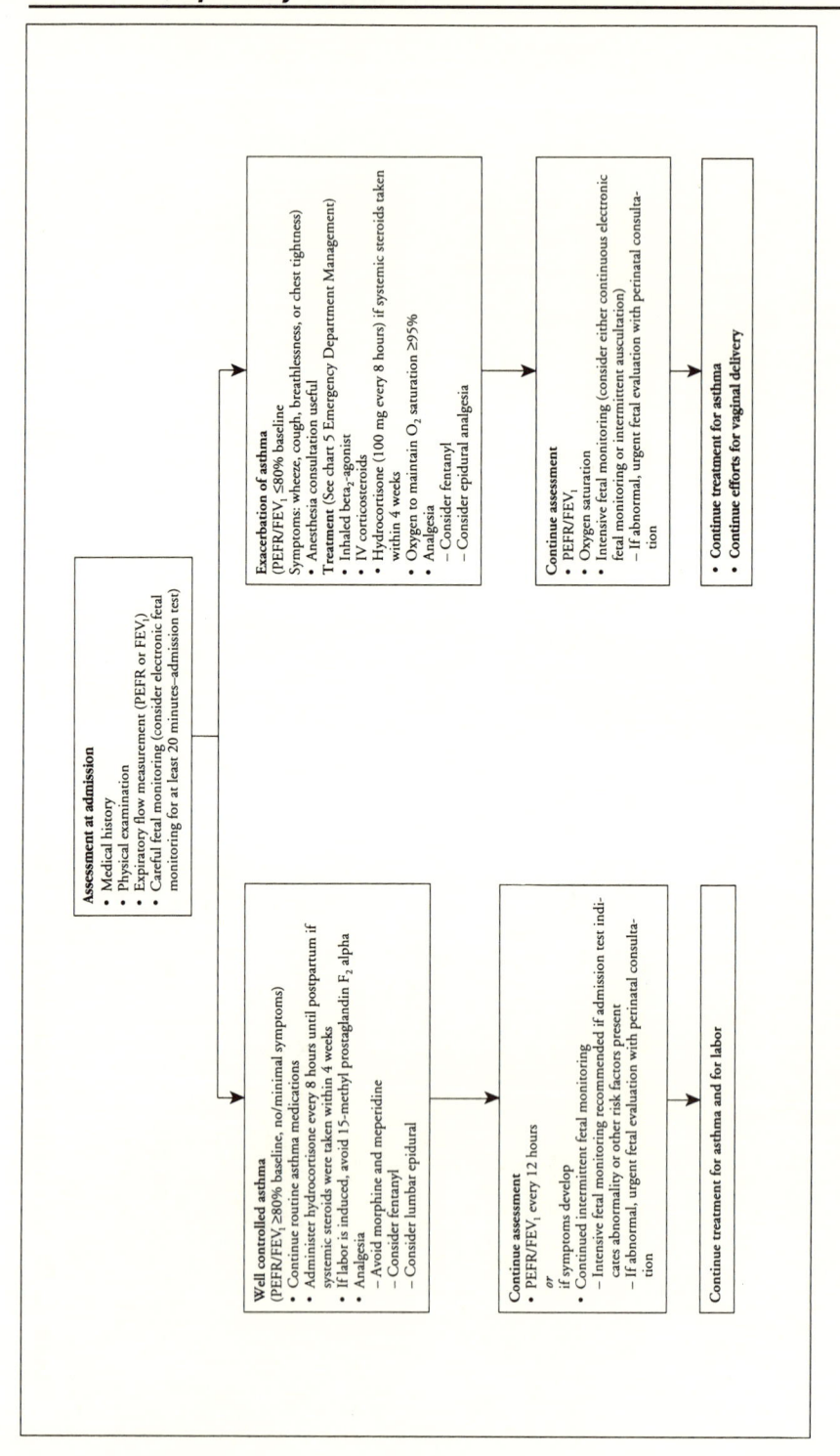

**Continue assessment**
- PEFR/FEV$_1$ every 12 hours
*or*
if symptoms develop
- Continued intermittent fetal monitoring
- Intensive fetal monitoring recommended if admission test indicates abnormality or other risk factors present
- If abnormal, urgent fetal evaluation with perinatal consultation

**Continue assessment**
- PEFR/FEV$_1$
- Oxygen saturation
- Intensive fetal monitoring (consider either continuous electronic fetal monitoring or intermittent auscultation)
- If abnormal, urgent fetal evaluation with perinatal consultation

**Continue treatment for asthma and for labor**

- Continue treatment for asthma
- Continue efforts for vaginal delivery

*Figure 12.16. Management of Asthma During Labor*

## Asthma

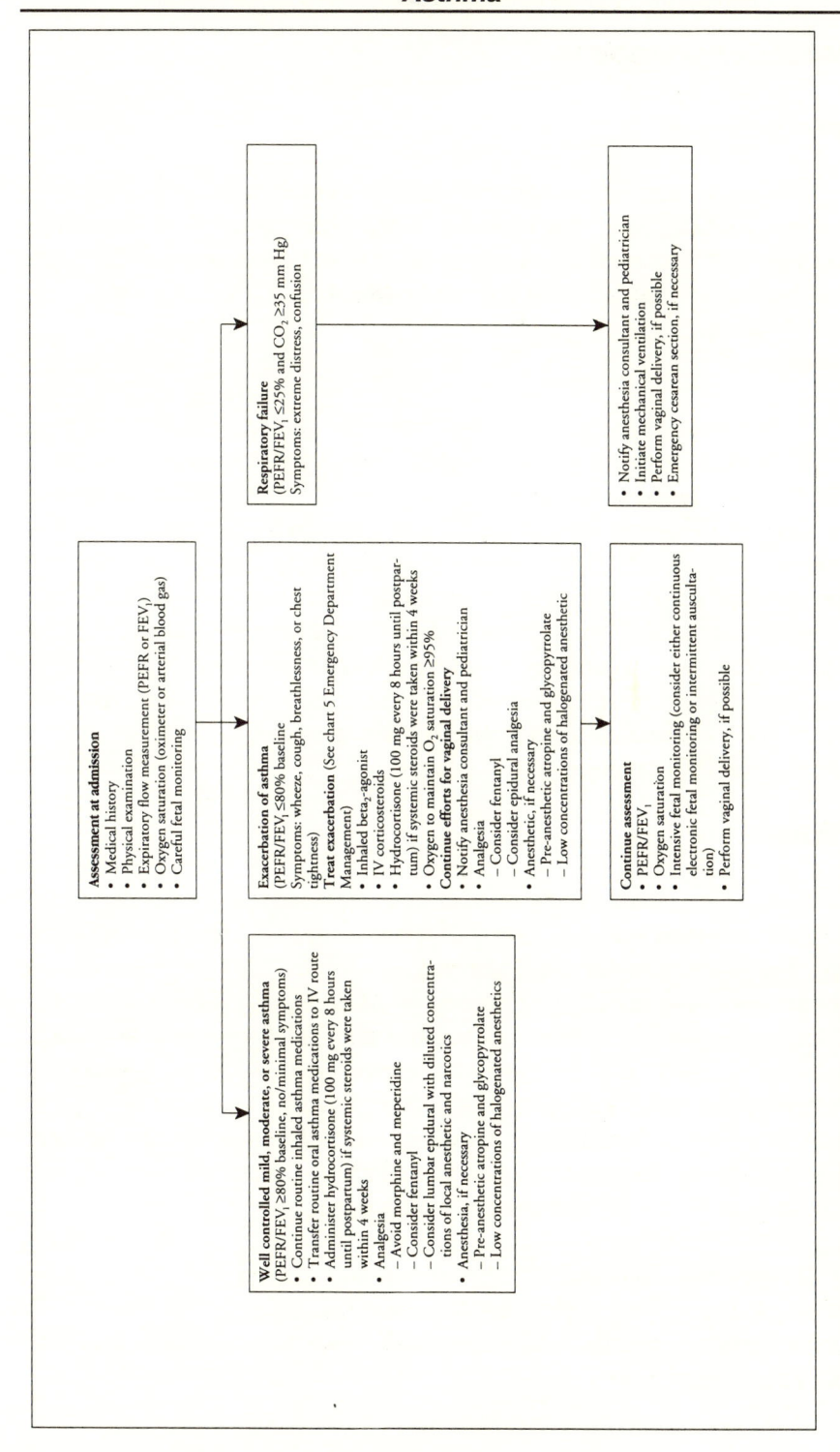

**Assessment at admission**
- Medical history
- Physical examination
- Expiratory flow measurement (PEFR or FEV₁)
- Oxygen saturation (oximeter or arterial blood gas)
- Careful fetal monitoring

**Well controlled mild, moderate, or severe asthma**
(PEFR/FEV₁ ≥80% baseline, no/minimal symptoms)
- Continue routine inhaled asthma medications
- Transfer routine oral asthma medications to IV route
- Administer hydrocortisone (100 mg every 8 hours until postpartum) if systemic steroids were taken within 4 weeks
- Analgesia
  - Avoid morphine and meperidine
  - Consider fentanyl
  - Consider lumbar epidural with diluted concentrations of local anesthetic and narcotics
- Anesthesia, if necessary
  - Pre-anesthetic atropine and glycopyrrolate
  - Low concentrations of halogenated anesthetics

**Exacerbation of asthma**
(PEFR/FEV₁ ≤80% baseline
Symptoms: wheeze, cough, breathlessness, or chest tightness)
- Treat exacerbation (See chart 5 Emergency Department Management)
  - Inhaled beta₂-agonist
  - IV corticosteroids
- Hydrocortisone (100 mg every 8 hours until postpartum) if systemic steroids were taken within 4 weeks
- Oxygen to maintain O₂ saturation ≥95%
- Continue efforts for vaginal delivery
- Notify anesthesia consultant and pediatrician
- Analgesia
  - Consider fentanyl
  - Consider epidural analgesia
- Anesthetic, if necessary
  - Pre-anesthetic atropine and glycopyrrolate
  - Low concentrations of halogenated anesthetic

**Respiratory failure**
(PEFR/FEV₁ ≤25% and CO₂ ≥35 mm Hg)
Symptoms: extreme distress, confusion

- Notify anesthesia consultant and pediatrician
- Initiate mechanical ventilation
- Perform vaginal delivery, if possible
- Emergency cesarean section, if necessary

**Continue assessment**
- PEFR/FEV₁
- Oxygen saturation
- Intensive fetal monitoring (consider either continuous electronic fetal monitoring or intermittent auscultation)
- Perform vaginal delivery, if possible

*Figure 12.17. Management of Asthma During Delivery*

## Special Considerations

### Hypertension

When a pregnant woman with asthma either has hypertension or develops hypertension, the pharmacologic management of the hypertension is best achieved by avoiding the use of beta-adrenergic antagonists (beta-blockers) because they may exacerbate the asthma.

### Diabetes

If diabetes, either insulin-dependent or gestational, and asthma coexist during pregnancy, the overall management may be complicated because asthma medication may impair carbohydrate tolerance and worsen diabetes. Specifically, systemic $beta_2$-agonists and systemic corticosteroids may cause hyperglycemia, which necessitates close monitoring of blood sugars and may increase the patient's insulin requirements. Although it would be best to avoid the use of these agents during the pregnancy of a woman with diabetes, asthma exacerbations may require systemic $beta_2$-agonists and/or systemic steroids. Close communication among the physicians managing the asthma, the diabetes, and the pregnancy is necessary.

### Rhinitis

Significant nasal symptoms occur in approximately 35 percent of randomly selected women. Few data exist regarding the interrelationships between rhinitis and pregnancy. In one survey, preexisting rhinitis worsened during pregnancy in 34 percent of the women, improved in 15 percent, remained unchanged in 45 percent, and could not be evaluated in 6 percent. It seems unlikely that gestational rhinitis would have any direct adverse effect on the course of pregnancy, but severe rhinitis can interfere with sleeping, eating, or emotional well-being. In addition, uncontrolled rhinitis or sinusitis during pregnancy may exacerbate coexisting asthma.

**Diagnosis.** Essentially, any of the recognized forms of rhinitis may occur during pregnancy, but the most common types appear to be allergic rhinitis, rhinitis medicamentosa, vasomotor rhinitis, and bacterial rhinosinusitis.

Allergic rhinitis is caused by an intranasal IgE-mediated reaction to inhaled allergens such as pollen, house-dust mites, mold spores, or animal dander. Prominent symptoms include sneezing, runny nose, nasal itching, and eye itching that may be exacerbated seasonably or by exposure to allergens (grass, house-dust mites, animal dander).

Rhinitis medicamentosa is the syndrome of rebound nasal congestion resulting from the overuse of topical vasoconstricting nose sprays. It may complicate another underlying cause of chronic rhinitis or a viral upper respiratory infection.

Vasomotor rhinitis of pregnancy is a syndrome of nasal congestion and vasomotor instability limited to the gestational period. Symptoms in these women with this condition tend to be most prominent in the second half of pregnancy and usually disappear within 5 days postpartum.

**Treatment.** Many women will be able to tolerate their nasal symptoms during pregnancy with little or no pharmacologic therapy. Although this may be desirable, especially during the first trimester, substantially bothersome symptoms warrant treatment.

For patients with allergic rhinitis, as with allergic asthma, environmental control measures are important to reduce antigen exposure. Pharmacotherapy is reasonable if environmental control measures do not provide sufficient control. Intranasal cromolyn may be considered first, based on its topical effects and reassuring gestational animal and human data. For patients with allergic rhinitis inadequately controlled by intranasal cromolyn, antihistamine therapy (tripelennamine or chlorpheniramine) should be considered. Many patients with eosinophilic rhinitis will respond better to a combination of an antihistamine and pseudoephedrine than to either drug alone.

An alternative to oral therapy for allergic rhinitis during pregnancy is intranasal corticosteroid therapy. Although there is no published experience on the use of these medications intranasally during pregnancy, some authors consider these medications to be preferable to oral medications for allergic rhinitis during pregnancy due to their topical application. Intranasal beclomethasone is recommended, beginning with two sprays in each nostril twice daily and then tapering to the lowest effective dose.

Although discontinuation of the topical vasoconstrictor is the most important treatment of rhinitis medicamentosa intolerable congestion frequently results. Addition of intranasal beclomethasone (two sprays in each nostril twice daily) usually allows comfortable discontinuation of the offending vasoconstricting spray. Two nonpharmacologic approaches may be useful for patients with vasomotor rhinitis during pregnancy. A buffered saline nose spray may be helpful for the nasal dryness, nasal bleeding, and vascular congestion associated with pregnancy. Exercise (commensurate with the pregnancy) may also be useful because exercise leads to physiologic nasal vasoconstriction. When pharmacologic therapy is required, pseudoephedrine is recommended.

## *Sinusitis*

Bacterial rhinosinusitis may complicate another underlying cause of rhinitis or may follow a viral upper respiratory infection. The incidence of sinusitis in pregnancy has been reported to be 1.5 percent, an apparent six-fold increased incidence over the non-pregnant population.

**Diagnosis.** The diagnosis of sinusitis during pregnancy is often made empirically based on clinical findings of posterior nasal drainage, sinus distribution pain, and purulent discharge lasting more than 5 to 7 days. A high index of suspicion must be maintained for bacterial sinusitis during pregnancy because as many as half of pregnant women with documented sinusitis may lack the classic clinical findings. Sinus radiographs should be used during pregnancy when indicated, such as when a clinically diagnosed sinus infection is not responding to antibiotic therapy or when a probable clinical diagnosis cannot be made without radiologic confirmation.

**Treatment.** Cultures of sinus aspirates obtained during pregnancy have shown the most common sinus pathogens to be Hemophilus influenza and Streptococcus pneumonae. Data on the use of antibiotics during pregnancy have been reviewed. Amoxicillin is the initial antibiotic of choice in the management of sinusitis during pregnancy in women who are not allergic to penicillin. Erythromycin is recommended for the penicillin-allergic patient with gestational sinusitis, and the addition of sulfisoxazole may be considered in early or mid-pregnancy if the patient is not responding in 5 to 7 days. Experience suggests that 3 weeks of therapy is superior to a 10- to 14-day course with regard to preventing the development of recurrent sinusitis during pregnancy. Oxymetazoline nose spray or drops (for up

## Asthma

to 5 days) and pseudoephedrine may also be helpful as adjunctive and symptomatic therapy of gestational bacterial rhinosinusitis.

An appropriate cephalosporin, amoxicillin/beta-lactamase inhibitor, erythromycin, or erythromycin plus sulfisoxazole (in early or mid pregnancy) may be considered for women with unequivocal clinical sinusitis who do not respond to amoxicillin. If improvement does not occur, sinus films should be obtained, and sinus irrigation may be necessary as both a diagnostic and therapeutic modality.

### Anaphylaxis

Any agent that can cause anaphylaxis in the non-pregnant state could potentially lead to anaphylaxis in the susceptible or sensitized pregnant patient. Maternal hypoxemia and hypotension caused by anaphylaxis may be catastrophic to the mother and the fetus. Thus management of anaphylaxis during pregnancy must be aggressive and expeditious, and all anaphylactic reactions should be considered potentially severe or life threatening until resolved.

**Treatment.** Because of the altered circulatory and respiratory physiology during pregnancy, adequate intravascular volume repletion and oxygenation are particularly important in the management of anaphylaxis during pregnancy to prevent both maternal and fetal complications. Epinephrine (0.3 cc of 1:1000 intramuscularly [IM]) is the initial pharmacologic treatment of choice and may be repeated every 10 to 15 minutes. If the reaction is due to a cutaneous injection or sting, a tourniquet should be placed above the site, 0.1 cc epinephrine should be injected at the site of the injection or sting, and 0.3 cc epinephrine should be injected into the opposite arm. Unless the reaction resolves promptly after the first epinephrine injection, diphenhydramine 50 mg IM (i.v. with hypotension) should be administered. For persistent symptoms, cimetidine 300 mg i.v. should be given. For persistent wheezing, nebulized $beta_2$-agonists may be administered, and for recalcitrant hypotension, plasma expanders are indicated. In cases of extreme hypotension where tissue perfusion may be inadequate, intravenous epinephrine (1:10,000) may be considered.

Section 2.9

## Good News and Great Tips for Pregnant Women with Asthma

Source: NIH Pub. No. 93-3279. September 1993. Extracted from the Report of the Working Group on Asthma and Pregnancy.

Congratulations. Your pregnancy is an exciting event, and your visit to the doctor shows you care about staying healthy. You are breathing for two now, and you need to keep your asthma under control. By taking the steps listed in this handout, you can control your asthma and protect your baby.

If you do not take these steps, you could lose control of your asthma. Asthma symptoms such as coughing, chest tightness, wheezing, and shortness of breath can keep your baby from getting enough oxygen to grow well. Your baby could be less healthy and smaller when born, or could even be born too early. But these things do not need to happen. Asthma can be controlled so you can have a normal pregnancy, labor, and delivery and a healthy baby.

Here are the steps you can take to control your asthma and protect your baby:

### Work with your doctor and other health care providers

- Keep your appointments.

- Ask all the questions you have. Writing them down before each visit is a good idea. It helps you remember them all.

- Tell your doctor about any wheezing, coughing, or shortness of breath that you have.

- Tell your doctor if you notice any changes in your asthma.

- Tell your doctor any concerns you have about your medicines or the other parts of your treatment plan.

## Asthma

- Make sure you know what your doctor wants you to do before you leave the office.

### *Take your medicines*

- Follow directions exactly about when to take your asthma medicines and how much medicine to take.

- Don't stop taking your asthma medicines unless your doctor directs you.

- Get your doctor's okay before you take ANY new medicines or over-the-counter drugs (drugs you choose yourself at the store, such as headache, cough, or cold medicine).

**Remember:** Using asthma medicine during pregnancy is much safer than letting your asthma get out of control. Such asthma medicines as inhaled beta-agonists, cromolyn, and inhaled steroids are safe for pregnant women when you take them as directed by your doctor. So, take your medicines and control your asthma.

### *Watch your asthma and treat symptoms fast*

Pregnancy is a time of change. Your asthma can change too and can get worse, better, or stay the same. If this is your first pregnancy, there is no way to predict what will happen with your asthma. If you have been pregnant before, your asthma is most likely to change or not change the same way it did with your last pregnancy. It is very important for you to watch your asthma closely.

- Use a peak flow meter each day so you can find any changes in your asthma and act early.

- Know how to tell if your asthma is getting worse. Make a list with your doctor of the ways you can tell if your asthma is getting worse.

- Make a plan with your doctor for dealing with any sign that your asthma is getting worse. Use it.

*Stay away from your asthma triggers*

Your asthma triggers are those things that you know make your asthma worse. House dust mites or damp places, animals, tobacco smoke, and very cold air are some examples of asthma triggers. You can stay away from some triggers. For other triggers, you can take action to keep them from bothering your asthma. See the "How to Control Asthma Triggers" handout for more information.

*Do not smoke or stay around people who smoke*

- Cigarette smoke makes it more likely that you will have asthma episodes.

- Smoking during your pregnancy makes it more likely that your baby will be born too early and too small. Your baby is more likely to be sick more often, too.

- If babies breathe in other people's smoke, the babies' lungs will not grow and work as well as they should. The baby is likely to have more colds and earaches.

- When babies live with people who smoke, they have a greater chance of developing asthma.

- If you smoke, now is the time to stop. Your doctor or nurse will help you. Ask the.

## Answers to Some Common Questions

**Are asthma medicines safe for pregnant women?** Yes, asthma medicines are safe when you take them as directed by your doctor. It is very important for your baby's health that you keep your asthma under good control.

**Can I exercise?** Yes. You can exercise. Exercise is important and you should be able to be physically active without having asthma symptoms. Talk to your doctor about this.

## Asthma

**Can I take allergy shots?** Yes. Allergy shots can be continued if you were getting them before you were pregnant. But allergy shots should not be started for the first time while you are pregnant.

**Should I get flu shots?** You can get flu shots. These are made from dead viruses that will not harm you or your baby. Flu shots are often recommended for people who have asthma. Ask your doctor.

**What happens if I get an asthma episode (or "attack") during labor or delivery?** Asthma episodes usually do not occur during labor and delivery. If asthma symptoms do occur, you will receive prompt treatment and you and your baby will be watched carefully. Your asthma will be controlled so you can have a normal labor and delivery.

**Will my breast milk be safe for my baby?** Yes. Very little asthma medicine will get to your baby through your breast milk. The small amount in breast milk will not harm your baby.

**Will my baby have asthma?** Perhaps. A child is more likely to have asthma when one or both parents have asthma or allergies.

Section 2.10

## How to Control Asthma Triggers

Adapted from National Asthma Education Program. *Teaching Your Patients About Asthma: A Clinician's Guide.* Washington. D.C.: U.S. Department of Health and Human Services, 1992.

Because you have asthma, your airways are very sensitive. They may react to things called triggers—these are things that can make asthma symptoms start. When you are near an asthma trigger your airways may become swollen, tighten up, and produce too much mucus. You may start to wheeze, cough, have congestion, itchy eyes, or a runny nose. It's important to find out what your asthma triggers are and figure out ways to control them.

Each person has different triggers. Here are common triggers and actions you can take to control them. Controlling your triggers will help you have fewer asthma symptoms and it will make your asthma treatment work better.

- Ask your doctor and other health care providers to help you find out what your asthma triggers are. You may need to keep a written record of your activities. For example, you write down what you were doing, and where, whenever you have symptoms. This will help you notice if your symptoms are caused by being near certain things. For example, if your symptoms are worse when you make your bed or vacuum, dust mites may be a trigger.

- Ask your doctor for help in deciding which actions will help the most to reduce your asthma symptoms.

- Number each action item in order of importance. Carry out the actions at the top of the list first. Once you have completed these actions, move on to actions that are of lesser importance.

- Discuss the results of these efforts with your doctor.

*Pollens and Molds (Outdoor)*

- Use air conditioning, if possible, during seasons when pollen and mold are highest.

- Keep windows closed during seasons when pollen and mold are highest.

- Avoid handling wet leaves or garden debris.

- Consider staying indoors during the middle of the day and afternoon when the pollen count is highest.

- If you are outside when the pollen count is high, it might help if you wash your hair before you go to bed.

## Asthma

*House Dust Mites*

**These are actions you should take to gain control of dust mites:**

- Put your mattress in an airtight, or plastic, cover.

- Put your pillow in an airtight cover or wash it once a week, every week, in hot water (130° F).

- Avoid sleeping or lying on upholstered furniture.

- Remove carpets that are laid on concrete.

- Wash your bed covers and clothes once a week every week in hot water (130° F).

**Some additional actions include:**

- Reduce indoor humidity to less than 50 percent. Use a dehumidifier if needed.

- Remove carpets from your bedroom.

- Use chemical agents to kill mites or to change mite antigens in the house.

- Avoid using a vacuum or being in a room while it is being vacuumed.

- If you must vacuum, one or more of the following things can be done to reduce the amount of dust you breathe in.

1. Use a dust mask.

2. Use a central vacuum cleaner with the collecting bag outside the home.

3. Use a vacuum cleaner that has powerful suction.

## Animal Allergy

All warm-blooded pets, including dogs, cats, birds, and rodents, can make your asthma worse. The flakes or scales from the skin, hair, or feathers of these animals and dried saliva or urine can make people start coughing, wheezing, or get itchy, watery eyes. This is called an allergy. The shortness of a pet's hair does not matter. There is no such thing as an allergy-free dog or cat.

- Remove the animal from the house.

- If you must have a pet with fur or feathers, keep the pet out of your bedroom at all times.

- If there is forced-air heating in the home and you have a pet, close the air ducts in your bedroom.

- Wash the pet once a week, every week.

- Avoid visits to friends or relatives who have pets with fur or feathers.

- Take asthma medicine (cromolyn or beta$_2$-agonist; cromolyn is often preferred) before visiting homes or sites where animals with fur or feathers are present.

- Choose a pet without fur or feathers.

- Avoid products made with feathers, for example, pillows and comforters. Also avoid pillows, bedding, and furniture stuffed with kapok (silky fibers from the seed pods of the silk-cotton tree).

## Cockroach Allergy

- Use insect sprays; but have someone else spray when you are outside of your home.

- Air out your home for a few hours after spraying.

- Use roach traps.

## Asthma

### *Indoor Molds*

- Keep bathrooms, kitchens, and basements well aired.

- Clean bathrooms, kitchens, and basements regularly.

- Do not use humidifiers.

- Use dehumidifiers for damp basement areas, with humidity level set for less than 50 percent but above 25 percent. Empty and clean the dehumidifier water tray regularly.

### *Tobacco Smoke*

- Do not smoke.

- Do not allow smoking in your home.

- Have household members smoke outside.

- Do not allow any smoking in your bedroom. Encourage family members to quit smoking. Ask your doctor for help on how to quit. Cigarette smoke can also harm your infant and young children. Studies show that children who breathe their mother's smoke have more lung diseases, such as asthma. Children with asthma who are around smoke have reduced lung function. They need more medicine and emergency room visits than children who are not around smoke.

### *Wood Smoke*

- Avoid using a wood-burning stove to heat your home.

- Avoid using kerosene heaters.

### *Strong Odors and Sprays*

- Do not stay in your home when it is being painted. Allow enough time for the paint to dry.

- Avoid perfume and perfumed cosmetics such as talcum powder and hairspray.

- Do not use room deodorizers.

- Use non-perfumed household cleaning products whenever possible.

- Reduce strong cooking odors (especially frying) by using a fan and opening windows.

## Colds and Infections

- Wash your hands frequently if people around you have a cold or flu.

- Be sure to get the right amount of rest, exercise, and nutritious food.

- Talk to your doctor about flu shots.

- Do not take over-the-counter cold remedies, such as antihistamines and cough syrup, unless you speak to your doctor first.

## Exercise

Exercise can make some people's asthma worse. But don't avoid exercise; it is important for your health. These things will help you exercise without bothering your asthma.

- Work out a medicine plan with your doctor that helps you to exercise comfortably.

- Take inhaled beta$_2$-agonist or cromolyn medicine before you start to exercise, if needed.

- Warm up before exercising and cool down afterwards.

## Weather

- Wear a scarf over your mouth and nose in cold weather.

- Pull a turtleneck over your nose on windy or cold days.

- Dress warmly in the winter or on windy days.

## Asthma

Remember: Following these suggestions will help keep asthma episodes from starting. It will help your asthma medicine work better. A plan to control your asthma triggers is an important part of controlling asthma.

## Section 2.11

## *How to Use a Metered-Dose Inhaler*

Source: NIH Pub. No. 93-3279. September 1993. Extracted from the Report of the Working Group on Asthma and Pregnancy.

Using a metered-dose inhaler is a good way to take asthma medicines. There are few side effects because the medicine goes right to the airways inside the lungs. It takes only 5 to 10 minutes for the medicine to have an effect compared to liquid asthma medicines, which can take 1 to 3 hours. A spacer or holding chamber attached to the inhaler can help make your inhaler easier to use. For patients taking inhaled steroids, a spacer may help prevent irritation to the mouth.

*Using the Inhaler*

Adapted from National Asthma Education Program, *Teaching Your Patients About Asthma: A Clinician's Guide*. Washington, D.C.: U.S. Department of Health and Human Services, 1992.

1. Remove the cap and hold the inhaler upright.

2. Shake the inhaler.

3. Tilt your head back slightly and breathe out.

4. Use the inhaler in any one of these ways. (A is the best way. B is useful for all patients. C is okay if you are having trouble with A or B.)

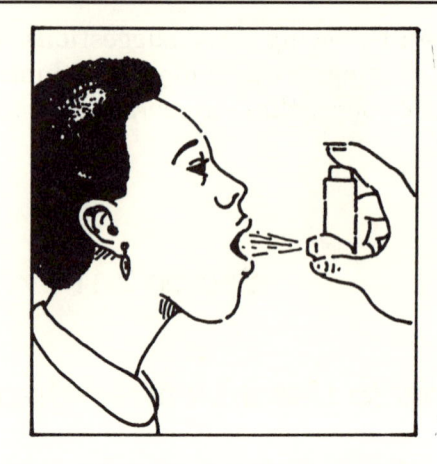

**Figure 2.18.** A. Open mouth with inhaler 1 to 2 inches away

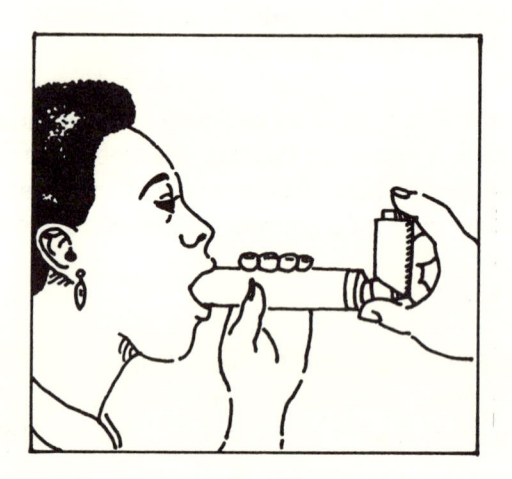

**Figure 2.19.** B. Use spacer

## Asthma

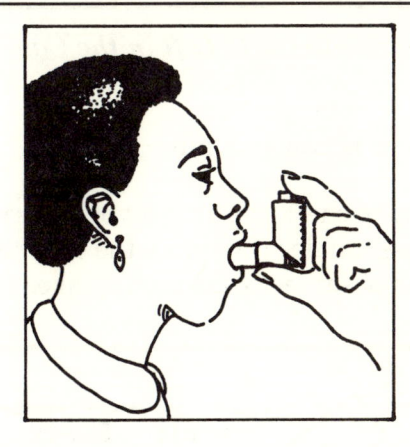

**Figure 2.20. C. In the mouth**

5. Press down on the inhaler to release the medicine as you start to breathe in slowly. 6. Breathe in slowly for 3 to 5 seconds.

7. Hold your breath for 10 seconds to allow the medicine to reach deep into your lungs.

8. Repeat puffs as prescribed. Waiting 1 minute between puffs may permit the second puff to go deeper into the lungs.

Note: Dry powder capsules are used differently. To use a dry powder inhaler, close your mouth tightly around the mouthpiece and inhale very fast.

### *Cleaning*

The inhaler should be cleaned often to prevent buildup that will clog the inhaler.

1. Once a day, clean the inhaler and cap by rinsing them in warm running water. Let them dry before you use it again.

2. Twice a week wash the plastic mouthpiece with mild dishwashing soap and warm water. Rinse and dry it well before putting it back.

# Respiratory Diseases and Disorders Sourcebook

*Checking How Much Medicine Is Left in the Canister*

1. If the canister is new, it is full.

2. An easy way to check the amount of medicine left in your metered-dose inhaler is to place the canister in a container of water and observe the position it takes in the water.

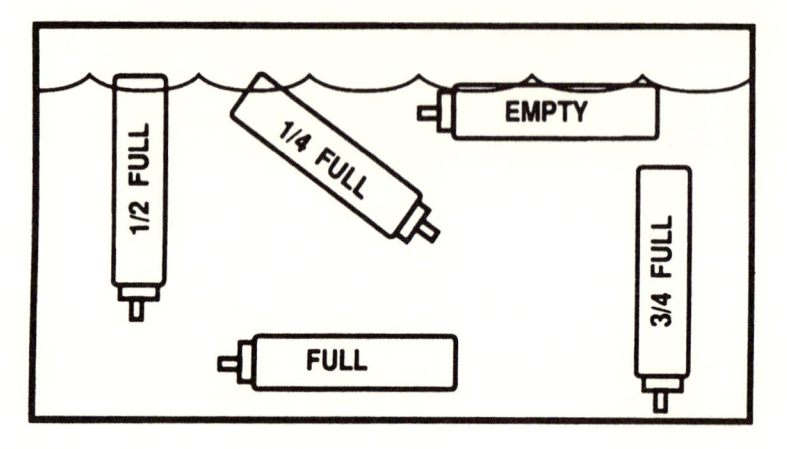

*Figure 2.21.*

Section 2.12

## *How to Use a Peak Flow Meter*

Adapted from National Asthma Education Program. *Teaching Your Patients About Asthma: A Clinician's Guide.* Washington. D.C.: U.S. Department of Health and Human Services, 1992.

It is very important during pregnancy to keep your lung function close to normal—that is, to make sure that your lungs are working as well as possible. Normal lung function is needed to provide enough oxygen to your growing baby.

## Asthma

A peak flow meter is a device that measures your lung function, that is, how well your lungs are working. This information will help you and your doctor to better control your asthma. For example, during an asthma episode the airways of the lungs get narrow and blocked. The peak flow meter can measure how much the airways are blocked hours or even days before you feel any chest tightness, coughing, or wheezing. By taking your medicine as soon as the peak flow measure changes, you may be able to stop the episode quickly and avoid a severe episode of asthma.

The peak flow meter can also be used to help you and your doctor:

- Decide if your medicine plan is working well.
- Decide when to add, reduce, or stop medicine.
- Decide when to seek emergency care.
- Identify triggers—that is, what causes your asthma to get worse.

Peak flow meters are used to check your asthma the way that blood pressure cuffs are used to check high blood pressure.

***How to Use a Peak Flow Meter:***

1. Place the arrow at the base of the numbered scale.
2. Stand up.
3. Take a deep breath.
4. Place the meter in your mouth and close your lips around the mouth piece. Do not put your tongue inside the hole. Do not bend your neck.
5. Blow out as hard and fast as you can.
6. Write down the number you get.

7. Repeat steps 1 through 6 two more times.

8. Write down the highest of the three numbers achieved.

*Find Your Personal Best Peak Flow Number*

Your personal best peak flow number is the highest peak flow number you can achieve over a 2-week period when your asthma is under good control—that is, when you feel good and do not have any coughing, wheezing, shortness of breath, or chest tightness.

Each patient's asthma is different, and your best peak flow number may be higher or lower than the average number for someone of your height, weight, and sex. This means that it is important for you and your doctor or nurse to find your own personal best peak flow number. Your own medicine plan needs to be based on your own personal best peak flow number.

To find out your personal best peak flow number, you will need to do these things:

- Use the peak flow meter every day for 2 weeks.

- Use the peak flow meter mornings and evenings (when you wake up and about 10 to 12 hours later).

- Use the peak flow meter before and after taking inhaled bronchodilator, if you take one.

- Write down the peak flow numbers on "My Weekly Asthma Symptom and Peak Flow Diary."

- Review the information in your diary with your doctor.

*Discuss With Your Doctor What to Do When Your Peak Flow Numbers Change*

The most important thing about measuring your peak flow number every day is to see how much it changes from your personal best number and from one reading to another. Your doctor will give you an "asthma control plan" that tells you what actions to take when there is a change in your peak flow numbers. For example, a fall in your peak flow of 20 to 30 percent of your personal best number may mean the start of an asthma episode. You need to follow your asthma control plan.

***Use the Peak Flow Zone System to Manage Your Asthma***

Peak flow zones are set up like traffic lights to help you know what to do when your peak flow number changes. Once you know your personal best peak flow number, your doctor will give you the numbers that tell you what to do in each zone. You or your doctor can write these on your Asthma Control Plan and "My Weekly Asthma Symptom and Peak Flow Diary." For example:

**Green zone** (80 to 100 percent of your personal best number) signals all clear. No asthma symptoms are present, and you may take your medicines as usual.

**Yellow zone** (50 to 80 percent of your personal best number) signals caution. An episode of asthma may be starting and you will need to take extra medicine for a while according to your doctor's directions. Or, your overall asthma may not be under good control, and the doctor may need to change your daily medicine plan.

**Red zone** (below 50 percent of your personal best number) signals a medical alert. You must take an inhaled $beta_2$-agonist right away, and call your doctor if your peak flow number does not return quickly to the yellow or green zone and stay in that zone.

Record your personal best peak flow number and peak flow zones on the upper left-hand corner of "My Weekly Asthma Symptom and Peak Flow Diary."

***Use the Diary to Keep Track of Your Peak Flow***

Adapted from National Asthma Education Program. *Teaching Your Patients About Asthma: A Clinician's Guide*. Washington. D.C.: U.S. Department of Health and Human Services, 1992.

Write down your peak flow number on "My Weekly Asthma Symptom and Peak Flow Diary" every day, or as instructed by your doctor.

Section 2.13

## My Weekly Asthma Symptom and Peak Flow Diary

Source: NIH Pub. No. 93-3279. September 1993. Extracted from the Report of the Working Group on Asthma and Pregnancy.

\_\_\_\_ My predicted peak flow number.
\_\_\_\_ My personal best peak flow number.
\_\_\_\_ My green zone (OK) 80-100% of personal best.
\_\_\_\_ My yellow zone (Caution) 50-80% of personal best.
\_\_\_\_ My red zone (Danger) less than 50% of personal best.

1. Take your peak flow reading every morning (a.m.) when you wake up and every night (p.m.) at bedtime. Try to take your peak flow readings at the same time each day. If you take an inhaled beta2-agonist medicine, take your peak flow reading before you take that medicine. Write down the highest reading of three tries in the box that says peak flow reading.

2. Look at the upper left corner of this sheet to see whether your number is in the green, yellow, or red zone.

3. In the space below the date and time, put an "X" in the box that matches the symptoms you have when you record your peak flow reading.

4. Look at your "Asthma Control Plan" for what to do when your number is in one of the zones and you have asthma symptoms.

5. Put an "X" in the box beside "medicine used" if you took extra asthma medicine to stop your symptoms.

6. If you made any visit to your doctor's office, emergency department, or hospital for treatment of an asthma episode, put an "X" in the box marked "urgent visit." Tell your doctor if you went to the emergency department or hospital.

## Asthma

| Date | a.m. | p.m. | a.m. | p.m. | a.m. | p.m. | a.m. | p.m. | a.m. | p.m. | a.m. | p.m. | a.m. | p.m. |
|---|---|---|---|---|---|---|---|---|---|---|---|---|---|---|
| Peak flow reading | | | | | | | | | | | | | | |
| No asthma symptoms | | | | | | | | | | | | | | |
| Mild asthma symptoms | | | | | | | | | | | | | | |
| Moderate asthma symptoms | | | | | | | | | | | | | | |
| Serious asthma symptoms | | | | | | | | | | | | | | |
| Medicine used to stop symptoms | | | | | | | | | | | | | | |
| Urgent visit to the doctor | | | | | | | | | | | | | | |

**Figure 2.22.** *My Weekly Asthma Symptom and Peak Flow Diary*

**No symptoms.** = No symptoms (wheeze, cough, chest tightness, or shortness of breath) even with normal physical activity.

**Mild symptoms.** = Symptoms during physical activity, but not at rest. Asthma symptoms do not keep you from sleeping or being active.

**Moderate symptoms.** = Symptoms while at rest; symptoms may keep you from sleeping or being active.

**Severe symptoms.** = Severe symptoms at rest (wheeze may be absent); symptoms cause problems walking or talking; muscles in neck or between ribs are pulled in when breathing.

Section 2.14

## *How to Take Your Medicine: Adrenergic Bronchodilators (Inhaled)*

Source: *FDA Consumer.* June 1991.

How you take a drug can affect how well it works and how safe it will be for you. Sometimes it can be almost as important as what you take. Timing, what you eat and when you eat, proper dose, and many other factors can mean the difference between feeling better, staying the same, or even feeling worse. This drug information section is intended to help you make your treatment work as effectively as possible. It is important to note, however, that this is only a guideline. You should talk to your doctor about how and when to take any prescribed drugs.

Adrenergic bronchodilators are most commonly used in metered-dose inhalers (small aerosol pumps). While doctors consider inhalers generally quite safe, these drugs can cause adverse effects if not used properly.

## Some Commonly Used Metered-Dose Inhalers:

*albuterol*
Proventil
Ventolin

*bitolterol*
Tornalate

*epinephrine*
AsthmaHaler
Bronkaid Mist
Medihaler-Epi
Primatene Mist

*isoetharine*
Bronkometer

*isoproterenol*
Isuprel
Medihaler-Iso

*metaproterenol*
Alupent

*pirbuterol*
Maxair

*terbutaline*
Brethaire

## Conditions These Drugs Treat

Adrenergic bronchodilators alleviate the symptoms of asthma, chronic bronchitis, and emphysema by opening air passages in the lungs to allow easier breathing.

While they are not a cure for asthma, adrenergic bronchodilators can temporarily relieve the classic symptoms of the disease: wheezing, coughing, shortness of breath, and tightness in the chest. They can also prevent bronchospasm when taken shortly before exercising.

## How to Take

There are several devices that administer adrenergic bronchodilators.

The metered-dose inhaler is the most common. A small aerosol pump, the inhaler sprays a controlled amount of medicated mist through a mouthpiece for the patient to inhale. The inhaler easily fits in a purse or bag to use anywhere.

Follow your doctor's directions for assembling and using the inhaler. For most brands, hold the inhaler bottle upside down and close your lips firmly over the mouthpiece. Press down firmly on the bottle as directed and inhale deeply. Then remove the mouthpiece and hold your breath a moment before exhaling slowly.

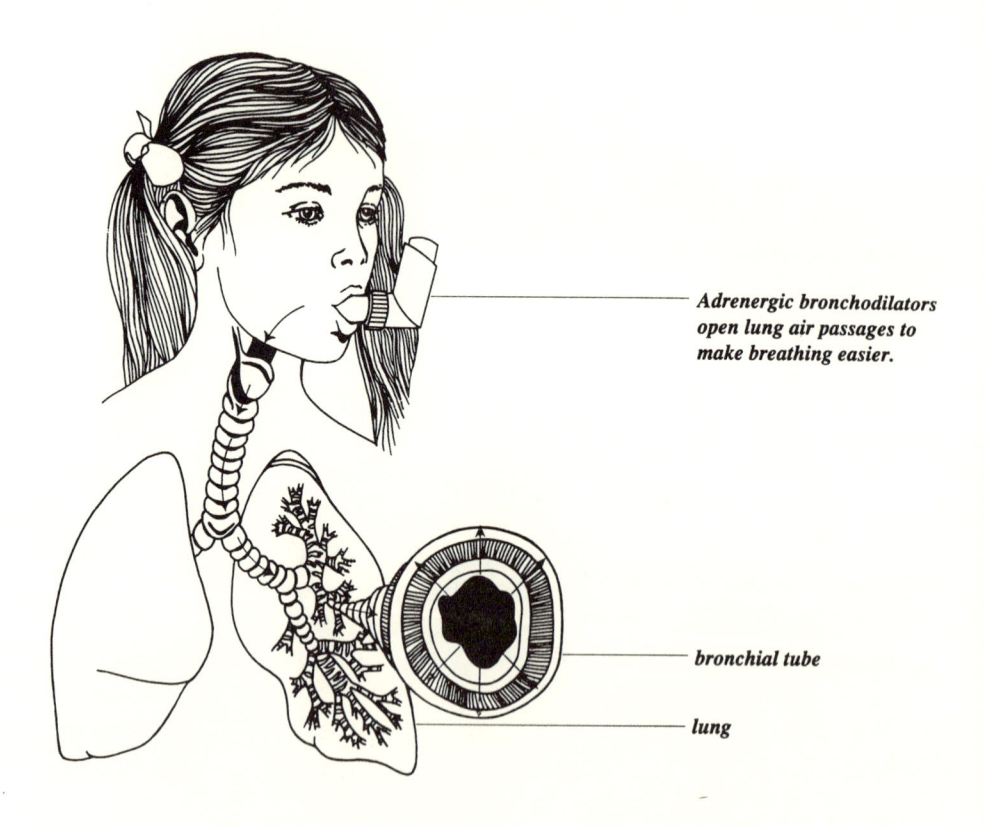

*Adrenergic bronchodilators open lung air passages to make breathing easier.*

*bronchial tube*

*lung*

**Figure 2.23.** Source: American Medical Association Encyclopedia of Medicine.

The prescribed dosage can vary, depending on the patient's symptoms and other factors. Always follow your doctor's instructions regarding the number and frequency of inhalations. Some patients are instructed to take two inhalations. Others are told to wait a minute or two and take another inhalation only if necessary.

Bronchodilators can also be taken using nebulizers or respirators to produce the spray, but these are almost always used only at a doctor's office or under strict medical supervision.

Most metered-dose inhalers require a doctor's prescription. Inhalers containing one type of bronchodilator, epinephrine, are available over the counter in brand names such as AsthmaHaler, Bronkaid, Primatene, and AsthmaNefrin. But do not use an over-the-counter inhaler unless your doctor recommends it and you have been diagnosed with asthma.

## Missed Doses

For adults using inhalers, a typical dose of the medicine is two inhalations, four times a day.

If you miss a dose, take it as soon as you remember, and consult your doctor about when to take the next dose. Be careful not to inhale more of the medicine than your doctor recommends. Large doses of bronchodilators might cause serious side effects.

## Relief of Symptoms

Bronchodilators may provide relief in as quickly as a few seconds or as long as 30 minutes after using.

## Side Effects and Risks

Side effects include nervousness, restlessness and trembling.

Less common side effects include coughing, dizziness, indigestion, irritated mouth or throat, pounding heartbeat, headache, increased sweating, an increase in blood pressure, muscle cramps or twitching, nausea or vomiting, sleeplessness, paleness, and weakness.

Seek immediate medical attention if any side effects develop, including the following: bluish skin, severe dizziness or faintness, continuous flushing or redness of face or skin, increased wheezing or difficulty in breathing, skin rashes, hives or itching, and swelling of the face, lips or eyelids.

Check with your doctor as soon as possible if you experience chest pain, irregular heartbeat, numbness in the hands or feet, or unusual breathing.

If the inhaler medicine leaves an unpleasant taste in your mouth or changes your sense of smell or taste, contact your doctor immediately.

## Precautions and Warnings

Check with your doctor at once if the bronchospasm continues after using an inhaler.

Also, tell your doctor if you are pregnant or breast-feeding, and ask about any additional risks under those circumstances.

Diabetics may find that their blood sugar levels rise after using this medicine. Diabetics who notice a change in their blood or urine sugar test results should tell their doctors.

## Before Taking This Medicine

Before using an inhaler, tell your doctor if you have had adverse reactions to any drugs, especially other adrenergic bronchodilators.

Also tell your doctor if you have any of the following medical problems:

- brain damage
- convulsions and seizures
- diabetes
- heart or blood vessel disease
- high blood pressure
- mental disease
- overactive thyroid
- Parkinson's disease

Inform your doctor of any prescription or over-the-counter drugs you are taking now or have taken in the last two weeks, especially any beta blockers, heart medicines, or mood-changing drugs.

Also, tell your doctor if you have ever used cocaine or other stimulants.

—*Rebecca D. Williams*

Section 2.15

# Asthma Education and Prevention Materials and Resources

Source: National Asthma Education and Prevention Program, National Heart, Lung and Blood Institute, November 1993.

## Introduction

### Who Should Use This Guide

Families and patients looking for sources of information about asthma and how to manage and control it will find this *Asthma Education and Prevention Materials and Resources* guide helpful. It includes organizations, educational programs, pamphlets, books, and audiovisual materials designed for children and adults with asthma or interested friends and relatives.

Leaders of asthma education programs can use this guide to locate sources of background and problem solving information needed as they plan and present programs. This guide may be duplicated and given to participants as an adjunct to other program handouts.

Physicians and other health professionals may also find the list of interest to their patients.

### How the Guide Is Organized and How to Get the Most Out of It

The *Asthma Education and Prevention Materials and Resources* guide has three major sections that describe various types of asthma resources that are currently available. It also provides information on how to locate specific resources such as asthma specialists and group education programs.

**Section 1: Family and Group Programs.** This section lists places to find family and group asthma education programs. Some specific programs are listed in Section 2.

**Section 2: Print Materials and Other Resources.** Materials described in this section include educational programs, pamphlets, workbooks, films, videos, slide-tape shows, puppets, books, and audiovisual materials for health professionals.

This section gives descriptions and ordering information for these educational materials. Materials from each source are grouped together. Please be aware that prices and availability are subject to change and that new materials are often produced from time to time. Materials from over 20 organizations are listed.

A limited number of audiovisual materials have been designed specifically for the education of health professionals. These are listed in a separate subsection.

**Section 3: Information Sources.** This section provides an alphabetical directory of organizations that can offer special services, education, or treatment to asthma patients and health professionals. Use this listing after you have reviewed Section 2 on materials and programs to see what you want to order. Several types of organizations are included in this section:

- Voluntary health and patient oriented organizations:

    American Lung Association and its local chapters
    Allergy and Asthma Network/Mothers of Asthmatics
    Asthma and Allergy Foundation of America
    American Allergy Association

- Professional societies of physicians who specialize in the treatment of lung disease and asthma:

    American Thoracic Society
    American Academy of Allergy and Immunology
    American College of Allergy and Immunology
    American College of Chest Physicians

- Professional society of physicians who specialize in the treatment of families:

    American Academy of Family Physicians

## Asthma

- Professional society of physicians who specialize in treatment of children:

    American Academy of Pediatrics

- Nationally known treatment centers that also produce educational materials:

    Foundation for Asthma/Tucson Medical Center—
    Tucson, Arizona
    National Jewish Center for Immunology and
    Respiratory Medicine—Denver, CO

- Federal Government agencies that fund research and produce educational materials on asthma:

    National Heart, Lung, and Blood Institute
    National Institute of Allergy and Infectious Diseases

- Federal Government agency that compiles national statistics on asthma:

    Centers for Disease Control and Prevention
    National Center for Health Statistics

You can also contact each organization to find what services, information, or treatment arrangements are currently offered to patients in general.

### *How To Contribute to This Guide*

What kinds of information would you like to see featured in the Asthma Education and Prevention Materials and Resources guide?
Do you know of any good local treatment centers or information sources?
What newsletters or other materials have we missed?
Please contact us with detailed information and how to locate and use these resources. To contribute information or ideas, write to:

Asthma Resource List Update
Attn: Christine Krutzsch
Building 31, Room 4A-21, NIH
Bethesda, Maryland 20892
(301) 496-4236

*Where To Get More Copies*

Contact:
National Asthma Education and Prevention Program
P.O. Box 30105
Bethesda, MD 20824-0105
(301) 251-1222

## Family and Group Programs

Family and group education programs on asthma provide the opportunity for asthma patients and their families to meet other persons in similar situations so that they can share their experiences and feelings. To locate asthma education programs, check your local telephone book under sponsor agencies. Try the following listings:

- Local Hospitals— Try the main number or try any of the following departments: public relations, respiratory therapy, patient education, community education, wellness centers, or cardiopulmonary rehabilitation.

- Local Chapters of the American Lung Association— Ask about family asthma programs or parent and child support groups. Also ask how to obtain the "Best of Superstuff" educational materials.

- Local Chapters of the Asthma and Allergy Foundation of America— Ask when the next ACT program is scheduled. Ask about other educational materials or programs in your area.

Specific programs for health professional, parents, and school health professionals are listed later in this chapter. You can begin by reading the descriptions about these programs.

## Asthma

### Print and Audiovisual Materials

#### Materials and Programs for Health Professionals

**Asthma Management Kit for Clinicians.** This kit contains valuable information and materials for use by clinicians in helping to teach patients about managing their asthma. It also contains reproducible handouts. Ordering information: National Asthma Education and Prevention Program (single copies free)

**Open Airways/Respiro Abierto.** This kit is designed for asthma leaders to teach inner-city or any low-income, low-education group. It includes a teaching manual, posters, teaching notes, and tips for leaders. Materials are in English and Spanish for sessions with three different groups: parents, older children aged 7—14 years, and younger children aged 4—6. Developed by Columbia University-College of Physicians and Surgeons. Ordering information: National Asthma Education and Prevention Program (single copies free)

**Air Power.** This booklet presents the basics of asthma management in four 1-hour sessions for children aged 9—13 years and their parents. Developed at the American Institutes for Research. Ordering information: National Asthma Education and Prevention Program (single copies free)

**Living With Asthma; Part 1: Manual for Teaching Parents, Part 2: Manual for Teaching Children.** In a series of lively and fun sessions, children learn the basics of asthma management. Parents focus on improving family and social dynamics that hinder good asthma management. Problem solving and self-assessment tools as well as helpful handouts and background materials are included. This set of books is an excellent reference for anyone who conducts asthma education programs. Ordering information: National Asthma Education and Prevention Program (single copies free)

**Air Wise.** This kit features assessment tools and reproducible materials to determine a child's status on 25 key asthma management skills. Each objective has a teaching script, criteria for mastery, and a behavioral goal. After each session, parents and the doctor meet with the leader and child to discuss what the child has learned. Developed by the American Institutes for Research. Ordering information: National Asthma Education and Prevention Program (single copies free)

**ACT (Asthma Care Training) for Kids.** ACT contains materials for teaching a program on asthma and asthma management to educate children with asthma, aged 6—12 years, about self-care. It also provides parents with information and support skills they need to help their children take charge of the disease. Ordering information: Asthma and Allergy Foundation of America (Free materials and leadership training are available to those interested in teaching ACT.)

**CALM: Childhood Asthma, Learning to Manage.** This series of manuals for home use features the basics of asthma management with a focus on the use of a peak flow meter. It includes a peak flow meter and manuals for use with very young children, preadolescent, and teenagers. Manuals for the attending physician and for parents are available. Ordering information: IOX Assessment Associates or Asthma and Allergy Foundation of America ($25.95 without meter or $35.95 with meter)

**Asthma Treatment Guidelines.** Ordering information: Asthma and Allergy Foundation of America ($1.00)

**Childhood Asthma: A Matter of Control.** This describes what asthma is, what causes it, its symptoms, what triggers it, asthma control, and treatment. It contains a useful chart of medications. It is designed for a fairly high reading level (ALA No. 6012). Ordering information: Local chapter of the American Lung Association (single copies free)

*Materials and Programs for Parents of Children With Asthma*

**Childhood Asthma.** Ordering information: American Academy of Allergy and Immunology ($0.50 each. Bulk prices available.)

**Best of Superstuff.** This is an activity booklet for kids, aged 6—8 years, designed to make learning about asthma fun. The activities are designed to help children and families with asthma management techniques at home and to enhance their coping skills as well as their self-esteem, self-awareness, and knowledge about asthma. Ordering information: Local chapter of the American Lung Association—call for price.

**Childhood Asthma Residential Treatment Centers.** Ordering information: Asthma and Allergy Foundation of America ($1.00)

**Your Child and Asthma.** This provides an accurate, up-to-date discussion of the disease; its causes; its triggers; physical and psychological effects of asthma on the family and patient; and drugs, their actions, and side effects. It is designed for the lay public. Ordering information: National Jewish Center for Immunology and Respiratory Medicine (single copies free)

**Children With Asthma: A Manual for Parents.** This book is known as the "asthma bible." It focuses on the importance of a parent's role in asthma management and teaches the basics of asthma and how medicines work. It was written by patients and their parents (Second edition, 296 pages). Ordering information: Pedipress, Inc. ($15.95 full-sized edition, $8.95 pocket-sized edition)

**A Parent's Guide to Allergies and Asthma.** This resource is comprehensive, up to date, and easy to read. It is essential reading for anyone new to asthma and allergies. Ordering information: Allergy and Asthma Network/Mothers of Asthmatics ($10.00)

**Family Asthma Programs.** This series of presentations by physicians and other health professionals includes topics of interest to parents of children with asthma. Often cosponsored by a local hospital, local physicians, and the local lung association chapter. Contact information: Local chapter of the American Lung Association

**Childhood Asthma: Infancy Through Adolescence** Ordering information: Asthma and Allergy Foundation of America ($1.25)

*Materials and Programs for School Health Professionals*

**Asthma and the Schoolchild.** This is a flyer from a series called *Tips to Remember* that provides practical advice to patients. Ordering information: American Academy of Allergy and Immunology ($0.50 each. Bulk prices available.)

**Open Airways for Schools.** This package of easy-to-use teaching materials for elementary schools includes a curriculum, instructors' guide, a poster, flip chart, and reproducible handouts for children and parents. It helps teach children and parents how to prevent asthma episodes and emergencies. This package is produced by the American Lung Association and can be obtained through two sources. Ordering information: Local chapter of the American Lung Association —or—Open Airways for Schools ($29.95)

**Asthma Alert Publications** These are quick and easy reference guides for school professionals to handle asthma episodes in the school setting. The following guides are designed to meet the needs of various staff:

- Physical Education Teachers—This guide includes facts about exercise, asthma, and ways to make gym classes a more positive experience for the child with asthma. It also has information folders for the child with asthma and for the teacher's file. (ALA No. 6015)

- School Administrators—This guide includes a reminder to keep current school medical records on all children. (ALA No. 6016)

- School Nurses—This guide includes a form to record specific details of the child's asthma history and medications. It gives guidelines to help the nurse assist other school personnel to interact supportively with the child with asthma. (ALA No. 6014)

- Teachers—This is a guide for the teacher to understand the special needs of the child with asthma in the school environment. (ALA No. 6013)

Ordering information: Local chapter of the American Lung Association (single copies free)

**Tips for Teachers: The Allergic Child.** This discusses asthma along with hay fever, skin allergies, and insect stings. It lists what to do in an asthma attack, reactions to medications, and allergy do's and don'ts. Intended for school teachers. Ordering information: Asthma and Allergy Foundation of America (Each copy costs $1.25. Bulk discounts are available.)

**Managing Asthma: A Guide for Schools.** This guide provides school personnel with the necessary information to begin an asthma management program. It contains basic guidelines that are presented through action steps for specific members of the school staff. Ordering information: National Asthma Education and Prevention Program (single copies free)

*General Materials for Patients*

**Asthma Fact and Fiction.** This book contains an illustrated list of triggers and lists myths and their explanations. It explains the five parts of asthma management: the doctor, medications, environmental control, personal care, and self-knowledge. It is intended for the lay public. Ordering information: Asthma Foundation of Southern Arizona (single copies free)

**Outpatient Treatment of Asthma.** This is a flyer from a series called *Tips to Remember* that provides practical advice to patients. Ordering information: American Academy of Allergy and Immunology. ($0.50 each. Bulk prices available.)

**Facts About Asthma.** This pamphlet provides a concise description of asthma episodes, who gets asthma, and how it is treated. It is intended for the lay public. (ALA No. 005C) Ordering information: Local chapter of the American Lung Association (single copies free)

**Controlling Asthma.** This is a series of feature articles in magazine format describing asthma and its treatment. (ALA No. 1125) Ordering information: Local chapter of the American Lung Association (single copies free)

**Understanding Asthma.** This presents an overview of what is known about the causes, diagnosis, and management of asthma. Ordering information: National Jewish Center for Immunology and Respiratory Medicine (single copies free)

**Management of Chronic Respiratory Disease.** This patient education booklet gives step-by-step instructions for managing lung disease, using a nebulizer, cleaning nasal passages, draining mucus, breathing effectively, and improving physical fitness. Ordering information: National Jewish Center for Immunology and Respiratory Medicine (single copies free)

**Learn Asthma Control in Seven Days.** This workbook teaches skills for the day-to-day management of asthma. Tracking forms are included. Ordering information: University of Alabama Hospital $6.95 (make check payable to "Asthma Handbook")

**The Asthma Organizer.** The organizer is a loose-leaf notebook with asthma management and educational materials. Divisions include a "home diary" with forms to help track daily activities, physician visits, medication and peak flow, and a management plan to make the most of physician appointments. Ordering information: Allergy and Asthma Network/Mothers of Asthmatics ($25.00 for book)

**What You Need to Know About Asthma.** This booklet explains the physiology, causes, triggers, diagnosis and treatment, and myths about asthma. Ordering information: National Institute of Allergy and Infectious Diseases (single copies free, multiple copies from U.S. Government Printing Office)

**Check Your Asthma "I.Q."** This is a one-page quiz with answers that explain the basic facts about asthma. Ordering information: National Asthma Education and Prevention Program (single copies free)

**Asthma Statistics: Data Fact Sheet.** This provides an overview of asthma prevalence, mortality, hospitalizations, and physician visits. Ordering information: National Asthma Education and Prevention Program (single copies free)

**Do You Have A Chronic Cough?** This discusses chronic cough as a symptom of asthma. Ordering information: National Asthma Education and Prevention Program (single copies free)

**Your Asthma Can Be Controlled: Expect Nothing Less.** This booklet helps patients work with their doctors to become free of asthma symptoms. Ordering information: National Asthma Education and Prevention Program (single copies free)

**"Hidden" Asthma...and Other Non-Classical Formats.** This explains "hidden" asthma and "cough" asthma (night cough) and how they are diagnosed and treated. It dispels the myth that asthma is psychological in origin. It is clearly written but somewhat technical. It is designed for health educators and the lay public. Ordering information: American Allergy Association (single copies $1.00)

**Facts About Asthma.** This provides basic information on asthma, its causes, asthma episodes, and treatments. It is available in English and Spanish. Ordering information: National Asthma Education and Prevention Program (single copies free)

**The Essential Asthma Handbook.** Following an overview of the physiological and epidemiological aspects of asthma, this book discusses finding a doctor and describes medications in detail. Other chapters address asthma and sex, pregnancy, exercise, and stress. Asthma in children, including its impact on family members, is also covered. Ordering information: Scribner's Publishing Company ($19.95)

**The Asthma Handbook.** This book is written for adults with asthma. It includes facts, practical information, asthma episode management techniques, and coping skills. (ALA No. 4002) Ordering information: Local chapter of the American Lung Association (single copies free)

**Asthma Resources Directory.** This directory is a comprehensive list of suppliers, resources, and organizations. Ordering information: Allergy and Asthma Network/Mothers of Asthmatics ($29.00)

**Primer on Allergic and Immunologic Diseases.** This book includes the biology of the immune response to rhinitis, asthma, and food allergy. It contains 26 chapters. Ordering information: American Academy of Allergy and Immunology ($15.00)

**One Minute Asthma: What You Need To Know.** This makes an ideal book for people starting to learn about asthma. It covers the basics of asthma and medicines used in the treatment of asthma. It is easy to read and available in English and Spanish. (40 pages) Ordering information: Pedipress, Inc. ($5.95)

**Asthma: The Complete Guide.** This is an excellent self-management guide for asthma and allergy patients and their families. (357 pages) Ordering information: Asthma and Allergy Foundation of America ($4.95)

**The Asthma Self Help Book.** This book provides a thorough, practical look at asthma that includes information from the National Heart, Lung, and Blood Institute's 1991 Asthma Guidelines. Ordering information: Asthma and Allergy Foundation of America ($18.95)

**Understanding Asthma: A Blueprint for Breathing.** •Each chapter is written by a nationally recognized asthma expert and caregiver. Ordering information: Asthma and Allergy Foundation of America ($7.00)

**What is Asthma?** Ordering information: Asthma and Allergy Foundation of America ($1.25)

*Materials for Children*

**Captain Wonderlung: Breathing Exercises for Asthmatic Children.** Captain Wonderlung uses a comic book format to teach children diaphragmatic or "belly" breathing. It is available in Spanish and French. Ordering information: American Academy of Pediatrics (single copies free)

**Asthma: Learn to Control It.** This is a three-fold brochure on asthma management. Ordering information: American Academy of Family Physicians (for free copy, ask for sample pack # 1523. 100 copies are $15.)

**So You Have Asthma Too.** This is a colorful book for children about a 7-year-old with asthma, explaining in simple terms what asthma is, what triggers asthma episodes, and how to cope with them. A video version is also available. Ordering information: Allergy and

Asthma Network/Mothers of Asthmatics ($5.00 for book, $10.00 for video, $13.00 for both)

**Winning Over Asthma.** This easy-to-read children's book tells the story of 5-year-old Graham. It describes asthma reactions, triggers, and medicines. It shows how parents and doctors can work together. Ordering information: Pedipress, Inc. ($7.95)

**All About Asthma.** This was written by a 10-year-old with asthma and clearly illustrates causes, symptoms, and ways to control asthma and lead a normal life. It is targeted to children in grades 2—6. (39 pages) Ordering information: Asthma and Allergy Foundation of America ($4.95)

**The Lion Who Had Asthma.** This is a beautifully illustrated hardback book encouraging preschoolers to use their imaginations and to take their asthma medications. (24 pages) Ordering information: Asthma and Allergy Foundation of America ($10.00)

**I'm A Meter Reader.** This is a sequel to *So You Have Asthma Too*. It teaches children how to use a peak flow meter. Ordering information: Allergy and Asthma Network/Mothers of Asthmatics ($5.00 for book, $10.00 for video, $13.00 for both) Materials

*About Special Topics*

**EXERCISE**

**Asthma and Exercise.** This book offers detailed advice and instruction on how adults and children with asthma can safely participate in exercise and sports activities. Ordering information: Allergy and Asthma Network/Mothers of Asthmatics ($10.00)

**Exercise and Asthma.** This summarizes the relationship between asthma and exercise. It tells which kinds of exercises are the best. It is suitable for the lay public. Ordering information: Asthma and Allergy Foundation of America ($1.25 per copy, bulk discount available.)

**Exercise Induced Asthma and Bronchospasm.** This is a flyer from a series called *Tips to Remember* that provides practical advice to patients. Ordering information: American Academy of Allergy and Immunology ($0.50 each. Bulk prices available.)

## ALLERGIES AND ASTHMA

**Hayfever and Rhinitis.** Ordering information: Asthma and Allergy Foundation of America ($1.25)

**Cat Induced Asthma.** Ordering information: Asthma and Allergy Foundation of America ($1.00)

**Cockroaches and Asthma.** Ordering information: Asthma and Allergy Foundation of America ($1.00)

**Food Allergies.** Ordering information: Asthma and Allergy Foundation of America ($1.00)

**Stinging Insect Allergy.** Ordering information: American Academy of Allergy and Immunology (Prices range from $0.50 to $0.75 each. Bulk rates are available.)

**Hints for the Allergic Patient.** Ordering information: American Academy of Allergy and Immunology (Prices range from $0.50 to $0.75 each. Bulk rates are available.)

**The Role of the Allergist.** Ordering information: American Academy of Allergy and Immunology (Prices range from $0.50 to $0.75 each. Bulk rates are available.)

**Allergy and Asthma, an Informational Brochure.** Ordering information: American Academy of Allergy and Immunology (Prices range from $0.50 to $0.75 each. Bulk rates are available.)

**Adverse Reactions to Foods.** Ordering information: American Academy of Allergy and Immunology (Prices range from $0.50 to $0.75 each. Bulk rates are available.)

**Dust 'n' Stuff.** This provides simple, easy-to-follow directions for ridding the house of house dust and otherwise allergy proofing the home. It is well illustrated and nontechnical. It is intended for the lay public. Ordering information: Asthma Foundation of Southern Arizona (single copies free)

**Weeds 'n' Things.** This is a simple guide to recognizing weeds, trees, and grasses that frequently cause allergic symptoms. The booklet also contains information on plants that are hypoallergenic and can be used in landscaping around the house. Ordering information: Asthma Foundation of Southern Arizona (single copies free)

**Allergy Plants.** This book describes allergenic plants, their characteristics, locations, and pollination times. Full color photographs help allergy sufferers recognize each kind of plant. Ordering information: American Academy of Allergy and Immunology ($12.00)

**Monograph on Insect Allergy.** This book provides information on insect allergies. Ordering information: American Academy of Allergy and Immunology ($14.00)

## ASTHMA MEDICATIONS

**What Every Patient Should Know About Asthma and Allergy Medication.** This is a flyer from a series called *Tips to Remember* that provides practical advice to patients. Ordering information: American Academy of Allergy and Immunology ($0.50 each. Bulk prices available.)

**Asthma and Allergy Medicines: What They Are and What They Do.** Ordering information: Asthma and Allergy Foundation of America ($1.25)

**Use of Steroids for Asthma and Allergy.** This is a flyer from a series called *Tips to Remember* that provides practical advice to patients. Ordering information: American Academy of Allergy and Immunology ($0.50 each. Bulk prices available.)

**Steroids.** Ordering information: Asthma and Allergy Foundation of America ($1.00)

**What Everyone Needs to Know About Theophylline.** Ordering information: Allergy and Asthma Network/Mothers of Asthmatics ($1.50 each)

**What Everyone Needs to Know About Corticosteroids.** Ordering information: Allergy and Asthma Network/Mothers of Asthmatics ($1.50 each)

**What Everyone Needs to Know About Bronchodilators.** Ordering information: Allergy and Asthma Network/Mothers of Asthmatics ($1.50 each)

**Theophylline Controversy.** Ordering information: Asthma and Allergy Foundation of America ($1.00)

**About Asthma/Allergy Medications.** This is a brochure intended for pharmacists to distribute with prescriptions. Short descriptions of medication categories are followed by questions to ask a pharmacist and helpful hints about taking and storing medications. Ordering information: American Academy of Allergy and Immunology

Asthma Information Sheets:

- Adrenergic Bronchodilators (Inhalation)
- Adrenergic Bronchodilators (Oral/Injection)
- Cromolyn (Inhalation)
- Cromolyn (Nasal)
- Xanthine Bronchodilators (Oral)

Written in an easy-to-understand language, each sheet covers key information for patients who take asthma drugs. Included are proper use of each medicine, what to do if you miss a dose, interactions with other drugs, side effects that do or do not require medical attention, how each drug works, and a list of the generic types in each class. Information is updated yearly by experts from key professional societies and academic institutions. Ordering information: U.S. Pharmacopoeia ($1.65 each copy, $9.90 for set)

## OTHER TOPICS

**Peak Performance.** This is a comprehensive peak flow reference. It is written for physicians, but anyone serious about peak flow monitoring will find it informative. Ordering information: Allergy and Asthma Network/Mothers of Asthmatics ($15.00)

**User's Guide to Peak Flow Monitoring.** This guide for children and adults teaches peak flow meter use. It is available in English and Spanish. Ordering information: Allergy and Asthma Network/ Mothers of Asthmatics ($5.00)

**Elderly and Asthma.** Ordering information: Asthma and Allergy Foundation of America ($1.00)

**Occupational Asthma.** Ordering information: Asthma and Allergy Foundation of America ($1.00)

**Peak Flow Meters.** Ordering information: Asthma and Allergy Foundation of America ($1.00)

**Pregnancy and Asthma.** Ordering information: Asthma and Allergy Foundation of America ($1.00)

**Psychological Aspects of Asthma.** Ordering information: Asthma and Allergy Foundation of America ($1.00)

**Traveling with Asthma and Allergy.** Ordering information: Asthma and Allergy Foundation of America ($1.00)

**Triggers and Asthma.** This is a flyer from a series called *Tips to Remember* that provides practical advice to patients. Ordering information: American Academy of Allergy and Immunology ($0.50 each. Bulk prices available.)

**Occupational Asthma.** This is a flyer from a series called *Tips to Remember* that provides practical advice to patients. Ordering information: American Academy of Allergy and Immunology ($0.50 each. Bulk prices available.)

**Asthma and Pregnancy.** This is a flyer from a series called *Tips to Remember* that provides practical advice to patients. Ordering information: American Academy of Allergy and Immunology ($0.50 each. Bulk prices available.)

**Asthma and Allergies in Seniors.** This is a flyer from a series called *Tips to Remember* that provides practical advice to patients. Ordering information: American Academy of Allergy and Immunology ($0.50 each. Bulk prices available.)

**Peak Flow Meter: A Thermometer for Asthma.** This is a flyer from a series called *Tips to Remember* that provides practical advice to patients. Ordering information: American Academy of Allergy and Immunology ($0.50 each. Bulk prices available.)

*Materials for Educating Health Professionals*

**Outpatient Management of the Child With Asthma.** (ALA No. 6034) slides/35-minute audio-cassette/workbook. This presents a systematic overview of actions, administration, and effects of the drugs presently available for the treatment of asthma. It is intended for physicians and medical students. Ordering information: Can be ordered or borrowed from local American Thoracic Society or American Lung Association chapters. ($65.00)

**Pharmacologic Therapy of Pediatric Asthma.** (ALA No. 6125) slides/35-minute audio-cassette/workbook. This describes the use of pharmacotherapy in the treatment of childhood asthma. It is intended for physicians and medical students. Ordering information: Can be ordered or borrowed from local American Thoracic Society or American Lung Association chapters. ($69.90)

**The Role of Allergy in Asthma.** (ALA No. 6074) 68 slides/34-minute cassette audiotape/workbook. Ordering information: Can be ordered or borrowed from local American Thoracic Society or American Lung Association chapters. ($65.00)

## Information Sources

**Allergy and Asthma Network/Mothers of Asthmatics**
3554 Chain Bridge Road
Suite 200
Fairfax, VA 22030-2709
(703) 385-4403
For phone orders only, call 1-800-878-4403

**American Academy of Allergy and Immunology**
611 East Wells Street
Milwaukee, WI 53202
(414) 272-6071

**American Academy of Family Physicians**
8880 Ward Parkway
Kansas City, MO 64114
(800) 944-0000

**American Academy of Pediatrics**
141 Northwest Point Boulevard
Box 927
Elk Grove Village, IL 60007
(708) 228-5005

**American Allergy Association**
P.O. Box 7273
Menlo Park, CA 94026
(415) 322-1663

**American College of Allergy and Immunology**
800 E. Northwest Highway, Suite 1080
Palatine, IL 60067-6516
(800) 842-7777
(708) 359-2800

**American College of Chest Physicians**
3300 Dundee Road
Northbrook, IL 60062
(708) 498-1400

**American Lung Association**
1740 Broadway
New York, NY 10019
(212) 315-8700

**American Thoracic Society**
1740 Broadway
New York, NY 10019
(212) 315-8700

**Asthma and Allergy Foundation of America**
1125 15th Street, NW
Suite 502
Washington, DC 20005
(202) 466-7643

**Asthma Foundation of Southern Arizona**
P.O. Box 42195
Tucson, AZ 85733
(602) 323-6046

**National Asthma Education and Prevention Program**
P.O. Box 30105
Bethesda, MD 20824-0105
(301) 251-1222

**National Center for Health Statistics**
Presidential Building
6525 Belcrest Road
Hyattsville, MD 20782
(301) 436-8500

**National Institute of Allergy and Infectious Diseases (NIAID)**
Building 31, Room 7A32
9000 Rockville Pike
Bethesda, MD 20892
(301) 496-4000

## National Jewish Center for Immunology and Respiratory Medicine
1400 Jackson Street
Denver, CO 80206
(303) 388 4461
800-222-5864 (Lung Line Newsletter)

## Open Airways for Schools
P.O. Box 1036
Evans City, PA 16033
800-292-5542 (credit card orders only)

## Pedipress, Inc.
125 Red Gate Lane
Amhurst, MA 01002
800-344-5864

## Scribner's Publishing
866 Third Avenue
New York, NY 10022
(212) 702-2000

## IOX Assessment Associates
11411 West Jefferson Boulevard
Culver City, CA 90230
(213) 822-3275

## University of Alabama Hospital
Marketing Department
619 S. 19th Street
Birmingham, AL 35233
(205) 934-5560

## U.S. Pharmacopoeia
12601 Twinbrook Parkway
Rockville, MD 20852-1790

Chapter 3

# Chronic Obstructive Pulmonary Disease (COPD)

*Chapter Contents*

Section 3. 1—Chronic Obstructive Pulmonary Disease .............. 160
Section 3. 2—Facts About Chronic Bronchitis ........................... 177
Section 3. 3—Facts About Chronic Cough ................................ 180
Section 3. 4—Facts About Emphysemia .................................... 182
Section 3. 5—Facts About ATT Deficiency-Related
          Emphysema ........................................................... 185
Section 3. 6—Around the Clock with COPD ............................. 188

Section 3.1

# Chronic Obstructive Pulmonary Disease (COPD)

Source: NIH Pub. No. 93-2020.

### What Is Chronic Obstructive Pulmonary Disease?

Chronic obstructive pulmonary disease (COPD), also called chronic obstructive lung disease, is a term that is used for two closely related diseases of the respiratory system: chronic bronchitis and emphysema. In many patients these diseases occur together, although there may be more symptoms of one than the other. Most patients with these diseases have a long history of heavy cigarette smoking.

COPD gets gradually worse over time. At first there may be only a mild shortness of breath and occasional coughing. Then a chronic cough develops with clear, colorless sputum. As the disease progresses, the cough becomes more frequent and more and more effort is needed to get air into and out of the lungs. In later stages of the disease, the heart may be affected. Eventually death occurs when the function of the lungs and heart is no longer adequate to deliver oxygen to the body's organs and tissues.

Cigarette smoking is the most important risk factor for COPD; it would probably be a minor health problem if people did not smoke. Other risk factors include age, heredity, exposure to air pollution at work and in the environment, and a history of childhood respiratory infections. Living in low socioeconomic conditions also seems to be a contributing factor.

More than 13.5 million Americans are thought to have COPD. It is the fifth leading cause of death in the United States. Between 1980 and 1990, the total death rate from COPD increased by 22 percent. In 1990, it was estimated that there were 84,000 deaths due to COPD, approximately 34 per 100,000 people. Although COPD is still much more common in men than women, the greatest increase in the COPD death rate between 1979 and 1989 occurred in females, particularly in black females (117.6 percent for black females vs. 93 percent for white

## Chronic Obstructive Pulmonary Disease

females). These increases reflect the increased number of women who smoke cigarettes.

COPD attacks people at the height of their productive years, disabling them with constant shortness of breath. It destroys their ability to earn a living, causes frequent use of the health care system, and disrupts the lives of the victims' family members for as long as 20 years before death occurs.

In 1990, COPD was the cause of approximately 16.2 million office visits to doctors and 1.9 million hospital days. The economic costs of this disease are enormous. In 1989, an estimated $7 billion was spent for care of persons with COPD and another $8 billion was lost to the economy by lost productivity due to morbidity and mortality from COPD.

### What Are Chronic Bronchitis and Emphysema?

Chronic bronchitis, one of the two major diseases of the lung grouped under COPD, is diagnosed when a patient has excessive airway mucus secretion leading to a persistent, productive cough. An individual is considered to have chronic bronchitis if cough and sputum are present on most days for a minimum of 3 months for at least 2 successive years or for 6 months during 1 year. In chronic bronchitis, there also may be narrowing of the large and small airways making it more difficult to move air in and out of the lungs. An estimated 12.1 million Americans have chronic bronchitis.

In emphysema there is permanent destruction of the alveoli, the tiny elastic air sacs of the lung, because of irreversible destruction of a protein in the lung called elastin that is important for maintaining the strength of the alveolar walls. The loss of elastin also causes collapse or narrowing of the smallest air passages called bronchioles, which in turn limits airflow out of the lung. The number of individuals with emphysema in the U.S. is estimated to be 2 million.

In the general population, emphysema usually develops in older individuals with a long smoking history. However, there is also a form of emphysema that runs in families. People with familial emphysema have a hereditary deficiency of a blood component, $alpha_1$-protease inhibitor, also called $alpha_1$-antitrypsin (AAT). The number of Americans with this genetic deficiency is quite small, probably no more than 70,000. It is estimated that 1 in 3,000 newborns have a genetic deficiency of AAT, and 1 to 3 percent of all cases of emphysema are due to AAT deficiency.

The destruction of elastin that occurs in emphysema is believed to result from an imbalance between two proteins in the lung—an enzyme called elastase which breaks down elastin, and AAT which inhibits elastase. In the normal individual, there is enough AAT to protect elastin so that abnormal elastin destruction does not occur. However, when there is a genetic deficiency of AAT, the activity of the elastase is not inhibited and elastin degradation occurs unchecked. If individuals with a severe genetic deficiency of $alpha_1$-protease inhibitor smoke, they usually have symptoms of COPD by the time they reach early middle age. Deficiency of $alpha_1$-protease inhibitor can be detected by blood tests available through hospital laboratories. People from families in which relatives have developed emphysema in their thirties and forties should be tested for AAT deficiency. If a deficiency is found, it is critical for these people not to smoke.

Some scientists believe that non-familial emphysema, usually called "smoker's emphysema" also results from an imbalance between elastin-degrading enzymes and their inhibitors. The elastase-AAT imbalance is thought to be a result of the effects of smoking, rather than inherited as in familial emphysema. Some evidence for this theory comes from studies on the effect of tobacco smoke on lung cells. These studies showed that tobacco smoke stimulates excess release of elastase from cells normally found in the lung. The inhaled smoke also stimulates more elastase-producing cells to migrate to the lung which in turn causes the release of even more elastase. To make matters worse, oxidants found in cigarette smoke inactivate a significant portion of the elastase inhibitors that are present, thereby decreasing the amount of active anti-elastase available for protecting the lung and further upsetting the elastase-anti-elastase balance.

Scientists believe that, in addition to smoking-related processes, there must be other factors that cause emphysema in the general population since only 15 to 20 percent of smokers develop emphysema. The nature and role of these other factors in smokers' emphysema are not yet clear.

## What Goes Wrong with the Lungs and Other Organs in Chronic Obstructive Pulmonary Disease?

The most important job that the lungs perform is to provide the body with oxygen and to remove carbon dioxide. This process is called gas exchange, and the normal anatomy of the lungs serves this pur-

## Chronic Obstructive Pulmonary Disease

pose well. The lungs contain 300 million alveoli whose ultra-thin walls form the gas exchange surface. Enmeshed in the wall of each of these air sacs is a network of tiny blood vessels, the capillaries, which bring blood to the gas exchange surface. When a person inhales, air flows from the nose and mouth through large and small airways into the alveoli. Oxygen from this air then passes through the thin walls of the inflated alveoli and is taken up by the red blood cells for delivery to the rest of the body. At the same time carbon dioxide leaves the blood and passes through the alveolar walls into the alveoli. During exhalation, the lung pushes the used air out of the alveoli and through the air passages until it escapes from the nose or mouth. When COPD develops, the walls of the small airways and alveoli lose their elasticity. The airway walls thicken, closing off some of the smaller air passages and narrowing larger ones. The passageways also become plugged with mucus. Air continues to get into alveoli when the lung expands during inhalation, but it is often unable to escape during exhalation because the air passages tend to collapse during exhalation, trapping the "stale" air in the lungs.

*Figure 13.1.* Gas exchange in the normal lung (top) and the emphysematous lung (bottom).

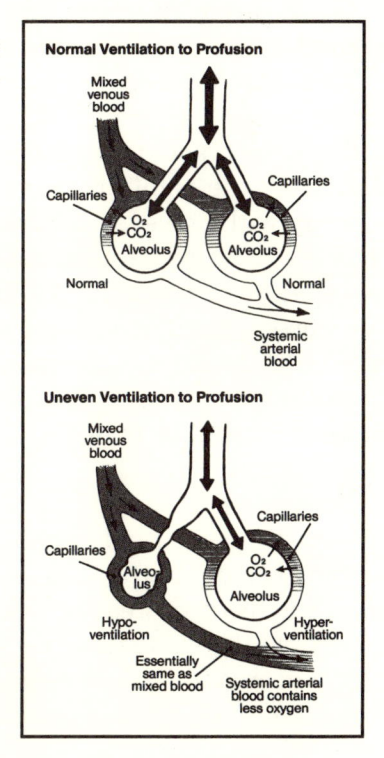

These abnormalities create two serious problems which affect gas exchange:

- Blood flow and air flow to the walls of the alveoli where gas exchange takes place are uneven or mismatched. In some alveoli there is adequate blood flow but little air, while in others there is a good supply of fresh air but not enough blood flow. When this occurs, fresh air cannot reach areas where there is good blood flow and oxygen cannot enter the bloodstream in normal quantities.

- Pushing the air through narrowed obstructed airways becomes harder and harder. This tires the respiratory muscles so that they are unable to get enough air to the alveoli. The critical step for removing carbon dioxide from the blood is adequate alveolar airflow. If airflow to the alveoli is insufficient, carbon dioxide builds up in the blood and blood oxygen diminishes. Inadequate supply of fresh air to the alveoli is called hypoventilation. Breathing oxygen can often correct the blood oxygen levels, but this does not help remove carbon dioxide. When carbon dioxide accumulation becomes a severe problem, mechanical breathing machines called respirators, or ventilators, must be used.

Pulmonary function studies of large groups of people show that lung function—the ability to move air into and out of the lungs—declines slowly with age even in healthy non-smokers. Because healthy non-smokers have excess lung capacity, this gradual loss of function does not lead to any symptoms. In smokers, however, lung function tends to worsen much more rapidly. If a smoker stops smoking before serious COPD develops, the rate at which lung function declines returns to almost normal. Unfortunately, because some lung damage cannot be reversed, pulmonary function is unlikely to return completely to normal.

COPD also makes the heart work much harder, especially the main chamber on the right side (right ventricle) which is responsible for pumping blood into the lungs. As COPD progresses, the amount of oxygen in the blood decreases which causes blood vessels in the lung to constrict. At the same time, many of the small blood vessels in the lungs have been damaged or destroyed as a result of the disease process. More and more work is required from the right ventricle to force

# Chronic Obstructive Pulmonary Disease

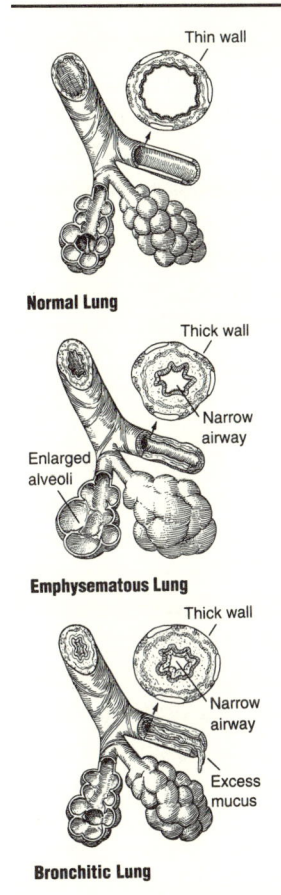

**Figure 13.2.** *Microscopic structure of terminal airways.*

blood through the remaining narrowed vessels. To perform this task, the right ventricle enlarges and thickens. When this occurs the normal rhythm of the heart may be disturbed by abnormal beats. This condition, in which the heart is enlarged because of lung problems, is called corpulmonale. Patients with corpulmonale tire easily and have chest pains and palpitations. If an additional strain is placed on the lungs and heart by a normally minor illness such as a cold, the heart may be unable to pump enough blood to meet the needs of other organs. This results in the inability of the liver and kidneys to carry out their normal functions which leads to swelling of the abdomen, legs, and ankles.

Another adjustment the body makes to inadequate blood oxygen is called secondary polycythemia, an increased production of oxygen-carrying red blood cells. The larger than normal number of red blood cells is helpful up to a point; however, a large overpopulation of red cells thickens the blood so much that it clogs small blood vessels causing a new set of problems. People who have poor supply of oxygen usually have a bluish tinge to their skin, lips, and nailbeds, a condition called cyanosis.

Too little oxygen and too much carbon dioxide in the blood also affect the nervous system, especially the brain, and can cause a variety of problems including headache, inability to sleep, impaired mental ability, and irritability.

## What Is the Course of Chronic Obstructive Pulmonary Disease?

Daily morning cough with clear sputum is the earliest symptom of COPD. During a cold or other acute respiratory tract infection, the coughing may be much more noticeable and the sputum often turns yellow or greenish. Periods of wheezing are likely to occur especially during or after colds or other respiratory tract infections. Shortness of breath on exertion develops later and progressively becomes more pronounced with severe episodes of breathlessness (dyspnea) occurring after even modest activity.

A typical course of COPD might proceed as follows. For a period of about 10 years after cigarette smoking begins, symptoms are usually not very noticeable. After this, the patient generally starts developing a chronic cough with the production of a small amount of sputum. It is unusual to develop shortness of breath during exertion below the age of 40, after which it becomes more common and may be well developed by the age of 50. However, although all COPD patients have these symptoms, not all cigarette smokers develop a notable cough and sputum production, or shortness of breath.

Most patients with COPD have some degree of reversible airways obstruction. It is therefore likely that, at first, treatment will lead to some improvement or stability in lung function. But as COPD progresses, almost all signs and symptoms except cough and sputum production tend to show a gradual worsening. This trend can show fluctuations, but over the course of 4 or 5 years, a slow deterioration becomes evident.

Repeated bouts of increased cough and sputum production disable most patients and recovery from coughing attacks may take a long time. Patients with severe lung damage sleep in a semi-sitting position because they are unable to breathe when they lie down. They often complain that they awaken during the night feeling "choked-up," and they need to sit up to cough.

Survival of patients with COPD is closely related to the level of their lung function when they are diagnosed and the rate at which they lose this function. Overall, the median survival is about 10 years for patients with COPD who have lost approximately two-thirds of their normally expected lung function at diagnosis.

## How Is Chronic Obstructive Pulmonary Disease Detected?

Researchers are still looking for accurate methods to predict a person's chances of developing airway obstruction. None of the current ways used to diagnose COPD detects the disease before irreversible lung damage occurs. While many measures of lung function have been developed, those most commonly used determine:

## Chronic Obstructive Pulmonary Disease

1. Air-containing volume of the lung (lung volume).

2. The ability to move air into and out of the lung.

3. The rate at which gases diffuse between the lung and blood.

4. Blood levels of oxygen and carbon dioxide.

**Lung volumes** are measured by breathing into and out of a device called a spirometer. Some types of spirometers are very simple mechanical devices which record volume changes as air is added to or removed from them. Other kinds are more sophisticated and use various types of electronic equipment to determine and record the volume of air moved into and out of the lungs. The three volume measures most relevant to COPD are forced vital capacity (FVC), residual volume (RV), and total lung capacity (TLC). The *forced vital capacity* is the maximum volume of air which can be forcibly expelled after inhaling as deeply as possible. Not all of the air in the lungs is removed when measuring the vital capacity. The amount remaining is called the *residual volume*. The *total lung capacity* is the combination of the forced vital capacity and residual volume. While most of the measured lung volumes or capacities change to some degree with COPD, residual volume usually increases quite markedly. This increase is the result of the weakened airways collapsing before all the normally expired air can leave the lungs. The increased residual volume makes breathing even more difficult and labored.

Because COPD results in narrowed air passages, a measure of the rate at which air can be expelled from the lungs can also be used to determine how severe the narrowing has become. In this test, the *forced vital capacity maneuver*, the patient is asked to inhale as deeply as possible, and on signal, exhale as completely and as rapidly as possible. The volume of air exhaled within 1 second is then measured. This value is referred to as the *forced expiratory volume in 1 second (FEV$_1$)*. When FEV$_1$ is used as an indicator of lung function, the average rate of decline in patients with chronic obstructive lung disease is observed to be two to three times the normal rate of 20-30 milliliters per year. This volume may also be expressed in terms of the percent of the vital capacity which can be expelled in 1 second. As COPD progresses, less air can be expelled in 1 second. A greater than expected annual fall in FEV$_1$ is the most sensitive test for COPD and a fairly good predictor of disability and early death.

Another measure of lung function is called *diffusing capacity*. For this, a more complicated test determines the amount of gas which can move in a given period of time from the alveolar side of the lung into the blood. A number of conditions can cause the diffusing capacity to decrease. However, in COPD the decrease is the result of the destruction of alveolar walls which leads to a significant decrease in surface area for diffusion of oxygen into the blood.

Because the primary function of the lung is to remove carbon dioxide from the blood and add oxygen, another indicator of pulmonary function is the blood levels of oxygen and carbon dioxide. As chronic obstructive pulmonary disease progresses, the amount of oxygen in the blood decreases and carbon dioxide increases.

In most cases, it is necessary to compare the results of several different tests in order to make the correct diagnosis, and to repeat some tests at intervals to determine the rate of disease progression or improvement. Measurement of $FEV_1$ and $FEV_1/FVC$ ratio should be a routine part of the physical examination of every COPD patient. It is hoped that current research will result in more accurate and earlier measures for detecting lung destruction and diminished function.

## How Is Chronic Obstructive Pulmonary Disease Treated?

*Monitored Respiratory Care Program*

Although there is no cure for COPD, the disease can be prevented in many cases. And, in almost all cases the disabling symptoms can be reduced. Because cigarette smoking is the most important cause of COPD, not smoking almost always prevents COPD from developing and quitting smoking slows the disease process.

If the patient and medical team develop and adhere to a program of complete respiratory care, disability can be minimized, acute episodes prevented, hospitalizations reduced, and some early deaths avoided. On the other hand, none of the therapies has been shown to slow the progression of the disease, and only oxygen therapy has been shown to increase the survival rate.

*Home Oxygen Therapy*

Home oxygen therapy can improve survival in patients with advanced COPD who have hypoxemia, low blood oxygen levels. This

## Chronic Obstructive Pulmonary Disease

treatment can improve a patient's exercise tolerance and ability to perform on psychological tests which reflect different aspects of brain function and muscle coordination. Increasing the concentration of oxygen in blood also improves the function of the heart and prevents the development of corpulmonale. Oxygen can also lessen sleeplessness, irritability, headaches, and the over-production of red blood cells. Continuous oxygen therapy is recommended for patients with low oxygen levels at rest, during exercise, or while sleeping. Many oxygen sources are available for home use; these include tanks of compressed gaseous oxygen or liquid oxygen and devices that concentrate oxygen from room air. However, oxygen is expensive with the cost per patient running into several hundred dollars per month, depending on the type of system and on the locale.

*Medications*

Medications frequently prescribed for COPD patients include:

- Bronchodilators help open narrowed airways. There are three main categories: sympathomimetics (isoproterenol, metaproterenol, terbutaline, albuterol) which can be inhaled, injected, or taken by mouth; parasympathomimetics (atropine, ipratropium bromide); and methylxanthines (theophylline and its derivatives) which can be given intravenously, orally or rectally.

- Corticosteroids or steroids (beclomethasone, dexamethasone, triamcinolone, flunisolide) lessen inflammation of the airway walls. They are sometimes used if airway obstruction cannot be kept under control with bronchodilators, and lung function is shown to improve on this therapy. Inhaled steroids given regularly may be of benefit in some patients and have few side effects.

- Antibiotics (tetracycline, ampicillin, erythromycin, and trimethoprim-sulfamethoxazole combinations) fight infection. They are frequently given at the first sign of a respiratory infection such as increased sputum production with a change in color of sputum from clear to yellow or green.

- Expectorants help loosen and expel mucus secretions from the airways.

- Diuretics help the body excrete excess fluid. They are given as therapy to avoid excess water retention associated with right-heart failure. Patients taking diuretics are monitored carefully because dehydration must be avoided. These drugs also may cause potassium imbalances which can lead to abnormal heart rhythms.

- Digitalis (usually in the form of digoxin) strengthens the force of the heartbeat. It is used very cautiously in patients who have COPD, especially if their blood oxygen tensions are low, because they are vulnerable to abnormal heart rhythms when taking this drug.

- Other drugs sometimes taken by patients with COPD are tranquilizers, pain killers (meperidine, morphine, propoxyphene, etc.), cough suppressants (codeine, etc.), and sleeping pills (barbiturates, etc.). All these drugs depress breathing to some extent; they are avoided whenever possible and used only with great caution.

- A number of combination drugs containing various assortments of sympathomimetics, methylxanthines, expectorants, and sedatives are marketed and widely advertised. These drugs are undesirable for COPD patients for several reasons. It is difficult to adjust the dose of methylxanthines without getting interfering side effects from the other ingredients. The sympathomimetic drug used in these preparations is ephedrine, a drug with many side effects and less bronchodilating effect than other drugs now available. The combination drugs often contain sedatives to combat the unpleasant side effects of ephedrine. They also contain expectorants which have not been proven to be effective for all patients and may have some side effects.

## Chronic Obstructive Pulmonary Disease

### Bullectomy

The surgical removal of large air spaces called bullae that are filled with stagnant air, may be beneficial in selected patients. Recently, use of lasers to remove bullae has been suggested.

### Lung Transplantation

This method has been successfully employed in some patients with end-stage COPD. In the hands of an experienced team, the one-year survival in patients with transplanted lungs is over 70 percent.

### Pulmonary Rehabilitation Programs

These programs, along with medical treatment, are useful for certain patients with COPD. The goals are to improve overall physical endurance and generally help to overcome the conditions which cause dyspnea and limit capacity for physical exercise and activities of daily living. General exercise training increases performance, maximum oxygen consumption, and overall sense of well-being. Administration of oxygen and nutritional supplements when necessary can improve respiratory muscle strength. Intermittent mechanical ventilatory support relieves dyspnea and rests respiratory muscles in selected patients. Continuous positive airway pressure (CPAP) is used as an adjunct to weaning from mechanical ventilation to minimize dyspnea during exercise. Relaxation techniques may also reduce the perception of ventilatory effort and dyspnea. Breathing exercises and breathing techniques, such as pursed lips breathing and relaxation, improve functional status.

### Keeping Air Passages Reasonably Clear

Keeping air passages reasonably clear of secretions is difficult for patients with advanced COPD. Some commonly used methods for mobilizing and removing secretions are the following:

- Postural bronchial drainage helps to remove secretions from the airways. The patient lies in prescribed positions that allow gravity to drain different parts of the lung. This is usually done after inhaling an aerosol. In the basic position, the patient lies on a bed with his chest and head over the side and his forearms resting on the floor.

- Chest percussion or lightly clapping the chest and back, may help dislodge tenacious or copious secretions.

- Controlled coughing techniques are taught to help the patient bring up secretions.

- Bland aerosols, often made from solutions of salt or bicarbonate of soda, are inhaled. These aerosols thin and loosen secretions. Treatments usually last 10 to 15 minutes and are taken three or four times a day. Bronchodilators are sometimes added to the aerosols.

## How Can Patients with Chronic Obstructive Pulmonary Disease Cope Best with Their Illness?

In most instances of COPD, some irreversible damage has already occurred by the time the doctor diagnoses the disease. At this point, the patient and the family should learn as much as possible about the disease and how to live with it. The goals, limitations, and techniques of treatment must be understood by the patient so that symptoms can be kept under control, and daily living can proceed as normally as possible. The doctor and other health care providers are good sources of information about COPD education programs. Patients and family members can usually take part in educational programs offered at a hospital or by a local branch of the American Lung Association.

Patients with COPD can help themselves in many ways. They can:

- Stop smoking. Many programs are available to help smokers quit smoking and to stay off tobacco. Some programs are based on behavior modification techniques; others combine these methods with nicotine gum or nicotine patches as aids to help smokers gradually overcome their dependence on nicotine.

- Avoid work-related exposures to dusts and fumes.

## Chronic Obstructive Pulmonary Disease

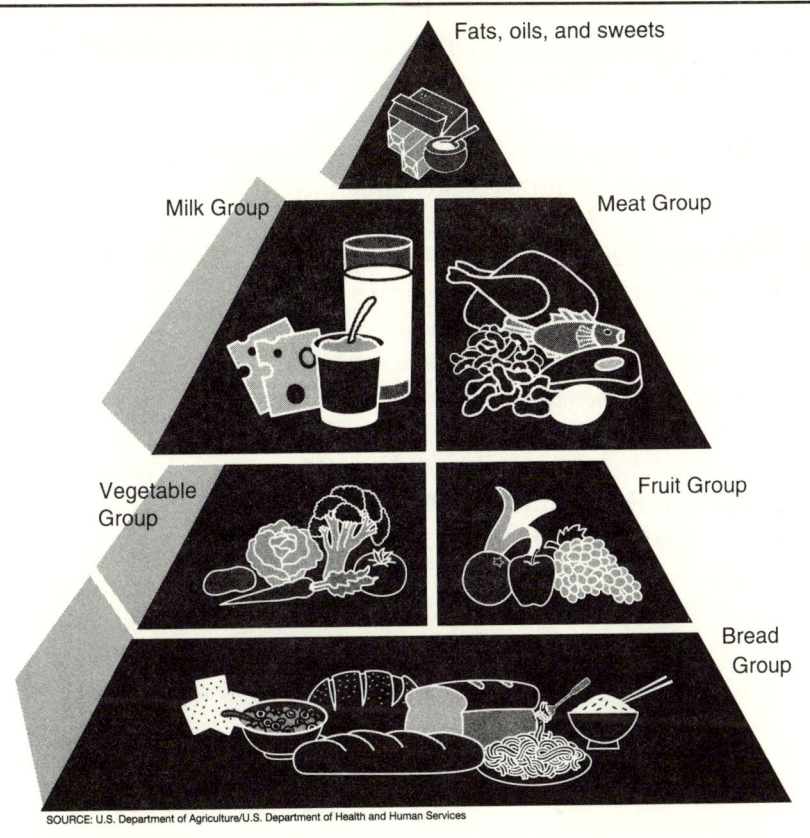

**Figure 3.3.** *A high protein diet is recommended for COPD patients.*

- Avoid air pollution, including cigarette smoke, and curtail physical activities during air pollution alerts.

- Refrain from intimate contact with people who have respiratory infections such as colds or the flu and get a one-time pneumonia vaccination (polyvalent pneumococcal vaccination) and yearly influenza shots.

- Avoid excessive heat, cold, and very high altitudes. (Note: Commercial aircraft cruise at high altitudes and maintain a cabin pressure equal to that of an elevation of 5,000 to 10,000 feet. This can result in hypoxemia for some COPD patients. However, with supplemental oxygen, most COPD patients can travel on commercial airlines.)

- Drink a lot of fluids. This is a good way to keep sputum loose so that it can be brought up by coughing.

- Maintain good nutrition. Usually a high protein diet, taken as many small feedings, is recommended.

- Consider "allergy shots." COPD patients often also have allergies or asthma which complicate COPD.

Of all the avoidable risk factors for COPD, smoking is by far the most significant. Cessation of smoking is the best way to decrease one's risk of developing COPD.

## What Types of Research on Chronic Obstructive Pulmonary Disease Is the National Heart, Lung, and Blood Institute Supporting?

The National Heart, Lung, and Blood Institute (NHLBI) is supporting a number of research programs on COPD with the following objectives:

1. To understand its underlying causes.

2. To develop methods of early detection.

3. To improve treatment.

4. To help patient's and their families better manage the disease.

A study completed several years ago examined the use of oxygen therapy for people who, because of COPD, cannot get enough oxygen into their blood by breathing air. This study has determined that continuous oxygen therapy is more beneficial in extending life than giving oxygen only for 12 hours at night.

Another clinical study compared inhalation therapy using a machine which administers medication to the lungs by intermittent positive pressure breathing (IPPB) with one that delivers the medicine by relying on the patient's own breathing. Although home use of IPPB machines is widespread, previous studies had not been able to show conclusively whether they were effective. In this study, 985 ambula-

## Chronic Obstructive Pulmonary Disease

tory patients with COPD were randomly assigned to a treatment group which received a bronchodilator aerosol solution by IPPB, or to a control group which received the medication via a compressor nebulizer. The only difference between the two groups was the positive pressure applied by the IPPB. There was no statistically significant difference between the two treatment groups in numbers of deaths, frequency and length of hospitalization, change in lung function tests, or in measurements of quality of life. This study suggests that the use of IPPB devices may be unnecessary.

An intervention trial called the Lung Health Study, which began in 1983, has enrolled approximately 6,000 smokers in a study to determine whether an intervention program incorporating smoking cessation and use of inhaled bronchodilators (to keep air passages open) in men and women at high risk of developing COPD can slow the decline in pulmonary function compared to a group receiving usual care. When this study is completed, it should help to determine the extent to which identification and treatment of asymptomatic subjects with early signs of obstructive lung disease would be useful as a preventive health measure. In addition, the study will test some of the current theories about behavior and smoking cessation. Early results indicate that cigarette smoking may be more harmful to women than to men. Furthermore. smoking cessation results in greater weight gain in women than in men, and to avoid weight gain women are less likely to quit smoking and more likely to revert to their smoking habit.

Because familial emphysema results from a deficiency of AAT in affected individuals, efforts to minimize the risk of emphysema have been directed at increasing the circulating AAT levels either by promoting or increasing the production of AAT within the individual, or augmenting it from the outside. One strategy for improving the production of AAT is by pharmacological means (e.g., by administration of drugs such as danazol or estrogen/progesterone combinations), but this has not been found to be effective. Genetic engineering to correct the defective gene or introduce the functional gene in the deficient individuals is being attempted by several NHLBI-supported investigators. The normal gene for AAT as well as the mutant genes causing AAT deficiency have been characterized and cloned, and animal models carrying the mutant gene have been developed. The resulting animals displayed many of the physical and histologic changes seen in human neonatal AAT deficiency. These studies should provide the groundwork for future development of gene replacement therapy for AAT deficiency.

In the meantime, attention is being focused on AAT augmentation therapy for familial emphysema. Studies have shown that intravenous infusion of AAT fractionated from blood is safe and biochemically effective, that is, the needed blood levels of AAT can be maintained by the continued administration of AAT at appropriate intervals.

Because of the practical and fiscal limitations to mounting a clinical trial for establishing the clinical efficacy of AAT augmentation therapy for emphysema, the NHLBI sponsored a national registry of patients with AAT deficiency to assess the natural history of severe AAT deficiency and to examine whether the disease course is altered by the augmentation therapy. This program is enrolling, at various medical centers both in the U.S. and Europe, at least 1,000 adult patients with AAT deficiency satisfying certain other eligibility criteria. The patients will be followed for 3 to 5 years (chest x-rays, lung function, blood and urine analysis, etc.) at one of 37 participating clinical centers. The evaluation of the data and the release of the conclusions are expected by early 1995.

Methods to treat emphysema before it becomes disabling remain an important research objective of programs supported by NHLBI. Since it is believed that either excess protease (elastase), or too little useful anti-protease, can lead to development of the disease, scientists have also been attempting to use other approaches to develop animal models which will mimic the human condition of inherited alpha-1-protease inhibitor deficiency and using such models to test if natural or synthetic anti-proteases can be used safely to prevent development of emphysema-like lesions in these animals. If found safe and effective in animals, these agents can be tried in humans.

*For More Information*

Additional information on COPD can be obtained from:

Office of the Director
Division of Lung Diseases
National Heart, Lung, and Blood Institute
National Institute of Health
9000 Rockville Pike
Westwood Building, Room 6A16
Bethesda, MD 20892
(301) 594-7430

## Section 3.2

# Facts About Chronic Bronchitis

Source: American Lung Association Pub. No. 0139. Used by permission.

## What Is Bronchitis?

Chronic bronchitis is an inflammation of the lining of the bronchial tubes.

These tubes, the bronchi, connect the windpipe with the lungs. When the bronchi are inflamed and/or infected, less air is able to flow to and from the lungs and a heavy mucus or phlegm is coughed up. This is bronchitis.

Many people suffer a brief attack of acute bronchitis with cough and mucus production when they have severe colds. Acute bronchitis is usually not associated with fever.

Chronic bronchitis is defined by the presence of a mucus-producing cough most days of the month, three months of a year for two successive years without other underlying disease to explain the cough. It may precede or accompany pulmonary emphysema.

## What Causes Chronic Bronchitis?

Cigarette smoking is by far the most common cause of chronic bronchitis. The bronchial tubes of people with chronic bronchitis may also have been irritated initially by bacterial or viral infections. Air pollution and industrial dusts are also causes.

Once the bronchial tubes have been irritated over a long period of time, excessive mucus is produced constantly, the lining of the bronchial tubes becomes thickened, an irritating cough develops, air flow may be hampered, and the lungs are endangered. The bronchial tubes then make an ideal breeding place for infections.

## Who Gets Chronic Bronchitis?

Chronic bronchitis is estimated to affect 5 percent of the population of the United States. Cough and mucus production are more common among men than women, which is also true of cigarette smoking. Chronic bronchitis symptoms are also more common among people over 40 than younger individuals.

No matter what their occupation or lifestyle, people who smoke cigarettes are those most likely to develop chronic bronchitis. But workers with certain jobs, especially those involving high concentrations of dust and irritating fumes, are also at high risk of developing this disease. Higher rates of chronic bronchitis are found among coal miners, grain handlers, metal molders, and other workers exposed to dust. Chronic bronchitis symptoms worsen when atmospheric concentrations of sulfur dioxide and other air pollutants increase. These symptoms are intensified when individuals also smoke.

## How Serious Is Chronic Bronchitis?

In 1990, about 12.6 million people suffered from chronic bronchitis. In 1989, bronchitis (not specified as acute, meaning short-term, or chronic, meaning long-term) ranked ninth among all causes of physician visits and was responsible for 11,160,000—or 1.6 percent of all visits to a doctor.

In 1989, 79,500 deaths were certified as due to chronic obstructive pulmonary disease (COPD) and related conditions, ranking as the fifth leading cause of death in the U.S. (The term "pulmonary" refers to the lungs.)

**Chronic obstructive pulmonary (lung) disease (COPD).** The term generally applies to chronic bronchitis and/or emphysema. COPD has increased by a dramatic 86 percent between 1970 and 1990.

Today, chronic bronchitis and emphysema combined constitute the most common chronic lung disease, affecting 14.6 million people in the U.S. The number of lives claimed by chronic lung disease has increased sharply, too. In 1979, it accounted for about 50,000 deaths. In 1982, the number rose to 59,000, and by 1989, the number of deaths reached 79,500.

Chronic bronchitis is often neglected by individuals until it is in an advanced state, because people mistakenly believe that the disease is not life-threatening. By the time a patient goes to his or her doctor the lungs have frequently been seriously injured. Then the patient may be in danger of developing serious respiratory problems or heart failure.

## Chronic Obstructive Pulmonary Disease

### How Chronic Bronchitis Attacks

Chronic bronchitis doesn't strike suddenly. After a winter cold seems cured, an individual may continue to cough and produce large amounts of mucus for several weeks. Since people who get chronic bronchitis are often smokers, the cough is usually dismissed as only "smoker's cough." As time goes on, colds become more damaging. Coughing and bringing up phlegm last longer after each cold.

Without realizing it, one begins to take this coughing and mucus production as a matter of course. Soon they are present all the time—before colds, during colds, after colds, all year round. Generally, the cough is worse in the morning and in damp, cold weather. An ounce or more of yellow mucus may be coughed up each day.

### Treatment For Chronic Bronchitis

The treatment of chronic bronchitis is primarily aimed at reducing irritation in the bronchial tubes. The discovery of antibiotic drugs has been helpful in treating acute infection associated with chronic bronchitis. However most people with chronic bronchitis do not need to take antibiotics continually.

Bronchodilator drugs may be prescribed to help relax and open up air passages in the lungs, if there is a tendency for these to close up. These drugs may be inhaled as aerosol sprays or taken as pills.

To effectively control chronic bronchitis, it is necessary to eliminate sources of irritation and infection in the nose, throat, mouth, sinuses, and bronchial tubes. This means an individual must avoid polluted air and dusty working conditions and give up smoking. Your local American Lung Association can suggest methods to help you quit smoking.

If the person with chronic bronchitis is exposed to dust and fumes at work, the doctor may suggest changing the work environment. All persons with chronic bronchitis must develop and follow a plan for a healthy lifestyle. Improving one's general health also increases the body's resistance to infections.

### *What Should You Do If You Have Chronic Bronchitis?*

A good health plan for any person with chronic bronchitis should include these rules:

*Respiratory Diseases and Disorders Sourcebook*

1. See your doctor or follow your doctor's instructions at the beginning of any cold or respiratory infection.

2. Don't smoke! Contact your local American Lung Association (check the white pages of the phone book) for information on how to quit smoking.

3. Follow a nutritious, well-balanced diet, and maintain your ideal body weight. Get regular exercise daily, without tiring yourself too much.

5. Ask your doctor about getting vaccinated against influenza and pneumococcal pneumonia.

6. Avoid exposure to colds and influenza at home or in public, and avoid respiratory irritants such as secondhand smoke, dust, and other air pollutants.

## Section 3.3

# Facts About Chronic Cough

Source: American Lung Association Pub. No. 0151. Used by permission.

### When a Cough Is Chronic

Has your cough been hanging around for a month or more? Then you have a chronic cough. It doesn't matter that you cough only in the morning when you get up, or only at night when you lie down. If you've been coughing for more than a month, your cough is chronic.

Maybe you cough only during winter and feel fine the rest of the year. That cough is a chronic

### What About Short-Term Coughs?

Just about everybody coughs from time to time. The common cold, for instance, is often followed by a cough that can last as long as

## Chronic Obstructive Pulmonary Disease

two or three weeks. But if your cough following a cold hangs on longer than usual, it may be developing into a chronic cough.

If there is shortness of breath with a cough, or any pain, or blood in the stuff you cough up, you should see your doctor immediately, even though your cough may not have lasted more than a few days.

Do you smoke a pack or more of cigarettes a day? If you do, you're considered a heavy smoker. Heavy cigarette smoking can cause a chronic cough.

But don't dismiss a cough that hangs on as "just a cigarette cough." That cigarette cough of yours is serious in itself. It means that your excessive smoking has already damaged your breathing passages. In fact, the smoker who coughs is the person most likely to get lung cancer. And more likely to get emphysema.

You may be so used to your cigarette cough that you can't tell when something new has been added. Are you coughing more than you used to? For longer at a time? Or has your cough changed its character? Maybe you're coughing up streaks of blood or more phlegm (mucus). Any of these happenings may be a sign that something is wrong.

### Chronic Cough Is a Symptom

A chronic cough is not a disease in itself. It is a sign of something g wrong with the breathing system. That's why it isn't smart to take cough medicine for more than a week or two unless your doctor tells you to. Medicine may help with the cough, but meanwhile the underlying illness can be getting steadily worse.

The most likely causes of chronic cough are: lung cancer, bronchitis (inflammation in the lung tubes), bronchiectasis (in which pus pockets form along the tubes), tuberculosis and other lung diseases.

The instant you realize you have a chronic cough, go to your doctor. The doctor can make a number of tests to find out if a lung disease is causing your cough. Then he can start treatment early in the game. That is when most lung diseases can be dealt with successfully.

If you're coughing too much, find out why. It may be something minor or it may be serious. Until you know for sure, it's nothing to fool around with or neglect.

Be sure—or you may be sorry.

Section 3.4

## Facts About Emphysema

Source: American Lung Association Pub. No. 0301. Used by permission.

### What Is Emphysema?

Emphysema is a condition in which there is over-inflation of structures in the lungs known as alveoli or air sacs. This over-inflation results from a breakdown of the walls of the alveoli which causes a decrease in respiratory function (the way the lungs work) and often breathlessness. Early symptoms of emphysema include shortness of breath and cough.

### How Serious Is Emphysema?

- Emphysema is a widespread disease of the lungs. In 1987, 2.0 million people in the US. had emphysema.

- It is estimated that 70,000 to 100,000 Americans living today were born with a deficiency of a protein known as alpha$_1$-antitrypsin (AAT) which can lead to an inherited form of emphysema.

- Emphysema ranks ninth among chronic conditions that contribute to lack of activity: over 42 percent of individuals with emphysema report that their daily activities have been limited by the disease.

- Many of the people with emphysema are older men but the condition is increasing among women. Males with emphysema outnumber females by 64 percent.

### Causes of Emphysema

It is known from scientific research that the normal lung has a remarkable balance between two classes of chemicals with opposing

## Chronic Obstructive Pulmonary Disease

action. The lung also has a system of elastic fibers. The fibers allow the lungs to expand and contract. When the chemical balance is altered, the lungs lose the ability to protect themselves against the destruction of these elastic fibers. This is what happens in emphysema.

There are a number of reasons this chemical imbalance occurs. Smoking is responsible for 82 percent of chronic lung disease including emphysema. Exposure to air pollution is one suspected cause. Irritating fumes and dusts on the job also are thought to be a factor.

A small number of people with emphysema have a rare inherited form of the disease called alpha$_1$-antitrypsin (AAT) deficiency-related emphysema or early onset emphysema. This form of disease is caused by an inherited lack of a protective protein called alpha$_1$-antitrypsin (AAT).

### How Does Emphysema Develop?

Emphysema begins with the destruction of air sacs (alveoli) in the lungs where oxygen from the air is exchanged for carbon dioxide in the blood. The walls of the air sacs are thin and fragile. Damage to the air sacs is irreversible and results in permanent holes in the tissues of the lower lungs. As air sacs are destroyed, the lungs are able to transfer less and less oxygen to the bloodstream causing shortness of breath. The lungs also lose their elasticity. The patient experiences great difficulty exhaling.

Emphysema doesn't develop suddenly—it comes on very gradually. Years of exposure to the irritation of cigarette smoke usually precede the development of emphysema.

A person may initially visit the doctor because he or she has begun to feel short of breath during activity or exercise. As the disease progresses a brief walk can be enough to bring on difficulty in breathing. Some people may have had chronic bronchitis before developing emphysema.

### Treatment for Emphysema

Doctors can help persons with emphysema live more comfortably with their disease. The goal of treatment is to provide relief of symptoms and prevent progression of the disease with a minimum of side effects. The doctor's advice and treatment may include:

- **Quitting smoking**—the single most important factor for maintaining healthy lungs.

- **Bronchodilator drugs**— (prescription drugs that relax and open up air passages in the lungs) may be prescribed to treat emphysema if there is a tendency toward airway constriction or tightening. These drugs may be inhaled as aerosol sprays or taken orally.

- **Antibiotics**—if you have a bacterial infection such as pneumococcal pneumonia.

- **Exercise**—Including breathing exercises to strengthen the muscles used in breathing as part of a pulmonary rehabilitation program to condition the rest of the body.

- **Treatment with Alpha$_1$-Proteinase Inhibitor (A1PI)**—only if a person has MT deficiency—related emphysema. A1PI Is not recommended for those who develop emphysema as a result of cigarette smoking or other environmental factors.

- **Lung transplantation**—Some recent reports have been encouraging. Experience at this point in time is limited.

Continuing research is being done to find answers to many questions about emphysema, especially about the best ways to prevent the disease.

Researchers know that quitting smoking can prevent the occurrence and decrease the progression of emphysema. Other environmental controls can also help prevent the disease.

If an individual has emphysema, the doctor will work hard to prevent the disease from getting worse by keeping the patient healthy and clear of any infection. The patient can participate in this prevention effort by following these general health guidelines:

1. Emphysema is a serious disease. It damages your lungs, and it can damage your heart. See your doctor at the first sign of symptoms.

2. DON'T SMOKE. A majority of those who get emphysema are smokers. Continued smoking makes emphysema worse,

especially for those who have AAT deficiency, the inherited form of emphysema.

3. Maintain overall good health habits, which include proper nutrition, adequate sleep, and regular exercise to build up your stamina and resistance to infections.

4. Reduce your exposure to air pollution, which may aggravate symptoms of emphysema. Refer to radio or television weather reports or your local newspaper for information about air quality. On days when the ozone (smog) level is unhealthy, restrict your activity to early morning or evening. When pollution levels are dangerous, remain indoors and stay as comfortable as possible.

5. Consult your doctor at the start of any cold or respiratory infection because infection can make your emphysema symptoms worse. Ask about getting vaccinated against influenza and pneumococcal pneumonia.

6. To receive more information about emphysema, contact your local American Lung Association office (check the white pages of your phone book).

Section 3.5

# Facts About AAT Deficiency-Related Emphysema

Source: American Lung Association Pun. No. 0426. Used by permission.

### What Is AAT Deficiency-Related Emphysema?

AAT deficiency-related emphysema is a relatively uncommon form of lung disease. Its technical name is "alpha$_1$-antitrypsin (AAT) deficiency-related emphysema." It is also sometimes called "early onset emphysema" or "familial emphysema" because it can appear when a person is as young as 30 or 40 years old and runs in families.

AAT deficiency-related emphysema is caused by an inherited lack of a protective protein called alpha$_1$-antitrypsin (AAT). In normal and healthy individuals, AAT protects the lungs from a natural enzyme (called neutrophil elastase) that helps fight bacteria and clean up dead lung tissue. However, this enzyme can also eventually damage lung tissue if not neutralized by AAT.

If the damage to lung tissue continues, emphysema develops and progresses. It can be fatal.

## Who Is Most At Risk?

It is estimated that there are 20,000 to 100,000 Americans today who were born with AAT deficiency. Of this group, an estimated 75-80 percent develop AAT deficiency-related emphysema. If AAT-deficient individuals also smoke, their risk of developing emphysema is much greater than the average person's.

## How Does Emphysema Develop?

While there are different causes of emphysema (such as smoking, the major cause, and AAT deficiency), the symptoms and the progression of the disease are similar.

Emphysema begins with the destruction of alveoli—small sac-like structures (resembling bunches of grapes) in the lungs where oxygen from the air is exchanged for carbon dioxide in the blood. The walls of the alveoli are thin and fragile, and are easily damaged. The damage is irreversible and results in permanent "holes" in the tissues of the lower lungs. As alveoli are destroyed, the lungs are able to transfer less and less oxygen to the bloodstream, causing shortness of breath. The lungs also lose their elasticity, so the patient experiences great difficulty exhaling.

## Protein-Enzyme Imbalance

One cause of damage to the alveoli is an enzyme in the body called neutrophil elastase. This enzyme, which is normally helpful, will attack the walls of alveoli if the lung is not protected by the protein AAT. People with AAT deficiency-related emphysema do not lack the protein, rather they do not have enough of that protein.

## What Are the Symptoms?

The first signs of AAT deficiency-related emphysema often appear between ages 30 and 40. The earliest symptom is usually shortness of breath during exertion; other symptoms are decreased exercise capacity and wheezing. Both the early age at which the disease is present and the fact that the disease most frequently appears in the lower rather than the upper lung regions helps distinguish AAT deficiency-related emphysema from other types of this disease.

## How Is AAT Deficiency Diagnosed?

A blood test can determine whether a person has low levels of the protective protein AAT. Approximately 1 in 2,500 people has this inherited deficiency; most of the people who have the deficiency are of Northern European descent. Testing is indicated by a family history of the disease, or when signs of emphysema appear at an early age or in the absence of smoking.

## Importance of Early Detection

It is very important to detect AAT deficiency as early as possible since early treatment is thought likely to slow or halt progression of the emphysema.

Individuals who know they have the deficiency should never smoke. Evidence shows that smoking significantly increases the risk and severity of emphysema in AAT-deficient individuals and may decrease their life span by as much as ten years.

## How Is AAT Deficiency-Related Emphysema Treated?

In December 1987, the US. Food and Drug Administration approved the first drug for treating AAT deficiency-related emphysema. The "generic" name of this drug is $Alpha_1$-Proteinase Inhibitor, or A1PI. It is an "orphan drug," meaning that it was developed under special federal guidelines that encourage research in the treatment of rare diseases.

A1PI raises levels of AAT in the body and provides the lung with a protective shield against neutrophil elastase, the destructive enzyme. The drug is derived from screened, viral-tested and heat-treated human plasma and must be taken throughout a patient's life.

A1PI is intended only for AAT deficient patients who have begun to show symptoms of emphysema. It is not recommended for those who develop emphysema as a result of cigarette smoking or other environmental factors.

Please consult your physician for additional information about testing, diagnosis and treatment. Your local American Lung Association also has additional materials and programs on emphysema. Contact them today.

Section 3.6

# Around the Clock with C.O.P.D. (Chronic Obstructive Pulmonary Disease): Helpful Hints for Respiratory Patients

Source: American Lung Association Pub No, 1230. 1992. Used by permission. Originally developed by the members of the Respiratory Club at Gaylord Hospital, Wallingford, Connecticut

*Pacing*

Pacing ourselves is one of the most important things we all have to learn. A prime consideration in regulating the tempo of daily living should be the awareness that your limits will fluctuate from day to day, or even hour to hour.

There will be times when you will wake up and know almost immediately it is a day for just loafing. Or, you may awake feeling super and up to a special task you have been saving for a good day. The important thing is to learn to trust your own feelings and go with them.

Don't take on more than you can handle comfortably and when you feel tired, QUIT. Remember, energy is like money in the bank—to be spent wisely. Repeated overspending puts one in debt physically as well as financially.

## Chronic Obstructive Pulmonary Disease

There will, of course, be many occasions when you may want to expend a little more physical energy than usual. These could range from washing windows to enjoying sex.

It is good for us to try to extend ourselves if it is done with a little common sense. Here are a few suggestions that will help:

1. Wait until an hour or more after eating. Digestion draws blood, with its oxygen, away from muscles leaving them less able to cope with extra demands. This is the very same reason that children are taught not to go swimming right after meals.

2. You may find you feel your best soon after taking your medicine or having a breathing treatment.

3. Those who have had an aerosol inhaler prescribed by their physician can use it to help a special effort, being careful NEVER to use more than prescribed.

4. Pace yourself and don't rush.

5. If you feel breathless, use pursed lip breathing. Remember—this really helps and you can do it any time, any place.

Don't permit yourself to be overburdened either by possessions or old habits. You will be amazed when you learn how many energy wasters you can eliminate with no noticeable loss.

It is important to remember that each COPD patient is unique. No two have exactly the same needs. You will find here some suggestions which will help you greatly and others which may seem nonsensical to you. All we can say is that each has helped one or more of us.

*To begin at the beginning...*

### WAKING UP

This is always a difficult moment for some folks and if you are not feeling up to snuff, it can be a real chore. Some hints:

- Soft music is much more pleasant than an alarm if you are easily startled.

- Try some stretching and relaxing exercises while still lying down. These do help to get your body in gear for the day as every cat in the world knows.

- Making a bed is one of the most demanding of household tasks, and if you must do it yourself, try this: half make your bed while you are still in it. Pull the top sheet and blanket up on one side and smooth them out. Exit from the unmade side, which is then easy to finish.

- If you find that a bedspread is an unnecessary frill which only adds work, leave yours off.

- An aid to making your bed while still in (or on) it is to mark the center of each sheet and blanket in a small permanent way, such as with a colored stitch or pen mark, on the top hem. While you are still sitting on your bed it is easy to line up the marks in the center. When you do get up everything will be in the right place.

- Before getting all the way up, however, it is a big help to do some of your dressing sitting on the edge of your bed. Every night leave your robe and slippers or shoes, socks and underwear where they are easy to reach in the morning. This will require less effort and help to keep you warm if your room is on the cool side.

- Incidentally, if you share quarters with another person, persuade him/her to let you have the bureau drawers which are easiest to reach—saves bending.

- If you have a room to yourself, make it a habit to put most often used items such as socks and underwear in the most convenient places and seldom used things in the far-away bottom drawers and top shelves.

## Chronic Obstructive Pulmonary Disease

## BATHING

- If for some reason you find a shower or tub bath too demanding, a great solution is to get a bath stool. This is waterproof and goes right into the tub. It can be removed easily and makes a nice seat when giving yourself a pedicure or just drying your feet and legs. For bathing, use a hand spray which may be attached to the tub faucet or shower head. You may find bathing this way so pleasant that you will wonder why you didn't always do it thus.

- A nice, long terry robe will eliminate the effort of drying altogether, just blot.

- When excess humidity bothers you, leave the bathroom door open and be sure to use your bathroom exhaust fan if you have one. If you feel weak, don't take a bath or shower when you are alone.

- It is not necessary to get wet all over, all at once, to be clean. A "basin bath" can be taken in place of a tub bath and is a lot less taxing.

- Those using oxygen through a long tube may find it makes bathing easier if the tube is passed over the shower curtain rod and thus out of the way.

- Shaving or making up is much easier if you have a low mirror so that you can sit down while doing either.

- Incidentally, it is OK to remove the nasal cannula briefly to wash your face, shave or apply makeup.

*Exiting from the bath is a good time to review a few...*

## Grooming Hints

- Many of us find that strong scents are irritating and unpleasant. Try to avoid toiletries that are too heavily perfumed. They may leave you and your friends gasping.

- Women are advised to avoid elaborate hairdos which will need tiresome setting and extended use of hand-held blowers and dryers. (Men too.)

- Also, MOST IMPORTANT, we are in agreement that the use of all kinds of aerosols and sprays, except those prescribed by a physician, is a bad idea. We all have sufficient respiratory problems without adding to them by inhaling unknown substances. Many sprays may be alright, but why take chances? There are many good liquid or gel type hair dressings, and the roll-on or solid deodorants are excellent. Some of these products are now available unscented.

- If you are troubled by occasional accidental loss of urine brought on by coughing, overexertion or stress, the new small flat sanitary pads with adhesive backs may be most useful in keeping neat.

*We've been standing around the bathroom long enough. It is time to think about...*

## Dressing

Quite a few of us feel that it is a good idea to finish dressing before breakfast. It gets the day off to a good start.

- We all have personal tastes in clothing but there is one consideration which affects most COPD people. It is a bad idea to wear anything which restricts chest and abdominal expansion. For this reason, belts, bras, and girdles that are tight should be avoided. Fortunately, we live in an era when "anything goes" clothing-wise; if a choice must be made between style and comfort, opt for comfort every time.

- Men may find that suspenders are more comfortable than a belt.

- Most women find that slacks and socks are much easier to put on than struggling into panty hose. Both sexes, however, should avoid socks and stockings having elastic bands which may bind the leg and restrict circulation.

## Chronic Obstructive Pulmonary Disease

- You can place your underwear inside your pants and put both on together.

- Almost all of us prefer slip-on type shoes—no bending over to tie shoelaces. Your favorite lace-up type shoes can be converted to slip-ons by the use of elastic shoe laces. Putting on any kind of shoe is made much easier if you use a long (12"-18") shoehorn.

- Women who have given up bras may find camisoles a comfortable and pretty substitute. If you are a woman who has given up girdles—ENJOY.

- Both men and women should avoid tight neck bands. Although some gentlemen still prefer neckties, an open neck with a loosely tied scarf, kerchief or bolo, is both attractive and much more comfortable. Another option is a colored T-shirt under an open neck sport shirt.

- Many of us are bothered by extremes of temperature and may find that cotton underclothing is more comfortable than synthetic. Some nationwide mail order houses carry complete lines of cotton undergarments including "vests" for women.

- "Long johns" are back in style for both sexes. Some of the new colored varieties, originally made for skiers, are quite attractive. They are most comfortable when worn under wide-legged slacks.

- If you are not too active and sit a lot, a large shawl is really great for occasional shivers. It is much easier to put on and take off than a sweater. The men should be reminded that President Lincoln often wore a shawl, even in public. After all, a shawl is nothing more than a loose cape (which F.D.R. often wore).

*Now that you are all bathed and comfortably dressed, it may be a good time to consider preparing your daily....*

## Medications

- Those of us who take pills and are also slightly forgetful have found a pillbox with a separate compartment for each day of the week most useful. Your druggist should carry them. However, if you are taking many pills, it will be better to lay out a day's supply each morning. There are several ways to do this and here is one.... Some fast food places have little one-ounce plastic cups with snap-on lids for ketchup, etc. in take-out orders. (Get friends to save some for you.) Have one cup for each pill-taking occasion during the day. Label or mark each cup with the time the contents are to be taken. Keep them in plain sight with a small clock nearby and a pad and pencil handy to keep score on your pill-taking. Other containers such as egg boxes or cleaned plastic pill bottles with original labels removed can be used in the same way. Something with a fairly snug cover is preferable. Whatever you put them in, it is important to keep pills away from heat and moisture.

- Whenever you get a new medicine or a refill from the drugstore, figure out how long it will last and mark on a calendar the time to reorder. This may save you from running out of a necessary medication in the middle of the night or on a holiday weekend.

- **NEVER USE ANYONE ELSE'S MEDICINE.** Nowhere is it more evident how different we all are than in the medicines which help each of us individually. Two people may have the same disease and the same symptoms and yet respond to the same medicine in entirely different ways.

This cannot be stressed too strongly. Never hesitate to ask for more information regarding your medicine or to tell your doctor when your medicine does not seem to be working for you. Never make changes in the dosage unless your doctor agrees. Keep a record of medicines that don't agree with you. It is easy to forget.

In addition to swallowing medicines many of us must also learn to inhale them.

*This is called....*

## Chronic Obstructive Pulmonary Disease

### *Respiratory Therapy*

- If it is necessary for you to take breathing treatments at home, try to get all of your equipment together in a convenient place where it can be left from treatment to treatment. Being near a bathroom or kitchen where it will be easy to clean equipment is helpful, but, of course, if you take treatments during the night, the first consideration may be to have your equipment near your bed.

- An ideal arrangement is to have a small table with a drawer or a flat topped desk in front of a window. Outside the window might be a good place to put a bird feeder. It is nice to have something to watch, read or listen to while taking a treatment. One word of caution, when you are finished, don't leave any medication sitting in the sun.

- You may find it difficult to listen to anything with a machine going. A radio or TV set with a small earphone attachment will solve this problem.

- Have a small clock handy to time your treatments.

- If you must measure a medication with an eye dropper, be sure there are no air bubbles in it before starting to measure.

- An excellent place to store small pieces of equipment such as tubes, medicine cups and mouthpieces is in one or two food storage boxes with lock tops. A good size is about 6"x 8"x 21/2". These will fit in a small drawer out of sight and parts that need sterilizing or soaking can be done right in the container.

- All equipment should be kept clean and should be sterilized as directed. Don't worry if your friend has been taught different methods to do this. It seems to be like making a mint julep—several different recipes but the same end result.

- When you disassemble your equipment to clean it after a treatment, you may find the plastic hose is difficult to pull loose. Try pulling it off while the machine is still running. The added "push" of the compressor will help loosen the hose.

- If you are using a mechanical nebulizer and feel you are not getting enough mist, check the hose coupling. Occasionally vibrations cause these to work loose. Just hand-tighten.

- Any small piece of equipment with a motor or compressor will be much quieter if you put some kind of a thick pad under it. Folded fabric or newspaper may suffice.

- Some of these machines have a small air filter which should be changed once in a while. Ask your supplier to give you some. They are easy to change.

- Last but not least—most medical equipment used at home can be purchased. In many cases this may be cheaper than monthly rental, but you will be responsible for repairs. Ask your supplier and compare.

*Many of our Respiratory Club members also use portable systems for supplying....*

## Oxygen

Those of us who use oxygen recommend your supplier come to visit you to explain all technical aspects of your equipment's operation. Get their emergency phone number and procedures to follow in case of technical questions or concerns about the equipment. However, since oxygen itself is a prescribed drug, questions about amount and usage are for your physician to answer.

- Some portable oxygen units (oxygen walkers) come equipped with a loose scale on the side for measuring the weight of the liquid oxygen. Those who use this type of system over a period of time often learn to estimate the weight fairly accurately. In this case the scale can be removed, leaving a leather loop with snap in place. The oxygen tubing can be threaded through this loop to eliminate some of the strain on the point of attachment of the tube to the pack. This helps prevent the tubing from being accidentally disconnected. The same method can be used to temporarily shorten the tube by looping it through several times.

## Chronic Obstructive Pulmonary Disease

- It is important to find out approximately how long each portable unit supply will last you specifically. Learn to time your outings so that you don't run short.

- If you have been out with a portable liquid unit and return home with no immediate plans to go out again soon, you can transfer your long house tubing to the portable unit to use up the remaining oxygen it holds. This utilizes oxygen which would otherwise only leak away.

- When using oxygen, try to inhale through your nose (a good idea anyway). Inhaling through your mouth can be very drying, and some of the oxygen may be wasted.

- Change nasal cannulas fairly often particularly if the prongs become soiled or uncomfortable. In many places they are free from your suppliers.

- Don't be embarrassed by the occasional attention your oxygen unit and tubing may attract. Most people know what they are and give them no more thought than a hearing aid. Others, who may not be familiar with this equipment, are interested in learning what it is. They appreciate your taking the time to explain what it does and why you must use it.

*By now you should be all set for the day ahead. Hopefully you feel like considering some . . .*

### Work at Home or Abroad

This is where some of us temporarily bog down. Each COPD person must find his or her own work ethic. Just remember this: nowhere is it written that any job must be finished as fast as possible. Many good books and paintings have been literally years in the making. If you don't feel like building a World Trade Center today, how about trying to lay a couple of bricks?

Most jobs, excluding prize fighting, call for some skill which may be useful in a less physical way than is common practice. Very few Respiratory Club members hold full-time jobs, yet here are some of the part-time jobs they do perform: management consulting; newspaper, radio and TV publicity; lobbying for a worthy cause; bookkeeping at home for a small neighborhood store; mechanical and electrical designing; handcrafting gifts to sell; telephoning and doing mailings for a political party—the list goes on. There are as many different things we can do as there are people. This includes you. Don't be afraid to start small. It sure beats not starting at all.

While you are planning a new mini-career, the housework piles up. Our Respiratory Club hints to make it easier fall into four general groups, the first of which is....

*Lifting and Toting*

- Get yourself a small utility cart, the kind with three shelves. As you move about doing chores, use your cart to carry everything needing transferral from one place to another.

- Pick up last night's newspaper, some soiled clothes for the laundry, a couple of used dishes, books to go back to the library, clean towels for the bathroom, etc. Try to travel in a circle and avoid going back and forth.

- Using a cart and working in a circle is very effective whether you live in a single room or a two-story house (have a cart on each floor).

- If you do live in a single room or a small apartment it is especially important to maintain reasonable order. Living in untidy quarters can be very depressing. Try to stay on top of things and create a pleasant ambience for yourself. It will make you feel better.

- Carrying things downstairs is not a problem for most of us. Carrying them up may be a different story. There is one way: On an exhale, lift your burden two or three steps and put it down, rest. Climb two or three steps, rest again. Repeat. This may be a little slow, but it is possible to do the job without knocking yourself out.

- If you live where you must climb stairs, you might consider a mechanical chair lift, but they are very expensive. In any case,

# Chronic Obstructive Pulmonary Disease

it is a good idea to have a chair to sit on or a table to lean on when you reach the top.

## Some Cleaning Tools

- One of the handiest of gadgets is a pair of pickup tongs (these look like giant scissors) used for retrieving things from hard-to-reach places. Most medical supply houses stock these.

- There is also a type of pickup tongs which expands in a criss-cross fashion. They are made of metal or wood and make it possible to pick up very small objects without bending. Marvelous, but hard to find. If you are lucky enough to find them, try slipping a small piece of rubber tubing over each end; this makes it easier to grasp things.

- Another pickup device is a magnet on a short string. This will stick to your cart so you will always have it with you. Great for thumbtacks, lost hairpins, etc., but no good, alas, for brass pins.

- If you must use a vacuum, which is not such a great idea, at least use a machine with a disposable bag and remove with extreme care. It is hard to imagine anything more irritating to lungs than shaking out a dust bag. A small hand vacuum is easy to use for spot cleanups and can stay on your cart.

- Sweeping and feather dusting are out, for obvious reasons, but if you do feel compelled to use a broom or dry mop, protect yourself by wrapping the working end in a damp cloth.

- A damp cloth for dusting is also good but if you hesitate to use one on wood furniture, here is a good disposable duster you can make for yourself. Get a roll of crinkly paper towels and a bottle of lemon oil from a hardware store. Tear towel in sections and fold in quarters, put about 4 or 5 coin-sized dots of oil on each towel and roll up tight. Store in a plastic bag or glass jar. Use and throw away.

- Even with precautions, housework is apt to stir up dust. If you find you must do a dusty job, the best idea is to use a mask.

- Around the house the "no aerosol" rule applies with no "ifs, ands or buts." Don't even think of inhaling oven cleaner or kitchen cleaner or bathroom cleaner, any of which may contain lye, ammonia or other "goodies."

- Avoid using anything harmful that can vaporize, such as kerosene, mothballs and solvents. Avoid, also, as far as possible, powders; if they must be used, handle with extreme care.

- Have good ventilation and an adequate supply of fresh air at all times.

## *In the Kitchen*

- Don't try to get everything done at once, set smaller goals. Almost all jobs can be divided into sections. For instance—clean the top shelf of the refrigerator today and the bottom shelf tomorrow or next week. Take comfort in the thought that the longer you put a job off, the longer it won't need redoing.

- Plan your meals when you are neither hungry nor tired. Light, well-balanced meals are too important to leave to impulse.

- The details of diet planning vary for each person and are too complex to go into here. One thing, however, is true for all of us with COPD. A number of small meals is always better than a few large ones. Common sense tells us that the more room the stomach takes up, the less room there is for air in the lungs. Also, as previously mentioned, prolonged digestion draws blood and oxygen to the stomach and away from other parts of the body which may need them more.

- Utilize convenience foods when desired, but remember that many packaged foods have high salt and sugar contents which may be banned if you are on a special diet. Learn to read labels.

- Keep plenty of water and/or fruit juices in the refrigerator.

## Chronic Obstructive Pulmonary Disease

- If you enjoy cooking, it is often almost as easy to make a double or triple amount of your specialties. Freeze the excess in meal-size containers and enjoy some cook-free meals when you feel like a day off.

- If you can afford one, a microwave oven may prove a boon in reducing kitchen time and temperatures. A slow-cooking electric crockpot may make things easier, too.

- When cooking, always use your exhaust fan, or make sure there is good ventilation.

- If you are bothered by the heat, try using a small portable fan when cooking or ironing. In fact such a portable fan is useful in any room, not only to cool you off but also to help overcome shortness of breath brought on by exertion or stress. It is also useful for blowing all sorts of offensive or irritating odors away from you, should the need arise. A portable fan may deserve a place on your "supply wagon."

- When tidying up after a meal, assemble all items which need putting away in the refrigerator in one spot. Then sit down and put them away.

- Put your most used pots and pans back on the stove and leave them there and instead of putting your dishes and silver away, reset the table for your next meal.

*Gardening*

- If you enjoy gardening (and have a yard), there are a number of ways to make it easier. The first is obvious—a riding mower, preferably with a self-starter. This can be a real morale booster.

- The second is old fashioned but good—a small floral or scuffle hoe. These are light and easy to handle. Cut down weeds while they are still small and leave them where they fall, good mulch.

- Some other easy-to-handle, lightweight tools are a floral rake which is about 7" wide; a three-pronged cultivator with a handle about 3' long and a nylon garden hose which rolls up flat on its own reel. One of these hoses, 50' long with its reel, weighs only 2 1/2 lbs. and can be carried in one hand.

- Another great boon to some gardeners is a folding stool. If bending over cuts off your wind, try gardening sitting down. Use a long-handled spear-type weeder, a clam rake about 18" long for leaves and your pickup scissors or tongs which are useful for removing garden debris from the ground. These few short hand-tools and the aforementioned folding stool can all be carried in a shallow garden basket.

- Here's how to make an easy flower garden. In the fall, gather as many seeds as possible from easy-to-grow hardy annuals. In the spring, sow (each kind separately), scattering by hand in prepared beds. Rake in and tamp lightly. When they come up, hoe down all but a few. What is left will give you a nice display without the hard work of transplanting seedlings.

- If you live where there is no space for your own garden, you may be able to have a window box or several shelves for plants inside the window. Even in a limited space, growing things can be one of the most rewarding pursuits there are.

*With all the house and yard work under control it may be time to make preparations for....*

## Going Out

- This is a good place to repeat that all COPD people are different in many ways. One way is in our reactions to weather. Some like it hot, some like it cold, some damp, some dry. The point is that if it is your kind of day—try to get out and enjoy.

- One thing which does bother us all considerably is air pollution. Find out where you can get a daily air quality report for your area and use it when making your plans for the day.

## Chronic Obstructive Pulmonary Disease

- Before going out, however, it is a good idea to make some preparations for your homecoming. Of course, we should learn to stop whatever it is we are doing before fatigue sets in, but sometimes this is easier said than done, particularly when away from home. At a time when you are most apt to be tired, it is lovely to come home and have nothing to do but relax. So....

- Before leaving, lay out your comfortable clothes and slippers, leave a drink in a handy thermos, set out whatever utensils you will need for your evening meal, even turn down your bed for a quick nap—whatever makes you feel good. Then homecoming can be more than just a relief, it can be a real pleasure.

- Try to get yourself a warm, lightweight coat for winter. Down is ideal. A heavy winter coat can wear you out before you are out the front door.

- In cold weather, also wear a nice long, warm I scarf, and if it gets too cold or windy, do not hesitate to wind it across your nose. Some of us, however, prefer a cold-weather mask. There is one being made now of soft sponge which is quite comfortable to wear. Mask or scarf is a personal choice, either has merit.

- Those of you who do considerable outdoor walking may find that a cane-seat or shooting stick is a real help. It gives you a cane to lean on and a small seat if you feel like resting.

### *Riding & Driving*

- If you have trouble getting from spot A to spot B, it matters not whether the problem arises in your legs or your lungs, you do have trouble walking and are entitled to a "handicapped" parking permit. It is simple to obtain in most places. Write to your State Motor Vehicle Department for an application. Get one and use it. When you use a "handicapped" parking space make sure you display your permit; not only is this required by law in many states, it may help persuade the weight lifters and other robust types that they are illegally parked in an area reserved for the handicapped.

- If you travel with someone else and know you may have to sit in the car for fairly long periods of time, make up a kit of helpful things for yourself and keep it in the car. In a shopping bag, for instance, include a small lap robe, pad and pencil, a paperback or two, (poetry is ideal if you like it), tissues, a package of pre-moistened wipes and whatever else suits your fancy. It also helps to carry a large piece of cardboard to use as a sunscreen if necessary.

- A coffee can with a snap-on plastic lid makes a dandy emergency urinal.

- If you do drive and find that you must put gas in your car yourself, try to get upwind from the pump so that you do not gas yourself as well as the car.

- It is an excellent idea for any driver to have a CB radio in the car to use if it is necessary to call for help in an emergency. For people with breathing problems it may be an absolute necessity. Try to imagine changing a tire, walking to the next off-ramp to call for help or hiking a long distance carrying a can of gas and you'll know why.

- When driving, practice doing breathing exercises while waiting for red lights to change—it beats fuming. Indeed, you should take a couple of minutes or even seconds to do breathing exercises whenever you come to a natural stopping place, a red light, a TV commercial, end of a chapter in a book or "whatever"—like now.

## *Traveling*

- If you plan an intercity trip, think of taking a bus. They do have advantages, including generally landing you in the middle of town where there is other local transportation available—not out in the boondocks somewhere. On interstate buses, the federal smoking laws are generally observed and

## Chronic Obstructive Pulmonary Disease

the drivers are most helpful. Sit in the front and if you have any special problems tell the driver.

- When you must travel alone—travel light. Get a small suitcase on wheels. There are also wheeled suitcase carriers. They are good but somewhat clumsy and just one more thing to carry around.

- Those of us who have had to travel on subways recommend staying out of them if at all possible. Most subways and elevated train lines can only be used by making long and exhausting stair climbs. This may be made many times more difficult by being caught in rush hour crowds which force you to move much faster than is comfortable.

- In addition, the air in many subway systems leaves a lot to be desired.

- All in all, subways can provide a very threatening environment for anyone with respiratory problems. We all strongly advise sticking to surface transportation wherever it is available.

- Whenever possible, avoid any kind of travel during rush hours. It is pleasant to be able to move at your own speed and with a little luck get a seat.

- Traveling with oxygen and traveling on planes are two subjects well covered in other places. Ask your local Lung Association or your oxygen supplier for information.

### *Shopping*

- If you are going shopping with an oxygen carrier, try to find a shopping cart on your way into the store. Put your oxygen pack into the cart while you shop.

- When you go shopping try to pick an off day and hour (not Friday or Saturday at high noon). This way you will be able to move at a leisurely pace and avoid being jostled.

- It is also helpful to stay out of all sorts of crowds, particularly indoors. Aside from the fact that the air may be smoky and generally unpleasant, you run a high risk of having someone sneeze or cough in your face.

- Don't be afraid to ask someone to stop smoking near you. We all have a right to breathe smoke free air, as most people are beginning to realize.

- In many areas there are "no-smoking" laws. Familiarize yourself with these and if you are in a store or restaurant where these laws are not observed, speak to the manager. Don't forget, you are the customer and are doing the proprietor a favor by being there.

- Shopping for clothing, especially dresses and slacks, can be exhausting even to one in the best of health. Know your measurements (write them down) and carry a small rolled-up tape measure with you. If you see something you like, check with the tape to see if it will fit before you buy. Have an understanding with the store that if it isn't satisfactory it can be returned.

- When you have a fairly large grocery order, have all the "spoilables," such as frozen foods, packed in a separate bag. When you get home, you can put away whatever needs refrigeration. Leave the rest for later when you feel more energetic or a "helper" can lend a hand.

- Incidentally, it won't hurt to wash your hands extra well when you get home. It is now known that colds are spread by hands as well as through the air.

*At the end of an afternoon out it is time to return home for a light supper, relax and enjoy some pleasant . . .*

## Rest and Recreation

We all seem to be in agreement that the most important and lasting pleasure any of us can have is the company of good friends. The mobile society we live in often makes it difficult to keep in touch with old acquaintances. Many of us live far from our birthplaces and early ties, and sometimes feel that after a certain age it is hard to start making new friends. THIS IS NOT TRUE.

- One of the best ways to make friends with whom you can share common interests and problems is to join a Respiratory Club. If you can't find such a group, get in touch with your local Lung Association or your hospital respiratory department.

This may be a good spot to stop for a moment and consider a matter of special concern to those of us who live alone—how to get help quickly when it may be needed.

- The buddy phone system can be a big help and provide a special feeling of security.

- Make arrangements to have a friend or relative call at the same time every day to make sure you are OK. If you plan to be out, let them know ahead of time to save needless concern.

- Get to know neighbors who can see your windows and arrange a signal they can see. For instance if a shade is pulled down every evening or a certain lamp is lit, it is a sign you are OK. If this isn't done, ask your neighbors to investigate.

- If you live in an apartment, let the neighbors on all sides of you know that if they hear you pounding you need help.

- Somewhere near you is someone who needs your friendship and help, too. Once you have gotten in touch with others, you will be amazed to find how rewarding it can be.

Alone or with company, there are many entertaining things to do at home besides watching TV. Many are also more fun; here are a few:

- Something that many of us have forgotten about are board games. There are probably some around your house that haven't been used in a long time—Checkers, Parcheesi, Monopoly, Scrabble, etc. There are also dominoes and many two- or-more-handed card games such as whist, pinochle, rummy or canasta.

- If you are a chess buff, you might enjoy joining a chess club. It is also fun to play games through the mail or over the phone.

- It may sound antisocial, but for many, solitaire can be very relaxing. There are several paperback books of solitaire games. Try learning a new game or two.

- Jigsaw puzzles can also while away many hours and provide a real sense of accomplishment when done.

- Do you like to read? Build up a supply of paperbacks for days when you can't get out to the library. Many libraries have a free paperback swap shelf. If yours doesn't, ask the librarian to start one. You can also often get good books cheaply at flea markets or garage sales. Also, try swapping with friends, neighbors and relatives. If you can't get out, find out if your library has a home delivery service—many do.

- Is there something you have always wanted to learn? Now is the time. Many local schools have adult classes in the evening on a staggering assortment of subjects. If you prefer to learn in the relaxing atmosphere of your home, there are literally hundreds of correspondence courses to choose from, from beekeeping to weather forecasting.

- If you have always wanted to learn a language there are good home-study courses with records. This is more fun if you find someone to practice your new language with. A telephone or pen pal might be just the thing.

- If you find your previous hobbies too demanding, try a scaled-down version for the time being. Cabinet makers may find

## Chronic Obstructive Pulmonary Disease

great pleasure in the growing hobby of making scale model furniture; machinists might enjoy making a scale model locomotive or assembling a clock; a dressmaker could make and dress period costume dolls.

- Is a super-active dog too much to handle? Try a small, quiet cat. If allergies forbid either, tropical fish, while not very affectionate, are beautiful and fascinating. A bird feeder near your favorite window can provide hours of pleasure. If, for some reason, all of these are out, a large, soft, stuffed critter has its uses as a confidant, punching bag or pillow.

- Needlework of all kinds gives many people both relaxation and pleasure. You men—don't forget Rosie Greer and his needlepoint. It is also a fact that at least half of the world's champion knitters and crocheters have been men. Try it, you may find you like it.

- If you like to paint, try watercolors for a change of pace. They are lightweight if you want to go sketching, odorless and dry fast. To develop a technique for using them, try some of the new coloring books for adults. These are really great fun for everyone, not just artists.

- This may be a good time to learn to play a musical instrument; piano or guitar for instance. The wind instruments are out—no tubas.

- Nowadays almost anything you could possibly want to buy can be purchased through the mail. So—"let your fingers do the walking"—not only through the phone book but also through a whole world of mail order catalogs. Many pleasant evenings can be spent sitting in your favorite (not too soft) easy chair and shopping.

- There are many, many other suggestions we could make, but the aforementioned will give you some ideas.

*And so....*

## To Bed

- Go to bed in easy stages so that you arrive there relaxed—not worn out. For example, put on your night clothes and a comfortable robe, then read or watch TV for a while.

- Plan your sleeping area so that everything you may need will be handy. The most important things being a light and telephone. Have any emergency numbers you think you might need taped to the phone and easy to read.

- Other helpful things are: a clock radio with an ear plug for late night listening if you have a sleeping companion; medication as need be; a glass of water and a small snack if you are so inclined; and a urinal in a safe and easy-to-reach place. (Little known fact—there are also urinals made for women.)

- An electric blanket is a must. No other blanket is necessary. They are lightweight, comfortable and make bed-making a cinch.

- Some sort of night light is a real necessity. It lessens the possibility of being disoriented if you waken suddenly and helps you locate things you may need in a hurry.

- There is now a light which throws the time on the ceiling and numerous small lamps which plug directly into a wall outlet. Watching a lava light may also serve to relax you and make you go to sleep. Best of all is a lighted aquarium which, in a darkened room, is absolutely enchanting.

- Some find this is a perfect time to do some muscle relaxing exercises.

- Pull your night cap (no kidding) down over your ears, say your prayers if so inclined—and so to sleep.

Pleasant dreams.

— *Katherine Meek Romanik and Natasha Lessnik*

Chapter 4

# Common Cold and Influenza

*Chapter Contents*

Section 4. 1—The Common Cold—Or Is It the Flu?..................... 212
Section 4. 2—How to Take Your Medicine: Antihistamines....... 221
Section 4. 3—Modern Pharmacy's Answer to Chicken Soup...... 224
Section 4. 4—How to Avoid the Flu ............................................... 231

Section 4. 1

# The Common Cold—or is it the Flu?

Source: National Institute of Allergy and Infectious Diseases November 1994.

## The Common Cold

Sneezing, scratchy throat, runny nose—everyone knows the first signs of a cold, probably the most common illness known to man. Although the common cold is usually mild, with symptoms lasting a week or less, it is a leading cause of doctor visits and of school and job absenteeism.

Scientists supported by the National Institute of Allergy and Infectious Diseases (NIAID) have made significant advances in understanding the structure and disease-causing mechanisms of the many viruses that can cause the common cold, with the goal of preventing and treating this troublesome and costly ailment.

## The Problem

In the course of a year, individuals in the United States suffer 1 billion colds, according to some estimates.

Colds are most prevalent among children, and seem to be related to youngsters' relative lack of resistance to infection and to contacts with other children in day-care centers and schools. Children have about six to eight colds a year. In families with children in school, the number of colds per child can be as high as 12 a year. Adults average about two to four colds a year, although the range varies widely. Women, especially those aged 20 to 30 years, have more colds than men, possibly because of their closer contact with children. On average, individuals older than 60 have fewer than one cold a year.

The economic impact of the common cold is enormous. The National Center for Health Statistics (NCHS) estimates that, in 1992, 65 million cases of the common cold in the United States required medical attention or resulted in restricted activity. In 1992, colds caused 157 million days of restricted activity and 15 million days lost from work, according to the NCHS.

Even when Americans don't call their doctors, they spend an estimated $700 million or more annually for over-the-counter medications for the treatment of respiratory infections.

## The Causes

### The Viruses

More than 200 different viruses are known to cause the symptoms of the common cold. Some, such as the rhinoviruses, seldom produce serious illnesses. Others, such as parainfluenza and respiratory syncytial virus, produce mild infections in adults but can precipitate severe lower respiratory infections in young children.

**Rhinoviruses** (from the Greek rhin, meaning "nose") cause an estimated 30 to 35 percent of all adult colds, and are most active in early fall, spring and summer. More than 110 distinct rhinovirus types have been identified. These agents grow best at temperatures of 33 degrees Celsius [about 91 degrees Fahrenheit (F)], the temperature of the human nasal mucosa.

**Coronaviruses** are believed to cause 10 to 20 percent of all adult colds. They induce colds primarily in the winter and early spring. Of the more than 30 isolated strains, three or four infect humans. The importance of coronaviruses as causative agents is hard to assess because, unlike rhinoviruses, they are difficult to grow in the laboratory.

Approximately 10 to 15 percent of adult colds are caused by viruses also responsible for other, more severe illnesses: adenoviruses, coxsackieviruses, echoviruses, orthomyxoviruses (including influenza A and B viruses), paramyxoviruses (including several parainfluenza viruses), respiratory syncytial virus and enteroviruses.

The causes of 30 to 50 percent of adult colds, presumed to be viral, remain unidentified.

The same viruses that produce colds in adults appear to cause colds in children. However, the relative importance of various viruses in pediatric colds is unclear because of the difficulty in isolating the precise cause of symptoms in studies of children with colds.

### Does Cold Cause a Cold?

Although many people are convinced that a cold results from exposure to cold weather, or from getting chilled or overheated, NIAID grantees have found that these conditions have little or no effect on the development or severity of a cold. Nor is susceptibility apparently related to factors such as exercise, diet or enlarged tonsils or adenoids.

On the other hand, research suggests that psychological stress, allergic disorders affecting the nasal passages or pharynx, and menstrual cycles may have an impact on a person's susceptibility to colds. For example, NIAID-funded experiments showed individuals under high levels of psychological stress are more prone to infection with any of five cold-producing viruses and more apt to experience respiratory symptoms than people experiencing less stress.

## The Cold Season

In the United States, most colds occur during the fall and winter. Beginning in late August or early September, the incidence of colds increases slowly for a few weeks and remains high until March or April, when it declines. The seasonal variation may relate to the opening of schools and to cold weather, which prompt people to spend more time indoors and increase the chances that viruses will spread from person to person.

Seasonal changes in relative humidity may also affect the prevalence of colds. The most common cold-causing viruses survive better when humidity is low—the colder months of the year. Cold weather also may make the nasal passages' lining drier and more vulnerable to viral infection.

## Cold Symptoms

Symptoms of the common cold usually begin two to three days after infection and often include nasal discharge, obstruction of nasal breathing, swelling of the sinus membranes, sneezing, sore throat, cough and headache. Fever is usually slight but can climb to 102° F among infants and young children. Cold symptoms can last from two to 14 days, but two-thirds of people recover in a week. If symptoms occur often or last much longer than two weeks, they may be the result of an allergy rather than a cold.

Colds occasionally can lead to secondary bacterial infections of the middle ear or sinuses, requiring treatment with antibiotics. High fever, significantly swollen glands, severe facial pain in the sinuses, and a cough that produces mucus may indicate a complication or more serious illness requiring a doctor's attention.

## How Cold Viruses Cause Disease

Viruses cause infection by overcoming the body's complex defense system. The body's first line of defense is mucus, produced by the membranes in the nose and throat. Mucus traps the material we inhale: pollen, dust, bacteria, viruses. When a virus penetrates the mucus and enters a cell, it commandeers the protein-making machinery to manufacture new viruses which, in turn, attack surrounding cells.

### Cold Syptoms: The Body Fights Back

Cold symptoms are probably the result of the body's immune response to the viral invasion. Virus-infected cells in the nose send out signals that recruit specialized white blood cells to the site of the infection. In turn, these cells emit a range of immune system mediators such as kinins. These chemicals probably lead to the symptoms of the common cold by causing swelling and inflammation of the nasal membranes, leakage of proteins and fluid from capillaries and lymph vessels, and the increased production of mucus.

Kinins and other mediators released by immune system cells in the nasal membranes are the subject of intensive research. Researchers are examining whether drugs to block these mediators, or the receptors on cells to which they bind, might benefit people with colds.

## How Colds Are Spread

Depending on the virus type, any or all of the following routes of transmission may be common:

- Touching infectious respiratory secretions on skin and on environmental surfaces and then touching the eyes or nose.
- Inhaling relatively large particles of respiratory secretions transported briefly in the air.
- Inhaling droplet nuclei: smaller infectious particles suspended in the air for long periods of time.

### Research on Rhinovirus Transmission

Much of the research on the transmission of the common cold has been done with rhinoviruses, which are shed in the highest concentration in nasal secretions. Studies suggest a person is most likely to transmit rhinoviruses in the second to fourth day of infection, when the amount of virus in nasal secretions is highest. Researchers have also shown that using aspirin to treat colds increases the amount of virus shed in nasal secretions, possibly making the cold sufferer more of a hazard to others.

NIAID grantees have found that rhinoviruses from nasal secretions can be transferred easily from the hands of an infected person to those of another—by shaking hands, for instance—or to a surface such as a doorknob or telephone that is then touched by another person. By touching one's eyes or nose with the fingers, something most people do many times a day, the susceptible person can be "self-inoculated." Other studies suggest rhinovirus colds can be transmitted through the air.

## Preventing Transmission

Handwashing is the simplest and most effective way to keep from getting rhinovirus colds. Not touching the nose or eyes is another. Individuals with colds should always sneeze or cough into a facial tissue, and promptly throw it away. If possible, one should avoid close, prolonged exposure to persons who have colds.

Because rhinoviruses can survive up to three hours outside the nasal passages on inanimate objects and skin, cleaning environmental surfaces with a virus-killing disinfectant might help prevent spread of infection.

### A Cold Vaccine?

The development of a vaccine that could prevent the common cold has reached an impasse because of the discovery of many different cold viruses. Each virus carries its own specific antigens, substances that induce the formation of specific protective proteins (antibodies) produced by the body. Until ways are found to combine many viral antigens in one vaccine, or take advantage of the antigenic cross-relationships that exist, prospects for a vaccine are dim. Evidence that changes occur in common-cold virus antigens further complicate development of a vaccine. Such changes occur in some influenza antigens and make it necessary to alter the influenza vaccine each year.

## Treatment

Only symptomatic treatment is available for uncomplicated cases of the common cold: bed rest, plenty of fluids, gargling with warm salt water, petroleum jelly for a raw nose, and aspirin or acetaminophen to relieve headache or fever.

**A word of caution:** several studies have linked the use of aspirin to the development of **Reye's syndrome** in children recovering from influenza or chickenpox. Reye's syndrome is a rare but serious illness that usually occurs in children between the ages of three and 12 years. It can affect all organs of the body, but most often injures the brain and liver. While most children who survive an episode of Reye's syndrome do not suffer any lasting consequences, the illness can lead to permanent brain damage or death. The American Academy of Pediatrics recommends children and teenagers not be given aspirin or any medications containing aspirin when they have any viral illness, particularly chickenpox or influenza. Many doctors recommend these medications be used for colds in adults only when headache or fever is present. However, researchers also have found aspirin and acetaminophen can suppress certain immune responses and increase nasal stuffiness in adults.

Nonprescription cold remedies, including decongestants and cough suppressants may relieve some cold symptoms but will not prevent, cure or even shorten the duration of illness. Moreover, most have some side effects, such as drowsiness, dizziness, insomnia or upset stomach, and should be taken with care. Antihistamines generally don't relieve cold symptoms, because the body makes inflammatory chemicals other than histamine when attacked by a cold virus.

Antibiotics do not kill viruses. These prescription drugs should be used only for rare bacterial complications, such as sinusitis or ear infections, that can develop as secondary infections. The use of antibiotics "just in case" will not prevent secondary bacterial infections.

## *Does Vitamin C Have A Role?*

Many people are convinced that taking large quantities of vitamin C will prevent colds or relieve symptoms. To test this theory, several large-scale, controlled studies involving children and adults have been conducted. To date, no conclusive data has shown that large doses of vitamin C prevent colds. The vitamin may reduce the severity or duration of symptoms, but definitive evidence is lacking.

Taking vitamin C over long periods of time in large amounts may be harmful. Too much vitamin C can cause severe diarrhea, a particular danger for elderly people and small children. In addition, too much vitamin C distorts results of tests commonly used to measure the amount of glucose in urine and blood. Combining oral anticoagulant drugs and excessive amounts of vitamin C can produce abnormal results in blood-clotting tests.

Inhaling steam also has been proposed as a treatment of colds on the assumption that increasing the temperature inside the nose inhibits rhinovirus replication. Recent studies found that this approach had no effect on the symptoms or amount of viral shedding in individuals with rhinovirus colds. However, steam may temporarily relieve symptoms of congestion associated with colds.

Interferon-alpha has been studied extensively for the treatment of the common cold. Investigators have shown interferon, given in daily doses by nasal spray, can prevent infection and illness. However, interferon causes unacceptable side effects such as nosebleeds and does not appear useful in treating established colds. Most cold researchers are concentrating on other approaches to combatting cold viruses.

## NIAID Research

In laboratories in Bethesda, Md., and at grantee institutions nationwide, NIAID supports basic research on the structure of viruses that cause colds and cold-like diseases, and on their disease-causing mechanisms. The institute provides rhinovirus research materials to investigators, and has made its nationwide network of Vaccine and Treatment Evaluation Units available for clinical studies of potential new treatments.

NIAID-supported researchers have pioneered the use of X-ray crystallography to look at the atomic structure of viruses. The ability to picture the rhinovirus at this level and study its three-dimensional structure has revolutionized the design and testing of new antiviral drugs.

The researchers have shown rhinoviruses all share a common structure—a rhinovirus canyon—required for attachment to susceptible cells. These canyons are not accessible to attack by antibodies. Investigators are using X-ray crystallography to develop new drugs that snugly fit into and change the shape of the rhinovirus canyon, making the virus non-infectious.

## Common Cold and Influenza

Also, scientists have identified the docking molecule on cells to which the rhinovirus canyon attaches. This molecule is known as the intracellular adhesion molecule-1 (ICAM-1). NIAID-supported studies suggest that ICAM-1, or ICAM-1 coupled to an antibody, might be used to disrupt rhinoviruses and prevent their replication.

NIAID-funded studies of kinins and other mediators released in the nasal membranes are underway to further illuminate the sequence of events that occur between infection with a cold virus and the onset of symptoms. Recently, for example, investigators found increased levels of interleukin-1 (IL-1) in the nasal secretions of people with experimentally induced rhinovirus colds. The researchers speculate that IL-1 could play a number of roles in the development of the common cold, including the recruitment of immune system cells to the nasal mucosa.

### *The Outlook*

Thanks to basic research, scientists know more about the rhinovirus than almost any other virus, and have powerful new tools for developing antiviral drugs. Although the common cold may never be uncommon, further investigations offer the hope of reducing the huge burden of this universal problem.

NIAID, a component of the National Institutes of Health (NIH), supports research on AIDS, tuberculosis and other infectious diseases as well as allergies and immunology. NIH is an agency of the U.S. Public Health Service, U.S. Department of Health and Human Services.

Figure 4.1 on the next page summarizes the symptoms of cold and flu.

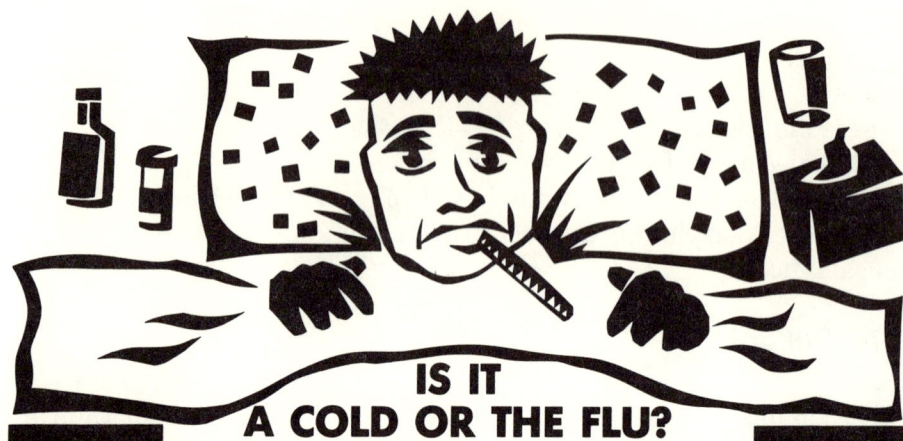

*Respiratory Diseases and Disorders Sourcebook*

## IS IT A COLD OR THE FLU?

| SYMPTOMS | COLD | FLU |
| --- | --- | --- |
| Fever | Rare | Characteristic, high (102-104°F); lasts 3-4 days |
| Headache | Rare | Prominent |
| General Aches, Pains | Slight | Usual; often severe |
| Fatigue, Weakness | Quite mild | Can last up to 2-3 weeks |
| Prostration (Extreme Exhaustion) | Never | Early and prominent |
| Stuffy Nose | Common | Sometimes |
| Sneezing | Usual | Sometimes |
| Sore Throat | Common | Sometimes |
| Chest Discomfort, Cough | Mild to moderate; hacking cough | Common; can become severe |
| COMPLICATIONS | Sinus congestion or earache | Bronchitis, pneumonia; can be life-threatening |
| PREVENTION | None | Annual vaccination; amantadine (an anti-viral drug) |
| TREATMENT | Only temporary relief of symptoms | Amantadine within 24-48 hours after onset of symptoms |

From the National Institutes of Health

*Figure 4.1.*

220

Common Cold and Influenza

Section 4.2

## How to Take Your Medicine: Antihistamines

Source: *FDA Consumer* September 1990.

How you take a medication makes a big difference in how well it works and how safe it will be for you. Sometimes it can be as important as what you take. Timing, what you eat and when you eat, proper dose, and many other factors can mean the difference between getting better, staying the same, or even getting worse. This drug information page is intended to help you make your medication work as effectively as possible. It is important to note, however, that this is only a guideline. You should talk to your doctor or pharmacist about how and when to take any prescribed drug.

Some antihistamines are available over-the-counter, or by prescription.

**Generic Names**
astemizole
azatadine
bromodiphenhydramine
*brompheniramine
carbinoxamine
*chlorpheniramine
clemastine
cecyproheptadine
*dexbrompheniramine
*dexchlorpheniramine
*dimenhydrinate
*diphenhydramine
diphenylpyraline
*doxylamine
phenindamine
*pyrilamine
terfenadine
tripelennamine
*triprolidine

* Starred drugs are in over-the-counter products.

Antihistamines work by temporarily blocking the action of a substance produced by the body called histamine, which can cause itching, sneezing, runny nose and eyes, and other symptoms. Most of these drugs can have a drying effect on the nasal mucous. They are structurally related to local anesthetics and can produce sedation. The reason why some antihistamines are effective against motion sickness and some symptoms of Parkinson's disease is not known.

## Conditions These Drugs Treat

- hay fever and other allergies

A few antihistamines have special uses, such as for treating:

- cough due to colds or inhaled irritants
- motion sickness
- sleeplessness
- hives
- stiffness and tremors in patients with Parkinson's disease

## How to Take

Extended-release tablets or capsules should be swallowed whole. The patient should follow directions on the container (or doctor's directions) on how often to take them.

Astemizole, one of the new relatively non-sedating antihistamines, is not absorbed well unless it is taken on an empty stomach, with no food one hour before and two hours after the medication.

Dimenhydrinate and diphenhydramine for motion sickness should be taken at least 30 minutes before travel and are most effective when taken one to two hours beforehand.

## Missed Doses

These drugs are for symptomatic relief, and a missed dose does not have any harmful consequences except for possible return of the symptoms. Too frequent dosing may cause increased sedation and other side effects.

## Side Effects and Risks

Common side effects such as drowsiness may decrease somewhat as your body adjusts to the medicine.

Notify your doctor as soon as possible if you notice any of these symptoms after taking antihistamines:

- blurred vision
- painful or difficult urination
- unusual tiredness or severe drowsiness
- weakness, clumsiness or unsteadiness
- marked dryness of the mouth, nose or throat
- fainting, seizures, or other loss of consciousness
- hallucinations
- shortness of breath.

Some of these may be due to overdose, others to individual intolerance to the medication.

## Precautions and Warnings

Most antihistamines cause some people to become drowsy. Make sure you know how you react to the drug you are taking before you drive or operate machinery. The elderly may be particularly susceptible to the sedative effect.

Do not give antihistamines to children under 6 years without consulting a doctor.

Antihistamines add to the effects of alcohol and other depressants. Therefore, avoid taking them close to the same time you drink alcohol or use drugs that slow down the nervous system, such as sedatives, tranquilizers, sleeping pills, narcotics, prescription pain medicines, seizure medications, muscle relaxants, or anesthetics.

Antihistamines may also mask nausea associated with overdose from other medicines you are taking or from other medical conditions. If you suspect such effects while taking antihistamines, be sure to inform your doctor.

When buying over-the-counter products, be sure to read the ingredient labels to make certain you are not taking more than one product containing antihistamines. If you are already taking a sedative or tranquilizer, do not take antihistamines, including those sold over-the-counter as sleep aids, without checking with your doctor.

If you get skin tests for allergies or are receiving allergy injections, tell your doctor if you are taking antihistamines because these drugs can distort test results and mask reactions.

For relief of dry mouth, nose and throat caused by antihistamines, use sugarless candy or gum or melt pieces of ice in your mouth. If dryness continues for two weeks or more, it may increase the chance of dental disease. Check with your doctor or dentist if the symptom persists.

## Section 4.3

## *Modern Pharmacy's Answers to Chicken Soup*

Source: Dept of Health and Human Services   Pub. No. (FDA) 93-1200

When cold or flu strikes, the suffering soul can hobble for help (or, better yet, wheedle someone else to go) to any nearby drugstore, supermarket, or convenience mart. There, a nose-clearing, cough-stopping, sinus-clearing, mind-boggling array of nonprescription medications offers, if not a cure, at least some symptomatic relief. Which to use depends on the specific symptoms that need relieving, whether other medical conditions rule out using certain ingredients, and whether the sufferer is willing to put up with the possibility of usually minor, but still bothersome and sometimes risky, side effects.

### *The Effectiveness of Nonprescription Drugs*

Several years ago, FDA called on a panel of nongovernment experts to study the safety and effectiveness of over-the-counter (OTC) cough and cold remedies and the accuracy of the claims made on the labels of those products. The panel (which also looked at drugs for allergies and asthma) was one of 17 set up by FDA to examine all nonprescription drugs marketed in the United States. The project,

## Common Cold and Influenza

mandated by a 1962 amendment to the Federal Food, Drug, and Cosmetic Act that requires all drugs to be proven effective as well as safe, will eventually establish federal standards on ingredients and labeling claims for all OTC drugs.

The panel found that proper use of nonprescription drugs can be effective in relieving cough, sinus congestion, runny nose, and some of the other symptoms associated with colds and flu. But it made clear that, although the products may relieve certain symptoms, they will not cure these conditions.

FDA then had its in-house experts review the panel's findings before it published proposed standards for these drugs. The proposals place the dozens of active ingredients into three categories:

- **Category I**—Generally recognized as safe and effective.

- **Category II**—Not generally recognized as safe and effective. These ingredients will be removed from products after FDA issues final standards.

- **Category III**—The available data are insufficient to allow FDA to decide whether the ingredient is safe and effective. More studies would need to be done, and unless the results show the ingredient is safe and effective, it could no longer be used after final standards are issued.

The accompanying table lists the active ingredients that FDA has proposed as Category I—safe and effective—for relieving certain symptoms of colds and flu. (The proposal for cough suppressants has been made final; the others are pending). These ingredients include:

*Decongestants*

Nasal decongestants, whether topical (sprays or drops) or oral (pills), open up the nasal passages. Topical decongestants clear up stuffy noses by constricting enlarged blood vessels. But if they are used for too long or too frequently, they can have the opposite effect: The effectiveness of each dose wears off sooner and sooner, and a "rebound effect" actually enlarges the blood vessels, producing more congestion. For that reason, FDA has proposed that topical decongestants carry instructions that warn users not to exceed the recommended dosage and not to use the product for more than three days. If symptoms persist, a physician should be consulted.

Oral decongestant labels should warn against use by persons suffering from high blood pressure, heart disease, diabetes, thyroid disease, or difficulty in urinating due to an enlarged prostate gland, unless directed by a doctor. The labels also should warn users that the product should not be taken for more than seven days, and that they should consult a doctor if symptoms do not improve or if they are accompanied by fever.

*Antihistamines*

Antihistamines, which are often used to relieve symptoms of hay fever-type allergies, also provide temporary relief from the runny nose and sneezing associated with the common cold. Although the antihistamine ingredients that are rated safe and effective have a low potential for side effects and toxicity, they may cause drowsiness, a fact that should be noted on the label along with a warning to avoid alcoholic beverages while taking the drug. The label also should include a warning against use by people who have asthma, glaucoma, emphysema, chronic pulmonary disease, shortness of breath, difficulty breathing, or difficulty urinating due to an enlarged prostate, unless directed by a doctor.

One antihistamine ingredient, doxylamine succinate, was added to category I only after an especially extensive review of safety data. The ingredient had been used in the prescription anti-morning sickness drug Bendectin, but concerns were later raised over a possible risk of birth defects in babies born to women who took the drug. (The drug is no longer marketed.) However, after its safety review, FDA concluded that the ingredient was unlikely to cause birth defects. The agency did not rule out the possibility that doxylamine succinate may have a weak teratogenic (birth-defect-causing) potential, but said it can be safely marketed as an OTC antihistamine if the label warns against use by pregnant and nursing women.

*Cough Suppressants*

Cough suppressants, also known as antitussives, include drugs taken orally (pills and syrups), as well as topical medications (throat lozenges and ointments to be rubbed on the chest or used in a vaporizer). They can temporarily relieve coughs due to minor throat irritation. But the labels should warn that a cough may be a sign of a serious condition and that a physician should be consulted if the cough lasts more than a week, tends to recur, or is accompanied by fever, rash, or persistent headache. Cough suppressants should not be used for persistent or chronic coughs such as those that occur with smoking, asthma and emphysema. (In such cases, coughing is essential to rid the bronchial airways of mucus and other secretions.)

Most nonprescription cough-cold remedies contain a combination of ingredients. In a proposed regulation published Aug. 12, 1988, FDA agreed that such combination products serve a useful purpose, since most cold and flu sufferers are not lucky enough to be afflicted with just one symptom.

In addition to decongestants, antihistamines and cough suppressants, these combination products may contain antipyretics to reduce fever and analgesics to relieve minor aches, pains and headaches that often accompany colds and the flu. The proposed rule listed the combinations that FDA has found safe and effective and the labeling that should accompany them. Most of the major cough-cold combination drug products contain ingredients rated safe and effective in the Aug. 12 proposal. Among them: *Comtrex, ChlorTrimeton Decongestant Tablets, Allerest, Sudafed Plus, Dristan, Nyquil, Vicks Vaporub, Vicks Inhaler, Co-Tylenol Cold Medication, and Formula 44 Cough Control Discs.*

Part of the proposal would permit a switch of the prescription antihistamine ingredient promethazine hydrochloride to nonprescription use in multi-ingredient cold products. (It would not be permitted as the sole active ingredient in OTC products labeled for relief of allergies, however. Promethazine is chemically related to the prescription antipsychotic drugs known as phenothiazines. FDA fears that allergy sufferers would be inclined to use such a product on a long-term basis, and such extended use could carry a risk of a rare but serious adverse reaction of the central nervous system known as tardive dyskinesia.)

The proposal would eliminate combinations using theophylline because there is no convincing evidence that such products can make good on their claims to ease labored breathing. If the standard becomes final as proposed, major products that would have to be reformulated to eliminate theophylline include *Primatene Tablets, Bronkotabs and Bronkolixir.*

Before taking any cough-cold product, no matter how much you're suffering from your miserable cold or the flu, take the time to read the label. There's information on dosing, warnings about who shouldn't take the medication, and special warnings and dosing instructions for children.

## Cold Medicines: FDA-Reviewed Ingredients

Here are the ingredients that FDA has proposed as safe and effective for use in over-the-counter (OTC) medications to relieve various symptoms of the common cold (The regulation on cough suppressant ingredients has been put into effect.)

*Antihistamines (relieve runny nose and sneezing)*

brompheniramine maleate
chlorcyclizine hydrochloride
chlorpheniramine maleate
dexbrompheniramine maleate
dexchlorpheniramine maleate
diphenhydramine hydrochloride
doxylamine succinate
phenindamine tartrate
pheniramine maleate
pyrilamine maleate
thonzylamine hydrochloride
triprolidine hydrochloride

*Antitussives (cough suppressants)*

**Oral:**
chlophedianol hydrochloride
codeine
codeine phosphate
codeine sulfate
dextromethorphan
dextromethorphan hydrobromide

**Topical:**
camphor
menthol

## Common Cold and Influenza

*Decongestants (relieve stuffy nose)*

**Oral:**
phenylephrine hydrochloride
pseudoephedrine hydrochloride
pseudoephedrine sulfate

**Topical:**
1-desoxyephedrine
ephedrine
ephedrine hydrochloride
ephedrine sulfate
racephedrine sulfate
racephedrine hydrochloride
naphazoline hydrochloride
oxymetazoline hydrochloride
phenylephrine hydrochloride
propylhexedrine
xylometazoline hydrochloride

*For more information, including labeling claims, dosages and warnings, see the proposed (or final, in the case of antitussives) standards published by FDA in the* Federal Register:

- Antihistamines: Jan. 15, 1985, and Aug.24, 1987
- Antitussives: Aug.12, 1987
- Decongestants: Jan.15, 1985
- Combinations: Aug. 12,1988

### Kids, Flu and Aspirin Don't Mix

Surely the most widely used cold and flu medicine is aspirin. In recent years, however, aspirin's use in youngsters suffering from such viral illnesses has been sharply curtailed. The reason: evidence that use of the drug in children and teenagers is linked to a rare but sometimes fatal condition called **Reye's syndrome**.

Reye's syndrome strikes children and teens who have the flu or chickenpox, but appear to be recovering. Symptoms include persistent vomiting, lethargy, sleepiness, violent headaches, and disorientation. Convulsions, coma and death can follow if Reye's syndrome is not treated immediately.

Although there is no cure, physicians have cut the death rate from Reye's syndrome from 80 percent to 20 percent by treating its symptoms. The key, says Dr. A.R. Colon, a pediatrician at Georgetown University Hospital in Washington, D.C., is to prevent brain swelling. A group of drugs called osmolar agents can control fluid buildup in the brain, ventilators can lower the body's carbon dioxide levels, and physicians and nurses can limit the patient's fluid intake.

What causes Reye's syndrome and how aspirin is linked to its onset are unknown. Retrospective studies, however, have shown that most Reye's syndrome victims took aspirin or a combination drug containing aspirin to reduce fever brought on by a case of the flu.

As a result, the U.S. Surgeon General, the Centers for Disease Control, and the American Academy of Pediatrics, among others, have advised parents not to give children aspirin if flu or chickenpox have been diagnosed or are even suspected. Further, FDA adopted a preliminary rule in 1986 requiring aspirin makers to add warnings about Reye's syndrome to their product labels. The rule became final in June 1988.

From these and other actions, the number of reported cases of Reye's syndrome dropped from 658 in 1980 to currently less than 25 a year.

As parents have gotten the word about not giving aspirin to their young children, teenagers have become the main victims of Reye's syndrome. David Perkins, executive director of the National Reye's Syndrome Foundation in Bryan, Ohio, blames the incidence on the fact that teenagers often take care of themselves when they have the flu or chickenpox, and often do so by taking aspirin, unaware that they— like younger children— are at risk of Reye's syndrome.

The overall news on Reye's syndrome is good. If treated early, most victims recover completely. Parents and physicians alike have become more familiar with Reye's syndrome and its symptoms. Still, about 15 percent of those who contract the illness suffer mental retardation, paralysis, or other neurological disorders. Parents need to know Reye's syndrome's symptoms and be on the alert.

—*Bill Rados*

Section 4.4

# How to Avoid the Flu

Source: Food and Drug Administration

Though flu is expected to make its usual rounds this winter, many Americans won't have to suffer its high fever, characteristic cough, and possibly serious complications. A safe, effective vaccine is available.

It was not always so.

In 1918-1919—during the worst flu epidemic of all time—doctors had meager resources to fight the disease. To relieve symptoms, they relied on aspirin and other simple remedies. An influenza vaccine and antibiotics to combat pneumonia and other flu complications were years away from development. It has been estimated that over 20 million people died and possibly half the world's population came down with the flu in this global epidemic, or pandemic.

Influenza epidemics spread quickly through large populations because flu viruses are highly contagious. During flu's acute phase, respiratory tract secretions are rich in infectious virus and the disease is transmitted easily by sneezing and coughing. The incubation period lasts one to three days. Then symptoms—such as chills and fever that develop within 24 hours, headache often accompanied by sensitivity to light, sore muscles, backache, weakness, and fatigue—appear suddenly. Respiratory tract symptoms may be mild at first with a dry, unproductive cough, scratchy sore throat, and runny nose. As the person's temperature rises— sometimes to as high as 104 degrees Fahrenheit—the muscle aches and headache get worse, and secondary bacterial infections, such as bronchitis and pneumonia, may move in. Ear infections are a common complication in children.

With no complications, acute symptoms usually subside after two or three days and the fever ends, although it may last as long as five days. Weakness and fatigue may persist for several weeks.

## Vaccine Most Important Defense

Today, we have several ways to defend people from influenza. The most important tool is immunization by a killed virus vaccine. Flu vaccines are licensed by FDA, and the exact composition of the vaccine varies each year, depending on the flu strains scientists expect to be most common.

Influenza viruses have the ability to change themselves, or mutate, thereby becoming different viruses. Having the flu once does not confer lasting immunity, as is the case with some childhood viral diseases. The antibodies people produce in response to the one flu virus don't recognize and, therefore, don't provide immunity to a different flu virus. Because the immunity conferred by a flu shot lasts for only about a year—and because different flu strains may circulate each season—individuals who want to be protected from flu should be vaccinated annually.

It takes two to four weeks for antibodies to develop after the vaccine is given. Therefore, the ideal time to get the flu vaccine is mid-October to mid-November, before the start of the flu season, which lasts from about December to March in the Northern Hemisphere. (Travelers should be aware that flu season lasts all year in some tropical climates, and in the Southern Hemisphere occurs from April to September.)

## Who Should Get the Vaccine?

Vaccination is available to anyone who wants it and whose doctor agrees it would be beneficial. The Public Health Service's Advisory Committee on Immunization Practices (ACIP) strongly recommends vaccination for:

**People age 65 or older.** (Effective May 1993, Medicare Part B pays for flu shots.)

**People over 6 months who have underlying medical conditions** that put them at increased risk for flu complications. These include:

- chronic cardiovascular disorders or lung disease, including asthma in children

- chronic metabolic diseases requiring hospitalization during the preceding year or regular checkups. These diseases include diabetes, kidney disorders, blood disorders, and impaired immune systems due to HIV infection or chemotherapy.

- Residents of nursing homes and other facilities that provide care for chronically ill persons of any age.

- Children and teenagers (6 months to 18 years of age) who have to take aspirin regularly and therefore may be at risk of developing Reye's syndrome after influenza. (Children who have symptoms of flu or chickenpox should not be given products containing aspirin or other salicylates without consulting a doctor.)

To reduce the risk of transmitting flu to high-risk persons, such as the elderly, transplant patients, and people with AIDS (who may have low antibody response to the flu vaccine)—and also to protect themselves from infection—ACIP recommends vaccination for doctors, nurses, hospital employees, employees of nursing homes and chronic-care facilities, visiting nurses, and home-care providers. Students, police, fire-fighters, and other essential workers and community service providers may also find vaccination useful.

In most cases, children at high risk for influenza complications may receive the flu vaccine when they receive other routine vaccinations, including DTP (diphtheria, tetanus and pertussis) and pneumococcal vaccines. Pregnant women who have a high-risk condition should be immunized regardless of the stage of pregnancy; healthy pregnant women may also want to consult their health-care providers about being vaccinated.

## Side Effects

The flu vaccine cannot cause flu because it contains only inactivated viruses. Any respiratory disease that appears immediately after vaccination is coincidental. However, the vaccine may have some side effects, especially in children who have not been exposed to the flu virus in the past.

The most commonly reported side effect in children and adults is soreness at the vaccination site that lasts up to two days. Fever, malaise, sore muscles, and other symptoms may begin 6 to 12 hours after vaccination and may last as long as two days.

People should be aware that they may test HIV-positive with the ELISA test after a recent flu shot, says the national Centers for Disease Control and Prevention. CDC recommends retesting with the more accurate Western Blot test to rule out false positives.

The vaccine is not for everyone. People allergic to eggs—the vaccine is made from highly purified, egg-grown viruses that have been made noninfectious—or other vaccine components should consult a doctor before getting a flu shot because they may develop hives, allergic asthma, difficulty breathing, and other allergic symptoms. The vaccine should not be given to any person ill with a high fever until the fever and other symptoms have abated.

## Drugs Help Some People

For these individuals, and persons expected to develop low levels of antibodies in response to the influenza vaccine because they have impaired immune systems, influenza-specific anti-viral drugs can be used for prevention during the flu season or after infection to relieve influenza symptoms.

The anti-viral agents Symmetrel (amantadine), approved by FDA in 1976, and Flumadine (rimantadine), a chemically similar drug approved by FDA in September 1993, are safe and effective in preventing signs and symptoms of infection caused by various strains of the influenza A virus in children over 1, healthy adults, and elderly patients. These drugs may also be used for family members or close contacts of influenza A patients and for elderly nursing home patients who have been vaccinated but may need added protection. When a vaccine is expected to be ineffective because an epidemic is caused by strains other than those covered by the vaccine. anti-viral drugs may be used to provide protection.

Either drug may be used following vaccination during a flu epidemic to provide protection during the two to four week period before antibodies develop. If an adult has already come down with the flu, treatment with Symmetrel or Flumadine has been shown to reduce symptoms and shorten the illness if administered within 48 hours after symptoms appear. Children with the flu can be treated with Symmetrel.

About 5 to 10 percent of people who take Symmetrel experience nausea, dizziness and insomnia. There have been reports of more serious neurological adverse events, including seizures and aggravations of psychiatric illnesses.

Flumadine has similar side effects, but at a lower rate.

Though many flu victims use over-the-counter preparations, such as decongestants and fever reducers, to make them feel more comfortable, none of these products affects the course of the disease.

## Prevention Worthwhile

Every year, about 20 percent of the U.S. population may become infected with flu, although each flu season is different. About 1 percent of those infected will require hospitalization because of complications, mostly bacterial pneumonia. Among those hospitalized, as many as 8 percent may die—about 20,000 people in an average year. But the 1957-1958 "Asian flu" caused 70,000 deaths, and the 1968-1969 "Hong Kong flu" carried off 34,000. The toll is usually greatest among the elderly.

The economic costs run high, too. From 15 million to 111 million workdays are lost each year, depending on the severity of the epidemic. Added to that are the costs of over-the-counter and prescription medicines, physician visits, hospitalization, and lost productivity.

It's no contest between the cost of a flu shot and the physical and other costs exacted by a bad case of the flu. A yearly vaccination early in the flu season is the best way to avoid this miserable disease.

## This Year's Vaccine

FDA's Vaccines and Related Biologicals Advisory Committee meets in late January each year to decide which strains of influenza virus should be incorporated into the vaccine for the coming flu season, based on reports from national and international surveillance systems. A World Health Organization panel meets in Geneva in mid-February to make final recommendations for the next season's flu vaccine.

The vaccine choices for the United States take into consideration the predominant strain(s) circulating among the population in the current season (November, December, January) and any "new" strains that may have appeared both here and in other parts of the world. Another important part of the decision process is the examination of antibody levels in people vaccinated with the current year's vaccine to determine if they had a good immune response. Equally important is examining antibody levels in the same people to see if the vaccine offered any protection against recently identified "new" strains.

"You have to make this decision [about which strains to include in the vaccine] a year in advance before the flu season starts," says Helen Regnery, Ph.D., chief, strain surveillance section, influenza branch, national Centers for Disease Control and Prevention. "There is an inherent problem; FDA's advisory committee must decide for a future event, based on past and current knowledge of circulating strains, as well as the appearance of new strains of influenza."

Flu viruses are divided into three types—A, B and C—though the C type is not common. Influenza A viruses cause the most severe and widespread outbreaks, while influenza B causes limited, milder illness.

Influenza A viruses are classified into subtypes on the basis of two surface antigens (substances that induce antibody formation) called hemagglutinin (H) and neuraminidase (N). Currently, the circulating subtypes of influenza A that have been identified as causing extensive human illness are influenza A (H3N2) and influenza A (H1N1). Influenza A (H3N2) viruses have been much more prevalent than influenza A (H1N1) during the last five years.

"Last year's flu season [1993-1994] was more severe than average," says Nancy Arden, chief, influenza epidemiology, CDC. "More than 99 percent of the influenza viruses isolated and characterized were type A(H3N2) and most were similar to the A/Beijing/32/92 strain. Although people of all ages are susceptible to type A(H3N2), compared with influenza type A (H1N1) and type B, the A(H3N2) viruses are associated with more illness, complications and deaths among the elderly."

The 1993-1994 influenza season began in November 1993 and peaked in late December 1993 and early January 1994. By early March, influenza activity was undetectable or had declined to very low levels in most of the United States. As in other seasons when the A(H3N2) strains have predominated, the proportion of influenza associated deaths was higher than average. Although it is still too early to estimate the actual number of such deaths during the 1993-1994 season, normally about 90 percent of these deaths occur among people 65 and older.

The trivalent influenza vaccine prepared for the 1994-1995 flu season will include A/Texas/36/91 (H1N1), A/Shangdong/9/93 (H3N2), and B/Panama/45/90, differing from the 1993-1994 vaccine only in the H3N2 component, which was A/Beijing/32/92 last season. The geographic name represents the place where the strain was isolated.

— *Evelyn Zamula*

Chapter 5

# Cystic Fibrosis

*Chapter Contents*

Section 5. 1—An Introduction to Cystic Fibrosis
    For Patients and Families ................................................. 240
Section 5. 2—Living with Cystic Fibrosis:
    Family Guide to Nutrition ................................................. 271
Section 5. 3—Teacher's Guide to CF ............................................. 291
Section 5. 4—Introduction to Chest Physical Therapy ............. 294
Section 5. 5—CF Gene: A Fifty-Year Search ............................. 315
Section 5. 6—Cystic Fibrosis: Tests, Treatments
    Improve Survival ................................................................. 320
Section 5. 7—FDA Licenses Cystic Fibrosis Treatment ............ 330
Section 5. 8—CF and DNA Tests: Implications of
    Carrier Screening ................................................................. 331

## Section 5.1

# An Introduction to Cystic Fibrosis for Patients and Families

Source: Cystic Fibrosis Foundation  Pub. No. N855B-3/93  PB480. Used by permission.

### What is Cystic Fibrosis?

Cystic fibrosis (usually called CF) is an inherited disease which causes glands in the body to fail to function normally. The affected glands are the exocrine (outward secreting) glands.

The exocrine glands normally produce thin, slippery secretions including sweat, mucus, tears, saliva, and digestive juices. These secretions are carried through ducts (small tubes) to the external surface of the body, or into hollow organs like the intestines or the airways. The exocrine glands and their secretions play an important part in maintaining the normal functions of the body.

In CF, the mucus-producing exocrine glands often produce thick, sticky secretions. These secretions may plug up ducts and other passageways. Mucus plugs most often occur in the lungs and intestines and can interfere with vital body functions, such as breathing and digestion.

The sweat glands are also affected in CF. The amount of salt (sodium and chloride) and potassium in the sweat is abnormally high. This may cause problems during periods of increased sweating.

These *exocrine* glands should not be confused with *endocrine* glands. Endocrine (inward secreting) glands produce hormones that pass into the bloodstream. They are usually not directly affected in CF.

### What CF Is Not

Many people have mistaken ideas about CF. It is important that you know what these common misconceptions are:

**CF is not contagious.** Because coughing is a frequent symptom of CF, many people are afraid that they might "catch" CF. CF is an in-

## Cystic Fibrosis

herited disorder. It is present at birth; no one "catches" CF. (More about how you get CF later.) You cannot catch CF, and you cannot give it to anyone else.

**CF is not caused by anything the mother or father did or did not do, before or during pregnancy.** Parents often feel responsible for everything that happens to their children. When their child is diagnosed with CF, many parents suffer feelings of guilt and responsibility. It is important that you understand that nothing you did during pregnancy caused this disease.

**CF does not impair intellectual ability.** People sometimes confuse CF with "CP" (cerebral palsy). Cystic fibrosis does not involve the brain and does not impair intellectual ability at all.

**CF is not curable at this time.** But with today's improved treatments, most people with CF grow up and lead active, productive lives. And a tremendous amount of time, energy, and money is being directed at finding new and better ways of treating CF, and at finding a cure.

### Is CF a New Disease?

Cystic fibrosis is not a new disease. Printed references as early as 1705 suggest that there were children who probably had CF. "Cystic fibrosis of the pancreas" was first reported in a scientific paper in 1936 by Dr. Guido Fanconi of Switzerland. The first comprehensive report of CF as a separate disease was written by Dr. Dorothy Andersen at Babies and Children's Hospital in New York City in 1938. Since that time, there has been an explosion of information and knowledge about CF.

### How Common Is CF?

CF is one of the most common inherited disorders of Caucasians (whites). CF occurs in about one of every 2,000 live-born Caucasian babies. It occurs in about one of every 17,000 black babies. CF is rare in Orientals and Native Americans. But CF does affect virtually every race. The disease occurs equally in male and female babies. In the United States, about 2,000 babies are born with CF every year.

There are about 30,000 people with CF in the U.S. today. The total number is increasing as more children are correctly diagnosed, treated earlier and living much longer.

### Genes, Chromosomes, and How Your Child Got CF

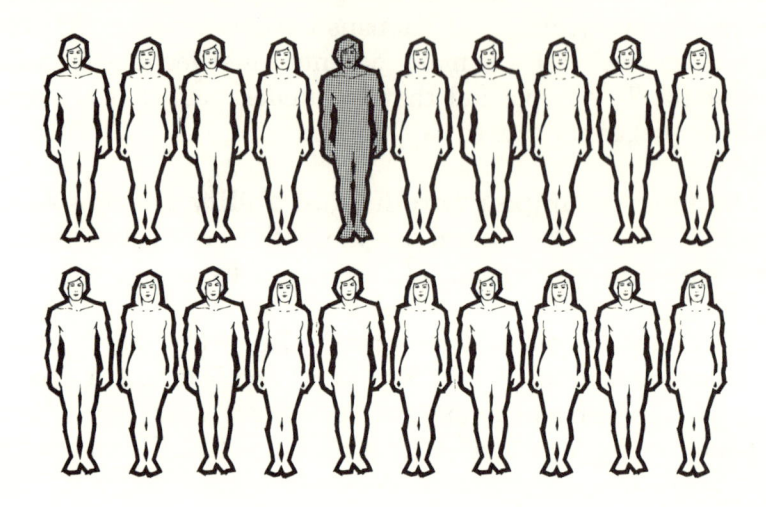

*Figure 5.1. One person in 20 carries the CF gene*

In the United States, about one person in every 20 carries the gene for CF. That means about 12 million people have the CF gene!

People who carry the CF gene have no symptoms typical of CF. In general, we can only detect some of these gene "carriers" at this time. Research is going on now to develop a test for all carriers.

Every child with CF was born with CF. It is an inherited (hereditary) disorder that begins at the moment of conception. The child's age when symptoms begin, the type of symptoms that occur, and the severity of the disease itself vary greatly from child to child.

For some children, the lungs are most affected. For others, the digestive system may have more problems. But the problems of CF may show up at any time. Despite the fact that it may take a while for the problems to appear, the disease actually begins at conception.

Conception occurs when the egg from the mother unites with the sperm from the father. Both the egg and the sperm contain thousands of genes. Genes are the basic units of heredity and determine physical and chemical characteristics such as eye and hair color, how tall the person will be, facial features, and many health conditions. Every person probably carries seven to eight genes which could be associated with serious health problems. CF is one such health problem. Genes are carried on chromosomes, the thread-like structures found in the nucleus of every cell in the body. Each chromosome carries thousands of different genes.

These genes are always present in pairs. Each parent gives one gene from his or her pair to make up a new pair for the child. In this way, genes pass on family characteristics from one generation to the next.

It is very important that you understand that parents cannot control which genes are passed on to their children.

### CF Is an "Autosomal Recessive" Disease

*Autosomal* means that the CF gene is not carried on the sex chromosome, so both male and female babies can get CF. Recessive means that, if the CF gene is paired with a normal gene, the normal gene will dominate (the CF gene will be recessive) and the person will not have cystic fibrosis. This person will, however, be a carrier of the CF gene.

So a carrier is a person with one CF gene and one normal gene, which dominates the recessive CF gene. A carrier has no symptoms and no disease.

When both parents are carriers and each contributes a CF gene, there is no dominant normal gene and the baby will be born with CF.

Both parents of a child with CF are carriers of a single CF gene. They inherited this gene from one of their parents, who in turn inherited the gene from one of their parents. Because the gene is common (remember, one in 20 Caucasian Americans carries the gene), marriages between carriers occur frequently (about one in every 400 marriages). And since a carrier has no symptoms of CF, we usually do not know the person is a carrier until he or she becomes the parent of a child with CF.

Remember, every child with CF got genes for this disease from both the mother and father. Therefore, CF genes are present on both sides of the family.

### More About the CF Gene

The specific gene responsible for CF has been identified. As you have learned, genes are the basic units of heredity. Genes are made up of small building blocks called base pairs. What makes the CF gene abnormal is a mutation, or change in the genetic material, resulting in a substitution or loss of one of the building blocks. Several different mutations can occur in the CF gene and new ones are still being discovered. Scientists are now actively studying the effects of this gene. Identifying the CF gene has been a big step toward understanding how and why this gene causes cystic fibrosis, and will be of great assistance in treating or curing the medical problems of CF.

### *Can CF Carriers Be Identified?*

At the present time, carriers of the cystic fibrosis gene can usually be determined if a family member has CF. This is done by testing the blood of the CF patient and identifying the specific mutation, or change, in the CF gene. The other family member's blood can then be tested for this same mutation to determine if he or she is a carrier.

Identifying carriers of the cystic fibrosis gene in the general public is more difficult. The currently known mutations can be looked for, but it would be impossible to know whether or not the person was a carrier of a different, as yet undiscovered, mutation. Therefore, routine screening of the general public for carriers of the CF gene is not recommended.

### *Prenatal Diagnosis*

Some genetic and chromosomal conditions can be detected before birth. This can be done by amniocentesis (taking out a small amount of fluid surrounding the fetus and examining the fluid biochemically and microscopically) or by chorionic villus biopsy (taking out a small piece of the placenta to study).

Cells obtained by amniocentesis or chorionic villus biopsy are used to study chromosomes. In this manner the CF gene can be examined for known mutations. Also, it is now possible to diagnose CF prenatally by measuring certain proteins in the amniotic fluid. However, this test is not 100 percent accurate.

More information on the genetics of CF can be obtained from the Cystic Fibrosis Foundation (CFF).

## Cystic Fibrosis

### What About the Risk of CF in Future Pregnancies?

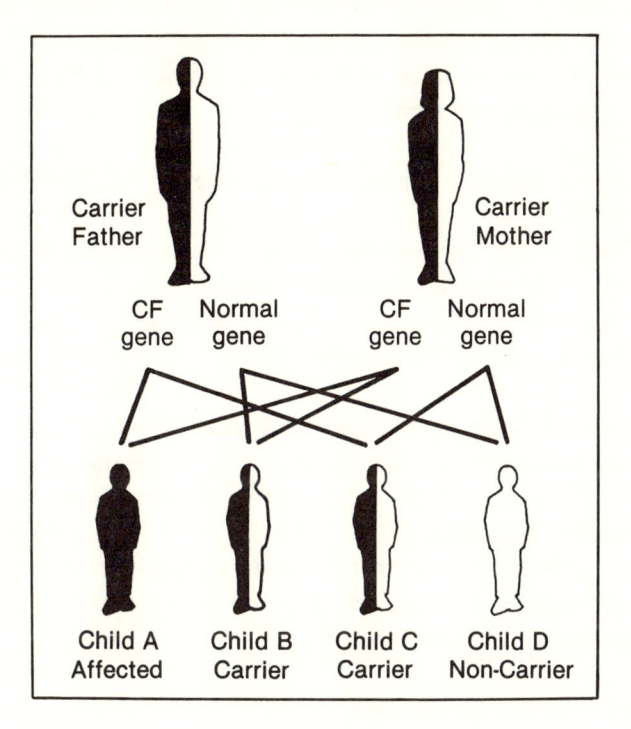

*Figure 5.2* The inheritance possibilities when both parents are carriers of the CF gene.

When both parents are carriers of the CF gene, their children will not automatically have CF. This is because the CF gene is carried by one-half of the father's sperm and by one-half of the mother's eggs.

This chart shows the possibilities when the egg and sperm of parents who carry the CF gene combine.

**Inheritance of CF.** The father's sperm with the CF gene can combine with the mother's egg that has the CF gene. This results in a child with two CF genes, so the child has cystic fibrosis.

A sperm without the CF gene can combine with an egg that has the CF gene, resulting in a child who is a carrier of the CF gene.

Another way for the child to become a carrier is when a sperm with the CF gene combines with an egg that does not have the gene.

If a sperm without the CF gene combines with an egg which also does not have the gene, the child does not inherit a CF gene from either parent, and will not be a carrier and will not have CF.

Therefore, when both parents are carriers of the CF gene, each and every pregnancy has a:

- One in four (25 percent) chance that the child will be born with CF.
- Two in four (50 percent) chance that the child will be a carrier of the CF gene but have no disease.
- One in four (25 percent) chance that the child will not carry the CF gene and not have CF.

**These odds apply to each pregnancy,** whether the parents already have children with CF or not. So a pregnancy that results in a child with CF does not mean that the next pregnancy will produce a child that does not have CF.

The egg and the sperm involved in fertilization are determined entirely by chance. There is no way to predict or control which genes will be passed on to your children.

*How Do CF Genes Cause CF?*

As you now know, CF is an inherited disease. But exactly how the CF gene causes the disease is not understood. In some unknown way, the CF gene causes problems in the mucous glands and the sweat glands.

**The sweat glands.** In CF, the sweat glands produce sweat that is much higher in salt content than normal. Perhaps the CF gene provides a faulty chemical pattern to the exocrine glands and causes their abnormal secretions. While we do not understand the exact mechanism, recent research indicates that an abnormality in the transport of certain ions—such as chloride ions—in cells exists in exocrine glands of CF patients. This abnormality is referred to as the "basic defect" in CF.

**The mucous glands.** Normal mucus is thin and slippery. In the airways, it helps to remove dust and germs so they cannot harm the lungs. It also lines the ducts and passageways of other organs, providing a lubricant.

In CF, mucus is thick and sticky and tends to block organ passageways. This blockage causes most of the symptoms of CF, and causes the two most serious aspects of CF:

- **Chronic lung disease.** At some point, virtually every person with CF develops chronic lung disease. It is the result of infections that develop when airways in the lungs are clogged by the thick mucous secretions.

- **Impaired digestion.** Digestive problems occur in about 85 percent of all people with CF. Thick mucous secretions block the flow of digestive enzymes from the pancreas into the intestines where the enzymes normally help to digest the food.

There is still a lot we don't know about cystic fibrosis and what causes it. But we have made tremendous strides in recent years. Scientists have recently identified the CF gene and are further defining the basic defect. These accomplishments will help us develop more effective prenatal diagnosis, easier identification of carriers, and better treatment.

### How CF Is Diagnosed

As with most diseases, the diagnosis of CF is based on the medical history, a physical examination, and laboratory tests.

**Medical History.** This is the patient's or family's "history" or description of the problems and symptoms. The medical history plays an important part in alerting the doctor to the possibility of CF, and guiding the doctor to an accurate diagnosis. And as you now know, CF is a hereditary disorder, so it is also important for the health-care team to get a medical history for each member of the family.

**Physical Examination.** The doctor must do a complete physical examination to look for signs of CF or other problems.

**Laboratory Tests.** Certain laboratory tests are necessary to confirm the diagnosis of CF and to look for effects of the disease in specific body organs. The sweat test is an important diagnostic test.

### When Does CF First Show Up?

As you have learned, CF is present at birth. However, the health problems caused by CF may not show up for a while. The time when symptoms caused by CF are first noticed varies greatly from person to person.

For most people with CF, the diagnosis is made in the first three years of life.

For a few people (about 10-15 percent of all people with CF) the earliest symptoms of CF show up at birth. These infants have an intestinal blockage called meconium ileus.

A few more babies with CF are identified before they develop symptoms-through routine screening done because there is a family history of CF.

Other children with CF do not develop symptoms until later in childhood or adolescence.

### What Are the Symptoms of CF?

Cystic fibrosis is a disease of many disguises. The exact symptoms and the severity of symptoms can vary greatly from person to person. And early CF symptoms are often similar to those of other childhood health problems. This can make CF difficult to diagnose. As a result, CF may often go undiagnosed—or misdiagnosed—for years.

Here is a list of the more common symptoms of CF:

- Recurrent wheezing
- Persistent cough and excessive mucus
- Recurrent pneumonia
- Failure to gain weight, often despite a good appetite
- Abnormal bowel movements (often chronic diarrhea; stools are frequent, bulky, greasy, and foul-smelling)
- Salty tasting skin
- Nasal polyps (small fleshy growths inside the nose)
- Clubbing (enlargement) of the fingertips and toes

None of these symptoms are unique to CF; they may appear in other illnesses. And, a person with CF may not have all of these symptoms. But when many of these symptoms are present, they provide clues to the doctor which help in making a prompt and accurate diagnosis.

## Cystic Fibrosis

Later, we will show how CF affects each organ system. You will learn what symptoms occur, why they occur, and how they are treated.

### The Sweat Test

CF is diagnosed by measuring the salt content in sweat. As you learned earlier, CF affects exocrine glands. The sweat gland is a type of exocrine gland. CF causes an abnormal amount of salt to be lost in the sweat. The total amount of sweat is usually normal, but the salt content is high. This characteristic is the basis for the test used to diagnose CF.

The sweat test is the simplest and most reliable method for diagnosing CF. Here is how the sweat test is done:

> A gauze pad or a piece of filter paper is placed on the child's forearm to collect sweat. Then the area—usually the arm or back—is wrapped in plastic. The sweat glands are stimulated to sweat using a harmless chemical called pilocarpine and a very small amount of electricity. (This is called pilocarpine iontophoresis. ) After several minutes, the plastic wrap is removed and the pad is sent to the laboratory for analysis.

If the child has CF, analysis of the sweat will show a high salt (sodium and chloride) level.

If the sweat test shows more than a normal amount of salt, the doctor will probably do a second sweat test to be certain of the diagnosis.

The sweat test is simple, painless, reliable, and inexpensive. However, to be accurate, it must be performed and interpreted correctly. The laboratory analysis requires specific procedures that must be done by experienced and trained technicians. So it is important to have the sweat test done by a medical laboratory that performs many of these tests each year.

### Other Facts About the Sweat Test

The sweat test can be used only to determine whether or not a person has CF. It cannot be used to predict how a patient will do or distinguish "mild" from more serious cases. There is no relationship between the salt level in the sweat and the severity of the disease.

The sweat test cannot be used for detection of carriers of the CF gene. Remember that carriers do not have CF themselves, so their sweat glands and sweat are normal.

## What About Testing Other Family Members?

Because of the genetic nature of CF, brothers and sisters of a child with CF should also be checked for the disease using the sweat test. This should be done whether or not symptoms of CF are present. Symptoms of CF can begin at different ages for different people.

In addition, any other family members (especially first cousins) should be checked with the sweat test if they have any of the symptoms of CF or if the family is worried.

## Testing Newborn Babies for CF

The sweat test may not work in newborns. Newborns often cannot produce enough sweat for a reliable test. Also, salt levels in the sweat of some babies that do not have CF may be high for the first few days of life. As a result, the sweat test is often not done until a baby is a few months old.

A method for screening newborns for CF has been developed. This method, called the immunoreactive trypsinogen test (IRT), is based on analysis of a blood sample usually obtained two to three days after birth. Positive tests are then confirmed by sweat testing. While widespread screening of all newborns remains controversial, this test may certainly be helpful to screen high risk infants (such as those with positive family histories of CF or meconium ileus) and to make difficult diagnoses.

## Remember

While the symptoms of CF may first appear at any age, most people have symptoms in the first few years of life. When symptoms appear, a sweat test is done to make a positive diagnosis of CF.

Because CF is inherited from the parents, brothers and sisters of a child with CF should also be tested.

Since both parents inherited CF genes from their parents, brothers and sisters of the parents may also carry the CF gene. So first cousins of the child should be tested if they have symptoms of CF.

As with any other disease, early diagnosis is important.

## The Respiratory System

Respiratory (breathing) problems are the most serious aspect of cystic fibrosis. Virtually every person with CF will eventually develop lung disease. Exactly when it occurs and just how severe it will be differs a lot from one person to another. But for most people with CF, lung disease is the factor that determines how well they function and how long they live. Normally, the germs and dust particles we inhale are trapped in the mucous layer and then carried up toward the throat where they can be coughed up or swallowed.

In CF, the mucus in the airways is thick and sticky. It traps particles, but it is so thick and sticky that the cilia cannot easily move the mucus to the throat. So instead of cleaning, the mucus itself clogs the breathing passages. When mucus blocks a small airway, it is called a mucous plug.

Mucous plugs keep air from getting into or out of some alveoli (air sacs), so they interfere with gas exchange.

The thick, sticky mucus in the small airways causes two problems:

- It can interfere with normal gas exchange by blocking the flow of air into and out of the alveoli.

- It makes removing particles and germs from the airways difficult. If not removed, the thick mucus and mucous plugs can lead to repeated lung infections and lung damage. Lung infections are especially dangerous to people with CF for two reasons:

- Repeated infections can damage the cilia and the airways, making them even less able to clear mucus, particles and germs from the lungs.

- Infections often cause more mucus to be produced. This can cause more mucous plugs and make an infection even harder to treat.

A cycle can develop that causes severe damage to the lungs. Mucous plugs block airways and provide an opportunity for germs to grow and spread infection. The lungs react by producing more mucus to clean the airways, but instead, the mucus blocks even more air passages. The infection spreads further and the cycle repeats itself.

Presumably because of this cycle, people with CF are very susceptible to certain types of lung infections. Two bacteria frequently cause lung infections in CF:

- Staphylococcus aureus (or simply Staph—pronounced "staff")
- Pseudomonas aeruginosa (or simply Pseudomonas—pronounced "soo-doe-mow-nas")

Often, it is not possible to completely remove these bacteria from the lungs. Chest physical therapy is used to help get rid of the thick secretions and make it easier to control the infection.

*The Symptoms*

Most of the respiratory symptoms of CF are caused by blockage of the airways with thick mucous secretions. There are many possible symptoms:

- Frequent or lingering cough
- Excessive sputum (phlegm) production
- Intermittent wheezing
- Repeated lung infections (frequent pneumonia or episodes of bronchitis)
- Difficulty breathing (or "catching" one's breath)
- Difficulty exercising

Indications of "flare-ups" or worsening of the lung disease include:

- An increase in cough and/or wheezing
- An increase in sputum production
- A decrease in exercise tolerance
- An increase in fatigue or feeling tired
- A barrel-shaped chest (due to air trapped in the lungs because airways are plugged)
- A decrease in lung function, as measured by pulmonary function tests (or "breathing" tests)
- Weight loss and/or poor appetite
- Fever (although fever is not always present during flare-ups)

## Tests

Your CF doctor learns a great deal by hearing your report of symptoms and how your child is feeling and acting. But sometimes your CF doctor may want to perform certain tests to get more specific information. There are four kinds of tests that help your CF doctor plan and follow the effectiveness of treatment.

**Chest X-ray.** The chest X-ray allows your doctor to look inside the lungs. It gives more information about how the disease may be affecting the lungs and helps to guide treatment decisions.

**Pulmonary Function Tests (breathing tests).** Your doctor may want to do one or more of these tests to measure how well the lungs are working. They provide information about any blockage of the bronchial tubes, and show how fast air can get into and out of the lungs. They also help the doctor evaluate changes in the lungs over a period of time. Pulmonary function tests are especially useful in making decisions about treatment, and measuring the success of treatment. However, it is difficult to do these breathing tests on infants and young children.

**Sputum Cultures (phlegm cultures).** These cultures check the sputum for evidence of an active infection in the lungs. A sample of mucus is placed in a dish that helps germs like staph and pseudomonas grow and multiply. Some time later, the dish is checked for these and other germs that can cause lung infections.

**Blood Test.** These are done periodically to identify other possible CF-related problems early on, so they can be treated before they become big health problems. A small sample of blood is usually taken with a syringe and then sent to a laboratory for testing.

## Treatment

Chronic (long-term) pulmonary disease is the most serious complication of CF. But for most people, proper therapy can slow down the damage to the lungs. The goal of treatment is to clear the airways of obstructions and to treat or prevent infections.

Because CF affects each person differently, treatment is designed specifically for the needs of each person. Your doctor will work with you to develop the best treatment plan for your situation.

There are four commonly used treatments for the lung problems of CF:

- Chest physical therapy
- Exercise
- Aerosols
- Antibiotics

**Chest Physical Therapy.** This is a form of physical therapy used to reduce and/or prevent blockage of the airways by the thick, sticky CF mucus. Some people call this chest physiotherapy.

Bronchial drainage (BD) is a specific component of chest physical therapy (CPT) that is frequently prescribed for people with CF. Bronchial drainage is also called postural drainage (PD) because the person lies in various positions (postures) that help to drain the thick mucus from the lungs.

In bronchial drainage, the child lies or sits in a position that allows a particular portion of the lung to drain toward the throat. With the aid of gravity, the thick mucus moves from the small airways into the larger airways where it can be coughed up more easily. At the same time, that region of the chest is usually percussed (clapped) and vibrated to help dislodge mucus and stimulate its movement. This is then repeated in different positions to drain different parts of the lung.

Parents, grandparents and older brothers and sisters can learn to help with bronchial drainage for regular home treatments. The positions to be used—as well as the frequency and duration of treatments—are tailored to your child's individual needs by your doctor. Most people with CF have these treatments done one to three times a day. Each bronchial drainage treatment takes about 20 to 30 minutes.

While it is usually more convenient to have another person to help with bronchial drainage, older people with CF can learn to perform effective chest physical therapy by themselves. Mechanical aids are also available, such as mechanical percussors (electric chest clappers) and vibrators. The Cystic Fibrosis Foundation provides a publication entitled *CHEST PHYSICAL THERAPY: Segmental Bronchial Drainage* which describes this therapy in greater detail.

**Exercise.** Physical exercise is important for all childen, and childen with CF are no exception. The child with CF should be allowed and encouraged to take part in exercises such as swimming, bicycling, running, sports and games. Most childen with CF can actively participate in almost any physical activity.

Exercise can be helpful in several ways:

- Exercise helps loosen mucus in the lungs so it can be coughed up more easily.

- Exercise stimulates coughing which helps clear the lungs.

- Exercise helps build up the strength and endurance of the breathing muscles.

- Exercise increases the general level of cardiovascular fitness (the strength of the heart muscle and breathing muscles).

Most doctors consider a regular exercise program very beneficial to their CF patients. Just remember, extra fluids and salt should be taken when exercising strenuously and when exercising in hot weather.

**Aerosols.** Aerosols are treatments in the form of a mist (made from liquid medication) which are inhaled through a mouthpiece or mask. Aerosol treatments are often combined with chest physical therapy to help clear mucus and secretions from the lungs.

Several types of medicine can be used in an aerosol treatment and inhaled into the lungs:

- **Bronchodilators**—widen the breathing tubes to make mucus removal and breathing easier. These are most often prescribed prior to chest physical therapy.

- **Mucolytics**—thin the mucus, making it easier to drain.

- **Decongestants**—reduce the swelling of the membranes that line breathing tubes.

- **Antibiotics**—help control infection. These are most often taken after chest physical therapy.

*These drugs are usually mixed with saline (a saltwater solution) and then turned into a mist that the person can breathe.*

**Antibiotics.** Antibiotics are drugs that kill infection-causing bacteria. Respiratory infections can occur frequently in CF, and antibiotics are an important part of the therapy. The type of antibiotic, how often it is taken, and over how long a time period it is taken vary for each person. Some people with CF need continuous antibiotics while others need antibiotics only to control flare-ups of infection. Your doctor will adjust antibiotic treatments to your child's individual needs.

Antibiotics can be given in three ways:

- *Oral antibiotics* are tablets or capsules that are swallowed.

- *Intravenous (IV) antibiotics* are liquid solutions that are put directly into the blood.

- *Aerosolized antibiotics* are liquids turned into a mist and inhaled.

Oral antibiotics are often used to treat mild flare-ups of lung infection. These are effective against staph and some other infections, but are not always effective against pseudomonas. Although oral antibiotics have not worked well against pseudomonas, new antibiotics are being developed that do work well. Your CF doctor will tell you if oral antibiotics are needed and which are best suited to your child's needs.

More serious lung infections may require intravenous (IV) antibiotics. There are several IV antibiotics which work well against pseudomonas and staph. A stay in the hospital is often part of this treatment, but many CFF care centers use home IV antibiotics with some of their patients.

Aerosolized antibiotics are generally those that do not work well when swallowed. An aerosol mist delivers the antibiotic directly into the airways. These antibiotics are still being studied to test the effectiveness of this type of treatment.

Bacteria sometimes develop resistance to certain antibiotics. For this reason, your doctor may change your child's antibiotics from time to time or use combinations of antibiotics.

## Cystic Fibrosis

*Prevention*

It is always better to prevent a health problem than to have to correct it after it has occurred. Immunizations are an important example of this. Your child should receive the usual childhood immunizations and an annual influenza (flu) shot. Many childhood illnesses and flu can affect the lungs, causing serious problems for the person with CF so prevention through immunizations is very important.

Like other children, your child should avoid unnecessary contact with anyone who has a cold or other contagious illness. But this does not mean that your child should be kept home from school or have activities limited because you are afraid your child will get sick or "catch something." It is just not possible to prevent exposure to all germs. Besides, your child's mental and emotional growth and development depend upon a normal, healthy interaction with the surrounding world.

**A special note about coughing.** Most people with CF cough frequently. Coughing helps to loosen mucus and to remove it from the air passages. This is a normal body defense mechanism. Coughing should always be encouraged. Your child should never be taught to suppress the cough or to be ashamed of it.

People tend to associate coughing with a contagious illness. It may take some effort on your part to educate the people around you. But remember, CF is not contagious! And since CF is not contagious, the cough is not spreading "CF germs" (there are no CF germs), so no one can catch CF in this way.

Cough suppressants should not be given to people with cystic fibrosis. Coughing is a healthy, natural mechanism for keeping the airways and lungs clear of excess mucus. If your child's cough becomes more frequent than usual, tell your doctor. It could mean there is an infection which should be treated while the child continues to cough effectively to help clear the lungs.

**A special note about climate.** The type of climate does not seem to affect CF. As long as the person with CF is receiving proper medical care, there is no reason to risk the social, emotional and financial hardships of moving just to avoid extremes of cold, heat or dampness.

**A special note about the upper respiratory tract.** CF also affects the upper respiratory tract—the nose and sinuses. While CF usually does not cause major problems there, two conditions may occur:

- Sinusitis
- Nasal polyps

Sinusitis occurs in most people with CF. The inflammation of the sinuses is caused by the thick, sticky mucus blocking the sinuses. This blockage may lead to sinus infections. Sinusitis can usually be treated by antihistamines and decongestants to open the sinuses, and by antibiotics to control infections. In rare severe cases, sinus irrigation (flushing) or other treatment may be needed.

Nasal polyps are small, fleshy growths inside the nose. These are less common than sinusitis. We are not sure what causes these polyps, but we think they are due to problems with the mucous glands in the nose. Most of the time they do not require treatment. If they cause nasal blockage or other problems, then special medications or surgical removal may be necessary.

*Possible Complications*

The effects of cystic fibrosis on the respiratory system may cause complications. Possible complications include:

**Clubbing.** Clubbing is an enlargement or rounding of the tips of the fingers and toes. It eventually occurs in nearly all people with CF. We do not know the exact cause, but it appears with the development of lung disease. Clubbing can change with pulmonary flare-ups and treatment, but it is not a reliable sign of the severity of lung disease. Clubbing also occurs in people born with heart disease and in people with other types of lung disease.

**Bronchiectasis.** In nearly all people with CF, the walls of the airways eventually become inflamed and damaged. This damage causes the airways (bronchi) to become stretched and floppy, a condition called bronchiectasis. This makes it more difficult to clear the mucus, particles and germs from the airways. It also causes a change in breathing patterns. Chest physical therapy and an effective cough help clear these floppy portions of the airways.

## Cystic Fibrosis

**Pneumothorax.** Pneumothorax is a rupture or break in lung tissue or airways that allows air to escape from the lung. This air becomes trapped between the lung and chest wall. As more air escapes, it may cause a partial or total collapse of a lung, and cause breathing difficulty. Pneumothorax occurs in about 4 percent of people with CF. In mild pneumothorax, the air may re-enter the lung and not require medical treatment, or require only oxygen therapy. Some cases require medical treatment to drain the trapped air and allow the lung to expand. For a few people, surgery is necessary to prevent pneumothorax from occurring again.

**Hemoptysis.** Hemoptysis means to cough up blood. In CF it may appear as small blood streaks in the sputum. This does not require any special medical care. It is caused by minor bleeding from the lining of an airway. This lining may become inflamed and more easily damaged. The thick, sticky mucus can then scrape or tear the lining and cause a small amount of bleeding. Less commonly, hemoptysis may occur when an artery ruptures and sends blood into an airway. This more serious type of hemoptysis may require medical therapy or surgery.

**Cor Pulmonale.** Extensive lung damage may cause the right side of the heart to become thicker and larger, a condition called cor pulmonale. The lung damage reduces gas exchange in the lungs, so less oxygen gets into the blood. To get the oxygen the body needs, the heart must work harder to circulate more blood through the lungs. At the same time, lung damage may increase the blood pressure of arteries going from the heart to the lungs. This also makes the heart work harder to pump blood to the lungs. The strain on the heart causes the right side of the heart to become larger. Cor pulmonale is treated by chest physical therapy to improve lung function. Supplemental oxygen and diuretics (medicines to get rid of extra fluid) may also help.

*Remember*

Your doctor is in the best position to know what kind of treatment your child needs at any given time. The effect of CF on the respiratory system will be different for each child, so treatment for CF may be different from one child to the next. Your child's treatment will also change as his/her condition changes and as newer methods of treatment are developed.

Your doctor is also the best source of information on any special precautions you need to take.

With good, comprehensive care, most people with CF can lead active and productive lives for long, long periods of time.

## Psychosocial Aspects of CF

CF is a serious chronic illness. Like any other chronic illness, CF can cause social, emotional, and psychological problems. This chapter will discuss some of these problems and offer suggestions on how to deal with them.

### Emotional Impact of CF

The diagnosis of cystic fibrosis showers a family with a whole host of feelings and emotions. These include:

- Concern—for the child's well-being
- Worry—about the future
- Guilt—for having a child who inherited this serious disease from his/her parents
- Fear—of the unknown (How will I cope? How sick will my child be? How long will my child live?)
- Anger—that this has happened to them
- Resentment—for the time and attention that the CF child requires

All of these feelings are perfectly normal. But it is important that you recognize them so that you can work through them. Talking openly about your feelings with your family, friends, and your health-care team can help.

### Your Child's Development

CF may cause problems that add to the already complicated process of normal childhood development. As with any chronic illness, how these problems are handled helps determine what other problems may arise in the future.

Several rules of thumb may help you in guiding your child's emotional and psychosocial development:

- Treat your child as normally as possible.
- Avoid being overly protective.
- Encourage your child to become self-reliant as he/she gets older.

All parents want to shelter and protect their children. It is important, however, for children to experience normal life events to grow up normally and be well-adjusted. Mental and physical health are closely related, so try not to be overly protective of your child. This brings up several issues which deserve special mention.

*Physical Activities*

Encourage your child to be as active as possible. Playing with other children makes him/her feel like a part of the group, and exercise stimulates coughing, which is a good way to clear mucus from the airways.

**Babysitters.** Time spent with a babysitter can be helpful to both you and your child. It will expose your child to a new and very normal experience and will provide you with an opportunity to get out of the house. Just do as you would with any child; instruct the babysitter about your child's special needs and leave a number where you can be reached.

**Nursery School.** Nursery school offers your child the chance to play and learn with other children of the same age. Very young children with CF should probably avoid day-care centers and nursery schools during outbreaks of viral infections such as the flu.

**Spending the Night Away.** Spending the night at a friend's house is fun and rewarding for children. If need be, chest physical therapy can be done before the child leaves home, but arrangements should be made for taking enzyme supplements or other regular medications.

*What About Discipline?*

Many parents of children with CF express a concern about discipline. Many are hesitant or even feel guilty about disciplining their child. But discipline is necessary for any child (including the child with CF) to be well adjusted and psychologically healthy.

It is important that you apply the same discipline and behavioral standards to all children in the family. If you have other children that do not have CF, they may resent what they see as special treatment for the child with CF.

Occasionally, your child may refuse treatments. Explain how necessary the treatments are to his/her health. Then, make treatments pleasant and fun by playing music or games or watching television during the treatments.

## *Education*

All children should be taught about CF as soon as they are able to understand. What you say to your child depends on his/her age, personality, and ability to understand. If you have questions, ask a member of your health-care team for guidance.

It is also very important to teach your other children and other members of the household about CF. They need to understand why the child with CF receives special attention.

## *The Teenager and Young Adult*

When your child gets older, he/she will begin to experience some of the special problems of the adolescent or young adult with CF. Two problems can be especially difficult: embarrassment at being different and resentment of dependency.

**Embarrassment at Being Different.** Teenagers with CF may be self-conscious about their cough. They may be shorter or thinner than their classmates. They may tire more easily during physical activity. They may have to take medications or treatment at school.

Your teenager's embarrassment can be eased if he/she understands what CF is, how it causes these problems, and why the treatments and medications are necessary. It will help a great deal if he/she understands and can explain to friends that the cough is not contagious and helps to clear the lungs; that medicines help to digest food, fight respiratory infection, or provide necessary vitamins. Removing the mystery will go a long way toward acceptance and understanding.

## Cystic Fibrosis

**Resentment of Dependency.** Teenagers and young adults want independence. They may rebel against schedules, treatments, medications, and limitations.

It is normal for adolescents to want to be independent of their parents. Learning independence and responsibility is an important part of growing up. Try to be patient, understanding, and flexible. Encourage your child to assume more responsibility for his/her own care as soon as possible.

Adolescence is a difficult time of life for anyone. For an individual with a chronic disease like CF, there are extra problems regarding education, achieving independence, sexual and social maturity, and career planning. The health-care team can help your teenager prepare for and deal with these problems of adolescence.

### *The Adult*

As CF patients are living longer and healthier lives, new issues develop relating to marriage, independent living, family planning and financial concerns. While the very existence of these issues represents a triumph for the adult with CF, they can, nonetheless, be difficult to deal with while managing a chronic illness. It is our hope and goal that many people with CF will be able to settle comfortably into an adult lifestyle. mixing good health care with independence, marriage, family and career. Your CFF care center will have special skills and resources to help you deal with these issues.

### *Siblings*

Remember that brothers and sisters of a child with CF may feel they are being ignored or left out because of the extra attention given to the child with CF. Be sure to explain why you are spending extra time with your CF child. And try to give your other children their own special times.

Often, siblings want to be included in providing care to the child with CF. Many older children become very protective of their brother or sister with CF and take responsibility for monitoring the child's needs and health.

## The Public

Despite the relatively common occurrence of cystic fibrosis, most people remain surprisingly uninformed about CF. This may make things a bit harder for you, as you may have to answer many questions from friends, family, and others about CF and your child. Think of each question as an opportunity to educate someone about CF and to promote the efforts for finding better treatments and a cure.

The Cystic Fibrosis Foundation and health-care professionals across the country are also actively trying to educate the public about CF.

## Financial Services

The medicines and home-care equipment for a child with CF can be quite expensive. Most states provide some type of financial assistance. Eligibility and the amount of support available frequently vary according to family income. Different types of help are available at the national, state, and local levels.

State-sponsored assistance is often given through the "Children with Special Health Needs" program, formerly known as "Crippled Children's Services" (this program may go by different names in different states). The Social Security Administration also has programs that may help.

You can get information about financial services from the social services department of your local hospital, your state health department, or the CFF care center nearest you.

## Remember

Even though CF affects a person physically and emotionally, people with CF can and do lead happy, active and fulfilling lives.

## The Future

Cystic fibrosis was first described in 1938. At first, nearly all children with CF were thought to die in the first six months of life. By the mid-1950's the median survival age was still just five years (meaning that about half of the people with CF lived to age five or older). By 1966, the median life expectancy for a person with CF was 11 years.

## Cystic Fibrosis

Due to rapid improvements in diagnosis and methods of treatment, the length and quality of life has greatly improved. Today, more than half of all people with CF live into their late 20's or older! Many are living into their 40's and 50's, and a few are over 60 years of age. Constant improvements in diagnosis and therapy, as well as careful follow up, are increasing the quality and length of life each year.

Because of the wide variation in the severity of the disease, it is not possible to predict the outlook for any specific individual with CF. But you have every reason to look to the future with optimism!

### *Research*

Researchers have made tremendous advances in understanding CF and developing better treatments. Here are a few important areas where researchers are making breakthroughs.

**Identifying the CF Gene.** Genetic researchers have located the gene that causes CF and have learned a great deal about what is wrong with the gene and how it causes CF. Additionally, in laboratories, scientists have replaced the defective gene in cells taken from CF patients. These discoveries are helping researchers better understand CF. This knowledge will lead to the development of new and better treatments for the disease. It already provides great hope for a cure. Finding the gene makes more effective prenatal diagnosis possible and allows detection of carriers of the gene.

**Improved Treatment Methods.** Many research studies are underway to find new and more effective antibiotics, new methods of chest physical therapy and new vaccines to help prevent dangerous infections. Other studies are investigating the importance of improved nutrition, exercise and muscle-training programs. Still others are looking at the role of medications (steroids and other anti-inflammatory drugs) that might slow the rate of lung damage in CF. Medications, such as amiloride, are being studied to try to thin the mucus in CF so that it does not block air passages. Several other agents, such as DNase and protease inhibitors, are being investigated for effectiveness in "digesting" or breaking up the thick, sticky mucus. Lastly, gene therapy may hold great promise as a cure for CF. As mentioned earlier, scientists have already been successful in the laboratory at inserting the normal gene in CF cells and correcting the basic defect.

**Heart-Lung and Double-Lung Transplants.** In recent years, both heart-lung transplants and double-lung transplants have become treatment options for some patients with severe lung disease. While these remain serious and complicated procedures, the growing success rate has made them a viable alternative for some people with CF and has helped these individuals to resume their roles in society.

*Remember*

Cystic fibrosis is a serious but far from hopeless disease. Early diagnosis, improved treatment, and careful follow up have greatly improved the outlook in recent years. With proper care, most people with CF are reaching adulthood and leading happy and productive lives. And we are learning more and more about CF—almost on a daily basis! We believe there is good reason to be optimistic about the future.

## The Health-Care Team

Care for the person with cystic fibrosis is complex and requires a comprehensive team approach for each individual. With the large number of people involved on the CF health-care team, patients and families can get confused about "who's who" and "who does what." The following is a brief description of each member of the CF health-care team.

*The CF Doctor*

The CF doctor heads up the health-care team that cares for people with CF. This physician provides directed patient care and teaches the family and the person with CF about the disease. The CF doctor also teaches other physicians, other health professionals, and the public about CF. He/she may also be involved in CF-related research. Your CF doctor will work closely with your pediatrician or family doctor to provide the best care for your child.

The CF doctor is the primary contact with the family and is directly responsible for diagnosis and treatment. The physician also acts as the coordinator of the health-care team and works with:

- The nurse—to direct day-to-day care

- The physical and respiratory therapist—to plan and carry out a respiratory-care program

- The dietician/nutritionist—to ensure proper diet and nutrition for the person with CF

- The social worker—to assure the child's and family's emotional well-being and help with other psychosocial issues

If your child is cared for at a CFF care center that has training programs, several other people may occasionally accompany your CF doctor. These may include physicians or medical students who are learning about CF and how best to treat the disease.

### Other Doctors

**Fellow.** A fellow is a physician who has completed medical school and residency and is obtaining sub-specialty training. In CFF care centers, this person is usually a pediatrician who is now sub-specializing in cystic fibrosis and diseases of the lungs. After several years of specialized training in CF and related conditions, the fellow often goes to another CFF care center where he/she will become the CF doctor for other people with CF.

**Resident.** A resident is a physician who has completed medical school, received a medical degree, and is obtaining specialty training (for example specialty training in pediatrics).

**Medical Student.** A medical student is studying to become a physician. These students may be learning about diagnosing illnesses and caring for patients, and learning how to evaluate and report about a patient's condition and progress.

In all cases, these other doctors are directly supervised by the primary or "attending" CF doctor.

### Other Team Members

The other important members of the health-care team include:

- Nurses
- Physical and Respiratory Therapists

- Dieticians/Nutritionists
- Social Workers

**Nurses.** Nurses in CFF care centers frequently specialize in CF care. The CF nurse plays a crucial role in coordinating the health-care team's daily activities. Besides providing direct patient care, the nurse works with the physician and:

- Helps coordinate and carry out health-care plans

- Facilitates communication between the health-care team and the patient and family

- Alerts other team members to psychological, social, and economic problems

- Educates the patient, the family, the public, and other health-care workers

- Acts as a source of support for the patient and family

**Physical and Respiratory Therapists.** Physical and respiratory therapists have direct responsibility for the respiratory care of people with CF. In the hospital, therapists usually provide direct care to patients, including chest physical therapy, bronchial drainage, and aerosol treatments. Therapists also instruct patients and families in how to do these treatments themselves at home. The respiratory therapist is also responsible for care and use of equipment such as nebulizers, compressors, and oxygen delivery systems. The therapist may also have direct responsibility for performing pulmonary function tests (breathing tests).

**Dieticians/Nutritionists.** Dieticians or nutritionists teach parents and patients the special importance of nutrition for a person with CF. These individuals provide information about:

- Special predigested baby formulas
- Supplemental vitamins
- High-calorie, high-protein diets
- Correct use of pancreatic enzymes supplements
- Use of dietary supplements

**Social Workers.** Social workers help the person with CF and the family deal with the social, emotional, and psychological impact of CF. The social worker helps to:

- Enhance communication between the family and the health-care team
- Teach the family ways to cope with the stress of chronic illness
- Obtain financial assistance for the family
- Prepare adolescents and young adults for independent living
- Identify stress within the family that may need professional attention

This team approach to health care may be confusing at first because many people are involved. But everyone is working together with a common goal—the best care possible!

## The Cystic Fibrosis Foundation

The Cystic Fibrosis Foundation (CFF) is a nonprofit organization dedicated to funding research to find a cure for cystic fibrosis and improving the quality of life for people with the disease. The Foundation works toward these goals in four areas:

- Research
- Medical Care
- Public Policy
- Education

### Research

Research is the Foundation's primary concern. Through its innovative approaches to cystic fibrosis research, there has never been a time of greater optimism for those fighting CF. Every day brings us one step closer to finding a cure.

The Foundation supports research in several ways. A network of CFF research centers, located at leading universities and medical schools around the country, is devoted exclusively to studying cystic fibrosis. Scientists at these centers work together, sharing ideas and information so the mysteries of CF can be resolved as quickly as possible.

The Foundation also offers a substantial number of research grants to the medical community. These grants range from student traineeships, which are available to undergraduate and graduate students in biomedical sciences as an introduction to the field of cystic fibrosis research, to research scholar awards, which encourage already established scientists to continue their studies of CF.

*Medical Care*

Medical care for those with CF is available through more than 120 CFF accredited care centers across the country. Doctors and other CF specialists at the centers are dedicated to providing the best care and treatment for those with cystic fibrosis. In addition, many care centers provide families with both educational and emotional support.

Through the newly created CFF Home Health and Pharmacy Services, the Foundation is saving money for people with CF while providing quality health-care services. The mail-order pharmacy stocks CF medications and ships them across the country, saving its members thousands of dollars. Call 1-800-541-4959 for details.

The Foundation's Home Health Services arranges quality nursing care with people who understand the special needs of individuals with CF. Providing medications and home care at a tremendous savings, CFF Home Health Services is already helping many people with CF. For details, call 1-800-342-6967.

*Public Policy*

Through its public policy programs, the Foundation provides information for governmental agencies and legislators on the national, state, and local levels and encourages them to devote their resources toward fighting cystic fibrosis.

The goals of the Foundation's public policy programs include increased funding for research, reducing the barriers to health care faced by many people with CF, and improving the educational and career opportunities for adults with CF.

*Education*

Education is carried out at levels for both the medical profession and the consumer. The Foundation supports training of medical students and residents at CFF care centers and sponsors conferences on

CF for scientists, physicians, and care-givers. For people with CF, their families, and the general public, the Foundation also produces a variety of publications including *Commitment*, a national newspaper devoted to supplying the most recent information about CF, *Consumer Fact Sheet*, which addresses financing care and topics affecting adults with CF, and brochures which cover specific topics regarding CF and the Foundation's programs.

In these ways, the Cystic Fibrosis Foundation is fighting for a bright future for everyone with cystic fibrosis.

If you'd like more information about the Foundation, any of its programs, or how to reach your local chapter, contact the Foundation Office at:

Cystic Fibrosis Foundation
6931 Arlington Road
Bethesda, Maryland 20814
Telephone: 1-800-FIGHT CF (outside Maryland)
OR 301-951-4422 (inside Maryland)

—*James C. Cunningham, M.D;*
*and Lynn M. Taussig, M.D.*

Section 5.2

## Living with Cystic Fibrosis: Family Guide to Nutrition

Source: McNeil Pharmaceutical Pub. No. N062A. Used by permission.

### Introduction

Cystic fibrosis (CF) is the most prevalent chronic, hereditary disease in the Caucasian population, occurring in one of 2,000 births. Cases of CF have been reported in Black Americans, Japanese, and American Indians, as well.

CF is characterized by impaired function of certain of the body's glands, resulting in recurrent lung disease, abnormal digestion, and elevated sweat salt concentration. However, great variation exists in the severity of CF among patients. Better treatments and earlier diagnosis are continually improving the outlook for people with CF.

Since nutritional deficits caused by poor digestion may occur at an early age in children with CF, it is important that proper nutrition be provided, starting at the time of diagnosis and continuing throughout life, as part of the daily routine. Good nutrition is vital to people with CF to prevent malnutrition, foster normal growth and weight gain, and help prevent lung problems.

Good nutrition for a child or adult with CF, however, means more than just eating a balanced, normal diet. A high-calorie diet without restriction on fat intake is recommended, along with pancreatic enzymes to control digestive symptoms.

## What Should You Eat to Stay Healthy?

Hardly a day goes by without someone telling us what we should and should not eat. The media gives us lots of advice, but much of it is confusing.

Some of the confusion exists because we do not know enough about nutrition to recommend a "perfect diet" for each individual. Nevertheless, dietary guidelines have been developed and, when followed, assure us that our nutritional needs may be met. However, no guideline can guarantee health and well-being. Health depends on many things, including heredity, lifestyle, personality traits, mental health and attitudes, and environment, in addition to diet.

While food alone cannot make you healthy, good eating habits can help keep you healthy and even improve your health. These guidelines are suggested for most Americans and will probably apply to some members of your family. People with certain conditions such as cystic fibrosis have special dietary requirements, which are covered later.

**Eat a variety of foods to assure yourself an adequate diet.** The human body requires more than 40 different nutrients for good health. Most foods contain several nutrients, but no single food supplies all the essential nutrients in the amounts that are needed. Therefore, eat a variety of foods selected from the major food groups as outlined in the Food Guide Pyramid (see figure 5.3).

**Maintain desirable body weight.** Obesity is associated with many chronic disorders such as high blood pressure, increased levels of cholesterol, heart disease, strokes, and certain cancers. Maintaining desirable body weight is, therefore, important. In order to lose weight, caloric intake must be decreased. A weight loss of one to two pounds a week is safe. Do not try to lose at a rate any faster than this. Avoid crash diets that severely restrict the variety of foods allowed, and keep in mind that exercising will help you burn off those calories. Conversely, do not attempt to reduce your weight below the desirable range. Severe weight loss may be associated with nutritional deficiencies. Establish your desirable weight and work at maintaining it. If you lose weight suddenly or for unknown reasons, see a physician. Unexplained weight loss may be an indication of an underlying disorder.

**Avoid too much fat, saturated fat, and cholesterol.** Several factors have been associated with an increased risk of heart attack including high blood pressure and cigarette smoking, but a high blood cholesterol level is clearly one of the major risk factors. Eating saturated fats and large amounts of cholesterol will increase blood cholesterol in many people. Therefore, it is sensible to reduce your daily consumption of cholesterol and saturated fat. Choose lean meats, fish, poultry, peas and beans as protein sources. Use skim or low-fat milk and eat moderate amounts of egg yolks and organ meats. When preparing foods, trim off the fat and instead of frying, whenever possible bake or broil. These guidelines refer only to family members who do not have CF. Fat requirements of people with CF will be discussed in the section, "Fat Intake."

**Eat foods with an adequate amount of starch and fiber.** Carbohydrates provide a major source of energy in the diet. An example of a simple carbohydrate is sugar; a complex carbohydrate is starch. Foods high in starch such as breads and other grain products, beans, and peas contain many more essential nutrients than do simple carbohydrates. Complex carbohydrates contain dietary fiber. Eating foods high in fiber has been found to reduce symptoms of chronic constipation and diverticular disease. Diets low in fiber may increase the risk of developing colon cancer. These factors suggest that a diet containing whole grains, breads, cereals, fruits, and other fiber-containing foods is essential.

**Avoid too much sugar.** Eating too much sugar has been associated with tooth decay. Not only is the amount of sugar of concern but how often it is eaten, as well. Sugar can be found in many forms. Common table sugar is called sucrose, but other forms include glucose, fructose, maltose, and lactose. Most foods contain sugar in one form or another, and therefore sugar cannot be avoided completely. Keep the amount of sugar and sweet foods that you eat to moderate levels.

**Avoid too much sodium.** Sodium chloride or table salt is essential to the diet. Often it is used as a preservative and is present in many beverages, processed foods, sauces, sandwich meats, and pickled foods. A major concern with high sodium intake is its association with increased blood pressure. In populations with a high sodium intake, high blood pressure is common. Since most Americans eat more sodium than needed, our sodium intake should be reduced. Use less table salt and eat sparingly those foods which contain a large amount of added sodium. Since people with CF lose more salt in their sweat than others, these restrictions should not apply to them.

**If you drink alcoholic beverages, do so in moderation.** Alcohol is a high-calorie beverage but is low in essential nutrients. Heavy drinkers often develop nutritional deficiencies as well as other serious diseases such as cirrhosis of the liver and certain forms of cancer. Consequently, it is suggested that if you drink, you do so in moderation. Pregnant women should refrain from alcohol consumption, since alcohol may cause birth defects and other problems during pregnancy.

**Vitamins.** The Recommended Dietary Allowances (RDA) of vitamins for family members can come from a balanced diet like the one outlined above or can be supplemented by taking one multivitamin per day to insure that 100% of each vitamin is included. Read the label on the multivitamin bottle to make sure that the supplement does not contain more than 100% of the RDA of vitamins or minerals. Remember that all of these vitamins and minerals are included in a balanced diet, but a multivitamin can provide the extra dietary insurance that some families feel they need.

**What's the best nutrition advice for a family?** It's following these Dietary Guidelines for Americans. Make the daily food choices as outlined in the Food Guide Pyramid. It's not a rigid prescription, but a general guide that lets you choose a healthful diet that's right for you.

**How many servings are right for me?** The Pyramid shows a range of servings for each major food group. The number of servings that are right for you depends on how many calories you need, which in turn depends on your age, sex, size and how active you are. But everyone should have at least the lowest number of servings in the ranges.

**How many servings for young children?** In order to grow and develop normally, preschool children need the same variety of foods as older family members do, but may need less calories. For fewer calories they can eat smaller servings. However, it is important that they have the equivalent of 2 cups of milk a day. But don't worry about how much your child eats at a single meal or even in a single day. Over a week, the choices should even out and provide a balance of nutrients that meet the child's needs.

## Food Guide Pyramid

### A Guide to Daily Food Choices

Fats, Oils, & Sweets
USE SPARINGLY

KEY
◻ Fat (naturally occurring and added)
◙ Sugars (added)

These symbols show fats, oils, and added sugars in foods.

Milk, Yogurt, & Cheese Group
2-3 SERVINGS

Meat, Poultry, Fish, Dry Beans, Eggs, & Nuts Group
2-3 SERVINGS

Vegetable Group
3-5 SERVINGS

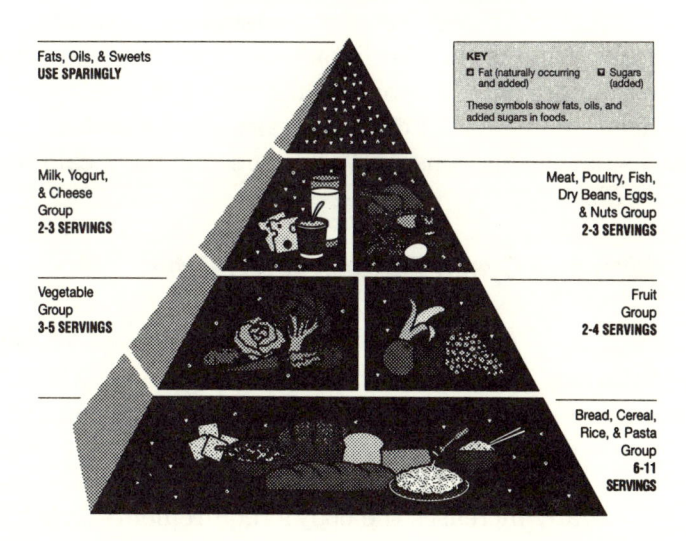

Fruit Group
2-4 SERVINGS

Bread, Cereal, Rice, & Pasta Group
6-11 SERVINGS

*Figure 5.3.*

**Getting everyone involved in family nutrition.** Feeding a family requires organization, which can be a shared responsibility. Planning weekly menus at a family meeting eliminates meals that are undesirable for some members. Having a weekly menu in mind also makes shopping easier because you know in advance what you need.

It can save time if you organize the shopping list according to the aisles in the grocery store, too. This way you can give the children a list for a specific aisle and let them find the products themselves. This gets them involved in the shopping, teaches them what to choose for a balanced diet, and gives you an opportunity to tell them why you chose to buy a certain product. In the kitchen, everyone can help out by doing some preparation work like cutting up vegetables for a salad or a stew, putting juice, milk, or water on the table, or toasting and buttering bread for breakfast. By including children in the different aspects of feeding a family, they gain information that they can use later in adolescence when they begin to take charge of themselves.

Just as individuals differ, so do individual needs. As stated before, food needs differ depending on age, sex, height, body size, physical activity, and other conditions such as pregnancy and illness. If one member of the family has cystic fibrosis, this does not mean that he or she must follow a completely different diet than the one consumed by the family. The basic guidelines still apply. What it does require is that the child with cystic fibrosis consume more calories than other family members. The CF child requires more energy for breathing, and for fighting infection and fever. The dietary needs of the child with CF do not require special foods or separate meals. As the next section will show, the need for increased caloric intake can be met by more frequent snacks, larger portions, and adding some extra calories to the usual family diet.

## How Nutrition and Cystic Fibrosis Are Related

Good nutrition is achieved when the diet provides adequate amounts of the nutrients the body requires for good health.

Cystic fibrosis can interfere with good nutrition in two major ways:

1. CF usually increases the body's requirements for nutrients used in energy production, growth, and maintenance.

2. CF usually makes it more difficult for the body to obtain these nutrients from food.

That doesn't mean that CF has to lead to poor nutrition. It simply means that proper nutritional management is a very important part of treatment for CF if the patient is to achieve optimal growth and development, and maintain the highest possible level of health. And because CF differs so widely from person to person, proper nutritional management will vary widely, too.

## Nutritional Concerns in Cystic Fibrosis

Digestion and absorption of nutrients. Cystic fibrosis affects the pancreas, a specialized organ (gland) in the abdomen. One of the major functions of the pancreas is to produce chemical substances known as digestive enzymes.

These enzymes normally are delivered to the small intestine in response to food coming down from the stomach. There the pancreatic enzymes partially digest food, that is, they break large nutrients—proteins, carbohydrates, and fats—into smaller nutrient particles. These particles are small enough to pass through the intestinal wall and into the body, a process called absorption.

In most patients, CF causes production of a thick mucus that plugs the duct leading from the pancreas to the small intestine. Consequently, not enough enzymes are present to properly digest food. If left untreated, one result is malabsorption, an inability to properly absorb nutrients. The other result is passage of these unabsorbed nutrients in the feces, leading to cramps, gas, and large, foul-smelling stools.

**Enzyme replacement therapy.** To compensate for this enzyme shortage, the majority of CF patients must take replacement pancreatic enzymes in tablet, powder, or capsule form. These enzymes must be taken to help digest every meal and snack, except for snacks that are virtually free of protein, starch, and fat, such as apple juice. Your nutritionist or physician can tell you more about foods that do not require enzymes.

Studies show that enzyme preparations are equally effective when taken anywhere from one-half hour before to one-half hour after eating. That way, the enzymes are in the small intestine when needed.

The amount of enzyme required varies greatly among patients, and depends largely on caloric and fat intake. For example, the amount of enzyme required to cover a high-calorie, high-fat meal will be greater than the amount required for a small snack. Another factor that affects dosage is the type of enzyme preparation used; because acid in the stomach destroys some of the enzymes taken in powdered and tablet form, a higher dosage may be required than for encapsulated enzymes, which have a special protective (enteric) coating that dissolves only in the small intestine. The correct enzyme dosage can be determined by a physician in several different ways, including fecal-fat studies (which compare fat intake to fat loss in the stools), blood levels of certain substances, an examination of frequency and type of stools, or even just observation of growth patterns in children.

The best type of enzyme to use will also vary among patients. For example, an individual with a high level of stomach acid production may have more acid than usual in the small intestine; since this can prevent the protective coating on encapsulated enzymes from dissolving, uncoated enzymes may be better utilized. Your physician will help you decide which type of enzyme preparation is most effective.

**Glucose Intolerance.** In CF, fibrosis of the pancreas can gradually lead to impaired function of specialized pancreatic cells, called islet cells. These cells produce chemicals responsible for regulation of blood glucose (blood sugar) levels. As a result, some CF patients may become glucose intolerant, that is, less able to clear glucose from the bloodstream.

Management of glucose intolerance usually includes dietary modification in order to regulate the types of food eaten and the timing of food intake. In addition, insulin may be given to lower blood sugar. Your physician can give you more detailed information on this topic.

**Caloric Requirements.** One of the major functions of food is to supply energy. The amount of energy a food provides is measured in calories, sometimes abbreviated as kcals.

Most CF patients have a higher caloric requirement than other individuals of the same age and sex for these reasons:

- More energy is used in breathing.
- Extra energy is used in fighting infections and during fevers.

- Fewer of the energy-producing nutrients in food are properly digested and absorbed into the body, even when treatment is optimal.

In order to meet his or her energy requirements, the typical CF child receiving enzyme therapy must consume approximately 120 percent to 150 percent of the United States RDA for calories for a healthy child of the same age and sex. This figure varies considerably from person to person, and may be as high as 200 percent of the RDA. Energy requirements are particularly high for children who are catching up on growth and development after a period of poor nutrition.

**How can an individual's calorie requirements be calculated?** Testing may be done by your child's nutritionist to establish the resting metabolic rate (the amount of energy required at rest) from which total energy requirements may be calculated. On a more practical level, adequate caloric intake can be defined as the level that promotes normal growth and development in children, and maintenance of desirable body weight in grown individuals.

See "How to Increase Intake" for a discussion of ways to increase caloric intake.

**Protein Requirements.** Protein is one of the three energy-producing types of nutrients in food, the other two are carbohydrates (made up of starches and sugars) and fats. In addition to being used for energy production, protein is necessary for growth and maintenance of body tissues, proper functioning of the immune system, and a number of other critical functions.

Most CF patients have higher than usual protein requirements, as well. People with CF who meet their increased caloric requirements by consuming a balanced diet usually meet their increased protein requirements at the same time.

Most high-protein foods are of animal origin, including milk and milk products, meats, poultry, fish, and eggs. Legumes, such as peas, beans, and lentils, are also good sources of protein, especially when eaten with grain products.

See "How to Increase Intake" for some examples of high-protein, high-calorie foods.

**Fat Intake.** In the past, CF patients were told to limit intake of fats and fatty foods. This was appropriate advice for that time, because replacement enzymes were not as effective as some of those available today, and malabsorption of fat was far harder to overcome.

However, today's replacement enzymes are more effective in promoting digestion and absorption of fats. In fact, it is now recommended that CF patients consume relatively high amounts of fat, for the following reasons:

- Ounce for ounce, fat provides more than twice as many calories as protein or carbohydrate.

- Conversion of fat to energy requires less oxygen than conversion of protein or carbohydrate to energy, therefore putting less of a burden on the respiratory system.

- Generally, individuals with CF have a low blood cholesterol level and therefore do not have to restrict the intake of saturated fat and cholesterol.

Adequate dietary fat is also required for provision of essential fatty acids, a group of nutrients which the body requires for normal functioning.

Does this mean that the whole family should increase its consumption of fat? No. The average healthy American consumes too much fat already. A balanced diet of normal foods should be prepared for the entire family. The CF patient can then increase fat intake by adding extra fats at serving time, eating larger portions of the fattier foods, and consuming additional high-fat foods.

See "How to Increase Intake" for suggestions on increasing dietary fat.

**Salt Intake.** CF patients lose more salt (sodium chloride) in their sweat than other individuals. Their need for additional salt is usually met simply by increasing intake of normal foods in order to meet caloric requirements. However, if you live in a very hot climate, your physician may advise adding extra salt to foods or increasing intake of salty foods.

**Vitamin and Mineral Intake.** CF patients who meet their caloric requirements by consuming a well-balanced diet, and whose fat absorption is well regulated, rarely develop vitamin and mineral deficiencies. However, because absorption is not optimal even at correct levels of enzyme replacement, supplementation is recommended.

Vitamins are absorbed most effectively when taken with fat-containing meals and pancreatic enzyme supplements. Infants and children up to 2 years old should take Polyvisol or a similar liquid multivitamin preparation, 1 mL per day. Children ages 2 to 8 years need a standard multiple vitamin providing 100% of the RDA for a healthy individual of the patient's age. Older children, adolescents, and adults need 1 to 2 tablets of a standard adult multiple vitamin preparation per day.

High potency multivitamin supplements are specially formulated to meet the needs of CF patients with poor dietary fat absorption. These supplements are indicated for use solely under medical supervision in patients who do not obtain sufficient fat-soluble vitamins A, D, E, and K.

Additional supplementation with any vitamin or mineral beyond this level is recommended only if a specific need is recognized by your physician.

### How to Increase Intake

Modifying intake of regular foods. Whenever possible, people with CF should meet their nutritional requirements by eating a balanced diet of everyday foods.

Start with a well-balanced diet for a healthy person of the same age (as outlined in this Family Guide to Nutrition). Then, if caloric and nutrient requirements are to be increased, modify intake by following these four steps:

1) Increase portion sizes
2) Add snacks and "mini-meals," especially at night. Good choices are:

- Dried fruit and nuts.
- Jam or jelly with toast or cheesecake, pudding, and other dessert food.
- Cold cuts, pizza, or left-overs.

3) Emphasize high-calorie, nutritious food at mealtime and snacktime. Serve as many high-protein, high-calorie foods as possible, including:

- Whole milk products, such as yogurt, cheese, custard, and pudding.

- Beverages made with whole milk, light cream, or undiluted evaporated milk, such as milkshakes, malteds, cocoa, egg nog, and instant breakfast.

- Nuts and nut butters, especially peanut.

- Meat, fish, poultry, or eggs prepared with added fat (see the hints on adding fat below) or in a mixed dish with another high-calorie, high-protein food (such as lasagna with meat and cheese).

At the same time, you may want to limit intake of foods that are filling but not very high in calories or needed nutrients. These include clear soups, tea, coffee, and low-calorie beverages.

4) Add extra fats. Remember, a little extra fat adds a lot of extra calories. Try these ideas:

- Put extra butter and margarine on bread products, cooked vegetables, hot cereals, pancakes, pasta, baked and mashed potatoes, rice, and other foods at serving time.

- Serve whipped cream or ice cream as a topping on desserts, cocoa, waffles, and other foods.

- Use extra mayonnaise on sandwiches and in salads such as tuna, potato, and macaroni.

- (Use sour cream as a topping for fruit, baked potatoes, fish, chili and other foods.

- Serve dips made from sour cream and mayonnaise with fresh vegetables and snack foods.

- Use extra salad dressing; avoid lo-cal or reduced-calorie dressings.

## Cystic Fibrosis

- Serve generous portions of gravies and sauces.

- Use creamed soups instead of clear bouillon broth.

Adding extra fats is especially important because fats provide more calories per unit than carbohydrates. Proteins and fats are also essential for the body to properly absorb vitamins A, D, E, and K.

Your nutritionist will be glad to give you further suggestions, as well as special recipes, for nutritious, high-calorie treats.

**Dietary supplements.** Several dietary supplements can be used to increase intake of calories and important nutrients.

Some common milkshake-like dietary supplements are Ensure®, Magnacal®, Sustacal®, Enrich®, Isocal®, and Osmolite®. These nutritionally balanced liquids are slightly different in composition, but each is high in calories, protein, and other important nutrients. Most come in two or more concentrations, providing anywhere from 240 to 480 calories per eight-ounce can. All are commercially available in a variety of flavors.

Sustacal® and Forta® puddings are similar in nutritional calories per five-ounce can. All of these pre-mixed, canned supplements require no refrigeration before serving. They can be served either with meals or as highly nutritious snacks, both at home and away.

Ask your nutritionist or physician for recommendations on which supplements to use and where to obtain them.

**Increasing intake when eating is not enough.** It is not always possible or practical for CF patients to meet their increased caloric and protein requirements by consuming table foods and food-like supplements. When eating is not enough to maintain good nutritional status and normal growth and development, your physician may suggest other types of feedings.

One option is tube feeding, which delivers liquid supplement directly to the stomach. Tube feedings may be given overnight as an adjunct to usual food intake.

Another option is delivery of nutrients directly to the bloodstream, through an intravenous tube.

If one of these options is necessary, your physician will suggest a route of feeding and a feeding formula that suits your special needs.

## Nutrition Through the Life Cycle.

At any stage in the life cycle, the goal of nutritional management is to help the individual realize his or her full potential. For a child, that means achieving optimal growth and development. For an adult, that means reaching and maintaining an ideal weight for height.

Guidelines for good nutrition of CF patients are very similar to those for the general population. Because increased nutritional requirements should be met by increasing intake of a well-balanced diet, feeding patterns for CF children are most often modifications of usual feeding patterns for healthy children of the same age. Moreover, much nutritional advice applies to all children, such as how to introduce new foods to infants, or how to progress to solid foods.

**Early infancy.** It is very important to assure adequate nutrition for the infant with cystic fibrosis. Your physician will advise you on the best feeding mode for your child.

**Breast feeding.** Life other infants, CF infants benefit from the physical and emotional advantages of breast feeding, but these two extra steps must be taken to assure adequate nutrition if the infant has malabsorption:

1. Enzymes must be provided to aid in digestion and absorption of breast-milk nutrients. Since infants cannot swallow capsules, enzymes must be given mixed in food. Capsules may be opened and the coated enzymes mixed with soft food such as applesauce, or a powdered form may be mixed in soft food.

2. If the child has increased requirements (especially for calories and protein), these may be met by providing formula in addition to breast milk. It may be a cow's milk-based formula, or a hydrolyzed (predigested) formula such as Pregestimil®. Both require extra enzymes for digestion and absorption, although hydrolyzed formulas require far less.

The decision of whether or not to continue breast feeding, and the choice of formula, will largely depend on the infant's ability to take the necessary enzymes. Coated enzymes are not effective unless the food in which they are mixed is completely consumed and swallowed. The

## Cystic Fibrosis

powdered form may cause irritation and sores in the mouth. Inability to take sufficient enzymes may necessitate discontinuation of breast feeding, with complete substitution of hydrolyzed formula.

**Non-breast fed infants.** As a rule, cow's milk-based formula is well tolerated when sufficient enzymes are provided, and is preferable to hydrolyzed formulas. However, some problems may arise, such as inability to take sufficient enzymes. (See section on Breast Feeding.) In such cases, a hydrolyzed formula, such as Pregestimil, is usually substituted.

**Toddlers.** CF toddlers usually have greater food requirements than other toddlers, but they don't always have larger appetites. Their small stomachs also limit the amount they can consume at mealtimes. One way to maximize the toddler's intake is to serve frequent meals and snacks in small to moderate portions, instead of serving a few large meals. Many parents also find it helpful to continue bottle feeding beyond infancy, in addition to providing solid foods and liquids in cups. It is common for toddlers and older children to refuse to eat certain foods, finish meals, or eat regularly. These behaviors can make mealtimes stressful for both parent and child, especially if intake appears inadequate. As a guideline, families should be encouraged to have regular mealtimes without distraction (TV watching) where the family sits together. Parents should establish clear rules and consequences for mealtimes and this should apply to their child with CF as well as to their healthy child. Increase in energy consumption for the child with CF is important and best done gradually over time. When a CF child just "plays" with the food, parents should be discouraged from nagging and keeping the child at the table beyond the time when other family members leave the table. A CF child's refusal to eat should be managed by consistent consequences that may be applicable to children in general, such as the main dish must be eaten before dessert.

It helps to praise a child when he/she eats well and as a reward let him/her watch a favorite TV program.

**School-Age Children.** As CF children enter school, they are faced with a desire to be "just like everybody else." At the same time, they have more freedom to choose when and what they eat.

Many CF youngsters are reluctant to take replacement enzymes in front of schoolmates and friends. Because enzyme therapy is essential to good nutrition, it is important to find an acceptable solution to this problem. Some children find it helpful to discuss CF with their friends. Other children prefer to hide the enzyme capsules inside a suitable food, such as a sandwich.

CF youngsters may also fail to eat all the food provided for them while at school. There are many reasons for this behavior, including difficulty in finding the time for snacks during the day, and the belief that increased intake will attract attention. School officials and health care providers may be of assistance in solving this common problem.

Some schools have restrictions on medications taken by students during school hours. In such cases, arrangements for taking enzymes and other necessary medications can usually be made with the school nurse.

**Teenagers.** The teen years are a time of increasing independence, sometimes characterized by rebellious behavior. They are also a time when CF patients must take increasing responsibility for their own good nutrition. A general rule is, whenever possible, plan a definite eating schedule and adhere to it as best you can. Family members and health care providers can work together to make this transition a smooth one.

*Throughout the life cycle, remember:*

- Every CF patient is unique. Nutritional management throughout life must be individualized.

- Your health care providers are always willing to discuss your nutritional concerns and problems.

## Sample Menus

The sample menus which follow include typical, nutritionally balanced menus for an average family. Along with each menu is a nutrient-and calorie-enriched version of the same menu for the child with cystic fibrosis. Notice that while the foods are basically the same, the meal for the CF child has been enriched with calories to provide for the child's additional requirements. Food preparation is the same and, with some practice, increasing calories in the diet will become second nature.

## Cystic Fibrosis

### Family Menu #1

| Breakfast: | Calories |
|---|---|
| 1 cup orange juice | 80 |
| ½ cup farina made with water | 70 |
| ½ cup skim milk | 40 |
| 1 soft-cooked egg | 75 |
| 1 slice toast | 70 |
| 1 tsp margarine | 45 |
| ½ banana | 40 |
| Total | 420 |

| Lunch: | |
|---|---|
| 1 cup skim milk | 80 |
| 1 slice whole wheat bread | 140 |
| 3 oz sliced turkey | 165 |
| 1 tsp mayonnaise | 45 |
| lettuce, tomato | 0 |
| ½ cup green beans | 25 |
| Total | 455 |

| Dinner: | |
|---|---|
| 1 cup skim milk | 80 |
| ⅛ honeydew melon | 40 |
| 3 oz rib steak | 165 |
| 1 baked potato | 70 |
| 1 tsp margarine or butter | 45 |
| ½ cup broccoli | 25 |
| ¾ cup strawberries | 40 |
| Total | 465 |

Total for 3 meals = 1440
Add snacks as desired.

### Nutrient- and Calorie-enriched Menu #1

| Breakfast: | Calories |
|---|---|
| 1 cup orange juice | 80 |
| ½ cup farina made with milk | 150 |
| 2 tsp margarine | 90 |
| 1 tbsp raisins | 30 |
| 1 cup whole milk | 160 |
| 2 scrambled eggs | 150 |
| fried in 2 tsp margarine | 90 |
| 1 tbsp catsup | 15 |
| 2 slices white bread | 140 |
| 2 tsp butter | 90 |
| 2 tsp jam | 60 |
| 1 large banana | 90 |
| Total | 1145 |

| Lunch: | |
|---|---|
| 1 cup whole milk | 160 |
| 2 slices white bread | 140 |
| 6 oz sliced turkey | 330 |
| 2 tsp mayonnaise | 90 |
| 2 tsp catsup | 30 |
| 15 potato chips | 250 |
| 1 cup ice cream | 270 |
| with chocolate fudge | 250 |
| Total | 1520 |

| Dinner: | |
|---|---|
| 1 cup whole milk | 160 |
| ¼ honeydew melon | 80 |
| 5 oz rib steak | 275 |
| broiled in BBQ sauce | 215 |
| 1 baked potato | 70 |
| 2 tbsp sour cream | 140 |
| ½ cup broccoli | 25 |
| in cheese sauce | 200 |
| ¾ cup strawberries | 40 |
| 3 tbsp cream | 165 |
| 2 tbsp sugar | 80 |
| 1 slice chocolate cake | 235 |
| Total | 1685 |

Total for 3 meals = 4350

### Snack Suggestions

| Snack: | Calories |
|---|---|
| ½ cup fruit salad | 55 |
| 5 crackers | 50 |
| 1 tbsp peanut butter | 95 |
| Total | 200 |

| Snack: | |
|---|---|
| 1 apple | 40 |
| 3 vanilla wafers | 50 |
| Total | 90 |

| Snack: | |
|---|---|
| ½ cup skim milk | 40 |
| 1 roll | 70 |
| 1 oz cheese | 75 |
| Total | 185 |

| Snack: | Calories |
|---|---|
| 2 slices white bread | 140 |
| 3 tbsp peanut butter | 270 |
| 3 tbsp jelly | 165 |
| 1 cup fruit juice | 80 |
| Total | 655 |

| Snack: | |
|---|---|
| 1 cup yogurt | 240 |
| 2 tbsp wheat germ | 50 |
| Total | 290 |

| Snack: | |
|---|---|
| 1 cup whole milk | 160 |
| 1 bran muffin | 125 |
| 2 tsp butter | 90 |
| Total | 375 |

*Figure 5.4.*

# Respiratory Diseases and Disorders Sourcebook

## Family Menu #2

| Breakfast: | Calories |
|---|---|
| ½ cup pineapple juice | 40 |
| 2 pancakes | 140 |
| 2 tbsp maple syrup | 90 |
| 1 cup skim milk | 80 |
| Total | 350 |

| Lunch: | |
|---|---|
| 1 cup skim milk | 80 |
| macaroni and cheese | |
| ½ cup macaroni | 70 |
| 1½ oz cheese | 110 |
| green salad | 0 |
| 2 bread sticks | 70 |
| 2 tbsp salad dressing, low-cal | 40 |
| Total | 370 |

| Dinner: | |
|---|---|
| 1 cup tomato juice | 40 |
| 4 oz fried chicken without skin | 210 |
| ½ cup rice | 70 |
| ½ cup green beans | 25 |
| 1 slice bread | 70 |
| 1 tsp butter | 45 |
| 1 cup fruit | 80 |
| Total | 540 |

Total for 3 meals = 1260
Add snacks as desired.

## Nutrient- and Calorie-enriched Menu #2

| Breakfast: | Calories |
|---|---|
| 1 cup pineapple juice | 80 |
| 3 pancakes | 210 |
| 4 tbsp maple syrup | 180 |
| 1 English muffin | 140 |
| 2 tbsp cream cheese | 120 |
| 2 tbsp jelly | 60 |
| 1 cup chocolate milk | 210 |
| Total | 1000 |

| Lunch: | |
|---|---|
| 1 cup whole milk | 160 |
| macaroni and cheese | |
| ½ cup macaroni | 70 |
| 2½ oz cheese | 185 |
| ½ cup milk | 80 |
| green salad | 0 |
| french bread | 140 |
| 2 tsp margarine | 90 |
| 2 tbsp salad dressing | 140 |
| 6 chocolate chip cookies | 200 |
| Total | 1065 |

| Dinner: | |
|---|---|
| 1 cup tomato juice | 40 |
| 6 oz fried chicken | 330 |
| ½ cup rice | 70 |
| 2 tsp margarine | 90 |
| ½ cup green beans | 25 |
| sauteed in mushrooms | 50 |
| 2 dinner rolls | 140 |
| 2 tsp margarine | 90 |
| 1 cup fruit cocktail | 200 |
| 3 tbsp whipped cream | 90 |
| Total | 1125 |

Total for 3 meals = 3190

## Snack Suggestions

| Snack: | Calories |
|---|---|
| 1 peach | 40 |
| Total | 40 |

| Snack: | |
|---|---|
| 1 tangerine | 40 |
| Total | 40 |

| Snack: | |
|---|---|
| 1 cup popcorn | 70 |
| ½ cup apple juice | 40 |
| Total | 110 |

| Snack: | Calories |
|---|---|
| 1 slice apple pie | 350 |
| 4 oz ice cream | 125 |
| Total | 475 |

| Snack: | |
|---|---|
| tuna sandwich | |
| 2 slices bread | 140 |
| ½ cup tuna | 110 |
| 2 tsp mayonnaise | 90 |
| Total | 340 |

| Snack: | |
|---|---|
| banana shake | |
| 1 cup yogurt | 240 |
| 1 banana | 90 |
| ½ cup whole milk | 80 |
| 2 tbsp raisins | 60 |
| Total | 470 |

*Figure 5.5.*

## Cystic Fibrosis

### Family Menu #3

| Breakfast: | Calories |
|---|---|
| ½ cup grapefruit juice | 40 |
| ½ cup bran flakes | 70 |
| 1 cup skim milk | 80 |
| Total | 190 |

| Lunch: | |
|---|---|
| 1 cup skim milk | 80 |
| 3 oz hamburger | 225 |
| 1 roll | 140 |
| lettuce, tomato | 0 |
| 10 french fries | 155 |
| 2 tbsp catsup | 15 |
| small banana | 60 |
| 8 oz diet cola | 0 |
| Total | 675 |

| Dinner: | |
|---|---|
| ½ cup cream of chicken soup | 90 |
| 3 oz salmon | 165 |
| ½ cup zucchini | 25 |
| ½ cup corn | 70 |
| 1 slice bread | 70 |
| 1 tsp margarine | 45 |
| 1 cup watermelon | 40 |
| Total | 505 |

Total for 3 meals = 1370
Add snacks as desired.

### Nutrient- and Calorie-enriched Menu #3

| Breakfast: | Calories |
|---|---|
| 1 cup grapefruit juice | 80 |
| 2 slices french toast | 230 |
| 2 tsp margarine | 90 |
| 1 cup sweetened cereal | 160 |
| ½ cup blueberries | 40 |
| 2 tbsp sugar | 80 |
| 1 cup whole milk | 160 |
| Total | 840 |

| Lunch: | |
|---|---|
| 1 cup whole milk | 160 |
| 3 oz hamburger | 225 |
| 1 roll | 140 |
| 2 slices american cheese | 215 |
| 2 tsp mayonnaise | 90 |
| lettuce, tomato, fried onions | 25 |
| 20 french fries | 310 |
| 4 tbsp catsup | 60 |
| banana with ice cream | 190 |
| 8 oz cola | 95 |
| Total | 1510 |

| Dinner: | |
|---|---|
| 1 cup cream of chicken soup | 180 |
| 5 oz salmon | 275 |
| cooked in 1 tsp butter | 90 |
| ½ cup creamed corn | 160 |
| ½ cup zucchini in | 25 |
| tomato sauce | 55 |
| 2 dinner rolls | 140 |
| 2 tsp margarine | 90 |
| 1 slice angel food cake | 135 |
| 1 cup whole milk | 160 |
| Total | 1310 |

Total for 3 meals = 3580

### Snack Suggestions

| Snack: | Calories |
|---|---|
| 10 cherries | 40 |
| Total | 40 |

| Snack: | |
|---|---|
| 5 pretzels | 70 |
| ½ cup orange juice | 40 |
| Total | 110 |

| Snack: | |
|---|---|
| 1 chocolate bar | 150 |
| 1 cup skim milk | 80 |
| Total | 230 |

| Snack: | Calories |
|---|---|
| 1 cup chocolate milk | 210 |
| 1 large danish pastry | 275 |
| Total | 485 |

| Snack: | |
|---|---|
| 1 slice pizza | 145 |
| with extra cheese | 100 |
| 1 cup chocolate pudding | 285 |
| Total | 530 |

| Snack: | |
|---|---|
| 2 oz chocolate-covered peanuts | 320 |
| 8 oz cola | 95 |
| Total | 415 |

*Figure 5.6.*

Here are some additional suggestions for high-calorie snacks:

### 250-Calorie Snacks

| | |
|---|---|
| 1 corn muffin | 125 |
| 2 tbsp jam | 120 |
| | 245 |

| | |
|---|---|
| chocolate malted | 235 |
| baked custard | 285 |
| 1 slice devil's food cake | 250 |
| 1 cup chocolate pudding | 285 |

### 500-Calorie Snacks

| | |
|---|---|
| 1 cup dry cereal | 160 |
| 1 banana | 90 |
| 1 cup whole milk | 160 |
| 1 slice toast | 70 |
| 1 tsp butter | 90 |
| | 570 |

| | |
|---|---|
| 6 graham crackers | 100 |
| 2 tbsp peanut butter | 190 |
| ½ cup dried fruit | 200 |
| | 490 |

| | |
|---|---|
| 8 saltine crackers | 100 |
| 1 oz cheese | 75 |
| 1 cup ice cream | 290 |
| | 465 |

| | |
|---|---|
| 8 oz yogurt | 240 |
| 4 tbsp raisins | 105 |
| 2 tbsp wheat germ | 50 |
| ¼ cup walnuts | 200 |
| | 595 |

### Greater than 750-Calorie Snacks

Ice cream sundae

| | |
|---|---|
| 2 scoops ice cream | 270 |
| 4 tbsp chocolate syrup | 250 |
| 3 tbsp whipped cream | 90 |
| ¼ cup chopped nuts | 200 |
| | 810 |

Roast beef sandwich

| | |
|---|---|
| 2 slices bread | 140 |
| 4 oz roast beef | 300 |
| 2 tsp catsup | 30 |
| 2 tsp mayonnaise | 90 |
| 6 chocolate chip cookies | 200 |
| | 760 |

| | |
|---|---|
| 2 slices pizza with extra cheese | 290 / 200 |
| 8 oz cola | 95 |
| 1 cup chocolate pudding | 285 |
| | 870 |

*Figure 5.7.*

*—Prepared under the professional direction of Elisabeth Luder, PhD, RD, Co-Director Pediatric Pulmonary Center, Mount Sinai School of Medicine, New York, New York.*

## Section 5.3

# A Teacher's Guide to CF

Source: Cystic Fibrosis Foundation 9/93. Used by permission.

The Cystic Fibrosis Foundation (CFF) has prepared this fact sheet for teachers to answer questions about students with cystic fibrosis (CF). In addition to reading the information provided here, talk with your student's parents or physician about the best ways to make the child comfortable, to maximize his or her learning experience. As a teacher, you play an important role in strengthening your student's self-image and in stimulating valuable relationships with other children.

### What Is Cystic Fibrosis?

Although many people with cystic fibrosis don't appear to be severely ill, CF is the most common fatal genetic disease, affecting 30,000 children and young adults in the United States alone. CF is a chronic disease, whereby the defective CF gene causes the formation of a thick, sticky mucus which leads to severe respiratory and digestive problems. One in twenty Americans-12 million people is a symptomless carrier of the defective CF gene. A child must inherit two such genes, one from each parent, to actually have the disease.

Cystic fibrosis is not contagious and affects each person differently. Therefore, it is difficult to make a generalization about an individual's physical and emotional health. If you have a student with CF in your class, he/she is in fair to good health to attend school, either on a full or even part-time basis. On the other hand, there are some individuals who are so severely affected that they are unable to attend school regularly.

When the CFF was founded in 1955, a child with CF was not expected to live much beyond the age of five. Today, dramatic advances in CF research and treatment, however, have greatly improved the chances of a child with CF living well into adulthood. As a teacher, you may help by understanding any special requirements a child with CF may have in planning for his/her future.

## What Are the Symptoms of CF?

Because CF produces various effects on the body, the disease may be confused with other conditions such as pneumonia, asthma, or "failure to thrive."

In many cases, people with CF don't appear to be suffering from a serious disorder. The only indications may be some physical symptoms:

- persistent coughing/wheezing;
- excessive appetite but poor weight gain;
- salty-tasting skin, sweat;
- recurrent respiratory infections such as pneumonia;
- thin body, small build;
- a slightly protruding abdomen;
- enlarged (clubbed) fingertips and,
- bulky, foul-smelling stools.

## Treating Cystic Fibrosis

As the teacher of a student with CF, it is helpful to understand the medical routines your student must go through. Treatment for CF varies, of course, depending on how far the disease has progressed and which organs are affected. Most current treatments are designed to either clear the lungs to make breathing easier, or to treat related digestive problems.

### Clearing the Lungs

The thick, sticky mucus produced in CF airways clogs breathing passages. If not removed, the mucus provides a breeding ground for chronic lung infections. Regular hospital visits to receive IV antibiotics is one way to minimize lung damage and improve the overall health of those with CF.

A treatment known as "chest physical therapy" may also be needed once or twice a day. During this therapy, the person with CF is clapped vigorously on the back and chest to help dislodge the mucus from the airways. In addition, a machine called a nebulizer is sometimes used to deliver aerosolized antibiotics to the lungs to help open up the airways and prevent or treat respiratory infections.

## Cystic Fibrosis

Coughing is the body's primary method of clearing the mucus that clogs CF lungs. Individuals with CF should not try to restrain coughing either physically or by taking cough suppressants. Your student may feel embarrassed to cough in front of others. Help your student feel comfortable by making it easy for him or her to slip out of the classroom for a drink of water. In addition, many children have been taught to expectorate the mucus into a tissue. Encourage your student to keep a box of tissues and a means of disposal at his or her desk.

Paying undue attention to coughing of course, will only embarrass the student. Classmates are likely to follow your lead as the teacher—if you accept the coughing as not that unusual—the rest of the class will usually do the same.

### Treating Digestive Problems

The thick CF mucus also obstructs the digestive system and prevents pancreatic enzymes from reaching the small intestine. Without treatment, the body cannot digest food properly. People with CF often need to take pancreatic enzyme supplements along with a high-calorie diet to help the body absorb the proper nutrients.

When eating meals and snacks, your student may take many capsules or tablets containing pancreatic enzymes, vitamins and antibiotics. It is not unusual for a person with CF to ingest more than 25 pills a day. Please note that these medications are not habit-forming and will not alter your student's mental or emotional behavior.

Some children prefer to take their medication privately just before eating. Others, unless supervised, may skip their dietary therapy by hiding, "forgetting," or throwing away their pills to avoid taking them in front of their classmates. Discuss with your student and his or her parents the most comfortable routine. You may want to suggest keeping the pills in your desk or in the nurse's office.

### Exercise

Exercise may be particularly beneficial to children with CF. Children with CF should always be encouraged to exercise and play as much as possible. Exercise helps loosen the mucus that clogs the lungs. Because of breathing difficulties, however, some children with CF may not have stamina and may become overly exhausted.

When exercising or in hot weather, your student may need to put extra salt on their food or take salt supplements and drink extra fluids.

Talking to the student and parents can help determine the appropriate physical activities. Try to include a child with CF in all games and activities in which they are physically able to participate. Aside from its obvious physical benefits, exercise helps to build self-esteem and to develop social interaction skills.

### Closing in on a Cure

The CFF supports cutting edge science which will someday lead to a cure for cystic fibrosis. Recently, an individual with CF received the first CF gene therapy treatment. This landmark research represents a milestone because it is the first time scientists have been able to attempt to treat the root cause of the disease, rather than treat the symptoms. Eventually, it is believed, gene therapy for CF will involve adding enough normal genes to CF airways to correct CF cells. The presence of normal genes should eventually override the effects of the defective CF genes and cure this deadly disease.

By understanding your student's illness, you can better provide the educational and emotional support needed for the child to carry on a meaningful and productive life.

## Section 5.4

# An Introduction to Chest Physical Therapy

Source: Cystic Fibrosis Foundation, 1992. Used by permission.

Chest physical therapy (CPT) is a widely accepted technique to help people with cystic fibrosis (CF) breathe with ease and stay healthy. CPT uses gravity and physical maneuvers to loosen the thick, sticky mucus in the lungs that is difficult to remove just by coughing. Unclogging the airways is critical to reducing the severity of lung infections.

## Cystic Fibrosis

CPT is easy to perform using the techniques you will learn here. For the child with cystic fibrosis, CPT can be performed by physical therapists, respiratory therapists, nurses, parents, siblings, and even friends. Many adolescents and adults with CF learn to perform these techniques on themselves.

CPT is often used in conjunction with other types of treatments, such as inhaled antibiotics and bronchodilators. For maximum effectiveness, bronchodilators should be taken before CPT to open the airways, and aerosolized antibiotics should be taken after CPT to treat the opened airways. Your doctor at your Cystic Fibrosis Foundation (CFF) care center will recommend an individualized routine for CPT and other treatments.

### Becoming Familiar with the Lungs

Learning more about the respiratory system and its relationship to internal organs can help you to understand why CPT treatments are effective and how each lung segment is drained.

*Draining the Lung Segments*

The goal of CPT is to clear mucus from each of the five lobes of the lungs by draining mucus into the larger airways so that it can be coughed out. The right lung is composed of three lobes: the upper lobe, the middle lobe, and the lower lobe. The left lung is made up of only two lobes: the upper lobe and the lower lobe.

The lobes are divided into smaller divisions called segments. The upper lobes on the left and right sides are each made up of three segments: **apical, posterior** and **anterior**. The lower lobes each include four segments: **superior, anterior basal, lateral basal** and **posterior basal**. The left upper lobe includes the **lingula**, which corresponds to the **middle lobe** on the right.

Each segment of the lung contains a network of air tubes, air sacs and blood vessels. These sacs allow for the exchange of oxygen and carbon dioxide between the blood and air. It is these segments which are being drained during segmental bronchial drainage. Note the position of each lung segment in [Figure 5.8 on the next page].

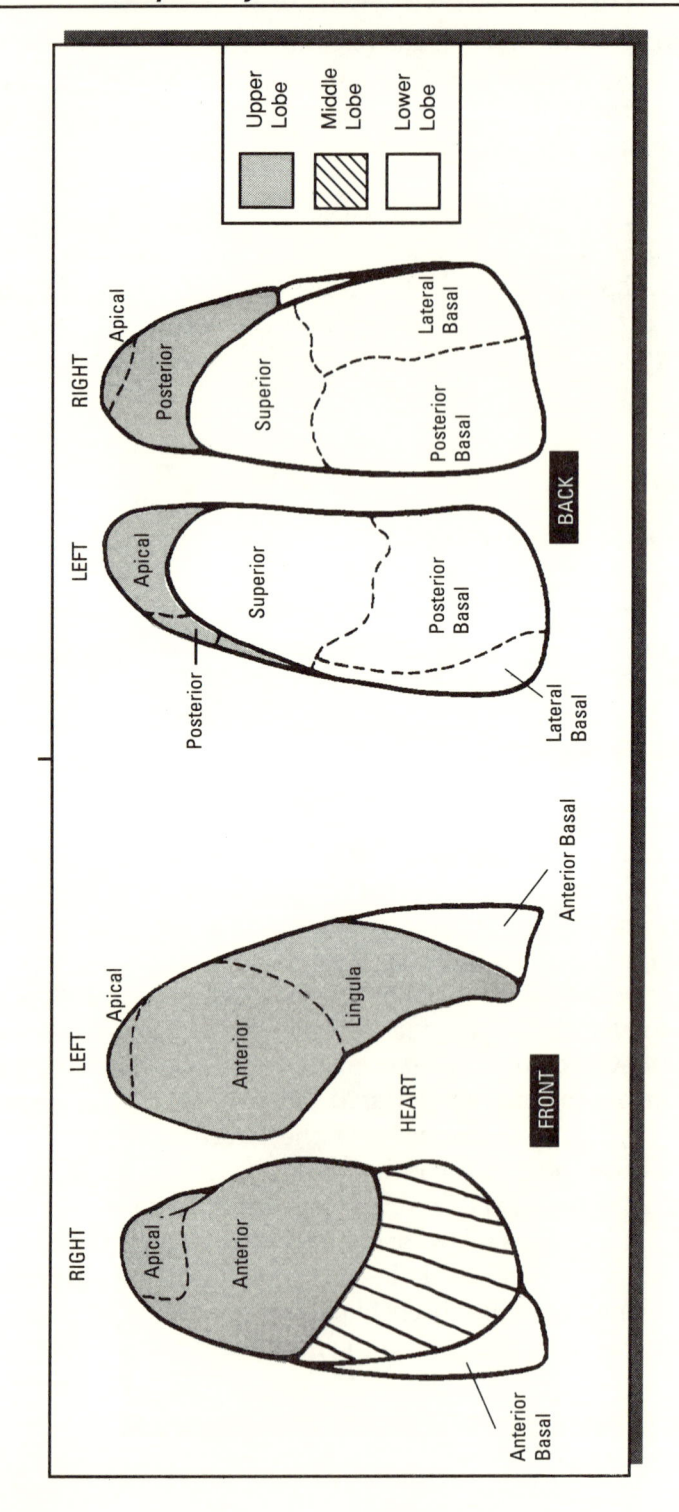

*Figure 5.8 External Anatomy of the Lung*

## Cystic Fibrosis

### Performing CPT

The performance of CPT involves a combination of techniques to remove secretions from the lungs, including: bronchial drainage positions, percussion, vibration, deep breathing and coughing.

Although individual CPT techniques will be further detailed, a brief summary of the complete treatment follows.

Once the patient is in one of several prescribed bronchial drainage positions, the care-giver performs percussion on the chest wall. This treatment is usually given for a period of one to five minutes and is sometimes followed by vibration over the same lung segment for approximately 15 seconds (or during five exhalations). The patient is then encouraged to cough vigorously and to expectorate, or swallow the loosened mucus, thus effectively clearing the lungs.

### Description of CPT Techniques

**Bronchial drainage**, or postural drainage, uses gravity to move secretions from the lungs upwards to the throat. The patient lies or sits in various positions so that the segment to be drained is uppermost on the patient's body. The segment is then drained using percussion, vibration and gravity. For a complete description of these positions, see Figures 5.12 through 5.22.

**Percussion**, or clapping, on the chest wall over the lung segment to be drained forces secretions into the larger airways. The hand is cupped as if to hold water but with the palm facing down as in Figure 5.9. The cupped hand conforms to the chest wall and traps a cushion of air to soften the clapping.

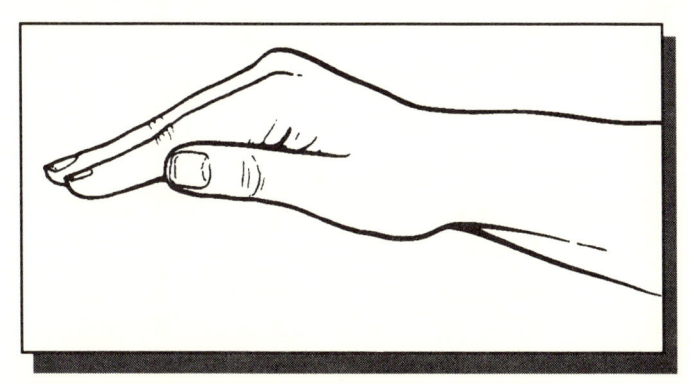

*Figure 5.9.* Cupped Hand

Percussion is done vigorously and rhythmically, but it should not be painful. Each percussion should have a hollow sound; it will not sting if the hand is cupped properly. The majority of the movement is in the wrist with the arm relaxed, making percussion less tiring to perform.

Percussion should be done only over the ribs. Special attention must be taken to avoid percussing over the spine, breastbone, stomach and lower ribs or back to prevent trauma to the spleen on the left, the liver on the right, and the kidneys in the lower back.

Various mechanical devices, powered either by electricity or compressed air, may be used as substitutes for the traditional cupped palm method for percussion. Consult your doctor or therapist for advice.

**Vibration** gently shakes secretions into the larger airways. The care-giver places a hand firmly on the chest wall over the appropriate segment and tenses the muscles of the arm and shoulder to create a fine shaking motion. Then, the care-giver applies a light pressure over the area being vibrated. (The care-giver may also place one hand over the other, then press the top and bottom hand into each other to vibrate.) Vibration is done with the flattened, not the cupped, hand as in Figure 5.10. The patient exhales, saying "FFF" or "SSS," when vibration is performed. Exhalation should be as slow and as complete as possible.

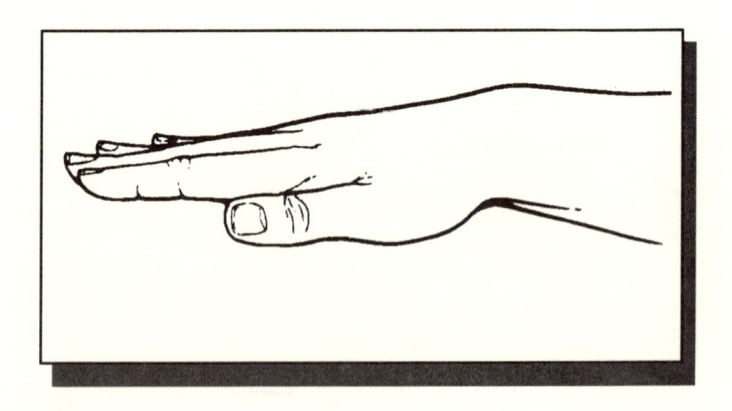

*Figure 5.10.* Flat Hand

## Cystic Fibrosis

**Deep breathing** moves the loosened secretions and may stimulate coughing. Diaphragmatic breathing, or belly breathing, is used to encourage deep breathing to move air into the lower lungs. The belly moves outward when the individual breathes in and sinks in when he or she breathes out.

**Coughing** is essential in clearing the airways. A forced but not strained exhalation, following a deep inhalation, may stimulate a productive cough. The sputum can be swallowed or preferably coughed out into a tissue or basin. To increase the cough's effectiveness while decreasing the strain to the patient, coughing may be assisted by supporting the sides of the lower chest with the hands or elbows.

At the end of each drainage position, the patient can take a deep breath, then expel it quickly in a "huff." This "huff" forces the air and mucus out, making the cough more effective.

### Timing of CPT

Generally, each treatment session can last for 20-40 minutes. CPT is best done before meals or one and a half to two hours after eating to minimize the chance of vomiting. Early morning and bedtime sessions are usually recommended. The duration of CPT and the number of treatment sessions may need to be increased if the patient is more congested. The recommended positions and duration of treatment are prescribed by the patient's doctor or therapist.

### Enhancing CPT for the Patient and Care-giver

Both the patient and the care-giver should try to be comfortable during CPT. Before beginning CPT, the patient should remove tight clothing, jewelry, buttons and zippers around the neck, chest and waist. Light, soft clothing, such as a T-shirt, may be worn and an extra towel or layer of clothing can be used to lessen any sting from percussion. Do not perform CPT on bare skin. The therapist or care-giver should remove rings and other bulky jewelry such as watches or bracelets. An ample supply of tissues or a receptacle for disposal of expectorated secretions should be provided.

### Performing CPT Comfortably and Carefully

The patient's head should be well supported when in a head-down position. The patient can bend at the hips and knees to allow for both a stronger cough and a more comfortable position.

The care-giver should not lean forward when treating the patient, but should remain in an upright position to protect his or her back. To achieve this, the table on which the patient lies should be positioned at a comfortable height for the care-giver.

### Purchasing Equipment

Equipment such as drainage tables, electrical and non-electrical palm percussors and vibrators may be helpful and can be purchased from medical equipment distributors. Older children and adults may find percussors useful when performing their own CPT, but younger children may be frightened by the noise of a percussor.

Ask your doctor or therapist at your CFF care center for recommendations on commercially available equipment. In addition, the CFF Pharmacy carries some discounted equipment. Call 1-800-541-4959 for details.

### Tips for Achieving the Proper Positions

To enable you to perform CPT more frequently and effectively, select a method of achieving the proper bronchial drainage angles that is easy to set up. Some families use a firm padded board or table. These tilt boards, or drainage tables, can be elevated at one end by placing blocks on the floor. Tables that adjust to various angles or heights can be constructed or obtained commercially.

Bed or study pillows, sofa cushions, bundles of newspapers under pillows for support, cribs with adjustable mattress heights/tilts, foam wedges and bean bag chairs work for many families. Infants can be positioned with or without pillows in the care-giver's lap.

### Insurance Coverage

Some insurance plans cover the cost of medical equipment; however, check with your insurance company before purchasing equipment. The company may require a prescription for the equipment from your doctor.

## Cystic Fibrosis

Some people find that occasionally using the services of a professional therapist can be helpful. Check with your insurance plan's coverage policies to learn if it will cover physical therapy. Coverage policies may vary if you receive therapy from a physical or respiratory therapist, or a nurse, depending on different state laws and licensing requirements. It is important to know what your plan covers before starting therapy. In addition, your doctor or therapist may have tips on getting your medical needs covered by your insurance policy.

### *Making CPT More Enjoyable*

An additional benefit of CPT is that it promotes a special time together for the parent and the child or the individual and spouse. On a regular basis, CPT offers a specific time for you to enjoy each other's company.

To enhance the time you spend with your child or spouse doing CPT, you can do one of the following:

- Schedule CPT around a favorite TV show.

- Play a favorite tape of songs or stories.

- Spend time playing, talking, or singing with your child before, during and after CPT.

- Encourage blowing or coughing games during CPT, such as blowing pinwheels or coughing the deepest cough.

- Ask willing and capable relatives, friends, brothers and sisters to perform CPT occasionally. This can provide a welcome break from the daily routine.

- Minimize interruptions by allowing other family members to take care of other chores.

Identifying ways that make CPT more enjoyable at all ages can help you to maintain a regular routine and obtain maximum health benefits.

*Respiratory Diseases and Disorders Sourcebook*

## Summary of Bronchial Drainage Positions

Lung segments are drained using gravity as the patient lies or sits in different positions. Percussion and vibration are performed on the front, back and sides of the patient's chest and are followed by deep breathing and coughing.

Figure 5.11 summarizes all positions used for bronchial drainage. Details and explanations are provided for patients of all ages in Figures 5.12 through 5.22.

## Instructions for Bronchial Drainage Positions

The following diagrams describe the bronchial drainage positions necessary to drain each lung segment. In the diagrams, shaded areas on the chest indicate the location of the segment that is to be drained in each position.

The maneuvers vary slightly with the patient's age. Here, the diagrams illustrate the first CPT position for 1) an infant with the care-giver holding the infant on his or her lap, 2) an older child or adult who performs CPT independently (assistance may be needed to treat some positions), and 3) a child or adult with the care-giver assisting with CPT. The remaining diagrams illustrate a care-giver giving CPT to a child, and can be adapted for infants and adults.

Instructions are shown using a drainage table, but alternatives are available. Pillows may be used for added comfort, but should not lessen the angle necessary for drainage. If the patient tires easily, the sequence of positions can be varied, but all segments should be treated regularly.

**Please remember to percuss and vibrate only over the ribs. Avoid percussing and vibrating over the spine, breastbone, stomach and lower ribs or back to prevent trauma to the spleen on the left, the liver on the right, and the kidneys in the lower back. Do not percuss and vibrate on bare skin.**

## Cystic Fibrosis

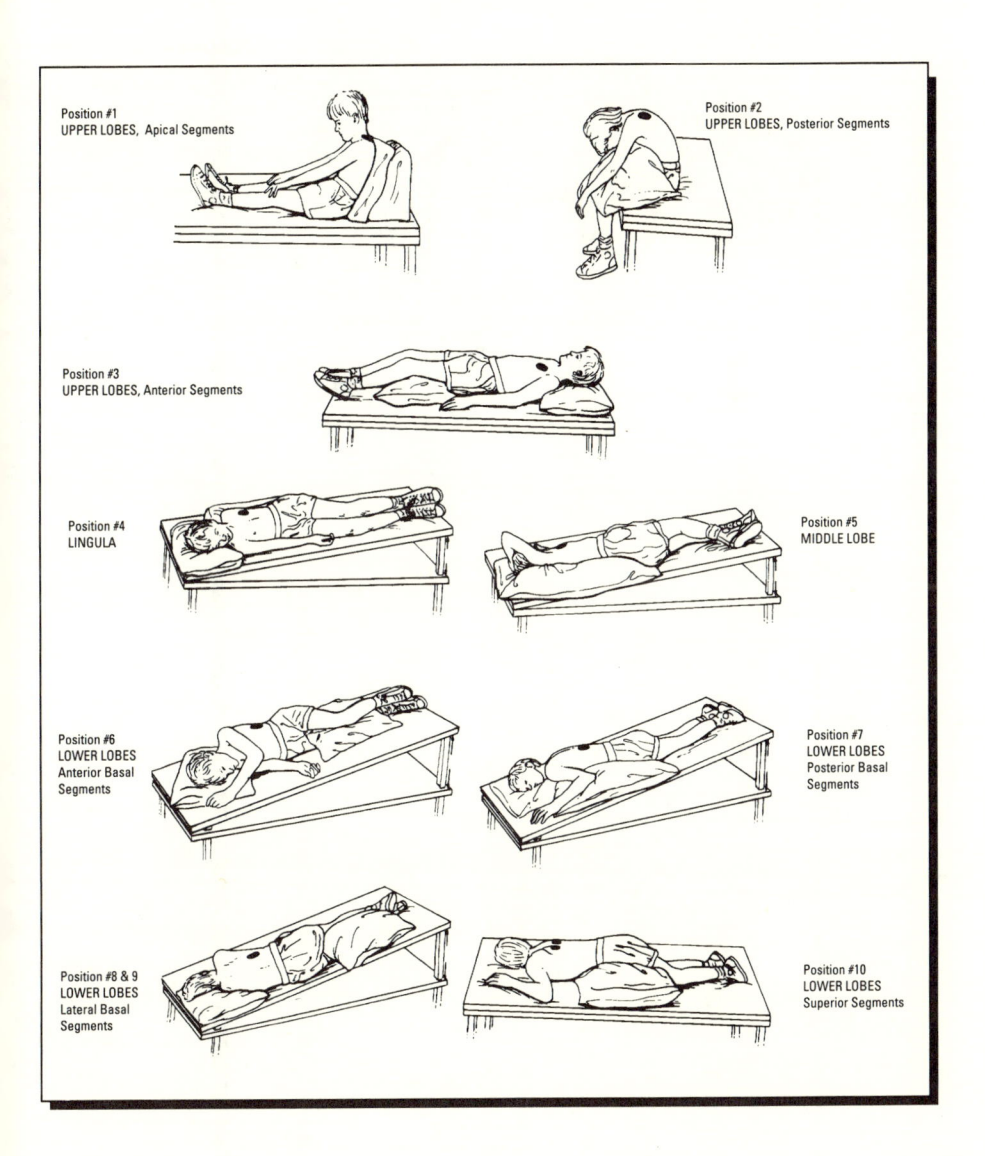

**Figure 5.11.** Summary of Bronchial Drainage Positions

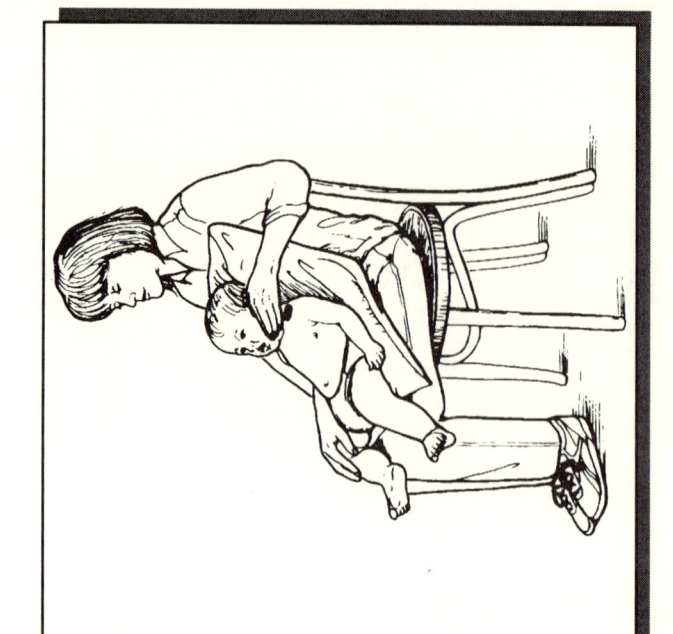

## Respiratory Diseases and Disorders Sourcebook

### INFANT

**Position # 1: UPPER LOBES**

**Apical segments**

Lean the infant back from a sitting position at a 30 degree angle on a pillow in your lap. Percuss and vibrate over the muscular area between the collarbone and the top of the scapula. Percuss and vibrate on both the **left** and **right** sides.

\* Infant shown without t-shirt for illustration purposes only.

*Figure 5.12.*

## Cystic Fibrosis

**ADULT**

**Position #1: UPPER LOBES**

**Apical segments**

Sit on a chair and lean backward on a pillow at a 30 degree angle. Percuss and vibrate over the muscular area between the collarbone and the top of the scapula on both the **left** and **right** sides of the chest.

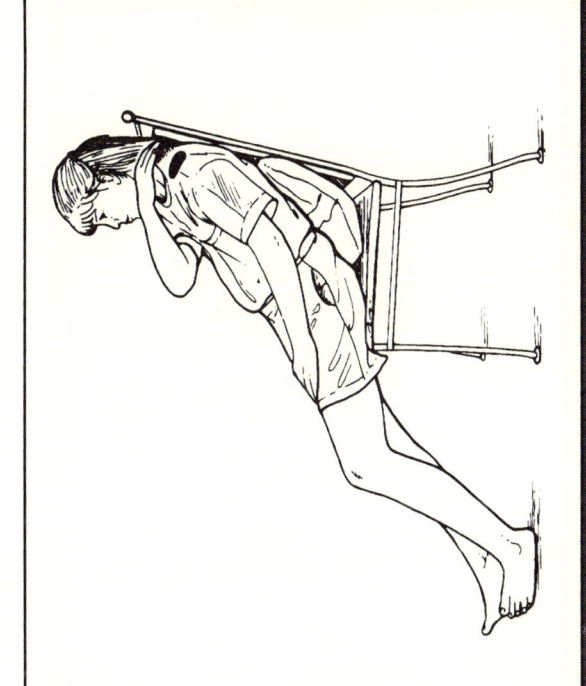

*Figure 5.13.*

**Respiratory Diseases and Disorders Sourcebook**

**CHILD**

**Position #1: UPPER LOBES**

**Apical segments**

The child sits on the flat drainage table and leans on a pillow at a 30 degree angle against the caregiver. Percuss and vibrate over the muscular area between the collarbone and the top of the scapula on both the **left** and **right** sides.

\* Child shown without t-shirt for illustration purposes only.

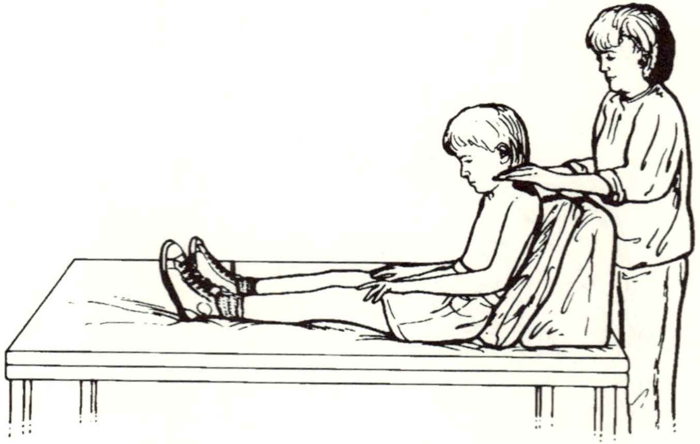

*Figure 5.14.*

## Cystic Fibrosis

**Position #2: UPPER LOBES**

**Posterior segments**

The child sits on the flat drainage table and leans forward over a folded pillow at a 30 degree angle. Stand behind the child and percuss and vibrate on the upper back on the **left** and **right** sides of the chest.

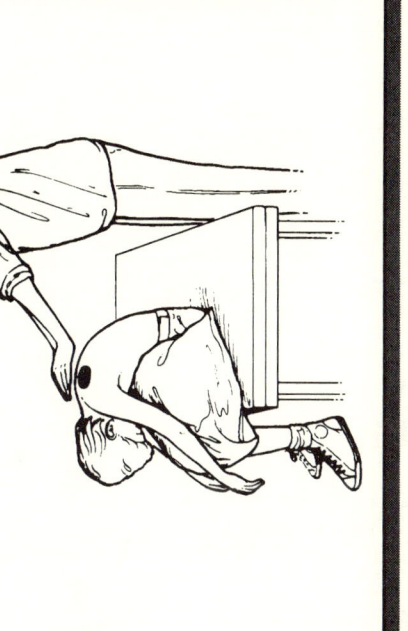

\* Child shown without t-shirt for illustration purposes only.

*Figure 5.15.*

# Respiratory Diseases and Disorders Sourcebook

**Position #3: UPPER LOBES**

**Anterior segments**

The child lies on his or her back on a flat drainage table. Percuss and vibrate between the collarbone and nipple on both the **left** and **right** sides of the chest.

\* Child shown without t-shirt for illustration purposes only.

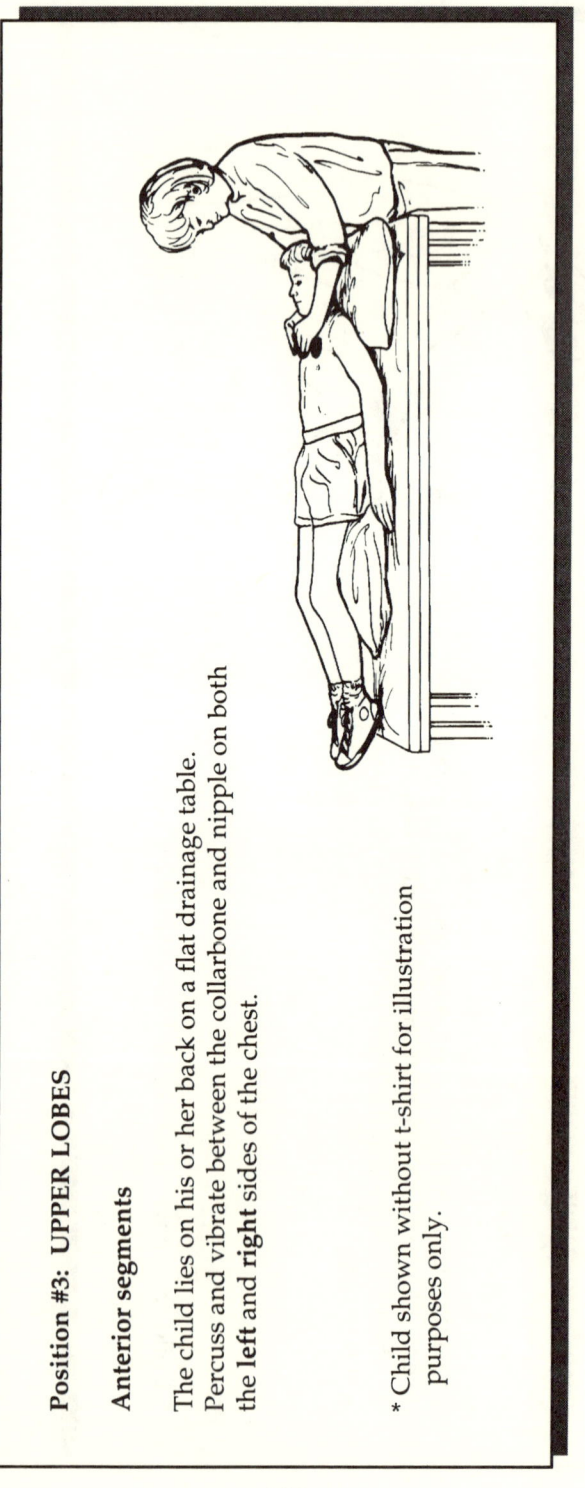

*Figure 5.16.*

## Cystic Fibrosis

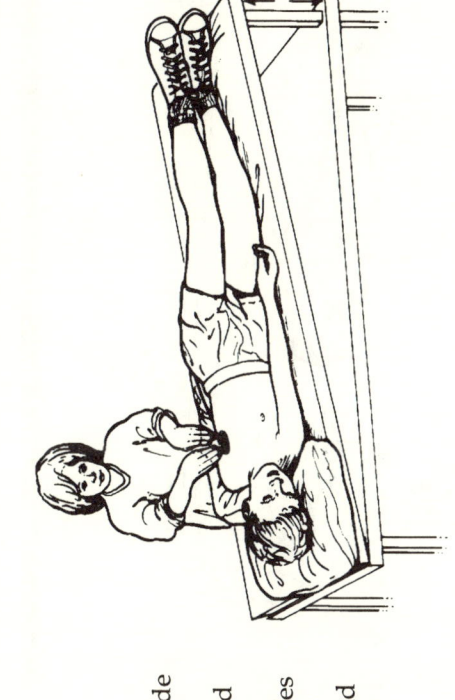

**Position #4: LINGULA**

Elevate the foot of the table 14 inches (about 15 degrees). The child lies head down on the right side and rotates 1/4 turn backward. A pillow may be placed behind the child (from shoulder to hip) and the child may flex his or her knees. Percuss and vibrate just outside the **left** nipple area. For females with tenderness around the breasts, percuss and vibrate with the heel of hand under the armpit and fingers extended forward beneath the breasts.

* Child shown without t-shirt for illustration purposes only.

*Figure 5.17.*

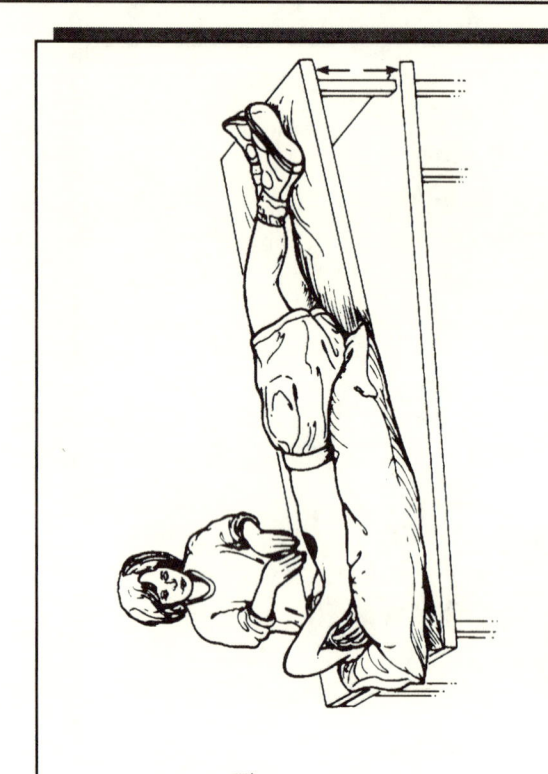

## Respiratory Diseases and Disorders Sourcebook

**Position #5: MIDDLE LOBE**

Elevate the foot of the table 14 inches (about 15 degrees). The child lies head down on the left side and rotates 1/4 turn backward. A pillow may be placed behind the child (from shoulder to hip) and the child may flex his or her knees. Percuss and vibrate just outside the **right** nipple area. For females with tenderness around the breasts, percuss and vibrate with the heel of hand under the armpit and fingers extended forward beneath the breasts.

\* Child shown without t-shirt for illustration purposes only.

*Figure 5.18.*

## Cystic Fibrosis

**Position #6: LOWER LOBES**

**Anterior Basal Segments**

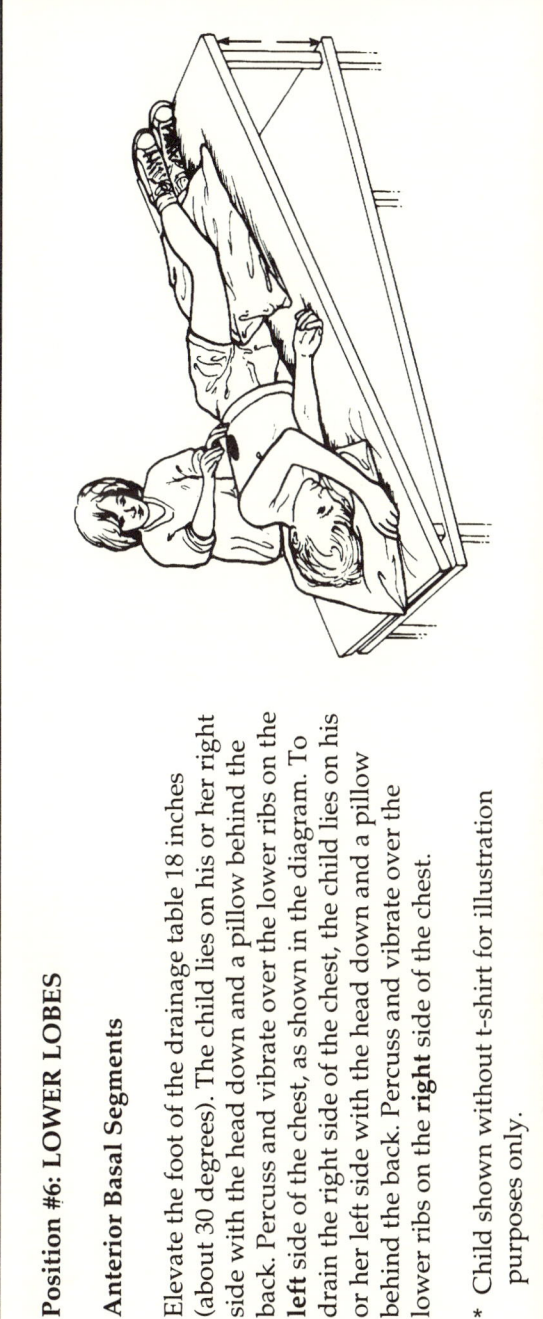

Elevate the foot of the drainage table 18 inches (about 30 degrees). The child lies on his or her right side with the head down and a pillow behind the back. Percuss and vibrate over the lower ribs on the **left** side of the chest, as shown in the diagram. To drain the right side of the chest, the child lies on his or her left side with the head down and a pillow behind the back. Percuss and vibrate over the lower ribs on the **right** side of the chest.

* Child shown without t-shirt for illustration purposes only.

*Figure 5.19.*

# Respiratory Diseases and Disorders Sourcebook

**Position #7: LOWER LOBES**

**Posterior Basal Segments**

Elevate the foot of the drainage table 18 inches (about 30 degrees). The child lies on his or her abdomen, head down, with a pillow under the hips. Percuss and vibrate over the lower ribs on both the **left** and **right** sides of the spine. Do not percuss or vibrate over the spine.

* Child shown without t-shirt for illustration purposes only.

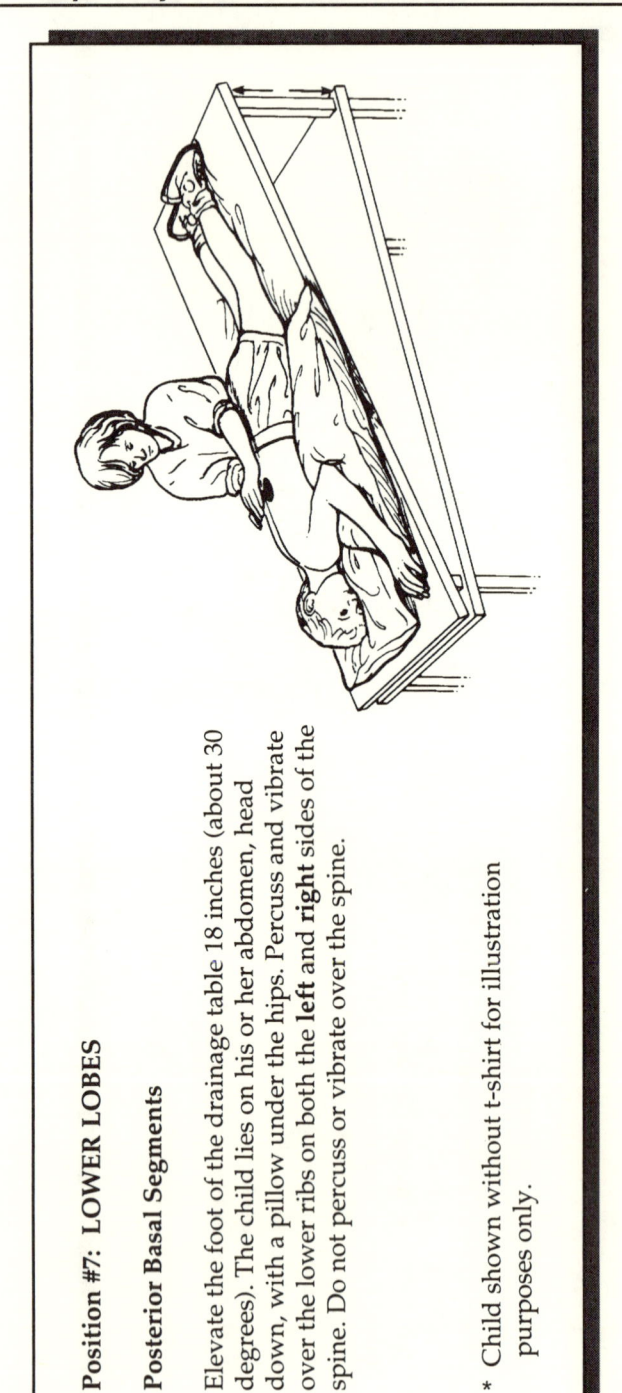

*Figure 5.20.*

## Cystic Fibrosis

**Position #8 & 9: LOWER LOBES**

**Lateral Basal Segments**

Elevate the foot of the table 18 inches (about 30 degrees). The child lies on his or her left side, head down, and leans 1/4 turn forward toward the table. The child can flex his or her upper leg over a pillow for support. Percuss and vibrate over the uppermost portion of the lower ribs to drain the **right** side, as shown in the diagram. To drain the left side, the child lies on his or her right side in the same position. Percuss and vibrate over the uppermost portion of the lower **left** ribs.

* Child shown without t-shirt for illustration purposes only.

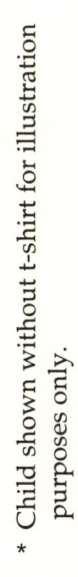

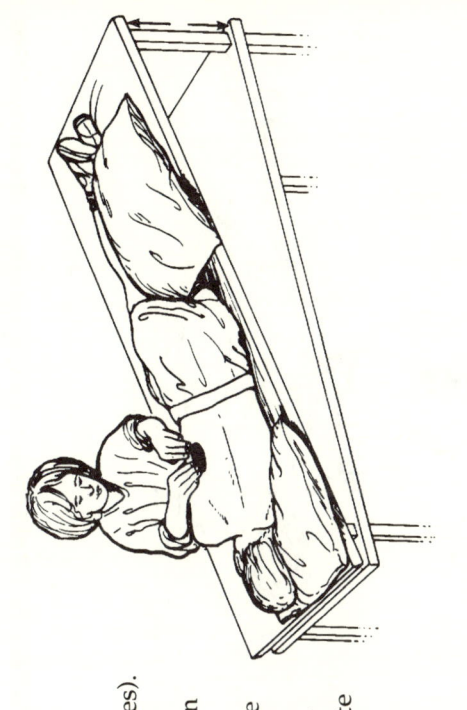

*Figure 5.21.*

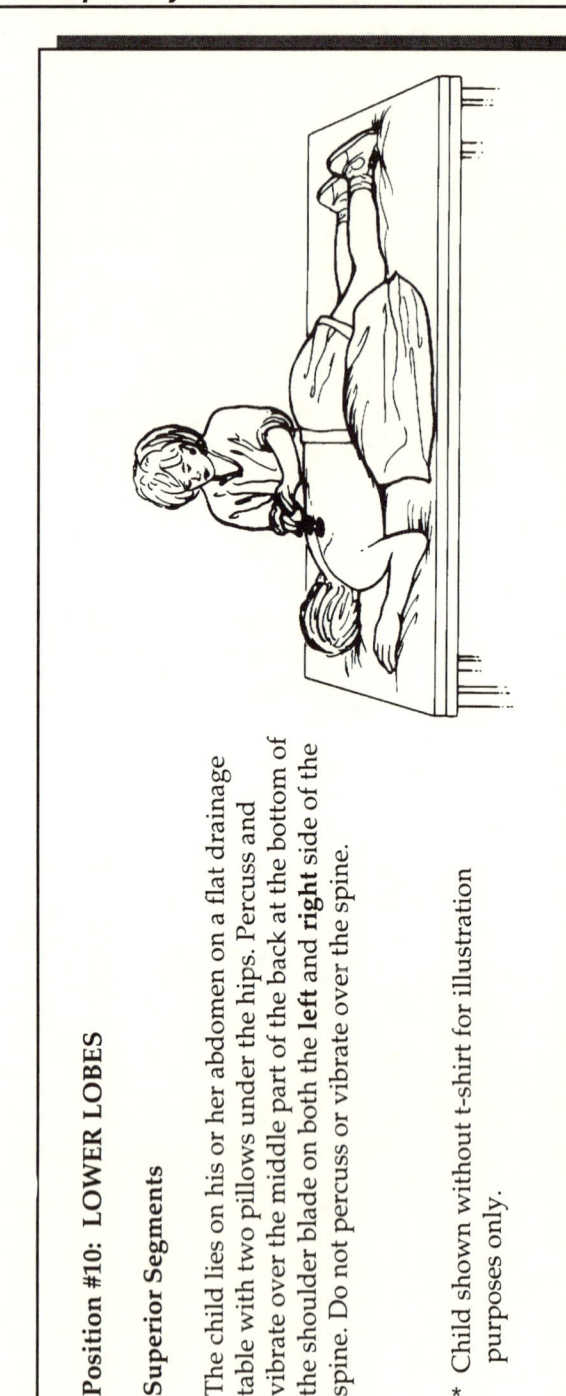

### Respiratory Diseases and Disorders Sourcebook

**Position #10: LOWER LOBES**

**Superior Segments**

The child lies on his or her abdomen on a flat drainage table with two pillows under the hips. Percuss and vibrate over the middle part of the back at the bottom of the shoulder blade on both the **left** and **right** side of the spine. Do not percuss or vibrate over the spine.

\* Child shown without t-shirt for illustration purposes only.

*Figure 5.22.*

Section 5.5

# The CF Gene: A Fifty-Year Search

Source: National Institute of Diabetes & Digestive & Kidney Diseases release, August 24, 1989.

The discovery of the cystic fibrosis (CF) gene epitomizes how basic research aimed at answering fundamental questions about the function of living organisms can provide the knowledge needed to solve long-standing medical puzzles. In identifying the CF gene, Dr. Francis Collins at the University of Michigan, Dr. Lap-Chee Tsui at the Hospital for Sick Children in Toronto, and their colleagues used and built on techniques developed over years of basic research in cell physiology and genetics.

Dr. Tsui's and Dr. Collin's work is supported by grants from the National Institute of Diabetes and Digestive and Kidney Diseases (NIDDK), a component of the Federal Government's National Institutes of Health (NIH). NIDDK Director Dr. Phillip Gorden said, "The CF gene is the key to understanding fully the underlying biochemical defect ln CF and to designing treatments aimed at correcting this defect rather than just treating the symptoms of the disease. This advance is an example of the rewards of basic research, which give scientists the tools they need to explore this disease at a molecular level."

## 50 Years of CF Research

For 50 years, CF has been the subject of a frustrating search for an underlying cause. Scientists first identified CF as a distinct syndrome in 1938. Since then, they have hunted for any cellular abnormality that could consistently explain the lung damage and digestive insufficiency caused by CF. Theories came and went. One hypothesis suggested that CF was a disorder of glycoprotein metabolism, another that CF resulted from a "factor" in blood that affected the motility of cilia, the fine hairs that move mucus along the trachea and lungs. Treatment remained limited to relieving the symptoms of CF. Doctors were helpless to control the disease process itself.

## Respiratory Diseases and Disorders Sourcebook

A major breakthrough in our understanding of CF came in 1953 when Dr. Paul di Sant-Agnese demonstrate abnormalities in the sweat of patients with CF. This discovery led to the most reliable diagnostic test for CF, the sweat test, and also provided a clue to the underlying pathophysiology. Dr. di Sant-Agnese, now scientist emeritus at NIDDK, has conducted CF research at the Institute since 1960 and is a leading authority on CF.

In the 70s and 80s basic research in key areas of biology—much of it supported by NIH-provided greatly refined techniques for culturing and studying cells and their function. In 1983, Dr. Paul Quinton, an NIDDK-supported researcher at the University of California, Riverside, used newly available methods of culturing and manipulating cells to identify for the first time a candidate for the underlying biochemical abnormality in CF. Dr. Quinton reported reduced permeability to chloride in the secretory ducts of epidermal (surface) tissues and sweat glands affected by CF. Other investigators observed similar ion transport defects in other tissues affected by CF.

At the same time, geneticists were making rapid advances in their ability to study and manipulate genes. Because genes serve as blueprints for protein, the structure of a putative CF gene could be inferred from the structure of an abnormal protein, and conversely, the defective protein could be identified if the gene were isolated. CF has a clear and consistent pattern of recessive inheritance. For that reason, scientists began to look for the CF gene, which, when located, would reveal a protein product that presumably affected ion transport.

### RFLP Analysis

The technique that laid the foundation for finding the gene was restriction fragment length polymorphism (RFLP) analysis. With this method, scientists use sites in the chain of genetic material, or DNA, which vary from person to person. The variations, known as markers, may mean nothing as far as health or appearance is concerned, but they serve as signposts for someone seeking a gene with an identifiable function. The closer a marker is to a specific gene, the more frequently the marker and the gene will be inherited together.

In RFLP analysis, scientists seek markers that are linked (close) to a gene. To do this, they use DNA probes, sequences of DNA that are artificially synthesized or cloned (copied) from an organism's DNA and radioactively labeled. DNA from individuals with and without CF is treated with restriction enzymes which recognize certain patterns in

## Cystic Fibrosis

the sequence of chemical bases that make up the steps in the ladder-like DNA structure. The restriction enzymes cut DNA at these sites. Variations in the lengths of fragments yielded by restriction enzymes reflect variable sites in the DNA sequence. Probes are sought that label these variable fragments, and testing is done to see whether the pattern of fragment lengths highlighted by any one probe seems to parallel the presence of the CF trait.

RFLP analysis and the other techniques used to trace the CF gene were borne of years of research that increased scientists' ability to manipulate genes and study how they work. RFLP is based on a knowledge of the structure of DNA and its role in heredity; the ability of enzymes to both cut DNA and stimulate its synthesis; the genetics of bacteria and viruses, which are essential to DNA cloning (copying); techniques and methods of DNA analysis; and methods of extracting DNA from cells of complex organisms and analyzing its structure.

### Linkages to CF

At first, scientists tested available genetic probes more or less at random to see if they identified DNA variations inherited with the CF trait. Their first success was finding a protein marker that was linked, or frequently inherited, along with CF. The marker is an enzyme called paraoxonase (PON). While PON did not provide information on the chromosomal location of the CF gene, it did indicate that CF was the result of a change (mutation) in a single gene.

The linkage with PON was announced in August 1985. In October of that year, NIDDK-supported scientists Dr. Lap-Chee Tsui in Toronto and colleagues working with scientists at Collaborative Research in Boston announced the linkage of CF to a marker found to be located on chromosome 7. In so doing, they vastly narrowed the location of the CF gene to one of the 23 chromosomes that compose the total complement of genetic information a human carries. The search for the gene gained momentum.

Within months, two new linkages with markers even closer to the CF gene were identified. Researchers from the National Cancer Institute and the University of Utah found that CF was linked to an oncogene—a cancer-related gene—called MET. European investigators also linked CF with a marker designated J3.11.

A collaboration among several U.S. centers established the order of these markers as MET-CF-J3.11, based on linkage studies of genetic samples provided by families with at least two members with CF.

(Linkage studies look at how often markers are inherited together or with certain physical traits.) Other markers were identified farther from the gene, and their order with respect to the CF gene was also established, providing additional information on the region in which the CF gene was located.

In spring of 1987, a British researcher announced a candidate gene for CF, but subsequently determined that this gene was not, in fact, responsible for the disease. The search continued.

Scientists estimated that the distance between MET and J3.11 was 2,000 kilobases (2 million base pairs). Base pairs are the steps in the ladder-like DNA structure. Their estimate was based on how often these markers were inherited together. The more often they are inherited together, the closer they are physically on the DNA chain.

## From Markers to a Physical Map

Rather than continue to screen new probes more or less at random (the shotgun approach), it was more systematic at this point to close in on the CF gene using physical methods of "walking" the chromosome. In gene walking, a method developed in the late 1970s, scientists cut a length of DNA under study into segments using restriction enzymes. The resulting collection of segments is called a gene library. Scientists then use DNA probes to identify a segment that overlaps one end of the DNA length under study, for example, the length between J3.11 and MET. Then they use this new segment as a probe to screen the library for a segment that overlaps it, but moves further along the DNA. Step by step, they "walk" the chromosome, making a collection of overlapping probes. The "steps" in gene walking, however, are only 20 or so kilobases (kb) in length, making walking too arduous a process to cover the distance involved between MET and J3.11. At this juncture, a physical map of some kind was needed to help determine distances involved between markers, based on physical data rather than on linkage frequencies. Dr. Collins and colleagues at the University of Michigan developed an important new approach analogous to gene walking that would cover 100 kb at a time. With the gene jumping technique, Dr. Collins' group identified a cloned DNA segment, designated CF63, about 100 kb away from MET towards the CF gene.

Using CF63, two other probes, and another new technique, pulsed field gel electrophoresis (PFGE), Dr. Collins' group made a restriction map of the CF gene region. Gel electrophoresis is the tech-

## Cystic Fibrosis

nique used to separate fragments of DNA created when the DNA is treated with restriction enzymes. Electrophoresis separates the resulting fragments based on their lengths. PFGE, developed in research aimed at increasing gene mapping capabilities, increased the versatility of electrophoresis by making it possible to separate much longer segments of DNA than was possible with conventional electrophoresis.

Dr. Collins' group treated a 3,000-kb section of DNA where the CF gene is likely to be with several different restriction enzymes, then analyzed the patterns of resulting fragments identified with the three probes. They could then make a gap of the positions of each length fragment on the region of DNA being studied, and how the fragments overlapped.

The physical map would provide the basis for narrowing the region of the CF gene to 200 to 300 kb, short enough to analyze with gene walking. At the same time, Dr. Tsui and colleagues at Toronto screened thousands of DNA segments from a chromosome 7 library to identify probes that would label the section of the chromosome near the CF gene. The combination of the probes and the restriction map could be used to narrow the candidate region to shorter ant shorter segments of DNA.

Simultaneously, these collaborating teams searched for segments of DNA that were expressed in the epithelial or surface tissue, the type of tissue that is affected by CF. While every cell in an organism has the same DNA, different sections of DNA—that is, different genes—serve as blueprints for (are expressed as) specific cellular proteins in different tissues. To look for DNA that is expressed in epithelial tissue, the investigators used RNA, a molecule with a structure similar to DNA which transmits the DNA messages into the cellular machinery. To determine which genes are expressed in CF-affected epithelial tissues, RHA that is expressed in epithelial tissues was used to screen segments of DNA from the region of the CF gene. This approach furnished another avenue towards narrowing the search.

Together these various techniques led scientists closer and closer to the gene.

### What Now?

Now that the gene has been identified, research will progress on a number of fronts. The precise function of the protein encoded by the CF gene must be determined. This will shed light on the pathophysiology of the disease and may allow development of drugs tailored to correct the defect. Different families with CF will be studied to see if variations in the genetic defect can account for the variable severity and manifestations of CF among families. The identification of the CF gene should allow improved screening for this disorder so that patients can be promptly diagnosed and treatment begun. Ultimately, finding the gene lays the groundwork for research on methods of genetic therapy to correct the gene that causes CF and thus to prevent or cure the disease.

Section 5.6

## Cystic Fibrosis:
## Test and Treatments Improve Survival

Source: Food and Drug Administration, June 1993.

Alex Deford had been ill almost from the moment of her birth on Oct. 30, 1971. Her frequent colds and ear infections coupled with her small size, despite a healthy appetite, prompted doctors to vaguely diagnose "failure to thrive." When Alex developed double pneumonia at 4 months, it was clear that something was very wrong.

That something turned out to be fibrosis, the most common inherited illness among white people of Northern and Western European ancestry, although it is seen in all ethnic groups. Symptoms include thick, sticky mucus clogging the lungs, impairing breathing and attracting infection; a blocked pancreas that can not release digestive enzymes, causing pain after eating; stubbed fingers from poor circulation; infertility; salty sweat; and other problems. Patients may have any or all of these symptoms—Alex had quite a list.

When she was diagnosed at Boston Children's Hospital early in 1972, Alex was so ill that she was expected to live only days. She survived eight years, but not easily.

Alex began each day by inhaling a decongestant. Then her parents took turns providing "postural drainage," a 30—60 minute pounding and pressing on 11 segments of the lungs, to loosen the mucus, which she coughed up. Alex would then take drugs—antibiotics to prevent lung infection and powdered digestive enzymes mixed into applesauce.

Despite this daily regimen, Alex died in January 1980. Her father, sportswriter and commentator Frank Deford, tells her story in his book, *Alex, the Life of a Child*.

Cystic fibrosis (CF) is inherited and affects 30,000 Americans. In 1989, scientists discovered the gene that causes cystic fibrosis. This discovery is enabling researchers to develop new diagnostic tests that will help identify those who can benefit from traditional as well as several new treatment approaches being evaluated by FDA.

## How CF Is Inherited

CF is typically passed from parents who each carry the gene, to children of either sex. Carriers have one faulty copy of the gene, which is responsible for the illness, plus one normal copy, which prevents symptoms. Each child of carrier parents has a 1 in 4 chance of inheriting CF; a 1 in 4 chance of being completely free of the mutant gene; and a chance of 1 in 2 of being a carrier, like the parents.

Couples usually learn that they carry CF when they have an affected child. By 1985, individuals who had a sibling with CF could find out if they carried the gene by taking a "genetic marker" (linkage analysis) test that spots a particular family's CF-carrying chromosome, but not the gene itself. Finding the CF gene makes it possible to detect most carriers, even if there are no affected relatives.

The Office of Technology Assessment estimates that 100 million to 200 million people in the United States might want to take a CF carrier test. About 8 million people in the United States, or 1 in 25 whites, may be carriers.

## Diagnosing CF

The same gene discovery that has led to developing carrier tests is expected to help more quickly diagnose CF, whose symptoms resemble those of other illnesses.

The most widely used and best-known CF test is the electrolyte sweat test. It detects the excess sodium, potassium and chloride (charged chemicals called electrolytes) found on the skin of many people with CF. A physician would perform a sweat test in a child with unexplained failure to gain weight, or with very frequent respiratory infections.

The sweat test evolved from the observations made by a physician, Dr. Paul di Sant'Agnese, during a 1953 heat wave in New York

City. He was curious why so many children with CF were being brought to Babies and Children's Hospital, where he worked, with heat prostration. The youngsters were unable to cope with the heat because too much salt exited their bodies in sweat. The fact that the sweat of a person with CF contains two to six times as much salt as normal sweat gave him the idea for the sweat test.

The sweat test became widely used by the mid-1950s, and is the only CF test cleared by FDA for marketing. (A forerunner of the sweat test was the observation that a child's brow was salty when kissed. At the turn of the century, this is how midwives identified babies with cystic fibrosis.)

Although the sweat test is a critical part of a CF diagnostic work-up, salty sweat can indicate any of several disorders. Other tests help focus the diagnosis. Some of these tests are based on methodologies developed by reference laboratories, which perform medical tests and send the results to physicians. According to Freda Yoder of FDA's Center for Devices and Radiological Health, methodologies developed in-house have not traditionally been regulated by the agency.

Explains Tom Tsakeris, director of the division of clinical laboratory devices at FDA, "FDA regulates products, not laboratories. As long as they are not marketing the test itself, we do not regulate the lab." However, he adds, the Clinical Laboratory Improvement Act, signed into law in 1988 but not yet fully implemented, will regulate reference laboratories.

One test developed by reference labs measures the amount of the protein trypsinogen in a newborn's blood. Trypsinogen is manufactured by the pancreas and sent to the intestine, where it is snipped to a shorter form, trypsin, which helps digest proteins. If the pancreas is clogged by the sticky mucus of CF, trypsinogen levels are elevated, because the longer protein cannot be cut down to size.

In one study conducted by researchers at the University of Colorado School of Medicine and Children's Hospital in Denver, the trypsinogen test identified 95.2 percent of infants with CF who did not have the earliest sign, a greenish discharge called meconium ileus indicating intestinal blockage. But in the study there were many false positives—of 96 infants who tested high for trypsinogen on two tests, only 31 had CF. So, although the trypsinogen test alone is not perfect, combined with a sweat test and observing symptoms it can begin to paint a portrait of CF.

Another test detects the level of certain fetal intestinal enzymes in the amniotic fluid (the liquid surrounding the fetus). Amniotic fluid is collected for testing by; procedure called amniocentesis. In a fetus with CF, these enzymes are decreased. Again, however, other disorders besides CF can produce this finding, and therefore it is not a specific disease marker. Researchers have turned to the genetic material to develop a definitive CF test.

## Genetic Testing

Developing a test to detect the gene that causes CF would provide a definitive diagnosis, because this mutant gene is the only cause of the disorder. The first step was to find out where the gene behind CF lies among the 23 pairs of chromosomes.

By 1985, several research teams had narrowed the search to a part of chromosome 7 (the seventh largest chromosome). Until the CF gene itself was isolated and characterized in 1989, relatives of patient could take an indirect test that uses linkage analysis. Because of the complexity of the interpretation, these tests are primarily performed at academic centers.

A genetic linkage test tracks a known DNA sequence (a genetic marker) that, within a family, always occurs in people with CF, and never in those who do not have the illness. A genetic marker and the gene responsible for the disorder behave like two inseparable friends. If you see one at a party, you know the other is nearby. Genetic linkage testing is based on the observation that genes carried close together on the same chromosome tend to be inherited together.

Ray White at the Howard Hughes Medical Institute at the University of Utah in Salt Lake City and Robert Williamson of St. Mary's Hospital Medical School in London each found a marker, one on either side of the CF gene. Using these two markers, a couple who already had a child with CF could have fetal chromosomes tested in a subsequent pregnancy. If the two markers on the two chromosome 7's in the fetus matched those of the affected child, then it, too, has likely inherited the disease.

A major limitation of linkage tests is that they only work on families known to have CF. Because people can carry CF without having symptoms, a disease-causing gene can be in a family without anyone in recent memory being ill. Finding the CF gene itself, however, may make possible a test useful on anyone, so that carriers could be detected in families where no one has CF.

Like other genetic tests, CF tests can be performed on any type of tissue, because all human cells (except red blood cells) contain two copies of all of the genes, and sperm and egg have one copy of each. The first CF tests used white blood cells. Then Williamson's group in London came up with a more pleasant alternative—a mouthwash! After swishing a saltwater solution in the mouth, the person spits into a bottle. The CF gene can be spotted in cells dislodged from the inside of the cheek.

Taking a cue from London, Genzyme Corp. (Cambridge, MA) developed a cheekbrush test for CF, which is investigational. A patient swabs cheek cells onto a brush, and the physician sends the sample to Genzyme. The presence of both normal and mutant CF genes indicates carrier status. If only mutant genes are there, CF is indicated (see Figure 5.23).

## To Test or Not to Test?

A carrier test provides information to couples who are not ill but whose children are at high risk of inheriting the condition.

Many experts predict that the day of universal CF screening is approaching, with several companies developing CF tests that simultaneously screen for several CF mutations.

Two factors contribute to the sensitivity of a CF carrier test. The first is the number of mutations that can be detected. The more mutations tested for, the more carriers will be spotted.

Ethnic background is the other important factor, says Marisa Ladoulis, a genetic counselor at Collaborative Diagnostic Services in Waltham, Mass. For example, a 12-mutation test that spots 84 percent of whites with a Northern or Western European background will detect 92 to 95 percent of Ashkenazi Jews, and the 16-mutation test finds 96 to 98 percent of them.

## All CF Mutations Are Not Equal

Checking for an errant CF gene may be easy, but interpreting the results may not be. Researchers are finding that different CF mutations cause different degrees of sickness. Alex Deford probably had two copies of delta F508, the most common and one of the more serious mutations that can cause CF. But a researcher in the laboratory of Francis Collins, the co-discoverer of the CF gene, has a milder case of CF because he inherited the delta F508 mutation as well as a different one.

## Cystic Fibrosis

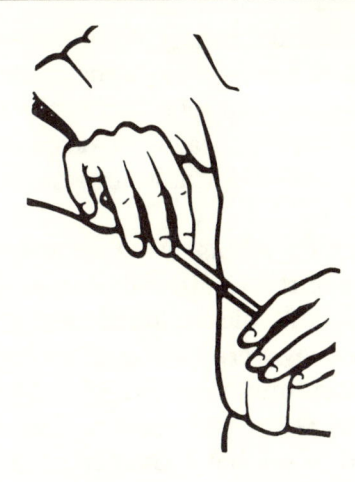

The health professional twists a tube containing a cheek brush and pulls it open, removing the cheek brush from the tube.

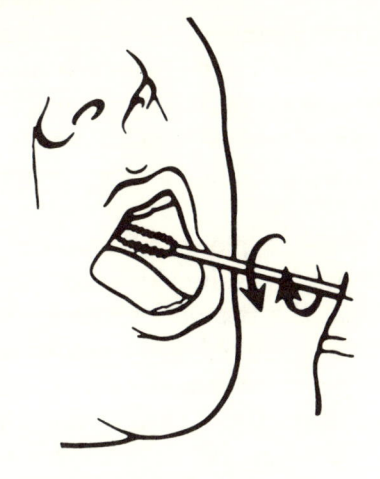

The cheek brush is inserted into the patient's mouth and twisted vigorously against the inside of the cheek for at least 30 seconds to collect cells containing DNA.

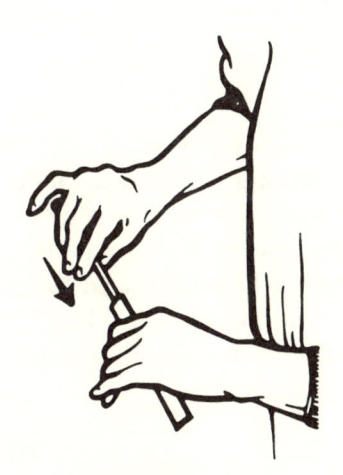

The professional then carefully places the cheek brush back into the original tube and replaces the cap.
(Artwork courtesy of Genzyme Corp., Cambridge, Mass.)

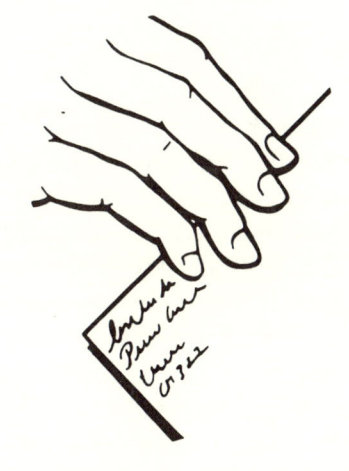

The cheek brush in its tube is mailed to the manufacturer for analysis.

*Figure 5.23.* Cheek Brush Test

This young man must perform postural drainage on himself and take antibiotics and digestive enzymes, but he also plays the trumpet, bikes, and sings. Still, a respiratory infection can send him to the hospital for a week or longer. Clinicians are finding that some people who have frequent bouts of pneumonia and other respiratory infections actually have CF.

Some people with CF may not even have lung or digestive symptoms. Aubrey Milunsky, D.Sc., Director of the Center for Human Genetics at the Boston University School of Medicine, found that some men who were referred to him because they were having difficulty fathering a child actually had CF. In examining x-rays that had been taken as part of a standard fertility work-up, Milunsky noticed the men lacked the vas deferens, the paired tubes that deliver sperm from the body. Knowing this is a symptom in 90 percent of men with CF, Milunsky tested their genes and found they had inherited CF.

"Cystic fibrosis is not a simple single mutation to look for," says Margaret Wallace, Ph.D., assistant professor in the division of genetics in the department of pediatrics at the University of Florida in Gainesville. "There will be a lot of problems in doing the diagnosis and giving an idea of what it means," she adds.

## *Treating CF*

CF symptoms are controlled with a number of drugs. Antibiotic drugs combat infections to which CF patients are prone, including *Pseudomonas aeruginosa* bacteria, a type of microbe that is attracted to the sticky mucus in the lungs. The combination of animal enzymes, called Viokase, that Alex Deford took regularly is still used today by CF patients. It is approved as a prescription digestive aid for CF patients and others with pancreatic insufficiencies. Combined with a high-calorie diet, this enzyme preparation aids digestion, helping the patient to maintain weight.

Many patients also take anti-inflammatory prescription drugs, such as ibuprofen (Motrin and others), prednisone (Deltasone, Winpred, Orason, and others), and naproxen (Anaprox, Naprosyn and others).

The drug amiloride (Midamor, Moduretic), introduced in 1967 and approved as an adjunct to treatment with some diuretic drugs, is now being tested as a treatment for CF. Scientists believe amiloride thins lung secretions by blocking sodium uptake by lung cells. Clinical studies are under way to assess amiloride as a CF treatment alone, and in combination with the biological products adenosine triphosphate (ATP) and uridine triphosphate (UTP). (ATP and UTP are components of the nucleic acids DNA and RNA.)

Other investigational products are aimed at tempering the body's immune response to lung infection, which can be excessive. One such product is deoxyribo-nuclease. The March 19, 1992, New England Journal of Medicine reported that in a pilot study, this protein biologic given in an aerosol helped clear the lungs of 16 adult CF patients. It is being tested in 900 CF patients at 50 medical centers in the United States.

## Gene Therapy

FDA has designated recombinant cystic fibrosis transmembrane conductance regulator (the gene's protein product, abbreviated CFTR) as well as gene therapy as orphan products. This gives their sponsors special incentives because they are developing products for a condition affecting relatively few people.

The first human gene therapy study of CF got under way last April 17 at the National Heart, Lung, and Blood Institute after FDA gave the go-ahead the previous day. An engineered cold virus (adenovirus) was introduced into the cells lining the nose and airways of a 23-year-old man with CF. The virus was altered to carry the normal CFTR gene and lacks the genes to cause a cold and to replicate.

The research was the first use of gene therapy for a common genetic disorder and the first use of a cold virus to transport genes. The study includes 10 patients 21 or older who have mild to moderate CF symptoms.

Previous experiments in rats indicated that replacing the CF genes in just 10 percent of the lung lining cells improves lung function. However, because the genes go to the patients' lungs but not their sex cells, CF can still be passed to the patients' children.

New knowledge of CF is coming so fast that the goals of carrier screening may change even before the tests are cleared for marketing.

Soon, detecting the gene for CF may be a way of finding who needs treatment, as early as possible, just as is presently done for high blood pressure and elevated blood cholesterol. Says Wallace, "CF research is moving so quickly, with a lot of hope for treatment in the near future. It will be treatable, and possibly easily."

## Advances and Stumbling Blocks

The symptoms of CF were first described in medical journals in 1938. The malady was attributed to a defect in the channels leading from certain glands—a remarkably accurate description, it would turn out. But the disorder was recognized before it was given a name, as illustrated by the 17th century saying, "A child that is salty to the taste will die shortly after birth."

In 1960, a CF patient rarely lived past the age of 12. By 1970, only half lived to see their 18th birthdays. In the 1970s, when postural drainage began to be implemented and FDA approved enzyme replacement and antibiotic therapy, the average lifespan began to creep upwards. Today, it is 29 years, according to the Cystic Fibrosis Foundation. New, more targeted therapies may raise survival age higher.

Cystic fibrosis researchers marked a medical milestone on Oct. 8, 1989, when *Science* magazine published a report by Francis Collins and his co-workers at the University of Michigan at Ann Arbor and Lap-chee Tsui at the Hospital for Sick Children in Toronto on precisely how a specific gene disrupts a certain protein to cause CF.

The researchers named the protein the "cystic fibrosis transmembrane conductance regulator," or CFTR for short. CFTR is normally manufactured inside cells lining glands in the respiratory passages, small intestine, pancreas and sweat glands. The protein travels to the cell's surface, where it controls the flow of salt in and out of the cell like a gateway in the cell membrane.

In the disorder, CFTR protein is abnormal in a way that prevents it from reaching the cell's surface. Without the gateway in the membrane, salt is trapped inside cells. Following a natural chemical tendency to try to dilute the salty interiors of cells, moisture is drawn inside them through other gateways. This dries out the surrounding secretions causing symptoms. In most people with CF, the protein is missing just one amino acid building block out of 1,480—a tiny but devastating glitch.

Almost as soon as Collins and Tsui described the mutation that causes CF, dubbed delta F508, a difficulty arose. Delta F508 was not the only way that the gene could be altered. (A gene consists of sequences of four types of building blocks. Just as a sentence can have an error in any of its letters, a gene can be altered in many ways. A person with CF inherits two abnormal forms.)

But within days of the publication of the *Science* report, several biotechnology firms were already devising carrier tests for delta F508.

A test for the disease-causing gene variant became available on an investigational basis by November 1989. But on February 1, 1990, Collins, Tsui, and several others reported in *The New England Journal of Medicine* that only 75.9 percent of white CF patients of Northern or Western European backgrounds had the delta F508 variant. How useful would a test for delta F508 be, researchers worried, if this wasn't the variant responsible for CF? At current count, more than 200 variants of the gene are known.

The multiple guises of the CF gene meant that a test to spot delta F508 would miss about 24 percent of Northern or Western European descended whites in the United States who do carry a CF gene. This, in turn, meant that the test would find only about half the couples in the United States who risk passing CF to a child this figure is derived by multiplying the chances of each parent having delta F508). But it would be too costly to develop a test for more than 200 different mutations when only a few of them are common.

Adding to the complexity is that different populations have different proportions of CF gene variants. For example, delta F508 occurs in only 35 percent of African-Americans and Jews of Central and Eastern European ancestry (called Ashkenazi) who carry CF, making the test for this mutation even less valuable than it is for non-Jewish whites. For Hispanics and Italians, the frequency of delta F508 is 50 percent.

The potential powder keg of a carrier test for a common genetic disease that would, at best, only work three-quarters of the time set off a flurry of statements by professional medical organizations. On Nov. 13, 1989, the American Society of Human Genetics urged caution in carrier testing until a greater percentage of the CF-carrying population could be identified, calling for pilot programs to test the tests. Meanwhile, they suggested the test only for those with a close affected relative.

In early March 1990, a panel of physicians, geneticists genetic counselors, and attorneys met at the National Institutes of Health in Bethesda, MD, to develop guidelines for CF carrier testing. This group echoed the earlier call for pilot programs, adding that widespread testing should wait until tests could detect 90 to 95 percent of carriers.

In December 1992, the American Society of Human Genetics reevaluated their 1989 statement, in light of the ability to detect many CF mutations. Their advice remains unchanged—for now, CF testing should be offered only to those with a relative who has the disorder. The organization calls for informed consent and genetic counseling, confidentiality of results, and quality control of the laboratory performing the test.

—*Ricki Lewis*

Ricki Lewis is a genetic counselor and is the author of textbooks on biology and human genetics.

## Section 5.7

## FDA Licenses Cystic Fibrosis Treatment

Source: Food and Drug Administration, June 1993.

Licensing of the first product in 30 years specifically developed to treat cystic fibrosis was announce in December 1993. The biologic product was licensed nine months after it was submitted for review by FDA. It was jointly reviewed with the Canadian Health Protection Branch and licensed simultaneously in both countries.

Dornase alfa, commonly called DNase, a product of recombinant DNA technology, reduces the frequency of respiratory infections and improves lung function in cystic fibrosis patients.

Cystic fibrosis, an inherited disorder that affects about 30,000 Americans, is characterized by thick mucous secretions in the lungs. The retention of this mucous in the airways contributes to reduced lung function and chronic lung infections. Respiratory complications are the major cause of death among patients.

In providing an expedited review, FDA followed procedures established to implement the Prescription Drug User Fee Act of 1992, which provides additional resources to FDA to speed up review of drugs and biologics submitted to the agency for approval.

Due to the relatively low incidence of cystic fibrosis, FDA has designated DNase an "orphan" product. This designation provides financial incentives for companies developing products for rare diseases—those affecting fewer than 200,000 people in the United States.

DNase was evaluated in a six-month, multi-center, placebo-controlled clinical trial of 968 cystic fibrosis patients 5 years and older. Daily doses of DNase, used in conjunction with standard therapies, reduced the risk of severe respiratory tract infections by 27 percent and increased patients' lung function.

No clinical trials were conducted to demonstrate safety and effectiveness of DNase in children younger than 5, in patients with breathing function measured at less than 40 percent, or in patients for longer than 12 months.

Side effects include inflammation of throat, chest pain, voice alteration, and laryngitis.

DNase is manufactured by Genentech Inc. of San Francisco, and is marketed under the trade name Pulmozyme.

Section 5.8

# Cystic Fibrosis and DNA Tests: The Implications of Carrier Screening

Source: Office of Technology Assessment, Congress of the United States. Pub. No. OTA-BA-532, August 1992.

### The Proliferation of Cystic Fibrosis in the United States

People want—expect—perfectly healthy babies. When a child is born with a genetic condition, parents suffer anxiety, endure anguish, and experience guilt: "This baby is sick because of us."

This chapter is about one of these inherited conditions: cystic fibrosis (CF). CF is a life-shortening disorder. It is a genetic condition—i.e., one that follows a clear pattern of inheritance in families—and is the most common, lethal recessive disorder in American Caucasians of European descent. Each year in the United States, about 1 in 2,500 babies is born with CF (i.e., about 1,700 to 2,000 babies with CF are born annually). Approximately 1 in 9,600 Hispanic, 1 in 17,000 to 19,000 African American and 1 in 90,000 Asian American newborns have CF.

| | |
|---|---|
| 1650. | Literature refers to now characteristic CF pancreatic and lung symptoms association with salty skin and early death. |
| 1705. | A book of folk philosophy states that a salty taste means a child is bewitched. |
| 1857. | *The Almanac of Children's Songs and Games*, Switzerland, quotes from Middle Ages: "Woe is the child who tastes salty from a kiss on the brow, for he is hexed, and soon must die." |
| 1938. | First reported description of disease, calling it "cystic fibrosis of the pancreas." |
| 1946. | Antibiotics found effective for treating CF-related lung infection. |
| 1946. | Inheritance pattern—autosomal recessive—suggested. |
| 1953. | Sweat abnormality in CF first described. |
| 1955. | First review of use of pancreatic enzymes to treat CF. |
| 1959. | Safe and accurate way to diagnose CF, "sweat testing," reported. |
| 1960 to present. | Accelerated improvement in survival. |
| 1968. | Mechanism underlying CF-related male infertility demonstrated. |
| 1981 to 1983. | Basis for sweat abnormality (i.e., electrolyte transport problems) described. |
| 1986. | CF gene localized to chromosome 7. |
| 1989. | CF gene and its most common mutation identified. |
| 1990. | CF mutation assays available from selected genetic laboratories, companies, and medical centers. |
| 1990. | CF mutation corrected in laboratory cells. |
| 1991. | Functions of CF gene described. |

SOURCE: Office of Technology Assessment, 1992, based on L.M. Taussig, *Cystic Fibrosis* (New York, NY: Thieme-Stratton, Inc., 1984).

*Table 5.24. History of CF: Selected Highlights*

Medicine has long recognized the consequences of CF (table 5.24) on several organ systems, particularly the lungs and pancreas. Only recently, however, have scientists pinpointed the most common change, or mutation, in the genetic material—DNA— that accounts for the majority of CF cases.

Because CF is a recessive trait, a child with CF must receive two mutant CF genes, one inherited from each parent, who are CF "carriers," but who do not have the disorder. Thus, while approximately 30,000 people in the United States have CF, as many as 8 million people could be carriers of one CF mutation. What are the implications of informing this latter pool of individuals—or a subset of those of reproductive age and younger—about tests that reveal CF carrier status?

## Why Is Cystic Fibrosis Carrier Screening Controversial?

Prospects of routine CF carrier screening polarize people. Everyone agrees that persons with a family history of CF should have the opportunity to avail themselves of CF mutation analysis, yet controversy swirls around using the same tests in the general population. What are the elements of the controversy? Can past experiences with other carrier screening initiatives and current research from CF carrier screening pilots resolve some issues?

### Today's Clinical and Social Tensions

For years, experts theorized about confronting the potential consequences of increased knowledge of human genetics. In the early 1990s, the CF mutation test moves the debate from the theoretical to the practical. Today, along with clinical tensions surrounding CF carrier screening, are legal, ethical, economic, and political considerations.

No mandatory genetic screening programs of adult populations exist in the United States; the Office of Technology Assessment (OTA) finds it highly unlikely that CF carrier screening will set a precedent in this regard. Nevertheless, people disagree about how CF carrier screening of the general population should be conducted.

Proponents of a measured approach to CF carrier screening express concern about several issues that might be raised if use of CF carrier tests becomes routine. Invariably, discussions about CF carrier screening raise concerns about the use of genetic information by insurance companies and become linked to broader social concerns about health care reform in the United States. Related to this are concerns about commercialization of genetic research, i.e., that market pressures will drive widespread use of tests before the potential for discrimination or stigmatization by other individuals or institutions (e.g., employers and insurers) is assessed. Also expressed are questions about the adequacy of quality assurance for DNA diagnostic facilities, personnel, and the tests themselves. Opponents of widespread CF carrier screening also wonder whether the current number of genetic specialists can handle a swell of CF carrier screening cases, let alone the cases from tests for other genetic conditions expected to arise from the Human Genome Project. Finally, the extraordinary tensions in the United States about abortion affect discussions about CF carrier testing and screening.

Those who advocate CF carrier tests for use beyond affected families are no less concerned about the issues just raised. Rather, proponents argue that individuals should be routinely informed about the assays so they can decide for themselves whether to be voluntarily screened. They assert that the tests are sensitive enough for current use and will, like most tests, continually improve. These voices believe that failing to inform patients now about the availability of CF carrier assays denies people the opportunity to make personal choices about their reproductive futures, either prospectively e.g., by avoiding conception, choosing to adopt, or using artificial insemination by donor—or by using prenatal testing to determine whether a fetus is affected.

*Lessons From Past Carrier Screening Efforts*

Carrier screening is not new to the United States. The 1970s and early 1980s saw a number of genetic screening efforts flourish throughout the country. Federal legislation—chiefly the National Sickle Cell Anemia, Cooley's Anemia, Tay-Sachs, and Genetic Diseases Act (Public Law 94-278; hereinafter the National Genetic Diseases Act) and its predecessors—fueled these programs. Today, what might work for CF carrier screening—and what will not work—can be gleaned from carrier screening for other genetic disorders, even though earlier screening occurred through more centralized efforts. In fact, some argue that creating a defined, federally funded program for CF carrier screening could avoid social concerns, although others assert the contrary.

Frequently considered a successful effort, Tay-Sachs carrier screening was initiated in 1971 at the behest of American Jewish communities. Tay-Sachs disease is a lethal, recessive genetic disorder that primarily affects Jews of Eastern and Central European descent and populations descended from French Canadian ancestors. It involves the central nervous system, resulting in mental retardation and death within the first years of life. Fourteen months of technical preparation, education of medical and religious leaders, and organizational planning preceded massive public education campaigns. Since screening commenced, over one-half million adults have been voluntarily screened; today, it is a part of general medical care.

In contrast, sickle cell programs in the 1970s are generally cited as screening gone wrong. The sickle cell mutation—which like the Tay-Sachs and CF mutations is recessive—affects hemoglobin, the oxygen-carrying molecule in blood. The sickle cell mutation is found predominantly in African Americans and some Mediterranean populations. Most individuals with sickle cell anemia live well into adulthood. Unlike Tay-Sachs screening, much sickle cell screening was mandatory. For the most part, Caucasians designed and implemented programs targeted toward African Americans, leading to proclamations of racist genocide. Even after elimination of most mandatory screening in the late 1970s, actual practice strayed from the stated goals of adequate genetic counseling, public education, and confidentiality of results.

Tay-Sachs carrier screening and sickle cell screening—along with carrier screening for other genetic conditions provide perspective for today's discussions about CF carrier screening. Two lessons in particular are clear:

- Participation should be voluntary and
- Public education is vital.

Disagreement exists, however, about the degree to which CF carrier screening can draw on the Tay-Sachs and sickle cell experiences to resolve other considerations (e.g. discrimination). Several factors contribute to questions raised about comparability, including: Today's political climate differs; CF carrier screening has the potential to involve larger numbers of people; and Tay-Sachs and sickle cell screening were implemented, in part, with explicit Government funding in a more programmatic fashion than will be likely for CF carrier screening.

*Cystic Fibrosis Carrier Screening Pilot Studies*

Opponents of routine CF carrier screening argue that historical perspectives fall short of adequately addressing potential adverse consequences raised by widespread utilization of CF mutation assays, including adequate education and counseling, and prospects for discrimination and stigmatization. They assert that until data are gathered from federally funded pilot projects specific to CF, carrier screening should not be routine. Proponents, on the other hand, argue that sufficient information is available from privately supported CF carrier screening projects, that much historical experience applies, and that any incremental gain that will be gleaned from federally funded studies is insufficient to a priori prevent routine CF carrier screening from proceeding.

## Federally Funded Studies

Despite pleas throughout the genetics community for the Federal Government to fund pilot projects to assess clinical and social considerations raised by the new CF mutation analyses, initial calls for funding of pilots went wanting. In the United Kingdom, the CF Research Trust actively funded and encouraged pilots unlike the CF Foundation in the United States, which has focused on investigations to find the CF gene and mutation, but divorces itself from CF carrier screening. Concern about abortion apparently played a major role in the later policy decision.

After some scrambling, the Ethical, Legal, and Social Issues (ELSI) Program of the National Center for Human Genome Research (NCHGR), National Institutes of Health (NIH), stepped forward to coordinate federally financed pilot studies. In October 1991 (fiscal year 1992), three units of NIH—the National Center for Human Genome Research, the National Institute of Child Health and Human Development, and the National Center for Nursing Research—launched a 3-year research initiative to analyze education and counseling methods related to CF mutation analysis.

Seven research teams, conducting eight studies, received support and will coordinate their efforts. Two of seven clinical studies focus on relatives of individuals with CF (CF carrier testing); the other five focus on the general population. One study involves theoretical modeling. Where appropriate, some features of the research, such as evaluation measures and tools, cost assessment, laboratory quality control procedures, and human subjects protection will be standardized across sites.

## Privately Funded Studies

Prior to the onset of federally sponsored pilot projects, several public and private institutions began to systematically offer CF carrier screening to subsets of the population; pregnant women and their partners, preconceptional adults, teenagers, and fetuses all have been target populations. Most privately funded efforts have been under way since early 1990, and most have collected, or are collecting, data on the incidence of carrier status and mutation frequencies. Some also follow psychosocial issues such as levels of anxiety and retention of information. Most studies can report results, and the various strategies used and different target populations reflect the lack of consensus on the best approach to CF carrier screening.

## What Factors Will Affect Utilization?

Initially, routine CF carrier screening will likely occur in the reproductive context; the prenatal population has been the traditional entry point into genetic services for many people. Preconceptional individuals are also a possible population, but for most individuals the first real opportunity for carrier screening takes place post-conception. A focus on pregnant women, however, is not without controversy. Reservations exist about abortion, as do concerns that prenatal testing negatively shapes perceptions of pregnancy, disability, and women. Nevertheless, the primary responsibility for providing CF carrier screening could come to reside with obstetricians, as has occurred with maternal serum alpha-fetoprotein (MSAFP) screening to detect fetuses with neural tube or abdominal wall defects or Down syndrome.

Based on the annual number of births (4.2 million) and spontaneous abortions (an estimated 1.8 million), there are approximately 6 million pregnancies per year for which CF carrier screening might be performed. Twenty-four percent of women giving birth receive no prenatal care until the third trimester, however, so CF carrier screening in the obstetric/prenatal context could initially involve, at most, 10 million men and women per year, depending on who is screened.

For some, the key question still hovering over carrier screening for CF is if, not when. For others, however, the debate has shifted to when. Several institutions already offer CF mutation analysis to individuals, regardless of family history. OTA projects approximately 63,000 individuals will be screened for their CF carrier status in 1992—about a 7-fold increase over 1991. This rapid upward trend is expected, given the nascent stage of the technology's movement into U.S. medical practice.

Without offering judgment on its appropriateness or inappropriateness, OTA finds that the matter of CF carrier screening in the United States is one of when, not if. Regardless of the number of individuals actually screened, it is clear that, increasingly, patients will be informed about the availability of CF carrier assays and a portion will opt to be screened. What is less clear is the timeframe for physicians to begin routinely informing patients about CF carrier tests. It could be within a year or two, but more likely will be a gradual process over several years. What factors affect—or will affect—routine carrier screening for CF? Eight aspects predominate:

- genetic services delivery and customs of care,
- public education,
- professional capacity,
- financing,
- stigmatization, classification, and discrimination issues,
- quality assurance of clinical laboratories and DNA test kits,
- automation, and
- costs and cost-effectiveness.

Of these issues, all but cost-effectiveness extend beyond CF to global concerns about future tests to assess other genetic risks.

## GENETIC SERVICES: STANDARDS OF CARE AND ENSURING QUALITY

One broad question expresses a facet of the current clinical controversy: Who serves as gatekeeper of a new technology? The degree to which large numbers of Americans opt to learn their CF carrier status depends first on their interaction with the genetic services system in the country. Utilization of DNA-based CF mutation analysis will depend on the extent to which physicians, genetic counselors, and other health professionals customarily inform individuals about the test's availability. In turn, moving from innovation to standard practice often depends on professional guidelines or statements. Disagreement exists about the applicability of CF carrier tests to individuals without positive family histories, which has led to tensions, with opposite sides questioning the motives of the other. Additionally, consumer acceptance will depend on perceptions that the professional services they receive with screening are of high quality.

### *Standards of Care*

Should all individuals be informed about tests to identify CF carrier status? Society has no definitive way of determining when physicians should routinely advise people about the availability of tests that could reveal their propensity to have a child with a genetic disorder. Physician practice might be driven by consumer demand, patient autonomy, liability fears, economic self-interest, or a combination of these factors. CF carrier screening presents a classic instance of the perennial problem of appropriately controlling the evolution of practice standards as a new technology becomes available. Thus, deciding the appropriate timing for routinely telling everyone about CF mutation tests is a contentious issue.

Physicians can now offer individuals with no family history of CF a test that can determine, with 85 to 95 percent sensitivity, whether they are CF carriers. With professional opinion in a state of flux—and knowledge of the assay's existence continuing to spread among patients—physicians might wonder whether they are obligated to inform patients of its availability, even before patients ask about it.

Some consumers are interested in genetic tests and CF carrier screening. A 1986 OTA telephone survey of a national probability sample of adult Americans reported that about 9 of 10 approved of making genetic tests available through doctors. Eighty-three percent said they would take a genetic test before having children, if it would tell them whether their children would probably inherit a fatal genetic disease. OTA's 1991 survey of genetic counselors and nurse geneticists found that 18.5 percent of respondents said they were "frequently" or "very frequently" asked by clients about DNA-based CF tests; about 71 percent said the number of inquiries increased from 1989 to 1991. On the other hand, some physicians report that actual willingness to undertake CF carrier screening is currently modest. In part, such reticence stems from the cost of CF mutation analysis, which patients must generally self-pay. It might also arise from a barrier common to many types of medical screening: lack of interest and reluctance to uncover what might be perceived as potentially unpleasant news.

Generally, physicians are obligated to inform patients of the risks and benefits of proposed procedures, so that patients themselves may decide whether to proceed. Where a patient specifically asks about a test, physicians would seem obligated to discuss the test, even if they do not recommend that it be taken. Whether physicians are obligated to query patients about their potential interest in a test the provider views as unwarranted by the patient's circumstances depends on the customary practice of similarly skilled and situated physicians.

Customary practice is often determined by the courts, and courts view statements issued by a relevant professional society as evidence of what a reasonably prudent physician might have done. In mid-1992, after extended discussion, the leadership of the American Society of Human Genetics (ASHG) approved a revised statement that CF mutation analysis "is not recommended" for those without a family history of CF. Some argue that the subtle change in language of the new statement retreats from the absoluteness of a 1990 ASHG statement that stated routine CF carrier screening is "NOT yet the standard of care." This view holds that the new statement reflects an evolution of debate within the society—that some believe CF carrier screening may now be offered to individuals without a family history of CF, although it might not be the "standard of care." Others argue that ASHG's position is unchanged—that the new statement is tantamount to restating that CF carrier screening should not be offered to individuals without a family history of CF. In either case, the statement cannot be interpreted to mean that CF carrier screening should be offered to all individuals. The 1990 and 1991 policy statements of professional societies and participants in an NIH workshop stated that CF carrier screening should not be the standard of care.

Today, some physicians take their cues strictly from the early guidelines; the extent to which the 1992 ASHG statement will affect physician practice remains to be seen. Others have concluded that a general population incidence of 1 child with CF per 2,500 births, coupled with the test's imperfect detection sensitivity, makes routinely informing patients about CF mutation analysis unnecessary. Additionally, some physicians might choose not to inform patients of the availability of CF mutation analysis because they judge that the test is too psychologically risky or too expensive to be worth the possible benefits for those without a family history of CF. Still other providers might be unaware of the test or its possible benefits.

Some physicians, however, disagree with existing guidelines and have already chosen to incorporate CF screening into their practices. They believe the assays are sufficiently sensitive for general use, and that even patients with unknown risks of conceiving a child with CF should now have the information to exercise choice in managing their health care. Still other physicians might be offering the assay out of concern that failing to could subject them to charges of medical malpractice if a couple has a child with CF and a court subsequently finds that CF carrier screening had become the standard of care—despite professional statements to the contrary. These practitioners might be concerned by the few cases where courts held that limited adoption of a practice by some professionals is sufficient to call into question the reasonableness of the defendant's practice—regardless of the extent to which that practice was accepted generally by the profession or suggested by professional societies. In fact, with respect to CF carrier screening, customary physician practice might evolve faster than that recommended by physicians' own professional societies, as has occurred for other practices such as amniocentesis.

## Duties of Care for Genetic Counseling

Once a decision is made to offer information about tests for CF carrier screening or to provide the assay itself—at least three important issues arise: what constitutes quality genetic counseling, confidentiality of information, and compensation for inadequate counseling or breach of confidentiality.

**Components of Genetic Counseling.** A genetics professional must understand enough about the patient's health, his or her reproductive plans, and available technologies so that an appropriate family history can be obtained and necessary analyses ordered. Less than this could give patients grounds to complain of a false assurance of safety. More than most aspects of medicine and counseling, genetic counseling involves family issues and family members. For a non-specialist, it might be enough to recognize the need for a referral.

Having elicited information and obtained test results, the provider must communicate the results in a meaningful way. Translating technically accurate information into understandable information is difficult, but essential. Effective communication also entails recognizing and understanding religious, psychosocial, and ethnocultural issues important to the client and his or her family. People interpret genetic risk information in a highly personal manner and can misperceive, misunderstand, or distort information. For CF carrier screening, an important aspect involves explaining the reproductive risks the client faces and what the condition involves. Perceptions of relative risk significantly affect qualitative decisions. Some consumers could mistake the assay's resolution and perceive that a negative result from use of the latest DNA technology means no risk.

No standard for genetic counseling exists. Some argue in favor of a standard based on what patients would want to know (modeled after informed consent requirements) because there is no fixed professional norm as an alternative, and because adequacy of the information conveyed turns more on the values of the patient being counseled than on professional norms. The prevailing approach in genetic counseling, however, appears to be based on a review of what most professionals do, rather than what an individual patient wants.

**Confidentiality.** Genetics professionals with information on the carrier status of a patient are legally obligated to keep that information confidential except under a few, specific circumstances. At least 21 States explicitly protect patient information pertaining to medical conditions and treatment; it is also part of the case law in many States without specific statutes. Offending physicians can have their licenses revoked or be subject to other disciplinary action. Patients whose confidential records have been revealed can also bring civil suit against the physician or facility.

Not all genetic information, however, must remain confidential. A provider might wish to reveal genetic information to interested third parties without a patient's permission. Health care professionals are not legally liable or subject to disciplinary action if a valid defense exists for releasing a patient's genetic or other medical information. With CF, the professional might desire to inform a patient's relatives that they also could be at higher than average risk of conceiving a child with CF. If the provider is persuaded that the relatives will not be notified after a patient has been advised to inform relatives that they too could carry a CF mutation—he or she might believe that breaching confidentiality would be appropriate.

The coming years will see a growing number of situations where health professionals will need to balance confidentiality of patients' genetic information against demands from relatives and other third parties for access to that information. Overall, the risk to the third party from non-disclosure must be balanced against the benefit of maintaining the expected confidentiality of the provider-patient setting. A provider contemplating disclosure to a patient's spouse must weigh the patient's own confidentiality against a spouse's interest in sharing decisions concerning conception, abortion, or preparation for the birth of a child with extraordinary medical needs.

**Compensation for Negligent Genetic Counseling.** Inadequate genetic counseling can result in a number of outcomes. Patients might forego conception or terminate a pregnancy when correct information would have reassured them. People might choose to conceive children when they otherwise would have practiced contraception, or they might fail to investigate using donor gametes that are free of the genetic trait they wish to avoid. Finally, they might lose the opportunity to choose to terminate a pregnancy.

The birth of a child with a genetic condition could result in malpractice claims of wrongful birth or wrongful life. For wrongful birth claims, most jurisdictions allow compensation for negligent failure to inform or failure to provide correct information in time for parents to either prevent conception or decide about pregnancy termination. With regard to CF, at least one court has ruled that parents may collect the extra medical costs associated with managing the condition. In this case, the couple maintained they would have avoided conceiving a second child had their physicians accurately diagnosed CF in their first child and thus identified each parent as a CF carrier. In wrongful life claims, the child asserts he or she was harmed by the failure to give the parents an opportunity to avoid conception or birth. Most U.S. courts have been reluctant to allow damages because they have been uncomfortable concluding that a child has been harmed by living with severe disabilities when the only alternative is never to have been born.

Practitioners who provide inadequate genetic counseling, including failing to recommend needed tests, might be subject to sanctions—from a reprimand to license revocation—by a regulatory body or a professional society. M.D.-geneticists, as physicians, are formally licensed by States. Ph.D.-geneticists and master's-level genetic counselors are not licensed by States, but until 1992 have been certified (along with physicians) by the American Board of Medical Genetics (ABMG). The continued certification of master's-level counselors by ABMG beyond 1992 is uncertain.

## PUBLIC EDUCATION

Both the way in which a provider communicates information about potential risk to the client (or risk to potential offspring) and the implications of the condition and prognosis influence a client's perception of the information. A person's subjective frame of reference, familiarity with genetics, and ability to understand statistical implications of genetic risks are also important.

Risk perception is always a more important determinant of decision making than actual risk. When confronting the risk of genetic disease in their offspring, and in making reproductive decisions, people tend to place greater weight on their ability to cope with a child with a disability or a fatal disease than on precise numerical risks. One study revealed that regardless of actual risk, parents overwhelmingly see situations as 0 or 100 percent—it will or will not happen—when they believe they cannot cope with the situation.

In addition to subjective factors that influence the interpretation of risk, most individuals have difficulty understanding risk in arithmetic terms, yet comprehending probabilities affects people's understanding of information provided by genetic tests. One study of predominantly Caucasian, middle-class women in Maryland found more than 20 percent thought that "1 out of 1,000" meant 10 percent, and 6 percent of respondents thought it meant greater than 10 percent. A 1991 national survey of public attitudes toward genetic tests reveals that belief in the accuracy of the technology is one of the strongest predictors of favorable attitudes toward genetic tests; that same survey of 1,006 Americans found that less than half were able to answer correctly four of five technical questions regarding genetic tests.

The need for better scientific literacy has been a topic of wide discussion in recent years, and mechanisms to achieve this goal apply equally to genetics education. Increased public education in genetics would benefit individuals' perceptions and understanding about genetic test results—likely reducing time needed for individual counseling.

Public education programs targeted to genetic diseases have been nearly nonexistent since those established under the National Genetic Diseases Act were phased out in 1981. The National Science Foundation (NSF) has supported teacher training programs in genetics for school teachers in Kansas, for example, but no NSF-funded, national effort exists. Teachers who participated in the Kansas program subsequently increased time devoted to genetics instruction at the high-school level by three-fold. Instruction in elementary schools increased 22-fold. More recently, the U.S. Department of Energy (DOE) began funding a 3-year project to prepare 50 selected science teachers per year to become State resource teachers.

Public education can go a long way toward preparing individuals for the decision of whether and when to be screened. Positive and negative experiences with large-scale Tay-Sachs, sickle cell, and α-and ß-thalassemia carrier screening programs—in the United States and abroad—demonstrate the value and importance of pretest community education.

## PROFESSIONAL TRAINING AND EDUCATION

Many types of health professionals perform genetic counseling: physicians, Ph.D. clinical geneticists, genetic counselors, nurses, and social workers. Critics of widespread CF carrier screening question whether the present genetics counseling system in the United States can handle the swell of cases if CF carrier screening becomes routine.

Currently, about 1,000 master's-level genetic counselors practice in the United States. An additional 100 nurse geneticists provide similar services. The ABMG has certified 630 professionals in genetic counseling, including master's-level genetic counselors, nurses, and M.D. and Ph.D. geneticists. If genetic counseling for CF carrier screening were to fall only to board-certified professionals, the available number of professionals might be short of what is needed. OTA's survey of genetic counselors and nurses in genetics also indicates that respondents believe routine CF carrier screening will strain the present genetic services delivery system. Respondents estimated that, on average, 1 hour would be needed to obtain a three-generational family history and to discuss CF carrier screening and genetic risks.

Skeptics of a personnel shortage assert that counseling about CF carrier assays is likely to take place in the general obstetric/prenatal context, however, and they believe 1 hour exaggerates the amount of time that suffices for all prenatal tests, let alone only CF carrier screening. Furthermore, counseling related to CF carrier screening is likely to extend beyond board-certified individuals to include other physicians and allied health professionals. For example, an unknown number of social workers, psychologists, and other public health professionals perform genetic counseling, often to minority and underserved populations.

Ultimately, the issue of adequate services and professional capacity could turn on the extent to which patients receive genetic services through specialized clinical settings, as they largely do now, versus access through primary care, community health, and public health settings. Overall, OTA cannot conclude whether increased numbers of genetic specialists are necessary—arguments exist pro and con. One finding is clear: Increased genetics education for all health care professionals is desirable. Routine carrier screening for CF—and tests yet to be developed for other genetic conditions—will require adequate training and education of individuals in the broader health care delivery system.

Increasing professional education in genetics will not be an easy task. The average 4-year medical school curriculum includes 21.6 hours of genetics instruction. Fifteen master's-level programs in genetic counseling exist, producing approximately 75 graduates per year. Of 200 U.S. universities that offer graduate nursing degrees, only 4 offer programs providing a master's-level genetics major. Only 9 of nearly 100 accredited social work graduate programs in the United States offer special courses on genetic topics. Few schools of public health offer genetics as part of their curriculum; none requires it.

Federal support for genetic services, education, and training has changed dramatically since 1981. Prior to 1981, genetics programs applied through their State for Federal funds under the National Genetic Diseases Act (Public Law 94-278). With creation of the Maternal and Child Health (MCH) Block Grant (Public Law 97-35), State genetic services now compete with other maternal and child health initiatives. Additionally, Federal spending on demonstration projects for service delivery, training, and education has declined after adjustment for inflation. Training support for master's level genetic counselors is minimal. The U.S. Department of Health and Human Services (DHHS) provides no financial support for training genetic counselors or for improving genetics education in medical schools. Through support to the Council of Regional Networks for Genetic Services (CORN), DHHS provides funds for some continuing professional genetics education programs for physicians, but not for other genetics professionals.

**FINANCING**

Health insurance in the United States is not monolithic. U.S. health care financing, which totaled more than $800 billion in 1991, is a mixture of public and private funds. Federal financing includes Medicare, Medicaid, and the Civilian Health and Medical Program of the Uniformed Services (CHAMPUS). Private funding mechanisms include self-funded plans, commercial health insurance plans, Blue Cross and Blue Shield (BC/BS) plans, health maintenance organizations (HMOs), self-pay, and non-reimbursed institutional funding. State high-risk pools—generally using public and private monies—are also an option in some States for people who cannot obtain private health insurance. Rules and regulations governing each sector vary. Thus, separating how the current financing paradigm might affect CF carrier screening—and vice versa—is difficult.

For the majority of Americans, access to health care, and the health insurance that makes such access possible, is provided through the private sector. Some acquire health insurance on their own through individual policies; 10 to 15 percent of people with health insurance have this type of coverage. Of group policies, about 15 percent have some medical underwriting—i.e., medical and genetic information are used to determine eligibility and premiums for health insurance. A large majority of insured individuals and their family members—163 million of the 214 million with health care coverage—obtain coverage via employer-offered large group policies with no medical underwriting. The employer, in turn, contracts with a commercial insurer, a BC/BS plan, an HMO, or is self-funded.

Self-funded health insurance plans are group policies that merit specific discussion, since they are features of Federal, not State, law. Since enactment of the Employee Retirement Income Security Act of 1974 (ERISA; 29 U.S.C. 1131 et seq.), many companies find self-funding beneficial because their employee benefit plans are not subject to State insurance regulation. With an ERISA plan, the employer directly assumes most or all of the financial liability for the health care expenses of its employees, rather than paying premiums to other third-party payors to assume that risk. Self-funded companies enjoy considerable latitude in designing employee coverage standards. Today, about 53 percent of the employment-based group market is self-funded, and therefore unregulated by the States.

In large measure, the number of people who opt to be screened could hinge on who pays, or will pay, for the cost of CF mutation analyses—the individual or a third-party payor. As mentioned previously, some physicians report that reluctance to undertake CP carrier screening seems to stem from the test's cost. Physicians seeing patients who rely on health insurance to cover part of their expenses usually inform them that their coverage probably precludes reimbursement for CF mutation analysis without a family history of CF, and so if they opt to be screened, they will likely need to self-pay. For laboratories that perform genetic tests, the issue of reimbursement also might be crucial to the ultimate volume of future business in this area.

*Private Sector Reimbursement*

Health insurance industry representatives assert that most companies will not pay for tests they consider screening assays. Thus, reimbursement for CF carrier tests in the absence of family history will likely remain on a self-pay basis unless they become part of routine pregnancy care again, as happened for MSAFP screening.

OTA's 1991 survey of commercial insurers, BC/BS plans, and HMOs confirms these policies for individual contracts or medically underwritten groups. OTA found carrier tests for CF, Tay-Sachs, and sickle cell would not be covered by 12 of 29 commercial insurers offering individual coverage for any reason—screening or family history. No company offering individual insurance or medically underwritten policies would cover CF carrier analysis if a patient requested it, but had no family history. If there is a family history, most companies would pay for carrier tests. Similar results were found for BC/BS plans and HMOs, although a few BC/BS plans and a few HMOs reported they would cover carrier tests performed for screening purposes.

As mentioned earlier, initial carrier screening for CF will likely take place in the context of obstetric/prenatal care. For all three respondent populations, prenatal screening tests for CF generally are not covered without a family history, although more would cover prenatal tests solely at patient request (without family history) than cover general carrier screening. Some respondents covered no prenatal tests.

Respondents were asked to indicate whether they agreed or disagreed with the following scenario:

> **Through** prior genetic testing, the husband is known to be a **carrier** for CF. Before having children, the wife seeks genetic **testing** for CF. The insurance company declines to pay for the **testing**, since there is no history of CF in her family.

For commercial insurers who write either individual policies or medically underwrite group policies, or both, 21 medical directors (41 percent) agreed strongly or somewhat with this scenario; 28 respondents (47 percent) disagreed somewhat or disagreed strongly. In part, these results reflect OTA's survey finding that several respondents would not cover any carrier tests, even when medically indicated by a family history. On the other hand, not all respondents who agreed with the scenario represented these companies. These individuals appeared not to understand that the situation was not a case of CF carrier screening, but one of testing to ascertain the couple's risk of conceiving an affected fetus in light of the male's family history.

OTA also found variation in how genetic counseling is covered by commercial insurers, BC/BS plans, and HMOs that offer individual policies or medically underwritten group coverage. OTA's survey of genetic counselors and nurse geneticists confirms these results: Reimbursement for genetic counseling by these professionals is more likely when a family history exists.

Finally, as stated earlier, most people obtain health care coverage through group policies. Determining how these thousands of policies would reimburse for CF carrier screening was not possible for this report. Nevertheless, information gathered informally indicates group policy coverage is unlikely to differ significantly from OTA's survey results—i.e., most policies will not cover CF carrier assays unless there is a family history. The Federal Office of Personnel Management, which oversees Federal employee health benefits, has denied reimbursement for preconception CF carrier screening because it views it as preventive, not therapeutic. On the other hand, one private institute's experience with reimbursement to clients for elective fetal CF carrier screening paints a different picture. In a small survey of clients, 16 of 27 reported they had been reimbursed for their tests. Eleven had been reimbursed fully—by either commercial insurers or BC/BS plans—and five had been partially reimbursed. It is likely that reimbursement occurs more frequently in this population than might be expected from OTA's survey because it occurs in the context of pregnancy management, not preconception.

*Public Sector Reimbursement*

Although access to CF carrier tests will largely depend on ability to pay because most private insurance does not cover them—at least to the extent that individual policies reflect group polices—some individuals will be Medicaid eligible. Reimbursement for their assays would be partially covered by this State-Federal partnership. In 1991, OTA surveyed directors of State Medicaid programs and found State to State variation in both the types of genetics and pregnancy-related services covered and the amounts reimbursed to providers for those services. Some States do not cover certain services at all. For all States and services, the dollars reimbursed fall short of the procedures' actual charges.

**STIGMATIZATION, CLASSIFICATION, AND DISCRIMINATION**

Concern is expressed that CF carrier screening might be sought or offered despite an uncertain potential for discrimination or stigmatization by other individuals or institutions (e.g., employers and insurers). Stigmatization of, or discrimination against, persons with certain diseases is not unique to illnesses with genetic origins. Yet as the number and scope of predictive genetic tests increase, so does concern about how perceptions of and behavior towards carriers (or individuals identified with predispositions) will develop.

*Stigmatization and Carrier Status*

While a relationship exists between a characteristic's visibility and the amount of stigma it induces, invisible characteristics (e.g., carrier status) are also stigmatized. Stigmatization of CF carriers will probably focus on the notion that it is irresponsible for people who are at genetic risk to knowingly transmit a condition to their children. A 1990 national survey of Americans reported 39 percent said "every woman who is pregnant should be tested to determine if the baby has any serious genetic defects." Twenty-two percent responded that regardless of what they would want for themselves, "a woman should have an abortion if the baby has a serious genetic defect." Nearly 10 percent believed laws should require a woman to have an abortion rather than have the government help pay for the child's care if the parents are poor.

Few empirical studies have examined stigmatization of CF carriers directly, but relevant research funded through the NE/DOE ELSI Programs of the Human Genome Project is under way. One study in Montreal, Canada, reports carriers generally expressed positive views about their newly determined carrier status. Most (68 percent) would want their partner tested, and 60 percent said if the partner were a carrier, it would not affect the relationship. Existing research on genetic carriers and stigmatization, generally for Tay-Sachs or sickle cell, have some bearing on carrier screening for CF—chiefly that public education is crucial to overcoming stigmatization.

How CF—as a condition—is viewed by Americans will affect perceptions and potential reproductive stigma of CF carriers. Of prime importance is a commitment to non-directive genetic counseling to reduce perceived biases so individuals can make informed choices about bearing children with CF. Such a professional commitment coupled with increased public awareness and education about CF carrier screening could reduce potential problems of stigmatization of CF carriers, as well as stigmatization for other disorders as genetic screening evolves through the 1990s and beyond.

## Health Care Coverage Access

One of the most frequently expressed concerns about CF carrier screening specifically, and genetic tests generally, is the effect they will have on health care access and risks classification in the United States. Consumers fear being excluded from health care coverage due to genetic and other factors. Such fears persist despite the fact that most contracts for individual health insurance coverage preclude blanket non-renewal. Similarly, an insurer cannot raise rates for an individual who has been continuously covered if the person develops a new condition. Of special import to small group policies is that it is legal for an insurer not to renew a group contract, or to renew with a steep premium increase, based on the results of one individual's genetic, or other medical, test. Group policies are rarely guaranteed renewable, and most people in the United States are covered by group policies. Many group policies have pre-existing condition clauses that preclude, for some period of time, reimbursement for expenses related to health conditions present on the policy's effective date.

One nationwide survey revealed 3 in 10 Americans say they or someone in their household have stayed in a job they wanted to leave mainly to preserve health care coverage. A 1989 OTA survey of Fortune 500 companies and a random sample of businesses with at least 1,000 employees found 11 percent of respondents assessed the health insurance risk of job applicants on a routine basis; another 25 percent assessed health risks sometimes. Nine percent of these respondents also took into account dependents' potential expenses when considering an individual's application. Forty-two percent of respondents said the health insurance risk of a job applicant reduced the likelihood of an otherwise healthy, able job applicant being hired.

OTA found the majority of respondents to its health insurers' survey "agree strongly" or "agree somewhat" that illnesses with genetic bases, such as CF or Huntington disease, are pre-existing conditions. Thus, insurers would exclude reimbursement for such conditions for a period of time if the person could obtain individual or medically underwritten insurance at all. More surprising, since carriers have no symptoms of the disorder, is the finding that respondents, collectively, are nearly evenly split on whether carrier status e.g., for CF or Tay-Sachs—is a pre-existing condition.

OTA's survey also revealed that genetic information is, for the most part, viewed no differently than other types of medical information. Personal and family medical histories were the most important factors in determining insurability, according to survey respondents. OTA found medical directors and underwriters felt less strongly about "genetic predisposition to significant conditions" as a facet of insurability than they did about medical history. Of significance to CF carrier screening, a minority of all types of insurers found carrier risk "very important" or "important" to insurability. Twenty-four percent (7 respondents) of medical directors at commercial insurers writing individual policies said "carrier risk for genetic disease" was "very important" or "important" to insurability; 18 percent (2 respondents) of HMOs responded similarly, as did 8 percent (2 respondents) of BC/BS chief underwriters.

Although an insurer might consider carrier status important to evaluating an application, carrier status does not appear to translate into difficulties for applicants in ultimately obtaining health care coverage from OTA's survey respondents. Ninety-three percent of respondents from commercial insurers and all HMOs offering individual coverage would accept the person with standard rates if the applicant was asymptomatic but had a family history of CF. For BC/BS plans, however, 55 percent would accept at standard rates, 21 percent would accept at the standard rate with an exclusion waiver, and 7 percent would decline to cover the CF carrier. For those who responded they would accept with an exclusion waiver or decline to cover, reluctance to offer standard insurance might stem from not wanting to pay for possible children or from a misunderstanding of the meaning of CF carrier status.

Overall, OTA's survey reveals genetic information is not viewed as a special type of information. In making decisions on insurability and rating based on genetics, what seems important is the particular condition (e.g., CF disease, diabetes, sickle cell anemia), not that the condition is genetically based. The increased availability of genetic information, however, adds to the amount of medical information that insurers can use for underwriting. The availability of this additional information leads to concern that risk assessments will become so accurate on an individual level as to undermine the risk-spreading function of insurance. This, of course, would have profound societal implications.

## Cystic Fibrosis

### Perspectives on the Future Use of Genetic Tests by Health Insurers

Commercial insurers, HMOs, and BC/BS plans already use genetic information in making decisions about individual policies or medically underwritten groups. People seeking either of these types of coverage reveal such information as part of the battery of questions to which applicants respond in personal and family history inquiries. OTA is unaware of any insurer who underwrites individual or medically underwritten groups and requires carrier or pre-symptomatic tests e.g., for Huntington or adult polycystic kidney diseases. Even a decade from now, OTA's survey data indicate the vast majority of respondents do not expect to require genetic tests of applicants who have a family history of serious genetic conditions, nor do they anticipate requiring carrier assays even if a family history exists.

Health insurers do not need genetic tests to find out genetic information. It is less expensive to ask a question or request medical records. Thus, whether genetic information is available to health insurers hinges on whether individuals who seek personal policies or are part of medically underwritten groups become aware of their genetic status because of general family history, because they have sought a genetic test because of family history, or because they have been screened in some other context.

OTA's survey reveals health insurers are concerned about the potential for negative financial consequences if genetic information is available to the consumer, but not them. Thirty-four medical directors (67 percent) from commercial insurers said they "agree strongly" or "agree somewhat" with the statement that "it's fair for insurers to use genetic tests to identify individuals with increased risk of disease." Thirty-eight respondents (74 percent) from commercial insurers agreed strongly or somewhat that "an insurer should have the option of determining how to use genetic information in determining risks."

### Access to Health Insurance After Genetic Tests

Existing information about how genetic test results currently affect individuals' health care coverage is largely anecdotal. One case from the Baylor College of Medicine (Houston, TX) illustrates why concern is expressed about health insurance and genetic screening and testing:

A couple in their 30s has a 6-year-old son with CF. Prenatal diagnostic studies of the current pregnancy indicate the fetus is affected. The couple decides to continue the pregnancy. The HMO indicated it should have no financial responsibility for the prenatal testing and that the family could be dropped from coverage if the mother did not terminate the pregnancy. The HMO felt this to be appropriate since the parents had requested and utilized prenatal diagnosis ostensibly to avoid a second affected child. After a social worker for the family spoke with the local director of the HMO, the company rapidly reversed its position.

Consumers and patient advocates maintain such situations represent the tip of an iceberg. They assert individuals who avail themselves of genetic tests subsequently have difficulty obtaining or retaining health insurance. Health insurance industry officials argue to the contrary. If the problem was prevalent, they assert, ample court cases could be cited because patients and their attorneys would not be passive recipients of decisions such as that just described.

To explore this issue, OTA asked third parties—nurses in genetics and genetic counselors—for their experiences. In 1991, at least 50 genetic counselors or nurses in clinical practice (14 percent of survey respondents) reported knowledge of 68 instances of patients who experienced difficulty with health insurance due to genetic tests.

It is important to note that most cases do not involve recessive disorders and carrier screening for conditions like CF, but involve situations in which genetic test results appear to have been treated the same as adverse test results for non-genetic conditions. Access to health care coverage for CF carriers presumably should not be an issue because CF carriers have no symptoms of the disorder, although OTA's survey of health insurers indicates otherwise in a small fraction of cases. For genetic testing or screening to detect genetic illness (or the potential for illness), however, the possibilities for problems are already unfolding.

The OTA data permit neither extrapolation about the actual number of cases that have occurred in the United States, nor speculation about trends. An estimated 110,600 individuals were seen in 1990 by the genetic counselors and nurses responding to OTA's survey, but OTA did not advise respondents to limit descriptions of clients' insurance difficulties to 1990; it is unlikely that all reported cases occurred in 1990.

## The Americans With Disabilities Act of 1990 and Genetics

In 1990, Congress enacted the Americans With Disabilities Act (ADA; Public Law 101-336), a comprehensive civil rights bill to prohibit discrimination against individuals with disabilities. The ADA encompasses private sector employment, public services, public accommodations, and telecommunications. It does not preempt State or local disability statutes.

Under the ADA, a person with a disability includes someone who has a "record" of or is "regarded" as having a disability, even if no actual incapacity currently exists. A "record" of disability means the person has a history of impairment. This provision protects those who have recovered from a disability that previously impaired their life activities (e.g., people recovered from diseases such as cancer who might still face discrimination based on misunderstanding, prejudice, or irrational fear). Additionally, individuals regarded as having disabilities include those who, with or without an impairment, do not have limitations in their major life functions, yet are treated as if they did have such limitations. This provision is particularly important for individuals who are perceived to have stigmatic conditions that are viewed negatively by society.

Examining genetics and the ADA from three broad categories — genetic conditions, genetic predisposition, and carrier status—sheds some light on how the ADA might interface with CF carrier screening and future genetic tests.

**Genetic Conditions.** Disability is defined only according to the degree of impairment and how severely the disability interferes with life activities, with no distinction between those with genetic origins and those without. A genetic condition that does not cause substantial impairment might not constitute a disability, unless others treat the person as disabled. Thus, significant cosmetic disfigurements (e.g., from burns or neurofibromatosis) could be classified as disabilities if public prejudices act to limit the life opportunities of people who have them. Congress and the courts have long recognized disabilities of primary or partial genetic origin, including Down syndrome, CF, muscular dystrophy, epilepsy, diabetes, and arthritis.

**Genetic Predisposition.** ADA judges disability not just by an objective measure of inability to perform tasks, but also subjectively by the degree to which the public makes the condition disabling through misunderstanding or prejudice. This latter definition might apply to individuals who are asymptomatic but predicted to develop disease in the future if the public perceives them as having a disability because they might or will get ill. Some argue the ADA's legislative history indicates genetic predisposition might be encompassed. One Congressman stated during the 1990 debate over the conference report that persons who are theoretically at risk "may not be discriminated against simply because they may not be qualified for a job sometime in the future." On the other hand, no further discussion on the issue occurred.

**Carrier Status.** Case law and the ADA's prohibition of discrimination generally hold that employment decisions must be based on reasonable medical judgments that show the disability prevents the individual from meeting legitimate performance criteria. For carriers of recessive conditions such as CF, sickle cell anemia, and Tay-Sachs, there is no disability per se; the ADA appears not to cover carriers. Such individuals are, however, at high risk of having an affected child if their partners also carry the trait and could be misunderstood to be affected by the disease. Discrimination against carriers could arguably constitute discrimination if based on a perception of disability.

**The Equal Employment Opportunity Commission (EEOC) Regulations.** In 1991, EEOC promulgated regulations for implementing the ADA. The regulations do not specifically prohibit discrimination against carriers or persons who are identified presymptomatically for a late-onset genetic condition (e.g., adult polycystic kidney disease or Huntington disease)—despite the fact that the NIH/DOE ELSI Working Group and the NIH/DOE Joint Subcommittee on the Human Genome urged EEOC to clearly protect these individuals. In its interpretive guidance, EEOC notes "the definition of the term 'impairment' does not include characteristic predisposition to illness or disease." From EEOC's perspective, carriers are not encompassed by the ADA's provisions. With respect to individuals diagnosed presymptomatically, EEOC concluded that "such individuals are protected, either when they develop a genetic disease that substantially limits one or more of their major life activities, or when an employer regards them as having a genetic disease that substantially limits one or more of their major life activities."

*The Americans with Disabilities Act and Health Insurance*

The ADA also might prohibit discrimination based on an employer's fear of future disability in an applicant's family that would affect the individual's use of health insurance and time away from the

## Cystic Fibrosis

job. Nevertheless, the ADA does not speak to this point directly, and so leaves open for future interpretation whether employers may discriminate against carriers who are perceived as more likely to incur extra costs due to illnesses that might occur in their future children. The ADA specifically does not restrict insurers, health care providers, or other benefit plan administrators from carrying out existing underwriting practices based on risk classification. Nor does the ADA make clear whether employers may question individuals about their marital or reproductive plans prior to offering employment or enrollment in an insurance plan. Furthermore, after a person is hired, ERISA-based, self-funded insurance plans can alter benefits to exclude or limit coverage for specific conditions; the ADA does not preempt ERISA.

## QUALITY ASSURANCE OF CLINICAL LABORATORIES AND DNA TEST KITS

Quality assurance for CF carrier screening means ensuring the safety and efficacy of the tests themselves, whether they are performed de novo in clinical diagnostic laboratories or via test kits. The quality of the laboratory's performance affects the quality of the counseling services. Ensuring that consumers receive high-quality technical and professional service is the responsibility of providers, under the shared oversight of the Federal Government, State and local governments, private entities (including professional societies), and the courts.

### The Clinical Laboratory Improvement Amendments of 1988

Quality assurance to assess clinical laboratory performance is still in flux, in largely because 1967 legislation governing regulation of clinical testing facilities was overhauled by Congress in 1988 with enactment of the Clinical Laboratory Improvement Amendments of 1988 (CLIA; Public Law 100-578). CLIA subjects most clinical laboratories to an array of accrediting requirements: qualifications for the laboratory director, standards for the supervision of laboratory testing, qualifications for technical personnel, management requirements, and an acceptable quality control program. CLIA authorizes the Health Care Financing Administration (HCFA) to police an estimated 300,000 to 600,000 physician, hospital, and freestanding laboratories to ensure they adhere to a comprehensive quality assurance program. HCFA may impose sanctions, if necessary.

CLIA clearly encompasses facilities performing DNA-based, clinical diagnostic analyses. But, while it details particular performance standards for several types of clinical diagnostic procedures, CLIA does not specifically address DNA-based tests. This lack of detailed directives for DNA-based diagnostics could be beneficial in the short-term, since the field is rapidly changing.

**State Authorities.** CLIA does not preclude States from regulating and licensing facilities within certain guidelines. After a pilot study, for example, the California State Department of Health Services intends to seek approval for State-specific licensing laws and regulations for DNA and cytogenetic laboratories. Similarly, New York has regulated clinical laboratories since 1964, and has established a genetics quality assurance program that includes requirements for licensing personnel, licensing facilities, laboratory performance standards, and DNA-based proficiency testing. Nevertheless, the principal State role in quality assurance for clinical facilities is licensure and certification of medical and clinical personnel, which are the sole provinces of States.

**The Role of Private Organizations.** While CLIA clearly expands the Federal role in clinical laboratory oversight, the law continues to permit, subject to DHHS approval, the involvement of other parties in regulating laboratory practices. Private organizations, including the Joint Commission on Accreditation of Health Care Organizations, may continue to accredit facilities. Private professional societies will likely have the greatest impact in the area of proficiency testing, one component of accreditation. Efforts by CORN and its regional networks, ASHG, and the College of American Pathologists (CAP) stand at the forefront of developing proficiency tests for DNA-based diagnostics.

In 1989, CAP established a committee to develop appropriate guidelines for all clinical tests involving DNA probes or other molecular biological techniques. The CAP committee has administered two DNA-based proficiency testing pilot programs, although their focus was not genetic disorders. CORN, which receives Federal funding and has been involved in quality assurance of genetics facilities since 1985, sponsored a DNA-based genetic test proficiency pilot of 20 laboratories in 1990. The Southeastern region has a regional proficiency testing program, and will be enlarging its planned second survey into a national test, to be completed in 1992; this effort includes CF mutation analysis. Full proficiency testing for DNA-based genetic diagnostics is planned by 1994. CORN and ASHG have liaisons with the others' efforts, and a joint ASHG/CAP DNA-based proficiency testing pilot for genetic diseases commenced in 1992.

Proficiency testing is widely viewed as a key measure of quality assurance. It can provide a reliable and identifiable benchmark to assess performance. In the past, professional societies' involvement in proficiency testing to ensure laboratory quality have predominated, and this situation is likely to continue. Cooperation among each of the groups will be essential, as professional-society-based programs could affect proficiency testing for CF mutations (and other DNA tests) long before HCFA proposes proficiency testing rules under CLIA.

## *Regulation of DNA Test Kits*

Increased use of CF mutation assays for carrier detection will depend, in part, on the development and availability of prepackaged kits. At least two companies—one in the United States and one in the United Kingdom—are testing such kits and anticipate their availability by 1994. Before marketing of the kits can occur, however, the U.S. Food and Drug Administration (FDA) must ensure the safety and efficacy of genetic diagnostic test kits, such as those under development for CF mutations. Since genetic diagnostic kits fall within the definition of devices, the extent to which CF mutation kits—or other DNA-based genetic test kits—become available will depend on FDA regulation of devices during development, testing, production, distribution, and use.

FDA's regulatory options range from registering an item's presence in the United States and periodically inspecting facilities to ensure good manufacturing practices, to setting performance and labeling requirements, to premarket review of a device. The agency also may engage in postmarketing surveillance to identify ineffective or dangerous devices. It may ban devices it deems unacceptable. Specific regulation depends on whether FDA classifies the device as Class I, II, or III, with Class III devices receiving the most stringent review.

Since no FDA-approved, DNA-based genetic diagnostic test kit comparable to those being developed for CF carrier analysis exists, it is difficult to predict the ultimate regulatory status of such kits. Preliminary indications are they will be regulated as Class III devices. In response to recent legislation and ongoing congressional concern, FDA appears to be increasing medical device regulation and postmarketing surveillance. If increased FDA scrutiny extends to DNA-based diagnostic test kits, developers can expect more stringent regulation of these products than of previous non-DNA-based genetic test kits. Increased regulation to provide greater assurance of safety and efficacy might, in turn, slow routine CF carrier screening.

## AUTOMATION

The extent to which costs for CF carrier tests decline depends, in part, on automation. Instrumentation will be especially crucial to the development of batteries of tests for multiple genetic disorders. Moreover, compared to most routine clinical tests, current DNA-based CF carrier assays are labor intensive.

Over the past few years, private industry and U.S. national laboratories have developed several instruments that increase the speed and volume of routine DNA diagnostic procedures. Goals for improved instrumentation for DNA analyses stem, in part, from the importance of rapid techniques to the Human Genome Project. Spin-off technologies from DNA mapping and sequencing appear amenable to applications for clinical diagnostics.

Currently, all but one step of what generally constitutes DNA diagnosis is automated or involves instrumentation under development. Most components of DNA analysis, however, are automated as individual units; efforts under way seek to coordinate sequential steps. Some machines are not faster than humans, but they can standardize the procedures and decrease human error.

Clearly, the crucial steps in DNA-based CF carrier assays are, or can be, automated. Advances in instrumentation indicate that automated, rapid carrier screening for CF—or other genetic conditions—is already technologically feasible. OTA finds the field of DNA automation is advancing at a pace that suggests entirely automated DNA diagnosis can be realized in the next few years.

## COSTS AND COST-EFFECTIVENESS

Perhaps the least examined facet of CF carrier screening is cost. Data for parts of OTA's analysis were often lacking and assumptions had to be made. Unlike the seven preceding factors, which in many cases will generically affect utilization of DNA-based tests for disorders other than CF, findings that pertain to cost-effectiveness do not

## Cystic Fibrosis

extend beyond CF carrier screening—although the approach used in this report could be applied to screening with other genetic tests.

While economic analyses can inform decisions surrounding resource allocation and access to genetic screening, they have limits. In the context of public policy and genetics, the 1983 President's Commission report on genetic screening articulates solid guidance about the benefits and limits of cost-effectiveness and cost-benefit analyses. These analytical approaches are tools to be used within an overall policy framework, not solely as a method of making or avoiding judgment. There is no intimation in OTA's analysis that something that saves or costs money is more or less desirable from a welfare standpoint.

*Cost of Cystic Fibrosis*

The cost of any illness is the answer to the hypothetical question: If the disease disappeared and everything else held constant, how many more dollars would be available to the economy? Many elements are needed to answer this question, but broadly speaking they fall into two categories: information about direct medical costs associated with CF and nonmedical direct costs related to the disease (i.e., family caregiving time).

Direct medical expenses for CF include costs of hospitalization, outpatient care, physical therapy, and drugs. These costs are not the same for everyone with the disease. Clinical symptoms of CF vary widely, although broad divisions in its severity can be drawn. Some individuals require only one inpatient visit every 2 years or so; others have problems so severe as to require four or more hospitalizations per year. Similar variation exists for other medical expenses. Overall, taking these several factors into account, average annual medical expenses for CF patients are estimated at $10,000. Assuming a median life expectancy in 1990 of 28 years, the present value of lifetime medical expenses is approximately $146,430 (1990 dollars using a 5 percent discount rate).

The main nonmedical direct cost associated with CF is parental time beyond the time required for a child without the illness. CF centers estimate that parents often must spend 2 hours per day on therapy for a child with CF. In addition, parents lose time from work when the person falls ill. Time is also spent on physician and clinic visits. OTA uses an estimate of 938 hours per year of extra caregiving to a person with CF, which is generally provided by family members. Assuming an estimated domestic/nursing wage of $10 per hour, the present value of CF-related lifetime nonmedical direct costs is $139,744 (1990 dollars using a 5 percent discount rate).

*Cost of Cystic Fibrosis Mutation Analysis*

Since CF is the most common, life-shortening, recessive disorder among Caucasians in the United States, commercial interest in the test is high. Currently, at least six commercial companies perform DNA-based CF mutation analyses, as do at least 40 university and hospital laboratories. The average price per sample was about $170 in 1992. With increased volume of tests and automation, however, many predict the cost per CF mutation assay will decrease. OTA uses a cost per test of $100 because the analysis focuses on the potential future of large-scale CF carrier screening and presumes economies of scale will apply.

Indirectly related to cost-effectiveness, but directly related to how much CF mutation analysis will cost in the future, is the issue of patents, licensing, and royalty fees for genetic diagnostics. A patent is pending for the CF gene, for example. Similarly, royalty licenses must be paid for the process—the polymerase chain reaction, or PCR—by which CF mutation analysis is performed. Thus, royalty licensing fees will be reflected in costs of the tests to consumers. Currently, debate is increasing on the issue of intellectual property protection and the Human Genome Project. A resolution of this controversy, if any, will affect costs of DNA-based diagnostic tests and hence cost-effectiveness of screening for genetic disorders.

*Costs and Cost-Effectiveness of Carrier Screening for Cystic Fibrosis*

Data about the cost of screening large numbers of individuals for CF carrier status do not exist. In estimating the cost of carrier screening for CF, OTA included costs of the CF mutation analyses, chorionic villus sampling for fetal testing, and costs for pretest education and post-test counseling. Taken together, these costs were analyzed in the context of several scenarios for preconception screening of women (and possibly their partners) and prenatal screening of pregnant women (and if necessary their partners and the fetus).

Regardless of the strategy or scale, CF carrier mutation analysis provides information to an individual about his or her likelihood of

## Cystic Fibrosis

having a child with CF should the partner also be a carrier. Hence, at its core, a cost-effectiveness analysis of CF carrier screening involves assumptions about reproductive behavior. A base case was established for the following six variables:

- 80 percent of women elect screening,
- 85 percent sensitivity of the CF mutation assay,
- 8.4 percent of +/+ couples are infertile,
- 10 percent of +/+ fertile couples choose not to conceive,
- 90 percent of +/+ fertile couples conceive, and 100 percent use prenatal testing, and
- 100 percent of CF-affected pregnancies detected are terminated.

As alternatives, other assumptions were made for several additional scenarios by varying the factors in turn (or combination) to yield a series of cost-effectiveness estimates. In evaluating costs and savings, changes in behavior were considered only for +/+ couples, and costs and savings were calculated for a hypothetical population of 100,000 eligible women (or couples). The economic costs include costs associated with CF carrier screening. The economic savings include avoiding the direct medical and nonmedical costs associated with having a child with CF. The base case and all scenarios were then compared to costs in the absence of screening.

One scenario, for example, assumed 50 percent of women chose to participate, another assumed all individuals elected screening. Another screened the woman and man simultaneously, rather than screening the man only when the woman was positive. Others used 50 percent as the frequency of affected pregnancies terminated. Overall, whether CF carrier screening can be paid for on a population basis through savings accrued by avoiding CF-related medical and caregiving costs depends on the assumptions used—including how many children people will have, average CF medical costs, and average time and cost devoted to caring for a child with CF, as well as variations in reproductive behaviors, costs of CF mutation analyses, and screening participation rates.

Eight of 14 scenarios examined by OTA result in a net cost over no screening. Under six cases, however, CF carrier screening is cost-effective, but most of these scenarios involve 100 percent participation, test sensitivity, or selective termination—all unlikely to be realized in the near term, if ever. Nevertheless, CF carrier screening can save money compared to no screening even under less absolute circumstances. The balance between net savings versus net cost in nearly all scenarios is fine. How many individuals participate in screening is relatively unimportant to cost-effectiveness, but it is clear the frequency of affected pregnancies terminated and the assay's price will ultimately affect this balance.

## Prenatal Diagnosis of Cystic Fibrosis

In addition to CF carrier screening of adults, prenatal diagnosis of CF can be performed. The type of test used to establish carrier status of the parents determines the DNA protocol for the fetus. The choice of technique to obtain a sample for DNA analysis involves consideration of timing, procedural risk, access to procedures, cost, and the presence or absence of other indications for prenatal diagnosis. Cells can be obtained via chorionic villus sampling (CVS) (performed at 9 to 12 weeks of pregnancy), amniocentesis (performed at 16 to 18 weeks), or through percutaneous umbilical blood sampling, also called cordocentesis (performed at 20 weeks). When CF mutation analysis is unavailable or inconclusive, microvillar intestinal enzyme levels can sometimes be measured in the amniotic fluid at 17 to 18 weeks, but this method suffers from a high false-positive and false-negative rate.

A new, experimental procedure, called blastomere analysis before implantation, or BABI, has been used to diagnose the CF status of an in vitro fertilized embryo before implanting it in the woman's uterus. The technique involves extracting a single cell from an embryo at about the eight-cell stage and analyzing its CF mutation status. Recently, an unaffected baby that had been tested with BABI was born to a couple in London at risk for CF.

For some families, prenatal diagnosis for CF is inconclusive. As in screening for carrier status, couples receive test results that yield percentages rather than certainties. There is speculation that this "restructuring of uncertainty" versus a "yes/no answer" will be confusing to individuals and cause undue stress; pilot studies to examine levels of anxiety in test populations before and after screening are under way. Assessments of anxiety levels of participants in other carrier screening programs are limited in what they offer to CF carrier screening because the levels of test uncertainty are not as great. Women offered hemoglobinopathy carrier screening, for example, were found to manifest appropriate levels of concern rather than undue

## Cystic Fibrosis

**Figure 5.25.** Prenatal Test Methods for CF

**Left:** Amniocentesis—the most widely used technique for prenatal diagnosis, generally at 16 to 18 weeks of a pregnancy. Cells shed by the developing fetus are extracted from a sample of amniotic fluid that has been withdrawn from the expectant mother's uterus by a hypodermic needle. The cells are cultured and then can be analyzed for chromosomal defects, such as Down syndrome. DNA analysis can also be performed (e.g., for CF mutation status).

**Right:** Chorionic villus sampling—a method of prenatal diagnosis that provides results as early as the 9th week of pregnancy. Fetal cells from the chorionic villi (protrusions of a membrane called the chorion that surrounds the fetus during its early development) are suctioned out through the uterine cervix and their DNA is analyzed. Preliminary results of this process can be obtained within a day.

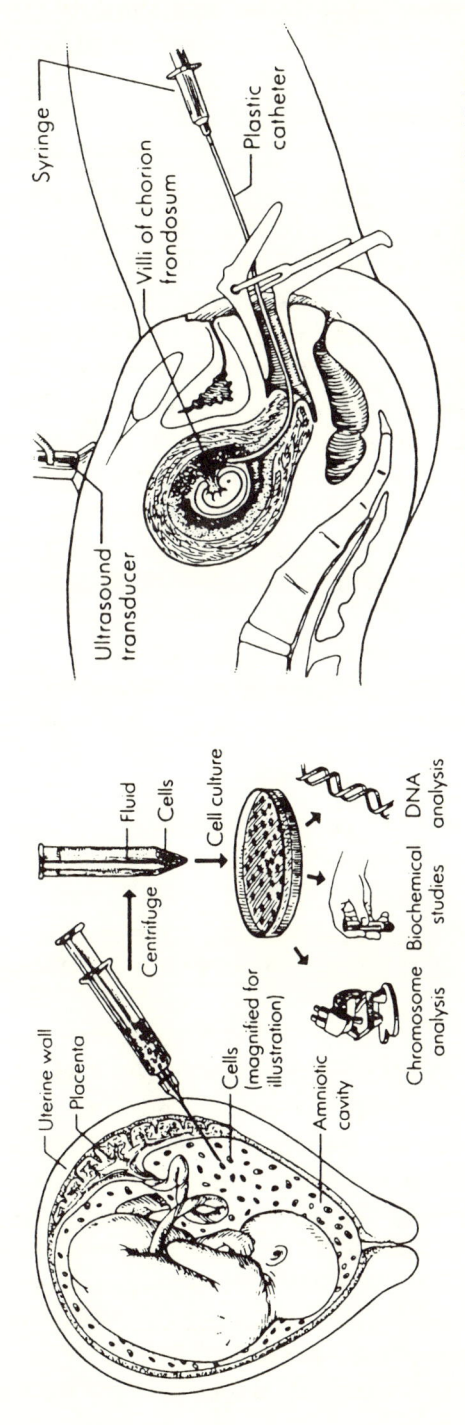

Photo credit: National Institute of General Medical Sciences

anxiety, but the test results were less ambiguous because the test is more sensitive.

## Gene Therapy and Cystic Fibrosis

Recent advances have moved gene therapy from theory to clinical and therapeutic experimental application. Protocols for gene therapy in humans must be approved by the Recombinant DNA Advisory Committee (RAC) of the National Institutes of Health (NIH), the NIH director, and the Food and Drug Administration in what can be a lengthy process, although the procedure has been streamlined. The first human gene therapy clinical trial was approved by the RAC and the NIH director in July 1990. By June 1992, nine other protocols for human gene therapy were in various stages of approval. For gene transfer—experiments that mark cells to trace the course of a treatment or the disease but are not therapeutic—an additional 15 protocols were in various stages of approval. Current human gene therapy trials include alteration of:

- white blood cells to treat a rare genetic disorder, severe combined immune deficiency due to adenosine deaminase deficiency, begun in September 1990;

- immune system cells to produce an anticancer agent, begun in January 1991; and

- liver cells to correct hypercholesterolemia, a genetic disorder of fatal cholesterol buildup, approved in October 1991, begun in June 1992.

The theory of gene therapy is straightforward: The normal gene is inserted into the cellular DNA either to code for a functioning protein product, or, in the case of cancer therapies, to confer disease-fighting properties. Experimentally, delivering normal genes into desired cells can be accomplished through physical or chemical means that disturb the cell membrane and allow DNA to enter, including specially modified viruses, liposomes (fatty materials able to transport drugs directly into cells), and direct injection. Somatic cell therapy—the only approach approved for human trials—changes only the DNA of the person receiving the therapy and cannot be inherited by offspring. In contrast, germ line gene therapy would alter the genetic material that is passed on to future generations. To date, no germ line therapy in humans has been proposed. For most conditions, cells are removed from the patient, genetically altered, and replaced.

Correction of abnormal Cl⁻ transport through insertion of the normal CF gene into defective cells suggested that gene therapy was a viable consideration for treating CF; currently, the respiratory deficits of the disease are being targeted for correction by gene therapy. Unlike the RAC-approved protocols in progress, however, lung cells are generally inaccessible for removal and redelivery after gene transfer, making other means of administering the DNA necessary. Several systems are under investigation for efficacy of delivery in vivo without side effects. In one system, DNA is removed from an adenovirus, the type of virus responsible for some forms of the common cold and other respiratory ailments, and the inactivated virus shell is used as a vector to deliver the CF gene directly into the lungs of rats. The CF gene has also been delivered into cells isolated from the lungs of CF patients by bronchial brushing. In vivo and in vitro, significant amounts of messenger RNA for the CF gene are still present 6 weeks later, suggesting that long-term expression of the gene will be feasible. It is not yet known, however, how frequently new doses of the CF gene would have to be administered. An alternative delivery mechanism, aerosolized liposomes, has been used to deliver alpha-1-antitrypsin genes into rabbit lungs. A similar system might be applicable to delivery of the CF gene to human lungs.

Many questions about the safety and efficacy of gene therapy for CF must be answered before it will be suitable for human trials. Scientists do not yet know how much corrected protein product is needed to restore normal function to a patient with CF. Neither do they know whether adverse health effects will result from placing too much CFTR in a patient. Further, even though the virus has been fully debilitated in theory, using a viral vector raises concerns about expression of contaminating normal virus. Crippled viruses could also join with genetic material already in the cell and allow expression of a new virus or activate cells to a cancerous state.

Ethical considerations are also raised by some. Because gene therapy involves altering the genetic makeup of an individual, some express concerns about eugenic overtones, although only somatic cell therapy is under consideration. The general public, however, is enthusiastic. A 1986 OTA survey found that 83 percent of the American public approved of human cell manipulation to cure usually fatal diseases, 78 percent would be willing to undergo gene therapy personally to correct a genetic proclivity to a serious or fatal disease, and 86 percent of respondents would be willing to have his or her child undergo gene therapy for a usually fatal disease.

Gene therapy clearly offers the promise of treatment for some disorders. On the other hand, heightened attention to genetics in general—and gene therapy in particular—in the popular press can raise false hopes for cures for diseases long before they will be feasible or readily available. For CF, critical steps have been made towards the first attempt at gene therapy in humans; clinical applications, however, are still on the horizon.

Chapter 6

# *Histoplasmosis*

## What Is Histo?

Histo used to be considered a fatal disease. Today, among the millions infected, there are very few fatalities. Histo is a masquerader. The "summer flu" that Midwesterners used to get often is now thought to have been histo. The disease is not "catching" from someone who has it, as tuberculosis is—but many times it has been mistaken for TB, as well as other diseases.

## What Causes Histoplasmosis?

Histo is caused by a fungus (mold), an extremely simple form of plant life. (Other familiar fungi are mushrooms, yeast and mildew.) The particular fungus, or plant, that causes this disease is known as Histoplasma capsulatum. It is tiny and light enough to float in the air when stirred up with dust.

Once it is breathed in, the fungus gets down into the lungs. In effect, it takes root there like a seed and continues to live. The tiny plants increase in number within the lungs simply by dividing themselves in two—over and over again.

---

"Facts About Histoplasmosis," American Lung Association Pub. No. 0619. Used by permission.

Although histoplasmosis is not as uniformly serious as was once believed, it infects millions of people all over the country, many of them living in the Mississippi, Ohio, Missouri and other river valleys.

It took years of detective work and the patient tracking down of clues to unmask and identify histo. There are still many mysteries about the disease, but certain facts are known.

## Where Histoplasmosis Is Found

Histo has gone to town. It used to be considered a rural Midwestern disease. But it has been discovered recently in small towns and even cities in the East and other parts of the country.

Because the histo seeds, called spores, are living things, they need certain conditions in which to flourish. There must be warmth, moisture, and preferably some darkness.

These conditions are found most often in accumulated droppings from chickens, pigeons, starlings, and other birds, as well as bats. Therefore, the place of infection for many people has often been old chicken houses, barns, belfries, pigeon lofts, caves and in parks under trees where many birds have roosted.

One outbreak of histoplasmosis involved a troop of Boy Scouts who had worked hard cleaning up an old city park in which many starlings roosted. The dank, damp undergrowth of the park was disturbed for the first time in years-and the boys breathed in a sufficient quantity of fungus-bearing dust to get the disease.

In one celebrated instance, a number of school children came down with what eventually was diagnosed as histoplasmosis. The source of the disease was painstakingly traced to a window of the school room. Several weeks before a load of coal had been dumped under the window. The coal, it is believed, came from a mine in which the histo fungus had grown.

## Who Gets Histoplasmosis

Most persons who come in contact with a heavy barrage of histo spores are infected. But fortunately in most persons the infection produces no symptoms. Usually people do not even know they have been infected, but some do get sick.

School children of both sexes are frequent victims. More men than women, however, get the disease as adults. Very young children

## Histoplasmosis

and old men are the most susceptible to the generalized form of histo that spreads from the lungs to other parts of the body.

### What Happens Within The Lungs

When the fungus-bearing dust is breathed in, the tiny histo spores are carried into the bronchial tubes (the air passages in the lungs). Some of the spores eventually reach deep down into the very tiny air sacs of the lung—where the air we breathe in finally winds up before it is exhaled. Then various things happen.

In the air sacs some of the spores are arrested by wandering police cells called phagocytes. They are taken to the lungs' lymph nodes, where they are trapped and held. But they may find the lymph nodes an excellent place in which to stay and multiply.

The lymph tissue reacts to this invasion. A sensitivity—actually an allergic reaction—develops. The area becomes inflamed. The tissues of the nodes may be damaged, as well as nearby lung cells. Scars and calcium deposits may form.

Others of the spores that reach the air sacs are attacked by the body's defenses right there. As it does tuberculosis germs, the body walls up most of these spores in calcified tubercles. (On an X-ray these look just like the tubercles of tuberculosis.) The little plants in their calcium prison become starved for oxygen and nutrition. Though remaining in the body, they are harmless and cannot multiply.

Spores that escape these defenses may damage lung tissue and even form cavities—also much like those of tuberculosis.

But, unless the spore invasion is enormous in quantity, these various reactions actually do the patient little harm in by far the majority of cases. Some feel no symptoms at all, others suffer a brief and relatively mild illness. Only when the spores spread throughout the body—as happens only rarely—is there real trouble. The "disseminated" form of histo is often fatal.

### What Histo Does

Depending on the number of spores the patient has taken in, the symptoms of histoplasmosis vary widely in intensity. The symptoms, when they appear, are usually almost identical with those of flu: fever, tiredness, sometimes a slight cough or chest pains. Actually, histo takes four possible forms:

**Mild infection.** This is often without symptoms. The patient may not ever know he has had it. It lasts from one to three days.

**Acute lung infection.** This is usually self-limiting and confined to the lungs. The patient feels fever, recurring chills, cough, chest pain and labored breathing. Even without treatment, this clears up in two weeks to three months.

**Chronic lung infection.** Looking much like TB on an X-ray, this form shows cavities, calcium nodules and other TB-like signs. Illness hangs on. Treatment, when indicated, usually helps.

**Disseminated form.** A large number of the fungus spores spreading outside the lungs mean more serious symptoms: loss of weight, extreme tiredness, anemia and weeks or months of convalescence. Without treatment, a great portion of these patients die within four to ten months after their exposure to the fungus. Fortunately, this is a rare form of the disease.

## How Histoplasmosis Is Diagnosed

There are both skin tests and blood tests that can reveal the presence of histo infection and disease.

Histo also shows up on chest X-rays, but since X-ray findings are almost indistinguishable from those of tuberculosis, this may be undependable. Healthy young men who once unknowingly had histo were kept out of military service during World War II because their X-rays suggested extensive tuberculosis scars.

Today there are a variety of specific skin tests—and also tests in which the organisms are examined under the microscope—that differentiate other fungus diseases and tuberculosis from histo.

## Treatment

Most cases of histo require little or no treatment. After their flu-like symptoms, patients recover of their own accord.

A drug, amphotericin B, has been found effective in the more severe cases of histo. Its use requires hospitalization, however, because the drug must be introduced into the bloodstream almost daily for a period of weeks or months. Side effects have to be carefully monitored.

## Histoplasmosis

Surgery—removal of sections of the lung that are imbedded with histo spores—may sometimes be indicated when there has been extensive damage.

## Prevention

Simple avoidance—of caves, belfries, old chicken houses, and the like—is one possible way to escape histo. But this may well be impossible, particularly for people in rural areas. And even if a real effort were made to stay away from places of suspected infection, there are so many areas of unknown infection that avoidance of histo would seem to be almost a matter of luck.

Here are a few simple rules that might—just might—help to prevent histoplasmosis or cut down its severity:

- Keep farm buildings as clean and dry as possible. But before sweeping them out, wet down the floor to prevent dust from rising.

- Always wet down chicken droppings before cleaning out chicken houses.

- Keep storm cellars clean and dry.

- Take care of minor illnesses; try to stay in as good general health as possible.

Chapter 7

# Pneumonia and Legionnaires' Disease

*Chapter Contents*

Section 7. 1—Facts About Pneumonia .......................................... 376
Section 7. 2—Pneumonia Prevention: It's Worth a Shot ............ 382
Section 7. 3—Questions and Answers on
  Legionnaires' Disease ............................................. 386
Section 7. 4—Legionnaires' Disease and Misters ....................... 388
Section 7. 5—Outbreak of Legionnaires' Disease Associated
  with a Cruise Ship ................................................. 389
Section 7. 6—Legionnaires' Disease Associated with Cooling
  Towers ...................................................................... 390

Section 7.1

# Facts About Pneumonia

Source: American Lung Association  Pub. No. 0029.  Used by permission.

## What Is Pneumonia

Pneumonia is a serious infection, or inflammation of your lungs. The air sacs in the lungs fill with pus, and other liquid. Oxygen has trouble reaching your blood. If there is too little oxygen in your blood, your body cells can't work properly—and may die.

## Pneumonia Is on the Rise

Until 1936, pneumonia was the No. 1 cause of death in the US. Then antibiotics brought it under control. Now this deadly enemy is making a comeback, in part because some bacteria can resist antibiotics. Pneumonia and influenza combined have ranked as the sixth leading cause of death since 1979.

## How Lungs Are Affected

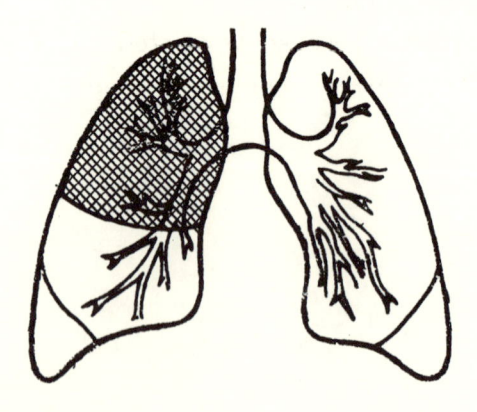

*Figure 31.1* Lobar *pneumonia affects a section (lobe) of a lung.*

# Pneumonia and Legionnaires' Disease

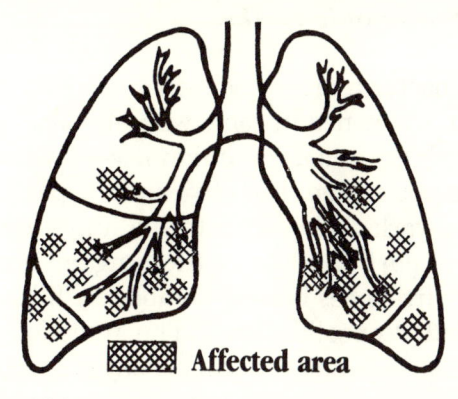

*Figure 31.2* Bronchial *pneumonia (or bronchopneumonia) affects patches throughout both lungs.*

## Causes of Pneumonia

Pneumonia is not a single disease. It can have over 30 different causes.

There are four main causes of pneumonia:

1. Bacteria

2. Viruses

3. Mycoplasmas

4. Others, such as pneumocystis

## 1. Bacterial Pneumonia

Bacterial pneumonia can attack anyone from infants through the very old. Alcoholics, the debilitated, post-operative patients, people with respiratory diseases or viral infections and people who are immuno-compromised are particularly vulnerable.

The *pneumococcus* is the most common cause of bacterial pneumonia. It is the only form of pneumonia for which a vaccine is available.

*How Bacterial Pneumonia Strikes*

Pneumonia bacteria are present in some healthy throats. When body defenses are weakened in some way—by illness, old age, malnutrition, general debility, impaired immunity—the bacteria can multiply and do serious damage. Usually when a person's resistance is lowered, bacteria work their way into the lungs and inflame the air sacs. The tissue of part of a lobe of the lung, an entire lobe, or even most of the lung's five lobes become completely filled with liquid matter. (This is called "consolidation.") The infection quickly spreads through the bloodstream and the whole body is invaded.

**Symptoms:** The onset of bacterial pneumonia can vary from gradual to sudden. The patient may experience shaking chills, chattering, severe chest pain, and a cough that produces rust-colored or greenish sputum. Temperature often shoots up as high as 105. The patient sweats profusely, and his breathing and pulse rate increase rapidly. From lack of oxygen in the blood, his lips and nailbeds may have a bluish cast. His mental state may be clouded or delirious.

## 2. Viral Pneumonia

Half of all pneumonias are believed to be of viral origin. More and more viruses are being identified as the cause of respiratory infection, and though most attack the upper respiratory tract, some produce pneumonia, especially in children. Most of these pneumonias are patchy and self-limiting, but primary influenza virus may be severe and occasionally fatal. The virus invades the lungs and multiplies, but there are almost no physical signs of lung tissue becoming filled with fluid. It finds most of its victims among those who have pre-existing heart or pulmonary illness or are pregnant.

**Symptoms:** The initial symptoms of viral pneumonia are those of influenza: fever, a dry cough, headache, muscle pain, and weakness. Within 12 to 36 hours, there is increasing breathlessness, the cough becomes worse and produces a scant amount of bloody sputum. There is a high fever and there may be blueness of lips. In the final stage, the patient has unbearable air hunger and breathlessness. Other viral pneumonias are complicated by an invasion of bacteria—with all the typical symptoms of bacterial pneumonia.

## 3. Mycoplasma Pneumonia

Because of its symptoms and physical signs, and because the course of the illness differed strikingly from those of classic pneumococcal pneumonia, mycoplasma pneumonia was once believed to be caused by one or more undiscovered viruses and was called "primary atypical pneumonia."

Identified during World War II, mycoplasmas are the smallest free-living agents of disease in man, unclassified as to whether bacteria or viruses, but having characteristics of both. They generally cause a mild and widespread pneumonia. It affects all age groups, occurring most frequently in older children and young adults. The death rate is low, even in untreated cases.

**Symptoms:** The most prominent symptom of mycoplasma pneumonia is a cough that tends to come in violent paroxysms, but produces only sparse whitish sputum. Chilly sensations and fever are early symptoms, and some patients experience nausea or vomiting. The patient's heartbeat is often slow, and in some extreme cases he may suffer from breathlessness and have a bluish cast to his lips and nailbeds.

## 4. Other Kinds of Pneumonia

*Pneumocystis carinii* pneumonia (PCP) is caused by an organism long thought of as a parasite but now believed to be a fungus. PCP is the first sign of illness in more than half of all persons with AIDS, and perhaps 80 percent (four out of five) will develop it sooner or later. It can be successfully treated in many cases. It may recur a few months later, but treatment can help to prevent or delay its recurrence.

Many of the less common pneumonias have a high death toll and are occurring more often. Various special pneumonias are caused by the inhalation of food, liquid, gases, dust, or a foreign body, by fungi, or by a bronchial obstruction such as a tumor. Rickettsia (also considered something between viruses and bacteria) cause Rocky Mountain spotted fever, Q fever, typhus, and psittacosis—diseases that involve the lungs to a greater or lesser extent. Tuberculosis pneumonia is an overwhelming lung infection and extremely dangerous unless treated early.

## Treatment of Pneumonia

If you develop pneumonia, your chances of prompt recovery are greatest under certain conditions: if you're young, if your pneumonia was caught early, if your defenses against disease are working well, if the infection hasn't spread, and if you're not suffering from other illness.

In the young and healthy, prompt treatment with antibiotics can cure bacterial and mycoplasma pneumonia, and a certain percentage of rickettsia cases. There is no effective treatment yet for viral pneumonia.

The drug or drugs used are determined by the germ causing the pneumonia and the judgement of the physician. After temperature returns to normal, medication must be continued according to physician's instructions—otherwise the pneumonia may recur. Relapses can be far more serious than the first attack.

Besides antibiotics, patients are given supportive treatment: proper diet, oxygen to relieve breathlessness and bluish cast to lips, medication to ease chest pain, and in the case of mycoplasma, some relief from the violent cough—anything that can produce and maintain in the patient the best possible conditions for recovery.

## Don't Rush Your Recovery!

The vigorous young person may lead a normal life within a week of his recovery from pneumonia. For the middle-aged, however, weeks may elapse before they regain their accustomed strength, vigor, and feeling of well being. A person should not be discouraged from returning to work or carrying out usual activities, but must be warned to expect some difficulties. Adequate rest is important to maintain progress toward full recovery and to avoid relapse.

## Prevention Is Possible

Because pneumonia is a common complication of influenza (flu), getting a flu shot every fall is good pneumonia prevention.

A vaccine is also available to help fight pneumococcal pneumonia—one type of bacterial pneumonia. Your doctor can help you decide if you—or a member of your family—needs the vaccine against pneumococcal pneumonia. It is usually given only to people at high risk of getting the disease and its life-threatening complications. Ask your doctor if you should be vaccinated. The greatest risk of pneumococcal pneumonia usually is among people who:

- Have chronic illnesses such as lung disease, heart disease, kidney disorders, sickle cell anemia, or diabetes.
- Are recovering from severe illness.
- Are in nursing homes or other chronic care facilities.
- Are age 65 or older.

The vaccine is generally given only once. Ask your doctor about re-vaccination recommendations. It is not recommended for pregnant women or children under age two.

Since pneumonia often follows ordinary respiratory infections, the most important preventive measure is for a person to be alert to any symptoms of respiratory trouble that linger more than a few days. Good health habits—proper diet and hygiene, plentiful rest, regular exercise, etc.—increase resistance to all respiratory illnesses. They also help promote fast recovery if the illnesses do occur.

## *If You Have Symptoms of Pneumonia*

1. Call your doctor immediately. Even with the many effective antibiotics, early diagnosis and treatment are important.

2. Follow your doctor's advice. If he says you should be in the hospital, go there. If he says you may stay at home if you stay in bed, be sure you STAY in bed.

3. To prevent recurrence of pneumonia—continue to take the medicine your doctor prescribes until he says you may stop.

4. Remember—even though pneumonia can be satisfactorily treated, it is an extremely serious illness.

Section 7.2

## Pneumonia Prevention: It's Worth a Shot

Source: National Institute on Aging Research Bulletin, June 1994 and Age Page, 1994.

### Fifth Leading Cause of Death in Older Americans

The National Institute on Aging (NIA) has developed a program to educate the public and health professionals about the importance of immunization against pneumococcal pneumonia in older people. What prompts this attention is that more than 200,000 cases of pneumococcal pneumonia occur every year in this country. About 40,000 of these cases end in death; of those, about 85 percent occur in older adults. In fact, pneumonia is the fifth leading cause of illness and death in older Americans.

NIA researchers recently confirmed that the pneumococcal pneumonia vaccine, available in the United States since 1977, is highly effective in preventing this disease. The Public Health Service recommends vaccinations for all people age 65 and older and other high-risk groups, such as those with a chronic illness (e.g., diabetes, lung or heart disease), a weak immune system (some cancers, HIV infection). Moreover, the vaccine is covered for all Medicare recipients. But despite the vaccine's proven clinical effectiveness, affordability, safety, and ease of administration, it remains under-used. Only about 10 percent of those people who should be immunized have received the vaccine.

### Age Page

*Who Should Get the Vaccine?*

According to the National Institute on Aging, one of the National Institutes of Health, everyone age 65 and older should get the pneumococcal vaccine. Some younger people should get it also. Ask a doctor for the vaccine if you:

- Are age 65 or older, or

## Pneumonia and Legionnaires' Disease

- Have a chronic illness, such as heart or lung disease or diabetes, or
- Have a weak immune system (this can be caused by certain kidney diseases, some cancers, HIV infection, organ transplant medicines, and other diseases).

Pneumococcal (pronounced new-moKOK-al) disease is an infection caused by bacteria. These bacteria can attack different parts of the body. When they invade the lungs, they cause the most common kind of bacterial pneumonia. When the same bacteria attack blood cells, they cause an infection called bacteremia (bak-ter-E-me-ah). And in the brain, they cause meningitis. Pneumococcal pneumonia is a serious illness that kills thousands of older people in the United States each year.

### Can Pneumonia Be Prevented?

The pneumococcal vaccine is safe, it works, and one shot lasts most people a lifetime.

People who get the vaccine are protected against almost all of the bacteria that cause pneumococcal pneumonia and other pneumococcal diseases as well. The shot, which is covered by Medicare, can be a lifesaver.

Some experts say it may be best to get the shot before age 65—anytime after age 50—since the younger you are, the better the results. They also say people should have this shot even if they have had pneumonia before. There are many different kinds of pneumonia, and having one kind does not protect against the others. The vaccine, however, does protect against 88 percent of the pneumococcal bacteria that cause pneumonia. It does not guarantee that you will never get pneumonia. It does not protect against viral pneumonia. Most people need to get the shot only once. However some older people may need a booster; check with your doctor to find out if this is necessary.

### Are There Side Effects?

Some people have mild side effects from the shot, but these usually are minor and last only a very short time. In studies, about half of the people getting the vaccine had mild side effects—swelling and soreness at the spot where the shot was given, usually on the arm. A few people (less than 1 percent) had fever and muscle pain as well as more serious swelling and pain on the arm. The pneumonia shot cannot cause pneumonia because it is not made from the bacteria itself, but from an extract that is not infectious. The same is true of the flu shot; it cannot cause flu. In fact, people can get the pneumonia vaccine and a flu shot at the same time.

*Key Facts*

- Everyone age 65 and older should get the pneumococcal vaccine.
- Anyone with a chronic disease or a weak immune system should also get the vaccine.
- Most people need to get it only once.
- Most people have mild or no side effects.
- It is covered by Medicare.

*About the Disease and the Vaccine*

There are two main kinds of pneumonia—viral pneumonia and bacterial pneumonia. Bacterial pneumonia is the most serious. One kind of bacteria causes pneumococcal pneumonia. In older people, this type of pneumonia is a common cause of hospitalization and death.

About 20 to 30 percent of people over age 65 who have pneumococcal pneumonia develop bacteremia. At least 20 percent of those with bacteremia die from it, even though they get antibiotics.

**People age 65 and older are at high risk. They are two to three times more** likely than people in general to get pneumococcal infections.

A recent, large study by the National Institutes of Health shows that the vaccine prevents most cases of pneumococcal pneumonia.

The U.S. Public Health Service, the National Foundation for Infectious Diseases, and the American Lung Association now recommend that all people age 65 and older get this vaccine.

*Resources*

More information about adult immunizations is available from the following groups:

## Pneumonia and Legionnaires' Disease

National Institute on Aging
P.O. Box 8057
Gaithersburg, MD 20898-8057
1-800-222-2225
1-800-222-4225 (TTY)

National Institute of Allergy and Infectious Diseases
9000 Rockville Pike
Room 7A50
Bethesda, MD 20892
(301) 496-5717

Centers for Disease Control and Prevention
National Immunization Program
1600 Clifton Road
Atlanta, GA 30333
(404) 639-1819

American Lung Association
1740 Broadway
New York, NY 10019-4374
1-800-LUNG-USA
1-800-586-4872

National Foundation for Infectious Diseases
Suite 750
4733 Bethesda Avenue
Bethesda, MD 20814
(301) 656-0003

## Section 7.3

# Questions & Answers on Legionnaires' Disease

Source: Center For Disease Control.

**Q. What is Legionnaires' disease?**

**A.** Legionnaires' disease is an acute respiratory infection caused by the bacterium *Legionella*. An outbreak of this disease in Philadelphia in 1976 largely among persons attending a state convention of the American Legion led to its name.

**Q. What are the usual symptoms of Legionnaires' disease?**

**A.** Patients usually develop fever, chills, and cough which may be dry or produce sputum. Other symptoms that may occur include abdominal pain diarrhea and confusion. It is difficult to distinguish Legionnaires' disease from other types of pneumonia by symptoms alone. The incubation period for Legionnaires' disease is two to ten days.

**Q. Is the illness always severe?**

**A.** Studies have shown that about 5 to 15% of known cases of Legionnaires' disease have been fatal. However many people may be infected with the bacterium causing Legionnaires' disease without developing any symptoms; others are treated without having to be hospitalized. Recent information suggests that many cases of Legionnaires' disease go undiagnosed.

**Q. How is the disease diagnosed?**

**A.** Your physician can order tests to confirm the diagnosis of Legionnaires' disease. The most useful tests include culturing the bacteria from sputum, detecting the presence of the bacteria in a urine sample, and comparing antibody levels in two blood samples collected three to six weeks apart.

**Q. Is there an effective treatment for Legionnaires' disease?**

A. Erythromycin appears to be effective in treating the disease and is currently recommended as the drug of choice. Other drugs are available for patients unable to tolerate erythromycin.

**Q. How is Legionnaires' disease spread?**

A. Most people contract Legionnaires' disease by inhaling mist that comes from a water source (e.g. showers, cooling towers whirlpool baths) contaminated with *Legionella* bacteria. In some cases the disease may be transmitted by other ways, such as aspirating contaminated water. There is no evidence for person-to-person spread of the disease.

**Q. Who gets Legionnaires' disease?**

A. People of any age may get Legionnaires' disease but the illness most often affects middle-aged and older persons particularly those who smoke cigarettes or who drink heavily. Also at extra risk are persons whose immune system is suppressed by diseases such as cancer, kidney failure requiring dialysis diabetes, AIDS, chronic lung disease or heart failure. Those who take drugs that suppress the immune system such as prednisone azathioprine or cyclosporine are also at higher risk.

**Q. Are air conditioning systems a potential source of spread?**

A. The bacterium has been found in cooling towers and evaporative condensers of large air conditioning systems. Such systems have been associated with outbreaks of disease.

**Q. Where is the disease found?**

A. Cases have been identified throughout the United States and in several foreign countries; it likely occurs worldwide.

**Q. How common is Legionnaires' disease in the United States?**

**A.** It is estimated that around 10,000 people develop Legionnaires' disease each year in the United States. An additional unknown number are infected with *Legionella* bacteria but have only a minor illness or no illness at all. The disease can occur in outbreaks or as single cases.

## Section 7.4

## Legionnaires' Disease and Misters

Source: *FDA Consumer,* April 1990.

An outbreak of Legionnaires' disease in Louisiana was linked to a supermarket's vegetable misting machine, according to the Louisiana Department of Health and Hospitals and the federal Centers for Disease Control.

There were 34 confirmed cases of Legionnaires' disease, a type of pneumonia, in October and November 1989 in Bogalusa, La. At least two people died from the disease. *Legionella pneumophila*, the bacteria that causes Legionnaires' disease, was found in a cultured sample from the machine's mist.

Louisiana public health officials said the mist machine found in the Bogalusa store was connected directly to a water supply line and had a small water reservoir tank. In a notice to all state health departments in January 1990, the FDA said reservoir tank-type misters should be checked immediately for contamination and then thoroughly cleaned and sanitized once a week.

Legionnaires' disease is transmitted by inhaling small droplets of water containing *L. pneumophila* bacteria. It cannot be transmitted from one person to another, and there is no evidence that the disease can be transmitted through food.

The disease got its name when American Legion members became ill while attending a 1976 convention in Philadelphia. That outbreak was traced to bacteria growing in standing water in an air-conditioning system and involved 221 illnesses, including 34 deaths.

(For more information on Legionnaires' disease, see "Still a Killer: Pneumonia Targets the Ill, the Elderly" in the June 1987 *FDA Consumer*.)

## Section 7.5

## *Outbreak of Legionnaires' Disease Associated with a Cruise Ship, 1994*

Source: *Morbidity and Mortality Weekly Report*, August 1994.

On July 15, 1994, CDC was notified by the New Jersey State Department of Health of six persons with pneumonia who had recently traveled to Bermuda on the cruise ship *Horizon*. In conjunction with local and state health departments, an investigation was initiated; as of August 10, a total of 14 passengers had Legionnaires' disease (LD) confirmed by either sputum culture (one patient), detection of antigens of *Legionella pneumophila* serogroup 1 (Lp-1) in urine by radioimmunoassay (seven patients), or fourfold rise in titer of antibodies to Lp-1 between acute and convalescent-phase serum specimens (six patients). Possible cases in 28 other passengers with pneumonia that occurred within 2 weeks after sailing aboard the *Horizon* are under investigation. Cases have occurred from nine separate week-long cruises during April 30—July 9, 1994.

To identify the source of *Legionella* sp., a case-control study was conducted, and environmental sampling of the ship's water system was performed. Exposure to the whirlpool baths was strongly associated with illness (odds ratio=16.4; 95% confidence interval 3.7—72.3). Cultures taken from a sand filter used for recirculation of whirlpool water yielded an isolate of Lp-1; this isolate and the clinical isolate had matching monoclonal antibody subtyping patterns.

A variety of interventions were completed, including hyperchlorination of the ship's potable water supply, removal of the whirlpool filters, and discontinuation of the whirlpool baths. Following completion of these interventions, on July 30 the *Horizon* resumed its weekly sailing schedule from New York City to Bermuda.

This outbreak represents the first documented instance of LD aboard a cruise ship docking in U.S. ports. Whirlpool spas previously have been associated with transmission of *Legionella*; hyperchlorination of water systems and replacement of filter devices have successfully terminated outbreaks of LD linked to whirlpool spas. CDC recommends post-intervention environmental sampling of whirlpool circulation systems in conjunction with ongoing surveillance for cases of pneumonia to ensure the efficacy of these interventions. Suspected cases of LD among *Horizon* passengers should be reported to CDC through state and local health departments.

Additional recommendations to reduce the transmission of *Legionella* sp. from whirlpool baths and aboard cruise ships will be the subject of a special meeting of public health officials, LD experts, and members of the whirlpool and cruise line industries; this meeting was tentatively scheduled for the fall of 1994 in Atlanta. Additional information about this meeting is available from CDC's Office of the Director National Center for Environmental Health, telephone (404) 488-7093.

Section 7.6

# *Legionnaires' Disease Associated with Cooling Towers—Massachusetts, Michigan, and Rhode Island, 1993*

Source: *Morbidity and Mortality Weekly Report*, July 1994.

From July through October 1993, outbreaks of Legionnaires' disease (LD) were reported from communities in Massachusetts and Rhode Island and from a state prison in Michigan. Cooling towers (CTs) were identified as the source of all three outbreaks. This report summarizes investigations by state and local health officials and CDC and efforts to control these outbreaks.

## Massachusetts

During July—August 1993, LD was diagnosed in 11 persons living in Fall River, Massachusetts. The mean age of patients was 59 years (range: 40-72 years); six were men. Three persons died. Three persons had *Legionella pneumophila* serogroup 1 (Lp-1) isolated from respiratory secretions, four had Lp-1 antigens detected in respiratory secretions by direct fluorescent antibody testing, three had fourfold rises in serum antibody titer to Lp-1, and one had both a fourfold rise in serum antibody titer and Lp-1 antigens detected in urine by radioimmunoassay.

A case-control study, matching the 11 patients and 22 controls by primary physician, age, sex, and underlying medical condition, indicated that patients were more likely than controls to have visited sites within a 0.04-square-mile (0.1-square-km) neighborhood of Fall River in the 2 weeks before onset of illness (matched odds ratio [ORl=14.0; 95% confidence interval [CI]=1.6-120.8); no other activities were significantly associated with acquiring LD.

Water samples from seven CTs within the neighborhood and from the homes of culture-positive patients were taken approximately 1 month after onset of the last identified case of LD in the community and cultured for legionellae. All samples from potable water taps in patients' homes were culture-negative. Five isolates were cultured from four CTs. Lp-1 was cultured from two conjoined CTs on a building within the neighborhood and had the same monoclonal antibody subtype (MAS) and pulsed-field gel electrophoresis (PFGE) patterns as all three clinical isolates.

The conjoined CTs were decontaminated on an emergency basis according to guidelines previously developed by a technical work group. The onset of the last identified case was August 10, and the CT was decontaminated on September 24. No additional cases were identified after decontamination.

## Michigan

During August—September 1993, LD was diagnosed in 17 persons with pneumonia at a state prison in Michigan; 16 patients were inmates, and one was an employee. One patient died. The mean age of the patients was 47 years (range: 29—81 years); all were men. One person had Lp-1 cultured from respiratory secretions and, for 11, LD was diagnosed by a fourfold rise in titer of antibodies to Lp-1; five patients with pneumonia had evidence of LD by single convalescent-phase antibody titers of 512 or more.

Water samples from wells and potable water taps in the prison and the prison hospital, from the prison hospital CT, and from a CT near the prison were cultured for legionellae. All of the potable water samples were culture-negative. Lp-1 was isolated from both CTs. The isolate from the CT located on the roof of the prison hospital had the same PFGE pattern as the single clinical isolate.

Fourteen (0.6%) of 2253 prisoners who used exercise yards each day adjacent (within 100 yards) to the prison hospital had LD, compared with two (0.1%) of the 2270 inmates who used yards at least 400 yards from the prison hospital (relative risk=7.1; 95% CI=1.6—31.0).

The CT on the prison hospital was shut down on September 17 and decontaminated according to published guidelines. No new cases of LD were identified with onset after September 1.

## *Rhode Island*

During August 30—October 20, 1993, LD was diagnosed in 17 patients who lived or worked in eastern Rhode Island. The patients' mean age was 54 years (range: 28—86 years); 11 were men. Two patients died. Seven patients had Lp-1 cultured from respiratory secretions and 10 had Lp-1 antigen detected in urine. A case-control study, matching the 17 patients with 33 controls by physician practice, age, sex, and underlying medical conditions, indicated that patients were more likely than controls to visit a 0.04square-mile (0.1-square-km) section of downtown Providence (matched OR=6.5; 95% CI=1.4—30.9) in the 2 weeks before onset of illness.

Water samples from the homes of six culture-positive patients were negative for legionellae by culture, but samples from 10 of 24 CTs and one of three decorative fountains in downtown Providence were positive for Lp-1. The environmental isolates were tested by MAS and PFGE; one isolate from a CT on a building located within the area had the same MAS and PFGE patterns as isolates cultured from four casepatients who reported visiting the LD-associated section of downtown Providence. No other sources of transmission were identified in the community. These Lp-1 isolates had MAS and PFGE patterns that were different than those from the Fall River outbreak (approximately 19 miies away); however, the PFGE patterns suggested that the isolates were genetically related.

The CT was shut down and decontaminated on an emergency basis on October 26. No additional cases of LD associated with the area were identified after decontamination of the CT.

Approximately 1000—1300 cases of LD are reported to CDC annually. However, because previous studies indicate that most cases are not diagnosed, the incidence of disease may be substantially higher. *Legionella* causes 1%—5% of community-acquired pneumonia in adults; most cases occur sporadically. The case-fatality rate of LD is 5%—30%.

Diagnosis of LD requires heightened clinical suspicion. Culturing respiratory secretions for legionellae and testing urine for presence of antigen are not routinely performed for patients with community-acquired pneumonia. Although not widely used, urinary antigen detection is a sensitive (60%—80%), highly specific (more than 99%), and rapid method for diagnosing infection caused by Lp-1 (the cause of 90% of cases of LD). In comparison, serial serum antibody titers require several weeks for definitive results. Single serum antibody titer results have low predictive value (positive and negative) and are not useful for diagnosing LD in nonoutbreak situations. However, they may be useful in identifying cases during outbreaks of LD when serial serum specimens are unavailable—as for some patients in the Michigan investigation—and when *Legionella* is suspected to be the cause of a substantial proportion of pneumonia under investigation.

Although most cases of LD are not associated with outbreaks, investigations of outbreaks have provided most of the knowledge about transmission of the disease. LD can be transmitted by aerosol-producing devices (e.g., CTs, evaporative condensers, whirlpool spas, humidifiers, and decorative fountains), and by potable water aerosolized by shower heads and tap-water faucets.

CTs and evaporative condensers have been identified as sources of transmission of LD since the late 1970s. Although legionellae can be cultured in up to 40% of CTs, these devices are rarely associated with outbreaks of LD. To reduce CT-related LD, CDC recommends maintenance of all CTs in accordance with published guidelines.

Although the attributable risk of CTs in sporadically occurring LD is unknown, the findings in this report indicate that CTs remain an important cause of outbreaks of LD. In each investigation, molecular typing of isolates confirmed the epidemiologic findings. CDC, in collaboration with other agencies, is establishing guidelines for prevention of LD, targeting CTs as well as other known sources of LD.

Chapter 8

# Pulmonary Disorders

*Chapter Contents*

Section 8. 1—Pulmonary Embolism ............................................. 396
Section 8. 2—Primary Pulmonary Hypertension ........................ 404
Section 8. 3—Facts About Idiopathic Pulmonary Fibrosis ......... 414

Section 8.1

## Pulmonary Embolism

Source: *FDA Consumer* November 1989.

### Difficult But Crucial Diagnosis

An 86-year-old man sails through gallbladder surgery like a champ, only to die a week later of a blood clot in the lung.

After completing long airplane flights in cramped economy class seats, two healthy, middle-aged physicians develop blood clots in the lung—within days of the flight in one case and a few weeks later in the other.

On New Year's Day, a 40-year-old bartender watches three consecutive bowl games on television while lying on the sofa and then goes right to bed, spending over 40 hours in a horizontal or near-horizontal position. Next day, he is hospitalized with a blood clot in the lung.

A 16-year-old breakdancer is admitted to the hospital with a swollen right arm and chest pain. His doctors discover a blood clot in the lung.

A 45-year-old U.S. senator and prospective candidate for the presidency develops a blood clot in the lung while recuperating from surgery to repair a weak spot in a brain artery.

With the exception of the octogenarian, all these people were correctly diagnosed and treated, and thus survived. They were the lucky ones. Each year there are about 630,000 cases of pulmonary embolism (the medical term for a blood clot that plugs the arteries supplying blood to the lungs) in the United States, and approximately 70,000 people die within an hour of their first symptoms. Of the 560,000 patients who survive longer than one hour, approximately 70 percent, or about 400,000, are misdiagnosed. Since about a third of this group dies, it is estimated that correct diagnosis and therapy could save more than 100,000 lives each year.

A blood clot in the lung is not formed there, but elsewhere in the body, a fact that puzzled doctors for centuries. The mystery was solved in 1845 when Rudolf Virchow, the German physician known as the father of pathology, described how the clot formed in a leg vein, then

## Pulmonary Disorders

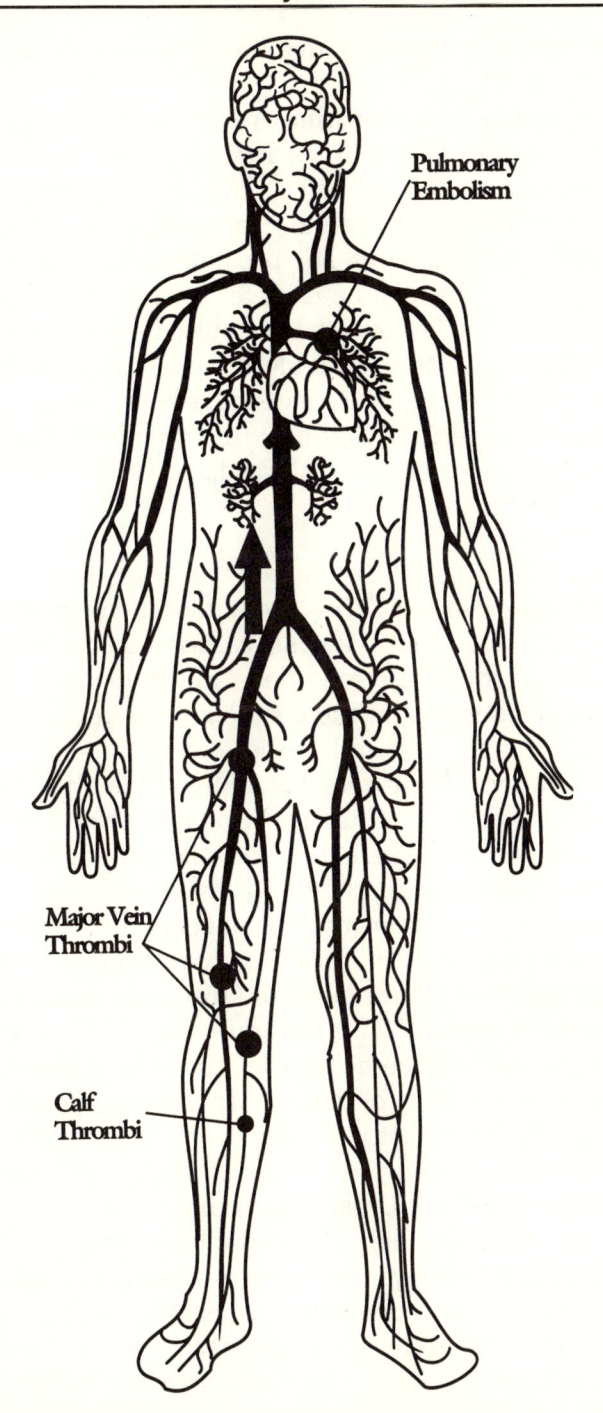

**Figure 8.1.** Blood clots that cause pulmonary embolisms can form in veins in arteries throughout the body.

flowed with the venous blood up to the right side of the heart where it was pumped to the lungs.

Further research proved him correct. About 95 percent of the time, clots that end up in the lungs develop in the large vein deep inside the muscles of the leg and pelvis. (Only about 1 to 2 percent originate in the upper extremities, usually in young, healthy men following strenuous exercise or activity. The breakdancer, for example, developed a blood clot in the arm he used for balancing and spinning.) A deep vein clot is not to be confused with blood clots that form on atherosclerotic plaque in arteries and block the flow of blood to the brain, causing a stroke, or to the heart, causing a heart attack. Nor are the affected veins the superficial leg veins that are visible under the skin, the ones that commonly become enlarged and twisted, or varicosed.

### *Virchow's Triad*

Virchow also postulated that three underlying conditions in the body, afterward called Virchow's triad, contributed to the formation of a vein clot. The first of these conditions, injury to a vein wall, can be caused by inflamed valves in the deep leg veins, an indwelling catheter, an injection or accident, or by other problems.

Normally, when a blood vessel is injured, a clot (thrombus) forms at the injured site to prevent further blood loss. Over a period of days or weeks, the blood vessel heals itself and the clot gradually dissolves. In certain instances, though, the blood clot doesn't stick to the damaged vein wall, but breaks away (or fragments of it break away) and is carried to the lungs via the bloodstream, causing pulmonary embolism. (A thrombus that breaks loose and travels is called an embolus.)

The second of Virchow's risk factors is sluggish blood flow. The circulatory system needs some help to get the venous blood back up to the heart against the force of gravity. (In very tall people, the blood must rise as high as five feet.) To keep the blood flowing in one direction, most leg veins are equipped with valves that prevent blood from flowing backward (reflux). Breathing in and breathing out creates a partial vacuum that also helps send the blood upward. More assistance comes from another quarter—the muscles of the legs, especially calf muscles, pump blood towards the heart by squeezing the deep veins in the leg during exercise and activity.

When the body is inactive, blood may stagnate in the veins (medically this is called venous stasis). Thickening and slowing of the blood flow tend to make the blood clot more readily. This condition may oc-

## Pulmonary Disorders

cur when people are bedridden because of a heart attack or congestive heart failure, are immobilized in a cast, or are recuperating from burns or surgery, especially oriopedic or prostate surgery. Stroke victims run as high as a 75 percent risk of developing deep vein clots in a paralyzed leg.

Virchow's third risk factor is blood that becomes hyper-coagulable (prone to clot excessively). Normally, circulating blood stays fluid through a kind of balancing act between clotting promoters and clotting inhibitors. If the clotting promoters increase, or if the activity of the clotting inhibitors decreases, the result may be blood that clots too readily.

People especially vulnerable to this hyper-coagulable state are those who have cancer, blood diseases such as polycythemia vera (characterized by an increase in red blood cells), some inherited diseases, and chronic ulcerative colitis. Women who use oral contraceptives, especially those who smoke, are also more likely to develop this condition. A rise in hormone levels may cause blood to coagulate more readily in pregnant women, who are five times more likely to develop deep vein clots than non-pregnant women in the same age group. Women who have just given birth are at increased risk if they are obese or have varicose veins, or if they've had deep vein clots or pulmonary embolism in the past.

### Finding a Clot

Obviously, there would be fewer deaths from pulmonary embolism if deep vein clots were treated with drugs before they broke loose and traveled to the lungs. Unfortunately, they don't always make their presence known. About half the people with deep vein blood clots have no symptoms. When symptoms do occur where the clot was formed, they may include slight swelling of the leg or calf, tenderness, cramp-like pain, chills, fever, a bluish discoloration of the skin in the area, and prominent superficial veins.

When deep vein clots are suspected, the best diagnostic test is a venogram. After a radiopaque contrast material is injected into a vein in the foot, the leg area is X-rayed. Clots show up as dark spots in the veins. Other tests, not as conclusive as a venogram, are available for those who are allergic to the contrast material.

Since it's important not to dislodge deep vein clots—and to prevent new ones from forming—people whose tests are positive may be hospitalized for a few days in bed with feet elevated and treated with blood thinners (anticoagulants) and painkillers. Anti-embolism elastic stockings, which function as a form of pressure on the leg veins, may be worn to aid circulation.

If untreated, about 50 percent of deep vein clots will travel to the lungs, where they cause death in about 10 percent of the cases, according to A.G. Turpie, M.D., and Jack Hirsch, M.D., writing in the October 1984 Hospital Medicine. Small emboli in the lungs may cause no symptoms at all. A large embolus can cause death within seconds if it lodges in the fork of the pulmonary artery where it divides into branches to each lung. More commonly, however, embolism is accompanied by shortness of breath, sometimes with wheezing, abnormally rapid and shallow breathing, anxiety, and restlessness. Other symptoms that may appear include chest pain, coughing up blood, rapid heartbeat, dizziness, fainting, and occasionally fever.

Since its symptoms imitate the symptoms of so many other chest and lung diseases, pulmonary embolism is often difficult to diagnose. Just as syphilis was known as the "great masquerader" in the past because of its ability to mimic other diseases, so pulmonary embolism is the medical mimic of our times. Its symptoms can be confused with pneumonia, heart attack, inflammation of the membrane lining the wall of the abdominal and pelvic cavity (peritonitis), inflammation of the sac that contains the heart (pericarditis), asthma, acute bronchitis combined with emphysema, lung cancer, and even an anxiety attack. Thomas A. Neff, M.D., chief of pulmonary service, Denver General Hospital, comments: "It is always essential to think of pulmonary thromboembolism [pulmonary embolism] in any acute, obscure, and, especially, serious lung disease."

Jan M. Orenstein, M. D., professor of pathology, George Washington University School of Medicine, and the director of the autopsy service at George Washington University Hospital, says: "Pulmonary emboli are a relatively common finding at autopsy, usually unsuspected and frequently the cause of death. We often find emboli in the lungs of the elderly, the obese, heavy smokers, and those with diabetes, but the most common underlying condition is heart disease."

Orenstein's observation is borne out by the results of a large multi-institutional study published in 1987. In all cases of pulmonary embolus identified at autopsy that caused or significantly contributed to a person's death, 46.8 percent were not diagnosed before death. "The autopsy is the only sure means of determining the incidence of pulmonary emboli. This is true for many problems in medicine, says Orenstein.

Physicians have a number of tests to help diagnose pulmonary embolism. Some tests are used to rule out other diseases; for example, an electrocardiogram will often distinguish between a heart attack and a pulmonary embolism. Other tests are more specific. Lung scans—which can show lung areas that are not receiving enough blood because of blockage by a clot—and measurement of the amount of oxygen in arterial blood are the most reliable screening tests. Pulmonary arteriography, a more invasive procedure, is performed when the diagnosis is in doubt. A flexible catheter containing a contrast material is passed into the pulmonary artery while the technician takes X-ray pictures. Emboli and obstructed pulmonary arterial branches can be seen on the X-ray screen.

## Treatment

Even though most blood clots resolve spontaneously in several days or weeks, once a diagnosis of pulmonary embolism has been made, patients are given anticoagulant drugs, usually heparin, through the vein for 7 to 10 days to prevent new clots from forming. After leaving the hospital, anti-clotting treatment may be continued at home with warfarin, which can be taken by mouth, for three to six months. Both prolonged sitting and standing, which encourage the pooling of blood in leg veins, should be avoided during this period. Because warfarin can cause birth defects, women who must be on prolonged or continuous anticoagulant therapy are advised against becoming pregnant.

Patients who have a dangerously large pulmonary embolus or who are at risk for recurring emboli and are in unstable condition because of poor pulmonary circulation are often given newer drugs—streptokinase, urokinase, and a genetically engineered drug called tissue plasminogen activator, or tPA. Given through the vein, these drugs actually dissolve clots, sometimes in a matter of hours. (Streptokinase and urokinase have been approved by FDA for the treatment of pulmonary emboli; FDA has approved tPA for dissolving blood clots that obstruct coronary arteries and cause heart attacks, but it is sometimes also used to dissolve lung clots.) These drugs are not used as frequently as heparin, because they can cause severe bleeding complications.

Physicians have another ace up their sleeves for those who can't be anticoagulated or who have had complications from previous anticoagulation. A small device called a filter can be inserted into the inferior vena cava, the large vein that leads directly into the heart. This device permits the flow of blood but traps any emboli that travel up from the leg or pelvic veins. The trapped clots gradually self-destruct. One of those most frequently used is the Greenfield filter, a stainless steel wire device that resembles an umbrella without the cloth cover. In April 1989, FDA approved another clot-catching device, the bird's nest filter, a tangle of wires that looks exactly like its name. Because filters can be inserted through a catheter introduced into a vein using local anesthesia, they provide safe and effective protection against pulmonary emboli without surgery.

Tests can confirm the diagnosis of acute pulmonary embolism in a patient who doesn't have the typical symptoms of the disease, and, in many cases, the disease can be effectively treated. The trick, however, is to suspect and diagnose the condition in the first place.

### People at High Risk for Pulmonary Embolism

- People immobilized for long periods due to illness or accidents
- Congestive heart failure patients
- Those with tumors, especially certain cancers of the gastrointestinal tract
- Post-surgical patients
- Pregnant women
- Women over the age of 30 using oral contraceptives
- Patients with intrinsic vein disease
- Those with certain blood disorders
- Chronic obstructive lung disease patients
- The obese

### An Ounce of Prevention

Keeping deep vein clots from forming is the best way to prevent pulmonary embolism, since most deaths due to the disease occur before treatment can begin. In individuals with predisposing factors, low-dose heparin may be given under the skin before and during certain surgical procedures—usually elective abdominal, pelvic and chest surgery—and is continued until the patient is up and about. The same treatment may be used in individuals who are recuperating from a heart attack, major burns, or acute paralysis, and in some bedridden

## Pulmonary Disorders

patients who have cancer and vein diseases or who are obese. Since anticoagulant drugs interfere with the clotting process throughout the body and may cause bleeding, patients must be carefully watched.

Intermittent pneumatic compression of the legs is also used on high-risk patients to prevent blood clots from forming. A plastic sleeve is fitted over each calf and inflated with air at regular intervals. Compression usually begins with surgery and continues until the patient can walk.

Patients at lesser risk are encouraged to get on their feet as soon as possible—ordinarily the day after surgery or childbirth. People who aren't allowed out of bed for a few days are usually told to move their feet and legs in bed as much as they safely can. Bending the knees and straightening the legs, contracting the muscles in the calf, pressing the balls of the feet against the footboard of the bed repeatedly, are some easy exercises that lower the risk of clot formation.

Healthy, active people don't usually have to worry about pulmonary embolism. Traveling, however, especially when sitting nearly immobile for long periods, has its dangers. For example, in a letter to The Lancet (Aug. 27, 1988), two doctors reported that over a three-year period at Heathrow Airport, an estimated 18 percent of 61 sudden deaths in passengers traveling long distances were due to pulmonary emboli. They advise air travelers not to smoke, as smoking thickens the blood, and recommend drinking plenty of non-alcoholic liquids to counteract the dehydrating effects of low humidity in the air cabins. Frequent walks around the plane will keep blood from pooling in leg veins and feet from swelling.

Other exercises that can be done in place are moving the feet up and down, toe-wiggling, and extending the lower legs. Contracting the muscles in the stomach and buttocks encourages blood flow in the pelvic veins, while deep breathing increases the flow of blood to the upper part of the body. Though the risk of blood pooling is slight in the upper extremities, people whose hands swell should do reaching exercises, or open and close the fingers occasionally.

The same goes for long trips in other vehicles. Walking up and down the train, or stopping the car occasionally to stretch the legs, helps the circulation. Wearing restrictive clothing in general is not sensible, but it is especially important to forego tight girdles or panty hose on the road, as they may act as tourniquets to the upper legs. If the doctor has advised wearing elastic stockings in the past, they should be worn while traveling.

People in sedentary jobs need to ambulate as well as eat during lunch hour, while devoted TV fans should make a habit of moving about during commercials and other dull spots.

Since there's not much we can do about some of the ills that are visited upon us, it's wise to do all we can about the ones we can prevent. The body requires activity to keep itself in good condition, and that's not really asking much.

— *Evelyn Zamula*

Evelyn Zamula is a free-lance writer in Potomac, Md.

Section 8.2

## Primary Pulmonary Hypertension

Source: National Institutes of Health   Pub. No. 92-3291.

### Introduction

Primary, or unexplained, pulmonary hypertension (PPH) is a rare lung disorder in which the blood pressure in the pulmonary artery rises far above normal levels for no apparent reason. The pulmonary artery is the blood vessel carrying oxygen-poor blood from the right ventricle, one of the pumping chambers of the heart, to the lungs. In the lungs, the blood picks up oxygen and then flows to the left side of the heart, where it is pumped by the left ventricle to the rest of the body through the aorta.

Hypertension is the medical term for an abnormally high blood pressure. Normal mean pulmonary-artery pressure is approximately 14 mmHg at rest. In the PPH patient, the mean blood pressure in the pulmonary artery is greater than 25 mmHg at rest and 30 mmHg during exercise. This abnormally high pressure (pulmonary hypertension) is associated with changes in the small blood vessels in the lungs, resulting in an increased resistance to blood flowing through the vessels.

This increased resistance, in turn, places a strain on the right ventricle, which now has to work harder than usual against the resistance to move adequate amounts of blood through the lungs.

## Incidence

The true incidence of primary pulmonary hypertension is unknown. The first reported case occurred in 1891, when E. Romberg, a German doctor, published a description of a patient who, at autopsy, showed thickening of the pulmonary artery but no heart or lung disease that might have caused the condition. In 1951, when 39 cases were reported by Dr. D.T. Dresdale in the United States, the illness received its name.

Between 1967 and 1973, a 10-fold increase in unexplained pulmonary hypertension was reported in central Europe. The rise was subsequently traced to aminorex fumarate, an amphetamine-like drug introduced in Europe in 1965 to control appetite. Only about 1 in 1,000 people who took the drug developed PPH. When they stopped taking the drug, some improved considerably; in others, the disease kept getting worse. Once aminorex was removed from the market, the incidence of primary pulmonary hypertension went down to normal levels.

In the United States it has been estimated that 300 new cases of PPH are diagnosed each year; the greatest number are reported in women between the ages of 21 and 40. Indeed, at one time the disease was thought to occur among young women almost exclusively; we now know, however, that males and females in all age ranges, from very young children to elderly people, can get PPH. Apparently it also affects people of all race and ethnic origins equally.

## Cause

There may be one or more causes of PPH; however, all remain unknown. The low incidence makes learning more about the disease extremely difficult. Studies of PPH also have been difficult because no animal model of the disease has been available. However, a strain of rats was recently identified in which pulmonary hypertension develops spontaneously. These rats may prove useful for the study of the causes and disease processes of PPH.

One thought is that some people with PPH may be hyper-reactors. This means they are unusually susceptible to agents that cause constriction, or narrowing, of blood vessels. Indeed, people with Raynaud's disease, a condition in which the fingers and toes easily turn blue when cold because of an extreme reaction of the blood vessels in their fingers and toes to cold, seem to be more likely than others to get PPH.

PPH sometimes occurs among close family members, suggesting there may be some inherited tendency toward hyper-reactivity. But even among brothers and sisters with PPH, the areas of the lung affected and the course of the disease may differ greatly.

## Course of the Disease

Researchers believe that one of the ways PPH starts is with injury to the layer of cells (the endothelial cells) that line the small blood vessels of the lungs. This injury, which occurs for unknown reasons, may bring about changes in the way the endothelial cells interact with smooth muscle cells in the vessel wall. As a result, the smooth muscle contracts more than normal and thereby narrows the vessel.

The process eventually results in the development of extra amounts of tissue in the walls of the pulmonary arteries. The amount of muscle increases in some arteries, and muscle appears in the walls of arteries that normally have no muscle. With time, scarring, or fibrosis, of the arteries takes place, and they become stiff as well as thickened. Some vessels may become completely blocked. There is also a tendency for blood clots to form within the smaller arteries.

In response to the extra demands placed on it by PPH, the heart muscle gets bigger, and the right ventricle expands in size. Overworked and enlarged, the right ventricle gradually becomes weak and loses its ability to pump enough blood to the lungs. Eventually, the right side of the heart may fail completely, resulting in death.

## Symptoms

In general, researchers find there is no correlation between the time PPH is thought to have started, the age at which it is diagnosed, and the severity of symptoms. In some patients, especially children, the disease progresses fairly rapidly.

The first symptom is frequently tiredness, with many patients thinking they tire easily because they are simply out of shape. Diffi-

## Pulmonary Disorders

culty in breathing (dyspnea), dizziness, and even fainting spells (syncope) are also typical early symptoms. Swelling in the ankles or legs (edema), bluish lips and skin (cyanosis), and chest pain (angina) are among other symptoms of the disease.

Patients with PPH may also complain of a racing pulse; many feel they have trouble getting enough air. Palpitations, a strong throbbing sensation brought on by the increased rate of the heartbeat, can also cause discomfort.

Some people with PPH do not seek medical advice until they can no longer go about their daily routine. The more severe the symptoms, the more advanced the disease. In these more advanced stages, the patient is able to perform only minimal activity and has symptoms even when resting. The disease may worsen to the point where the patient is completely bedridden.

### Diagnosis

PPH is rarely picked up in a routine medical examination. Even in its later stages, the signs of the disease can be confused with other conditions affecting the heart and lungs. Thus, much time can pass between the time the symptoms of PPH appear and a definite diagnosis is made.

PPH remains a diagnosis of exclusion. This means that it is diagnosed only after the doctor finds pulmonary hypertension and excludes or cannot find other reasons for the hypertension, such as a chronic obstructive pulmonary disease (chronic bronchitis and emphysema), pulmonary emboli, or some forms of congenital heart disease.

The first tests for PPH help the doctor determine how well the heart and lungs are performing. If the results of these tests do not give the doctor enough information, the doctor must perform a cardiac catheterization. The procedure, discussed below, is the way the doctor can make certain that the patient's problems are due to PPH and not to some other condition.

#### Electrocardiogram

The electrocardiogram (ECG) is a record of the electrical activity produced by the heart. An abnormal ECG may indicate that the heart is undergoing unusual stress.

In addition to the usual ECG performed while the patient is at rest, the doctor may order an exercise ECG. This ECG helps the doctor evaluate the performance of the heart during exercise, for example, walking a treadmill in the doctor's office.

### Echocardiogram

In an echocardiogram, the doctor uses sound waves to map the structure of the heart by placing a slim device that looks like a microphone on the patient's chest. The instrument sends sound waves into the heart, which then are reflected back to form a moving image of the beating heart's structure on a TV screen. A record is made on paper or videotape. The moving pictures show how well the heart is functioning. The still pictures permit the doctor to measure the size of the heart and the thickness of the heart muscle; in the patient with severe pulmonary hypertension, the still pictures will show that the right heart is enlarged, while the left heart is either normal or reduced in size.

### Pulmonary Function Tests

A variety of tests called pulmonary function tests (PFTs) evaluate lung function. In these procedures, the patient, with a nose clip in place, breathes in and out through a mouthpiece. The patient's breathing displaces the air held in a container suspended in water. As the container rises and falls in response to the patient's breathing, the movements produce a record, or spirogram, that helps the doctor measure lung volume (how much air the lungs hold) and the air flow in and out of the lungs. Some devices measure air flow electronically.

A mild restriction in air movement is commonly seen in patients with PPH. This restriction is thought to be due, in part, to the increased stiffness of the lungs resulting from both the changes in the structure and the high blood pressure in the pulmonary arteries.

### Perfusion Lung Scan

A perfusion lung scan shows the pattern of blood flow in the lungs; it can also tell the doctor whether a patient has large blood clots in the lungs. In the perfusion scan, the doctor injects a radioactive substance into a vein. Immediately after the injection, the chest is scanned for radioactivity. Areas in the lung where blood clots are blocking the flow of blood will show up as blank or clear areas. Two patterns of pulmonary perfusion are seen in patients with PPH. One

## Pulmonary Disorders

is a normal pattern of blood distribution; the other shows a scattering of patchy abnormalities in blood flow. A major reason for doing a perfusion scan is to distinguish patients with PPH from those whose pulmonary hypertension is due to blood clots in the lungs.

### Right-Heart Cardiac Catheterization

In right-heart cardiac catheterization, the doctor places a thin, flexible tube, or catheter, through an arm, leg, or neck vein in the patient, and then threads the catheter into the right ventricle and pulmonary artery. Most important in terms of PPH is the ability of the doctor to get a precise measure of the blood pressure in the right side of the heart and the pulmonary artery with this procedure. It is the only way to get this measure, and must be performed in the hospital by a specialist.

During catheterization, the doctor can also evaluate the right heart's pumping ability; this is done by measuring the amount of blood pumped out of the right side of the heart with each heartbeat.

### Functional Classification

Once PPH is diagnosed, most doctors will classify the disease according to the functional classification system developed by the New York Heart Association. It is based on patient reports of how much activity they can comfortably undertake.

- Class 1—Patients with no symptoms of any kind, and for whom ordinary physical activity does not cause fatigue, palpitation, dyspnea, or anginal pain.
- Class 2—Patients who are comfortable at rest but have symptoms with ordinary physical activity.
- Class 3—Patients who are comfortable at rest but have symptoms with less-than-ordinary effort.
- Class 4—Patients who have symptoms at rest.

### Treatment

Some patients do well by taking medicines that make the work of the right ventricle easier. Anticoagulants, for example, can decrease the tendency of the blood to clot, thereby permitting blood to flow more freely. Diuretics decrease the amount of fluid in the body, further reducing the amount of work the heart has to do.

Until recently, nothing more could be done for people who have primary pulmonary hypertension. However, today doctors can choose from a variety of drugs that help lower blood pressure in the lungs and improve the performance of the heart in many patients.

Some patients also require supplemental oxygen delivered through nasal prongs or a mask if breathing becomes difficult; some need oxygen around the clock. In severely affected cases, a heart-lung, single lung, or double lung transplantation may be appropriate.

## Drugs

Doctors now know that PPH patients respond differently to the different medicines that dilate, or relax, blood vessels and that no one drug is consistently effective in all patients. Because individual reactions vary, different drugs have to be tried before chronic or long-term treatment begins. During the course of the disease, the amount and type of medicine may also have to be changed.

To find out which medicine works best for a particular patient, doctors evaluate the drugs during cardiac catheterization. This way they can see the effect of the medicine on the patient's heart and lungs. They can also adjust the dose to reduce the side effects that may occur—for example, systemic low blood pressure (hypotension); nausea; angina; headaches; or flushing.

To determine whether a drug is improving a patient's condition, both the pulmonary pressure and the amount of blood being pumped by the heart (the cardiac output) must be evaluated. A decrease in pulmonary pressure alone, for example, does not necessarily mean that the patient is recovering; cardiac output must either increase or remain unchanged. The most desirable response is a decrease in pressure and an increase in cardiac output. Once the patient has reached a stable condition, he or she can go home, returning every few weeks or months to the doctor for follow-up.

At present, results with calcium channel blocking drugs are encouraging. By relaxing the smooth muscle in the walls of the heart and blood vessels, these calcium blockers improve the ability of the heart to pump blood.

A new vasodilator, prostacycline, is helping some severely ill patients. The drug, which is now being studied in clinical trials, imitates the natural prostacycline that the body produces on its own to dilate

## Pulmonary Disorders

blood vessels. Prostacycline also seems to help prevent blood clots from forming.

Prostacycline is administered intravenously by a portable, battery-operated syringe pump. The pump is worn attached to a belt around the waist or carried in a small shoulder pack. The medicine is then slowly and continuously pumped into the body through a catheter placed in a vein in the neck.

Prostacycline seems to improve pulmonary hypertension and permit more physical activity. Currently limited in supply, it is sometimes used as a bridge to help those patients waiting for a transplant. It may become long-term treatment for more patients once it is released for general distribution

### *Transplantation*

The first heart-lung transplant was performed in this country in 1981. Many of these operations were performed for patients with primary pulmonary hypertension. The survival rate is the same as for other patients with heart-lung transplants, about 60 percent for 1 year, and 37 percent for 5 years.

Meanwhile, the single lung transplant is becoming another method of transplant used in cases of PPH. This newer procedure, in which one lung—either the left or right—is replaced, was first performed in 1983 in patients with pulmonary fibrosis. Double lung transplants have also been done to treat PPH, but are less common than the single lung transplant for treatment of PPH.

There are fewer complications with the single lung transplant than with the heart-lung transplant, and the survival rate is on the order of 70 to 80 percent for 1 year. A surprising finding is the remarkable ability of the right ventricle to heal itself. In patients with lung transplants, both the structure and function of the right ventricle markedly improve.

### *The Primary Pulmonary Hypertension Patient Registry 1981-1988*

In 1981, the National Heart, Lung, and Blood Institute (NHLBI) established the first PPH-patient registry in the world. The registry followed 194 people with PPH; over a period of at least 1 year and, in some cases, for as long as 7.5 years. Much of what we know about the illness today stems from this study.

At the time the patients enrolled in the registry, 75 percent were in functional classes 3 or 4. They had an average mean pulmonary artery pressure three times the normal, an abnormally high pressure in the right side of the heart, and a reduced cardiac output. In making the diagnosis of PPH, investigators found no complications arising from cardiac catheterization.

The study findings show that pulmonary artery pressure in patients who had symptoms for less than 1 year was similar to that in patients who had symptoms for more than 3 years. Researchers also found that patients whose only symptom was difficulty in breathing upon exercise already had very high pulmonary artery pressure. This suggests that the pulmonary artery pressure rises to high levels early in the course of the disease.

No correlations could be found between the cause of PPH and cigarette smoking, occupation, place of residence, pregnancy, use of appetite suppressants, or use of prescription drugs, including oral contraceptives. This study was designed to serve only as a registry, so it was not possible to evaluate the effectiveness of treatment.

Because we still do not understand the cause or have a cure for PPH, NHLBI remains committed to supporting basic and clinical studies of this illness. Basic research studies are focusing on the possible involvement of immunologic and genetic factors in the cause and progression of PPH, looking at agents that cause narrowing of the pulmonary blood vessels, and identifying factors that cause growth of smooth muscle and formation of scar tissue in the vessel walls. Most important is finding a reliable way to diagnose PPH early in the course of the disease and that does not require cardiac catheterization.

### *Living with Primary Pulmonary Hypertension*

With the cause of primary pulmonary hypertension still unknown, there is at present no known way to prevent or cure this disease. However, many patients report that by changing some parts of their lifestyle, they can go about many of their daily tasks. For example, they do relaxation exercises, try to reduce stress, and adopt a positive mental attitude

People with PPH go to school, work at home or outside the home part-time or full-time, and raise their children. Indeed, most patients with PPH do not look sick, and some feel perfectly well much of the time as long as they do not strain themselves physically.

## Pulmonary Disorders

Walking is good exercise for many patients; others choose swimming. Some patients with advanced PPH carry portable oxygen when they go out; patients who find walking too exhausting may use a wheelchair or motorized scooter. Others stay busy with activities that are not of a physical nature.

For the patient who lives at a high altitude, a move to a lower altitude—where the air is not so thin, and thus the amount of oxygen is higher can be helpful. Medical care is important, preferably by a doctor who is a pulmonary vascular specialist. These specialists are usually located at major research centers. PPH patients can also help themselves by following the same sensible health measures that everyone should observe. These include eating a healthy diet, not smoking, and getting plenty of rest. Pregnancy is not advised because it puts an extra load on the heart. Oral contraceptives are not recommended, and other methods of birth control should be used.

Most doctors and patients agree that it is important for both patient and family to be as informed as possible about PPH. In this way everyone can understand the illness and apply that information to what is happening. In addition to family and close friends, support groups can help the PPH patient.

*For More Information*

If you are interested in receiving more information on primary pulmonary hypertension, contact:

Office of the Director
Division of Lung Diseases
National Heart, Lung, and Blood Institute
National Institutes of Health
Bethesda, MD 20892
(301) 496-7208

## Section 8.3

## Facts About Idiopathic Pulmonary Fibrosis

Source: National Institutes of Health Pub. No. 93-2997.

### What Is Idiopathic Pulmonary Fibrosis (IPF)?

Idiopathic Pulmonary Fibrosis (IPF) is a disease of inflammation that results in scarring, or fibrosis, of the lungs. In time, this fibrosis can build up to the point where the lungs are unable to provide oxygen to the tissues of the body.

Doctors use the word "idiopathic" (from the Greek "idio" meaning "peculiar" or "unusual" and "pathy" meaning "illness") to describe the disease, because the cause of IPF is unknown. Currently, researchers believe that IPF may result from either an autoimmune disorder, a condition in which the body's immune system attacks its own tissues, or the after-effects of an infection, most likely a virus.

Whatever the trigger is for IPF, it appears to set off a series of events in which the inflammation and immune activity in the lungs—and, eventually, the fibrosis processes, too—become uncontrollable. In a few cases, heredity appears to play a part, possibly making some individuals more likely than others to get IPF.

In studies of patients with IPF, the average survival rate has been found to be 4 to 6 years after diagnosis. Those who develop idiopathic pulmonary fibrosis at a young age seem to have a longer survival.

### How Common Is IPF?

The exact number of people who develop idiopathic pulmonary fibrosis each year is not known. It is known, however, that equal numbers of men and women get the illness and that most cases of IPF are diagnosed when patients are between the ages of 40 and 70.

### What Are the Symptoms of IPF?

Early symptoms of idiopathic pulmonary fibrosis are usually similar to those of other lung diseases. Very often, for example, pa-

## Pulmonary Disorders

tients suffer from a dry cough and dyspnea (shortness of breath). As the disease progresses, dyspnea becomes the major problem. Day-to-day activities such as climbing stairs, walking short distances, dressing, and even talking on the phone and eating become more difficult and sometimes nearly impossible. Enlargement (clubbing) of the fingertips may develop. The patient may also become less able to fight infection. In advanced stages of the illness, the patient may need oxygen all the time.

IPF can lead to death. Often the immediate cause is respiratory failure due to hypoxemia, right-heart failure, a heart attack, blood clot (embolism) in the lungs, stroke, or lung infection brought on by the disease.

### What Is the Course of IPF?

Although the course of idiopathic pulmonary fibrosis varies greatly from person to person, the disease usually develops slowly, sometimes over years.

The early stages are marked by alveolitis, an inflammation of the air sacs called alveoli, in the lungs. The job of the air sacs is to allow the transfer of oxygen from the lungs into the blood and the elimination of carbon dioxide from the lungs and out of the body.

As IPF progresses, the alveoli become damaged and scarred, thus stiffening the lungs. The stiffening makes breathing difficult and brings on a feeling of breathlessness (dyspnea), especially during activities that require extra effort.

In addition, scarring of the alveoli reduces the ability of the lungs to transfer oxygen. The resulting lack of oxygen in the blood (hypoxemia) may cause increases in the pressure inside the blood vessels of the lungs, a situation known as pulmonary hypertension. The high blood pressure in the lungs then puts a strain on the right ventricle, the lower right side of the heart, which pumps the oxygen-poor blood into the lungs.

### How Is IPF Diagnosed?

The first suspicion that a person may have idiopathic pulmonary fibrosis is usually based on the patient's symptoms and medical history. The doctor will try to confirm or rule out any suspicion by ordering one or more of the following tests:

- **Chest X-ray**—A simple chest x-ray is a picture of the lungs and surrounding tissues, most often taken while the patient is standing up. In an IPF patient, the x-ray usually reveals shadows, mostly in the lower part of the lungs. In addition, lung size tends to appear smaller than normal.

- **Computed Tomography (CT)**—A computed tomography scan of the chest is a series of x-rays that provide a view of the lungs that looks almost as if a slice had been made through the chest. During a CT scan, the patient lies inside a long, oval-shaped machine that permits x-ray beams to pass through the top, sides, and back of the body. A computer is used to combine all the pictures taken from these positions and thus gives the doctor a good look at what's going on inside the lungs and chest.

- **Blood Tests**—When IPF is suspected, the doctor will also analyze the patient's blood. A low level of oxygen in the arterial blood may reveal that the alveoli are not taking up enough oxygen.

- **Pulmonary Function Tests**—Pulmonary function tests (PFTs) require the patient to breathe into a mouthpiece. The mouthpiece, in turn, is connected to a machine that measures the amount of air the patient breathes in and out over a specific period of time. The results tell the doctor how well the air passages in the lungs are functioning and how well the lungs are expanding.

- **Bronchoalveolar Lavage**—Lung washings (bronchoalveolar lavage) are also helpful in arriving at a diagnosis of IPF. In this procedure, the doctor inserts a long, narrow, flexible, lighted tube called a bronchoscope down the windpipe and into the lungs to remove fluid (lavage) and other materials from inside the lungs. The amounts of certain cells and proteins found in the materials are measured to determine the stage of the lung disease.

Even if some or all of the results from such tests are abnormal, they are rarely sufficient to make a specific diagnosis of IPF. The only

## Pulmonary Disorders

way the doctor can confirm a diagnosis of IPF is by examining the lung tissue; such tissue is usually obtained by an open lung biopsy.

- **Open Lung Biopsy**—In an open lung biopsy, a chest surgeon makes cuts between the ribs in the chest and removes small pieces of tissue from several places in the lungs. The material is examined in the laboratory to determine how much inflammation and fibrosis are in the lungs. It is the only way to confirm whether the patient has IPF. If IPF is present, the biopsy results are also the best way to find out how far the disease has progressed and what the outlook is.

In a patient with no other significant illness, recovery from an open lung biopsy is relatively quick. The hospital stay is usually 4 to 7 days; some newer procedures require less surgery, bringing hospital stays down to 1 to 3 days.

### Can IPF Be Treated?

The best chance of slowing the progress of IPF is by starting treatment as soon as possible. Most IPF patients require treatment throughout life, usually under the guidance of a lung specialist. Some major medical centers and large teaching hospitals do research on the disease and provide consultation and treatment to patients.

Treatment for idiopathic pulmonary fibrosis may vary a great deal. It depends on many things, including the age of the patient and stage of the disease. The aim of treatment is to reduce the inflammation of the alveoli and stop the abnormal process that ends in fibrosis. Once scar tissue has formed in the lung, it cannot be returned to normal.

### How Is IPF Treated?

Drugs are the primary way that IPF is treated. They are usually prescribed for at least 3 to 6 months. This gives the doctor time to see if a particular treatment is effective. A combination of tests is used to monitor how well a particular medicine is working. The dose may have to be adjusted so that the medicine gives the best possible results with the least side-effects. Most side-effects are reduced when the dose is made smaller or the drug is stopped. Commonly used drugs are prednisone and cytoxan. Oxygen administration and, in special cases, transplantation of the lung are other choices.

- **Prednisone**—A corticosteroid, prednisone, is the most common drug given to patients with idiopathic pulmonary fibrosis. About 25 to 35 percent of all patients respond favorably to this medicine. No one knows exactly how corticosteroids work or why some patients do well on prednisone while others do not.

  Patients take prednisone by mouth every morning, starting with a high dose for the first 4 to 8 weeks. As they improve, they gradually take smaller amounts. Changes in mood are one of the more common side effects of prednisone; most patients, however, can handle the mood changes—anxiety, depression, or sleeplessness—once they know what is causing the problem. A less common side effect is a rise in blood-sugar levels.

- **Cytoxan-Cyclophosphamide**—Also referred to as cytoxan, may be taken together with prednisone, or instead of it. Like prednisone, cytoxan is swallowed each day.

  One of the more serious side effects of cyclophosphamide is leukopenia, a condition in which the number of white blood cells drops to a dangerously low level. Leukopenia can be controlled by regularly checking the blood count and adjusting the dose of cytoxan if necessary.

- **Other Medicines**—Azathioprine, penicillamine, chlorambucil, vincristine sulfate, and colchicine have been used in a few patients with idiopathic pulmonary fibrosis. Their effectiveness in treating IPF, however, has not been adequately tested.

- **Oxygen**—In addition to treatment with medicine, some patients may need oxygen, especially when blood oxygen becomes low. This treatment helps resupply the blood with oxygen. As a result, breathlessness is reduced, the patient can be more active, and the severity of pulmonary hypertension decreases.

- **Exercise**—Regular exercise may be useful for patients with IPF. A daily walk or regular use of a stationary bicycle or treadmill can improve muscle strength and breathing ability and also increase overall strength. If needed, supplemental oxygen should be used; sometimes it is the only way a patient is able to do a reasonable amount of activity.

- **Lung transplantation**—Either of both lungs or only one, is an alternative to drug treatment for patients in the severe, final stages of IPF. It is most often performed in patients under 60 years of age who do not respond to any other form of treatment. The 1-year survival rate is approximately 60 percent.

### How Will IPF Affect a Patient's Lifestyle?

Many IPF patients, particularly those in the early stages of the disease, respond to drug treatment and can continue to go about most of their normal activities, including working. Some patients with advanced IPF need to carry oxygen with them.

In addition to getting proper treatment, IPF patients can help themselves by following the same sensible health measures that everyone should observe. These include eating a healthy diet, maintaining proper weight, exercising regularly, and getting enough rest. Above all, IPF patients should not smoke. Pregnancy is not advised because the illness puts an extra load on the heart and lungs.

As with many chronic illnesses, emotional support and psychological counseling can be of much help to the patient. Most doctors and patients agree that it is important for both patient and family to be as informed as possible about IPF. In this way, everyone involved can understand the illness and apply that information to what is happening in his or her own life.

### Can a Patient Participate in the IPF Research Programs at the National Institutes of Health (NIH)?

Some people with idiopathic pulmonary fibrosis may be eligible to participate in an experimental clinical trial at the Warren Grant Magnuson Clinical Center of the National Institutes of Health in Bethesda, Maryland. Participants must meet the specific requirements of the study. For more information on these trials, the patient's doctor should contact:

NIH Patient Referral Service
(301) 496-4891

*Or the doctor may write to:*

National Heart, Lung, and Blood Institute
Pulmonary Branch
Building 10, Room 6D03
9000 Rockville Pike
Bethesda. MD 20892

*For Additional Information, Contact:*

American Lung Association
(Contact your local chapter listed in the phone book.)

Chapter 9

# Respiratory Distress Syndrome (RDS)—Infants

*Chapter Contents*

Section 9. 1—Preterm Babies Get a Double Breath of Life ........ 422
Section 9. 2—Antiviral Drug Benefits Infants with Severe
 Respiratory Disease ................................................. 428
Section 9. 3—Calf Extract Benefits Premature Infants.............. 431

## Section 9.1

# Preterm Babies Get a Double Breath of Life

Source: *FDA Consumer*, April 1992.

When Benjamin McClatchey was born almost three months premature on July 27, 1990, he weighed only 2 pounds, 13 ounces, and his underdeveloped lungs struggled for every breath.

Benjamin's parents, Steve and Trillis McClatchey of Lafayette, Ind., got only a glimpse of their son before doctors whisked him off to another hospital an hour away. They called Trillis McClatchey at 5 o'clock the next morning for her permission to give Benjamin a pulmonary surfactant, a new lifesaving drug, to help him breathe.

"[They] told us it worked best if given in the first six hours of life," McClatchey remembers. "I said, 'He was born at 11:10 last night—you have 10 minutes!'

The doctor laughed. He said, 'Everything's going to be fine.'"

Benjamin received the drug and is indeed fine today. But at birth he developed respiratory distress syndrome, or RDS, a life-threatening lung condition that strikes about 65,000 infants each year. RDS has become more treatable in recent years because of surfactant and new ventilators recently approved by FDA.

RDS is common among the approximately 380,000 premature infants born in the United States each year. About 3,000 infants died of RDS in 1988, making it the fourth most common cause of all infant deaths.

RDS is also called hyaline membrane disease. In 1963, a baby boy born to then President and Mrs. John F. Kennedy died of the condition.

But neonatal medicine has improved since then, reducing deaths from RDS steadily over the last 15 years. Preliminary statistics indicate they may have fallen even further—more than 30 percent between 1987 and 1990. FDA's recent approval of several new ventilators and two kinds of surfactant to treat RDS has contributed to premature infants' chances of survival.

## Respiratory Distress Syndrome (RDS)—Infants

### Lubricating Lungs

Short for "surface-active agent," a pulmonary surfactant is perhaps the most beneficial new treatment RDS patients like Benjamin can receive. FDA has approved two kinds of surfactant, the first in July 1990 and the second a year later.

A pulmonary surfactant is a foamy liquid produced naturally in human and animal lungs. It reduces the surface tension between the wet lung tissue and dry air to keep the tiny air sacs in the lungs, called alveoli, from collapsing between breaths.

Without lung surfactant, every breath requires tremendous force, like blowing up a new balloon.

Because surfactant production is one of the last processes a fetus develops in the womb, preterm infants often don't have it. Commercially prepared surfactants replace the missing natural lung surfactant until the infant can produce his or her own a few days after birth.

"Surfactant has made a dramatic difference in the survival of very low birth-weight infants," says Dr. K.N. Siva Subramanian, the chief of the Division of Neonatology at Georgetown University Hospital in Washington, D.C.

Georgetown has been using a surfactant in clinical trials for more than three years, and doctors say babies who get it require less intensive medical care and less time on ventilators because of it.

The first FDA-approved surfactant was Exosurf Pediatric, a synthetic compound made by Burroughs Wellcome Co. of Research Triangle Park, N.C. The second approved surfactant, Survanta, is a compound made from cow lungs. It was developed in Japan and is distributed by Ross Laboratories of Columbus, Ohio.

Both drugs are passed down the infants' lungs through a ventilator tube. They can be given as "rescue" treatments to babies who have already developed RDS, or "prophylactic" (preventive) treatments to infants at risk of developing RDS.

In either case, studies show that surfactants reduce RDS deaths by about half. They also shorten the time infants need to be on ventilators.

Pulmonary surfactant has been a lifesaver to children born unexpectedly early. It has also given hope to parents who know their unborn children are at high risk for prematurity.

For example, in 1990, Leslie and Matthew Carter of Carmel, Ind., chose to have their children at the Indiana University Medical Center in part because they knew the hospital had surfactant.

Leslie Carter was carrying quadruplets, and she knew she would probably deliver early, as is often the case with multiple births.

Surfactants were not approved for general use at the time, but the Indiana hospital had one through an FDA treatment program that allows lifesaving drugs to be used in certain hospitals before they receive approval.

"We were aware of the drug called surfactant," Leslie Carter remembers, "and we were really glad to be in a hospital where they could use that."

Katelin, Katherine, Abigail, and Elizabeth Carter were born nearly 10 weeks early on Jan. 30, 1990, weighing less than 3 pounds each. They all developed respiratory distress syndrome, were treated with a surfactant, and placed on ventilators. At first their progress was slow, but after about two months in the hospital, all were home and doing well.

"We've been very fortunate," their mother says. "They're really healthy."

The Indiana University Medical Center has participated in clinical trials of both approved pulmonary surfactants for about four years, according to associate professor of pediatrics William A. Engle, M.D., who treated the Carter quadruplets and Benjamin McClatchey.

He says his colleagues have used both kinds, with promising results.

"I think the major benefit of surfactant is that it reduces the risks associated with respiratory distress syndrome," Engle says, "and we know that about 50 percent of the babies less than 1,500 grams [3.3 pounds] will have severe hyaline membrane disease."

### Bellows for Baby

A surfactant is no miracle cure for respiratory distress syndrome, however. Like Benjamin McClatchey and the Carter quadruplets, infants born too early may still spend months hooked to ventilators to help them breathe.

The newest kind of respirator for newborns is called a "high-frequency ventilator," which works very differently from the older, conventional ventilators.

Conventional ventilators have been used on infants for years and are largely responsible for the drastic drop in infant deaths from RDS throughout the 1970s. The high-frequency concept, a modification of conventional ventilation, was first described in 1959 but wasn't tested on infants until the early 1980s or approved by FDA until 1987.

Conventional ventilators force air down an infant's lungs with pressures high enough to expand them, sometimes damaging the delicate airways in the process.

A high-frequency ventilator, however, supplies oxygen to the baby through tiny, rapid puffs of air that barely move the lungs. It creates a vibrating column of air in the lungs without forcing them to expand in the traditional manner.

While a conventional ventilator "breathes" only about 14 times per minute, a high-frequency ventilator puffs at least 150 times per minute.

It's still not scientifically proven, however, whether high-frequency ventilators are better in the long run than the older machines for all premature infants. Doctors use them mostly when conventional ventilation isn't successful.

Since 1987, FDA has approved for use on infants three high-frequency ventilators made by Bunnell Inc. of Salt Lake City, UT, Infrasonics Inc. of San Diego, CA, and SensorMedics Corp. of Yorba Linda, CA.

Despite the benefits of both surfactants and high-frequency ventilators, problems remain.

Neither the surfactant drugs nor the high-frequency ventilators seem to reduce the incidence of a chronic lung condition stemming from long-term ventilator use called bronchopulmonary dysplasia, or BPD.

"That's kind of disappointing," says Dorothy Gail, Ph.D., chief of the Cell and Developmental Biology Branch at the National Heart, Lung, and Blood Institute. "Surfactant's great for RDS, but as far as the more chronic lung diseases go, it's not what everyone had hoped."

Benjamin McClatchey, for example, developed BPD. He still requires oxygen fed to his nose from a portable tank at home.

Babies on high-frequency ventilators develop other common side effects found with conventional ventilation, such as high blood pressure, a rise in heart rate, brain hemorrhaging, and a condition called pneumothorax, in which air blows out the side of the lungs and into the chest cavity.

"High-frequency ventilation is just not natural, so the body perceives it as something different and reacts to it," says Jim Dillard, a review scientist at FDA. "Over time, more light will be shed on the overall survival improvements with high frequency ventilators, if any."

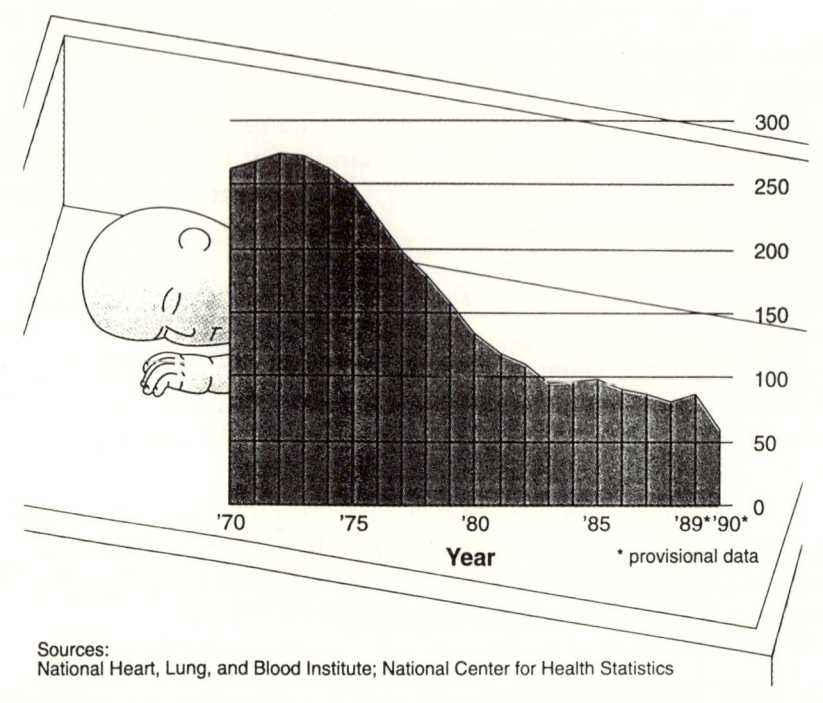

**Figure 9.1.** *Infant mortality from neonatal RDS per 100,000 live births in the United States, 1970-1990*

At Indiana University's Riley Hospital for Children, where Benjamin and the Carter quadruplets were treated, doctors use high-frequency ventilators in the severest cases.

Two of the Carters' daughters developed more serious lung problems, and one of them, Abigail, was placed on a Bunnell high-frequency ventilator. The other, Katelin, had similar problems but was placed on a conventional ventilator.

"Abigail's lungs healed a lot better and she did a lot better than Katelin did. And their problems were very, very similar," Carter says. "We felt the [high-frequency ventilator] really helped."

"I think it's been moderately successful," says Engle, of the Riley Hospital program. "Babies that would have had less than a 20 percent chance of survival [on conventional ventilation] now have a 50 to 60 percent chance."

## Looking for Tomorrow's Cures

In the future, scientists hope to provide even better chances for premature infants like Benjamin and the Carter quadruplets.

Last October, a scientist from The Scripps Research Institute in La Jolla, CA, described in the journal *Science* a new kind of surfactant he manufactured with synthetic human proteins. He said the synthetic human surfactant, if successful in humans, could be more like human surfactant than those presently on the market. It has not been tested in humans to show effectiveness and safety, however, one requirement for FDA approval.

According to the National Heart, Lung, and Blood Institute, scientists are examining human surfactant in a number of studies, researching its basic genetic makeup and how it is produced and used by lungs.

In clinical settings, doctors are still testing for the best possible dose and time to give a surfactant to newborns, as well as ways to use the drug to treat adult lung disorders.

For many premature children, new technologies have already eased their untimely transitions from the womb to the world.

The Carter quadruplets, for example, are still not as physically mature as other 2-year-olds, but in other ways they have developed normally. "They're doing just wonderfully," their mother says.

Benjamin McClatchey also is doing well. Now nearly 2 years old, he talks as well as any child his age, even though he too, is catching up to his peers physically.

"I don't let that get me down," says his mother. "He spent a total of seven months in the hospital out of his first 10 months of life, and a baby can't develop in a hospital bed."

"But he's made a lot of progress since we've had him home. He's doing just great."

*—Rebecca D. Williams is a staff writer for* FDA Consumer.

## Section 9.2

## Antiviral Drug Benefits Infants with Severe Respiratory Disease

Source: *Research Resources Reporter*, June 1992.

Infants receiving the antiviral medication ribavirin as treatment for a common and often dangerous respiratory disease caused by respiratory syncytial virus (RSV) require less time on ventilators and have shorter hospital stays than do infants who do not receive the drug, according to researchers at Stanford University School of Medicine in California.

Dr. David W. Smith, former associate professor of pediatrics at Stanford, and his colleagues studied 28 infants with RSV infections severe enough to necessitate mechanical ventilation, breathing assistance. They found that the average ventilation time for infants receiving ribavirin was half of the ventilation time for those on placebo. The study is the first to demonstrate that ribavirin can reduce the length of hospitalization and the need for supportive therapy among infants with the most severe cases of RSV disease, the researchers say.

Dr. Smith, now associate director of the pediatric intensive care unit at Sutter Memorial Hospital in Sacramento, California, notes that RSV infection represents the major winter respiratory disease affecting infants and young children. The virus often attacks the lower respiratory tract, causing bronchiolitis, an inflammation of the small airways of the lungs.

"It's a serious problem for intensive care units and resources, both in terms of space and staff," Dr. Smith explains.

"By age 2 or 3, almost every child will have contracted an RSV infection," says coinvestigator Dr. Charles G. Prober, professor of pediatrics, medicine, microbiology, and immunology at Stanford. "Only a small percentage of these children require hospitalization, but RSV can cause significant morbidity and even mortality in certain high-risk groups or in very young infants." According to Dr. Prober, about 10 percent of infants hospitalized for RSV end up in the intensive care unit, where many need mechanical ventilation.

The researchers point out that although previous studies had shown ribavirin to be effective for RSV infected infants who were able

## Respiratory Distress Syndrome (RDS)—Infants

to breathe spontaneously, there had been no placebo-controlled study of the drug's efficacy in ventilated patients. "With the two principal questions of safety and efficacy in mind, we decided to pursue a clinical investigation of the treatment of infants with the most severe infection—those requiring mechanical ventilation," says Dr. Smith.

Some researchers have questioned the safety of administering ribavirin to mechanically ventilated infants. The drug is delivered to the lungs as an aerosol mist; reportedly it can crystallize within the respiratory equipment and impair the air supply to the patient.

To overcome this problem Dr. Smith and Dr. Lorry R. Frankel, director of pediatric critical care services at Lucile Salter Packard Children's Hospital at Stanford, worked with respiratory therapists to develop a safe system for delivering aerosolized ribavirin to infants on assisted ventilation. The researchers prevented crystallization of the drug by placing heated wires in the ventilator tubing and by frequently inspecting the apparatus and changing the filters.

Using this delivery system the researchers administered aerosolized ribavirin to 14 RSV-infected infants for 7 days; an equal number of control infants received a placebo of sterile aerosolized water. The infants given ribavirin required mechanical ventilation for an average of only 5 days, compared to 10 days for control infants, the researchers report. Time on supplemental oxygen also declined by an average of about 5 days for infants treated with ribavirin.

Slightly greater differences between the ribavirin and control groups appeared when the researchers considered only those infants who were healthy before they contracted RSV. Three infants treated with ribavirin and four in the placebo group had previous underlying conditions, primarily heart and lung disorders. Previously normal infants treated with ribavirin had an average hospital stay of 9 days, as opposed to 15 for the placebo group. When infants with underlying conditions were included in the comparison, however, the difference in average hospital stay was less than 2 days.

"The evidence indicates the drug is effective for mechanically ventilated children who were normal prior to RSV infection," says Dr. Smith, "and I believe it should be used for those patients." He emphasizes, however, that more work needs to be done to determine the drug's efficacy in children with chronic underlying diseases. "Very few infants with such underlying problems have been studied," he says.

The shorter hospital stay and mechanical ventilation time for ribavirin treated infants with no underlying disease translates into substantial savings in hospital bills, the researchers point out. "The intensive care unit is an expensive place to live," notes Dr. Prober.

Ribavirin is expensive—approximately $600 per day, according to Dr. Prober—but the researchers say the money saved on intensive care far outweighs the cost of the drug. "It's just not cost effective to keep somebody in an intensive care unit bed for 10 days when you can get them out in 5 or 6," explains Dr. Frankel.

Although the investigators feel that ribavirin should be administered to previously normal infants placed on mechanical ventilation, they refrain from broader recommendations. "I do not think every infant with an RSV infection should be treated with ribavirin," says Dr. Prober. "We focused our study on ventilated patients. For children who are not on mechanical ventilation, or who are not at high risk of ultimately needing mechanical ventilation, use of ribavirin is much more controversial and unclear."

Dr. Frankel notes that the care of patients with RSV has improved in recent years, and mortality has dropped. "Many physicians believe the disease is self-limiting," he says. "They question the validity of exposing children with less severe cases to this expensive antiviral drug."

Dr. Smith will soon begin a study at Sutter Memorial Hospital to test ribavirin's effectiveness on RSV patients with underlying heart and lung problems. "It's tempting to say that because ribavirin works in previously normal infants, it should also work in infants with underlying diseases, but that's not a fair conclusion," says Dr. Smith. "Infants with underlying diseases probably react very differently to the effects of the infection.

"Another principal question that needs to be answered is: What happens to these children after their RSV infection?" Dr. Smith points out that infants with severe RSV bronchiolitis run a greater risk of developing asthma in early childhood. "It remains to be seen whether ribavirin will in fact make these children less vulnerable to such health problems later on," he says. "Long-term follow-up of children who receive ribavirin will be necessary to sort out this question."

Since the study the researchers have continued to administer aerosolized ribavirin to mechanically ventilated infants with RSV infection. "We have continued to deliver the drug with no substantial problems at all," Dr. Smith reports. "My impression is that the efficacy of the drug is consistent, and the children require mechanical ventilation for about the same period of time as in the study."

# Respiratory Distress Syndrome (RDS)—Infants

"I think ribavirin will be used more often in the future to treat infants with severe RSV infection," says Dr. Prober. Financial considerations and the need for skillful administration of the drug represent the primary barriers to its use, he says.

*The research described in this chapter was supported by the General Clinical Research Centers Program of the National Center for Research Resources, the Stanford University Medical Center Technology Transfer Program, and the National Institute of Allergy and Infectious Diseases.*

—Scott J. Brown

## Section 9.3

## *Calf Extract Benefits Premature Infants*

Source: *Research Resources Reporter*, January 1992.

Calf-derived surfactant—a substance that helps the lungs expand smoothly during breathing—introduced into the lungs of premature infants immediately at birth improved survival rates despite the continuing risk of a life-threatening lung disorder known as hyaline membrane disease. The immediate, or "prophylactic," treatment was superior to calf surfactant "rescue therapy" given several hours later, according to investigators who evaluated 479 premature babies born at three New York medical centers.

Dr. James W. Kendig, associate professor of pediatrics at the University of Rochester School of Medicine in New York and a principal investigator in the randomized clinical study, says that 88 percent of the premature infants given surfactant prophylactically at delivery survived and were discharged to go home without ventilatory assistance. This was in contrast to 80 percent survival of infants whose calf surfactant treatment began several hours later, when x-ray films and monitoring devices showed signs of moderate-to-severe respiratory distress, he says. The survival advantage of the prophylactic approach was particularly striking in a subgroup of infants whose gestational age was estimated to be 26 weeks or less, Dr. Kendig says.

Hyaline membrane disease (HMD), often called respiratory distress syndrome, is a disorder in which the alveoli, or air sacs, tend to collapse because the premature infant's lungs are not producing enough surfactant.

Dr. Kendig explains that the surfactant is a complex combination of fats and proteins that coats the surface of the alveoli and lowers their surface tension, facilitating expansion and deflation during breathing.

For premature infants deficient in surfactant, various approaches to surfactant replacement therapy have been studied during the past 15 years, Dr. Kendig says. Preparations of human, bovine, swine, and synthetic surfactant have been administered in a variety of dosage schedules in efforts to lubricate the "stiff" lungs of these babies and to ease their labored breathing. In addition to surfactant treatment of the newborn, glucocorticoid drugs such as betamethasone may be administered to the mother a few days before delivery to enhance maturation of the fetal lungs and their production of surfactant.

Dr. Kendig and coinvestigators at Albany Medical College and the Westchester Medical Center of New York Medical College in Valhalla administered a calf lung surfactant extract to the newborns via a small plastic tube inserted through the mouth to the trachea. All the premature infants in the study also received supplementary oxygen. One criterion for an infant to receive surfactant therapy in the rescue arm of the study was a requirement for at least 40 percent oxygen—a relatively high level considering that ordinary room air consists of 21 percent oxygen, Dr. Kendig says. He estimates that despite oxygen therapy, without supplementary surfactant the infant mortality would probably reach about 30 percent.

By random assignment, 235 of the infants received the prophylactic dose of surfactant at the time of delivery; the other 244 infants were initially treated 4 to 6 hours after delivery at the same dose level if chest x-ray evaluation and either oxygen requirements or ventilator pressures indicated clinically severe disease. Infants in both groups received additional doses of surfactant at 12 to 24-hour intervals as required.

The higher survival rate of the infants whose initial dose of surfactant was given prophylactically, Dr. Kendig says, was due primarily to the longer survival of the most premature infants—those of 26 weeks gestation or less. Seventy-five percent of those very premature

## Respiratory Distress Syndrome (RDS)—Infants

infants receiving prophylaxis survived, in contrast to 54 percent of rescue therapy recipients. Pneumothorax, a disastrous accumulation of air in the pleural space surrounding the lungs that often leads to total lung collapse and death, occurred in 7 percent of the very premature infants in the prophylaxis group and in 18 percent of those receiving rescue therapy.

"We saw an inverse correlation between the number of weeks of gestation and the differential survival advantage to the newborn," Dr. Kendig says. As gestation time increased, the benefits of prophylaxis lessened with each successive week, gradually leveling off at about the 30th week. The usual length of gestation is 40 weeks.

"No evidence of an immune reaction against the calf preparation has been seen," Dr. Kendig says. "Immune complexes related to the bovine surfactant have not been detected. Children now aged 7 and 8 who received the calf preparation as premature infants have had no higher incidence of allergies and immunologic problems than average children."

The Rochester neonatologist says that the calf preparation contains phospholipid as well as two components called surfactant proteins B and C that are essential to spreading surfactant throughout the alveoli. "Phospholipid alone won't move the surfactant through the lungs," he says. "Fortunately, the process we use to extract surfactant from bovine lungs retains both of those important proteins, and they remain throughout its production."

One disadvantage of administering calf surfactant prophylactically to all premature babies is that 30 to 40 percent of those receiving it do not need it, according to Dr. Kendig. "They would not all develop HMD but we cannot identify which infants would," he says. "However, we do not know of any harmful side effects of our surfactant instillation."

Other sources of replacement surfactant, particularly natural human amniotic fluid, require a great deal of time and effort to obtain, Dr. Kendig says. He notes that a completely synthetic compound, with organic chemicals substituted for the proteins B and C, has been approved by the U.S. Food and Drug Administration. "Also on the horizon is the possibility—or probability—of a genetically engineered surfactant within the next 10 years," he adds. "The genes for human surfactant proteins B and C have already been cloned. I think there will eventually be a biosynthetic surfactant consisting of lipids plus the human cloned-gene-derived proteins."

To improve on their current calf surfactant regimen, Dr. Kendig and his colleagues are exploring an alternative schedule of administering surfactant prophylactically. "We delay its administration 5 to 10 minutes until the infant's ventilatory tubing is in place, and we have monitored the heart rate. By the time breath sounds tell us that the ventilatory tube is in the right position, the baby's color usually has improved, and we go on to instill the surfactant. We are now conducting a randomized trial to compare immediate prophylactic surfactant therapy and the poststabilization surfactant administration," he says.

*Dr. Kendig acknowledges the research contributions of Dr. Robert H. Notter and the late Dr. Donald L. Shapiro. The research described in this chapter was supported by the General Clinical Research Centers Program of the National Center for Research Resources and by a Specialized Center of Research (SCOR) grant from the National Heart, Lung and Blood Institute.*

—Jane Collins

Chapter 10

# *Sarcoidosis*

Sarcoidosis is a disease due to inflammation. It can appear in almost any body organ, but most often starts in the lungs or lymph nodes.

No one yet knows what causes sarcoidosis. The disease can appear suddenly and disappear. Or it can develop gradually and go on to produce symptoms that come and go, sometimes for a lifetime.

As sarcoidosis progresses, small lumps, or granulomas, appear in the affected tissues. In the majority of cases, these granulomas clear up, either with or without treatment.

In the few cases where the granulomas do not heal and disappear, the tissues tend to remain inflamed and become scarred (fibrotic).

Sarcoidosis was first identified over 100 years ago by two dermatologists working independently, Dr. Jonathan Hutchinson in England and Dr. Caesar Boeck in Norway. Sarcoidosis was originally called Hutchinson's disease or Boeck's disease. Dr. Boeck went on to fashion today's name for the disease from the Greek words "sark" and "oid," meaning flesh-like. The term describes the skin eruptions that are frequently caused by the illness.

---

NIH Pub. No. 91-3093. Nov. 1991.

## Usual Symptoms

Shortness of breath (dyspnea) and a cough that won't go away can be among the first symptoms of sarcoidosis. But sarcoidosis can also show up suddenly with the appearance of skin rashes. Red bumps (erythema nodosum) on the face, arms, or shins, and inflammation of the eyes are also common symptoms. It is not unusual, however, for sarcoidosis symptoms to be more general. Weight loss, fatigue, night sweats, fever, or just an overall feeling of ill health can also be clues to the disease.

## Who Gets Sarcoidosis?

Sarcoidosis was once considered a rare disease. We now know that it is a common chronic illness that appears all over the world. Indeed, it is the most common of the fibrotic lung disorders, and occurs often enough in the United States for Congress to have declared a national Sarcoidosis Awareness Day in 1990.

Anyone can get sarcoidosis. It occurs in all races and in both sexes. Nevertheless, the risk is greater if you are a young black adult, especially a black woman, or of Scandinavian, German, Irish, or Puerto Rican origin. No one knows why.

Because sarcoidosis can escape diagnosis or be mistaken for several other diseases, we can only guess at how many people are affected. The best estimate today is that about 5 in 100,000 white people in the United States have sarcoidosis. Among black people, it occurs more frequently, in probably 40 out of 100,000 people.

Overall, there appear to be 20 cases per 100,000 in cities on the east coast and somewhat fewer in rural locations. Some scientists, however, believe that these figures greatly under-estimate the percentage of the U.S. population with sarcoidosis.

Sarcoidosis mainly affects people between 20 to 40 years of age. White women are just as likely as white men to get sarcoidosis, but the black female gets sarcoidosis two times as often as the black male.

Sarcoidosis also appears to be more common and more severe in certain geographic areas. It has long been recognized as a common disease in Scandinavian countries, where it is estimated to affect 64 out of 100,000 people. But it was not until the mid-1940's—when a large number of cases were identified during mass chest x-ray screening for the Armed Forces—that its high prevalence was recognized in North America

## What Sarcoidosis is Not

Much about sarcoidosis remains unknown. Nevertheless, if you have the disease, you can be reassured about several things.

Sarcoidosis is usually not crippling. It often goes away by itself, with most cases healing in 24 to 36 months. Even when sarcoidosis lasts longer, most patients can go about their lives as usual.

Sarcoidosis is not a cancer. It is not contagious, and your friends and family will not catch it from you. Although it can occur in families, there is no evidence that sarcoidosis is passed from parents to children.

## Some Things We Don't Know About Sarcoidosis

Sarcoidosis is currently thought to be associated with an abnormal immune response. Whether a foreign substance is the trigger; whether that trigger is a chemical, drug, virus, or some other substance; and how exactly the immune disturbance is caused are not known.

Researchers supported by the National Heart, Lung, and Blood Institute are trying to solve some of these mysteries. Among the research questions they are trying to answer are:

- Does sarcoidosis have many causes, or is it produced by a single agent?

- In which body organ does sarcoidosis actually start?

- How does sarcoidosis spread from one part of the body to another?

- Do heredity, environment, and lifestyle play any role in the appearance, severity, or length of the disease?

- Is the abnormal immune response seen in patients a cause or an effect of the disease?

- How can sarcoidosis be prevented?

## Course of the Disease

In general, sarcoidosis appears briefly and heals naturally in 60 to 70 percent of the cases, often without the patient knowing or doing anything about it. From 20 to 30 percent of sarcoidosis patients are left with some permanent lung damage. In 10 to 15 percent of the patients, sarcoidosis can become chronic.

When either the granulomas or fibrosis seriously affect the function of a vital organ—the lungs, heart, nervous system, liver, or kidneys, for example—sarcoidosis can be fatal. This occurs 5 to 10 percent of the time.

No one can predict how sarcoidosis will progress in an individual patient. But the symptoms the patient experiences the doctor's findings, and the patient's race can give some clues.

For example, a sudden onset of general symptoms such as weight loss or feeling poorly are usually taken to mean that the course of sarcoidosis will be relatively short and mild. Dyspnea and possibly skin sarcoidosis often indicate that the sarcoidosis will be more chronic and severe.

White patients are more likely to develop the milder form of the disease. Black people tend to develop the more chronic and severe form.

Sarcoidosis rarely develops before the age of 10 or after the age of 60. However, the illness—with or without symptoms—has been reported in younger as well as in older people. When symptoms do appear in these age groups, the symptoms are those that are more general in nature, for example, tiredness, sluggishness, coughing, and a general feeling of ill health.

## Diagnosis

Preliminary diagnosis of sarcoidosis is based on the patient's medical history, routine tests, a physical examination, and a chest x-ray.

The doctor confirms the diagnosis of sarcoidosis by eliminating other diseases with similar features. These include such granulomatous diseases as berylliosis (a disease resulting from exposure to beryllium metal), tuberculosis, farmer's lung disease (hypersensitivity pneumonitis), fungal infections, rheumatoid arthritis, rheumatic fever, and cancer of the lymph nodes (lymphoma).

## Signs and Symptoms

In addition to the lungs and lymph nodes, the body organs more likely than others to be affected by sarcoidosis are the liver, skin, heart, nervous system, and kidneys, in that order of frequency. Patients can have symptoms related to the specific organ affected, they can have only general symptoms, or they can be without any symptoms whatsoever. Symptoms also can vary according to how long the illness has been under way, where the granulomas are forming, how much tissue has become affected, and whether the granulomatous process is still active.

Even when there are no symptoms, a doctor can sometimes pick up signs of sarcoidosis during a routine examination, usually a chest x-ray, or when checking out another complaint. The patient's age and race or ethnic group can raise an additional red flag that a sign or symptom of illness could be related to sarcoidosis. Enlargement of the salivary or tear glands and cysts in bone tissue are also among sarcoidosis signals.

**Lungs.** The lungs are usually the first site involved in sarcoidosis. Indeed, about 9 out of 10 sarcoidosis patients have some type of lung problem, with nearly one-third of these patients showing some respiratory symptoms—usually coughing, either dry or with phlegm, and dyspnea. Occasionally, patients have chest pain and a feeling of tightness in the chest.

It is thought that sarcoidosis of the lungs begins with alveolitis (inflammation of the alveoli), the tiny sac-like air spaces in the lungs where carbon dioxide and oxygen are exchanged. Alveolitis either clears up spontaneously or leads to granuloma formation. Eventually fibrosis can form, causing the lung to stiffen and making breathing even more difficult.

**Eyes.** Eye disease occurs in about 20 to 30 percent of patients with sarcoidosis, particularly in children who get the disease. Almost any part of the eye can be affected—the membranes of the eyelids, cornea, outer coat of the eyeball (sclera), retina, and lens. The eye involvement can start with no symptoms at all or with reddening or watery eyes. In a few cases, cataracts, glaucoma, and blindness can result.

**Skin.** The skin is affected in about 20 percent of sarcoidosis patients. Skin sarcoidosis is usually marked by small, raised patches on the face. Occasionally the patches are purplish in color and larger. Patches can also appear on limbs, face, and buttocks.

Other symptoms include erythema nodosum, mostly on the legs and often accompanied by arthritis in the ankles, elbows, wrists, and hands. Erythema nodosum usually goes away, but other skin problems can persist.

**Nervous system.** In an occasional case (1 to 5 percent), sarcoidosis can lead to neurological problems. For example, sarcoid granulomas can appear in the brain, spinal cord, and facial and optic nerves. Facial paralysis and other symptoms of nerve damage call for prompt treatment.

## Laboratory Tests

No single test can be relied on for a correct diagnosis of sarcoidosis. X-rays and blood tests are usually the first procedures the doctor will order. Pulmonary function tests often provide clues to diagnosis. Other tests may also be used, some more often than others. Many of the tests that the doctor calls on to help diagnose sarcoidosis can also help the doctor follow the progress of the disease and determine whether the sarcoidosis is getting better or worse.

**Chest x-ray.** A picture of the lungs, heart, as well as the surrounding tissues containing lymph nodes, where infection-fighting white blood cells form, can give the first indication of sarcoidosis. For example, a swelling of the lymph glands between the two lungs can show up on an x-ray. An x-ray can also show which areas of the lung are affected.

**Pulmonary function tests.** By performing a variety of tests called pulmonary function tests (PFT), the doctor can find out how well the lungs are doing their job of expanding and exchanging oxygen and carbon dioxide with the blood. The lungs of sarcoidosis patients cannot handle these tasks as well as they should; this is because granulomas and fibrosis of lung tissue decrease lung capacity and disturb the normal flow of gases between the lungs and the blood.

One PFT procedure calls for the patient to breathe into a machine, called a spirometer. It is a mechanical device that records changes in the lung size as air is inhaled and exhaled, as well as the time it takes the patient to do this.

**Blood tests.** Blood analyses can evaluate the number and types of blood cells in the body and how well the cells are functioning. They can also measure the levels of various blood proteins known to be involved in immunological activities, and they can show increases in serum calcium levels and abnormal liver function that often accompany sarcoidosis.

Blood tests can measure a blood substance called angiotensin-converting enzyme (ACE). Because the cells that make up granulomas secrete large amounts of ACE, the enzyme levels are often high in patients with sarcoidosis. ACE levels, however, are not always high in sarcoidosis patients, and increased ACE levels can also show up in other illnesses.

**Bronchoalveolar lavage.** This test uses an instrument called a bronchoscope—a long, narrow tube with a light at the end—to wash out, or lavage, cells and other materials from inside the lungs. This wash fluid is then examined for the amount of various cells and other substances that reflect inflammation and immune activity in the lungs. A high number of white blood cells in this fluid usually indicates an inflammation in the lungs.

**Biopsy.** Microscopic examination of specimens of lung tissue obtained with a bronchoscope, or of specimens of other tissues, can tell a doctor where granulomas have formed in the body.

**Gallium scanning.** In this procedure, the doctor injects the radioactive chemical element gallium-67 into the patient's vein. The gallium collects at places in the body affected by sarcoidosis and other inflammatory conditions. Two days after the injection, the body is scanned for radioactivity.

Increases in gallium uptake at any site in the body indicate that inflammatory activity has developed at the site and also give an idea of which tissue, and how much tissue, has been affected. However, since any type of inflammation causes gallium uptake, a positive gallium scan does not necessarily mean that the patient has sarcoidosis.

**Kveim test.** This test involves injecting a standardized preparation of sarcoid tissue material into the skin. On the one hand, a unique lump formed at the point of injection is considered positive for sarcoidosis. On the other hand, the test result is not always positive even if the patient has sarcoidosis.

The Kveim test is not used often in the United States because no test material has been approved for sale by the U.S. Food and Drug Administration. However, a few hospitals and clinics may have some standardized test preparation prepared privately for their own use.

**Slit-lamp examination.** An instrument called a slit lamp, which permits examination of the inside of the eye, can be used to detect silent damage from sarcoidosis.

## Management

Fortunately, many patients with sarcoidosis require no treatment. Symptoms, after all, are usually not disabling and do tend to disappear spontaneously.

When therapy is recommended, the main goal is to keep the lungs and other affected body organs working and to relieve symptoms. The disease is considered inactive once the symptoms fade. After many years of experience with treating the disease, corticosteroids remain the primary treatment for inflammation and granuloma formation. Prednisone is probably the corticosteroid most often prescribed today. There is no treatment at present to reverse the fibrosis that might be present in advanced sarcoidosis.

Occasionally, a blood test will show a high blood level of calcium accompanying sarcoidosis. The reasons for this are not clear. Some scientists believe that this condition is not common. When it does occur, the patient may be advised to avoid calcium-rich foods, vitamin D, or sunlight, or to take prednisone; this corticosteroid quickly reverses the condition.

Because sarcoidosis can disappear even without therapy, doctors sometimes disagree on when to start the treatment, what dose to prescribe, and how long to continue the medicine. The doctor's decision depends on the organ system involved and how far the inflammation has progressed. If the disease appears to be severe—especially in the lungs, eyes, heart, nervous system, spleen, or kidneys—the doctor may prescribe corticosteroids . Corticosteroid treatment usually results in improvement. Symptoms often start up again, however, when it is stopped. Treatment, therefore, may be necessary for several years, sometimes for as long as the disease remains active or to prevent relapse.

Frequent checkups are important so that the doctor can monitor the illness and, if necessary, adjust the treatment. Corticosteroids for example can have side effects—mood swings, swelling, and weight gain because the treatment tends to make the body hold on to water; high blood pressure; high blood sugar; and craving for food. Long-term use can affect the stomach, skin, and bones. This situation can bring on stomach pain, an ulcer, or acne, or cause the loss of calcium from bones. However, if the corticosteroid is taken in carefully prescribed, low doses, the benefits from the treatment are usually far greater than the problems.

Besides corticosteroids, various other drugs have been tried, but their effectiveness has not been established in controlled studies. These drugs include chloroquine and D-penicillamine.

Several drugs such as chlorambucil, azathioprine, methotrexate, and cyclophosphamide, which might suppress alveolitis by killing the cells that produce granulomas, have also been used. None have been evaluated in controlled clinical trials, and the risk of using these drugs is high, especially in pregnant women.

Cyclosporine, a drug used widely in organ transplants to suppress immune reaction, has been evaluated in one controlled trial. It was found to be unsuccessful.

## Research Status in Sarcoidosis: Goals of the National Heart, Lung, and Blood Institute

There are many unanswered questions about sarcoidosis. Identifying the agent that causes the illness, along with the inflammatory mechanisms that set the stage for the alveolitis, granuloma formation, and fibrosis that characterize the disease, is the major aim of the National Heart, Lung, and Blood Institute's program on sarcoidosis. Development of reliable methods of diagnosis, treatment, and, eventually, the prevention of sarcoidosis is the ultimate goal.

Originally, scientists thought that sarcoidosis was caused by an acquired state of immunological inertness (anergy). This notion was revised a few years ago, when the technique of bronchoalveolar lavage provided access to a vast array of cells and cell-derived mediators operating in the lungs of sarcoidosis patients. Sarcoidosis is now believed to be associated with a complex mix of immunological disturbances involving simultaneous activation, as well as depression, of certain immunological functions.

Immunological studies on sarcoidosis patients show that many of the immune functions associated with thymus-derived white blood cells, called T-lymphocytes or T-cells, are depressed. The depression of this cellular component of systemic immune response is expressed in the inability of the patients to evoke a delayed hypersensitivity skin reaction (a positive skin test), when tested by the appropriate foreign substance, or antigen, underneath the skin.

In addition, the blood of sarcoidosis patients contains a reduced number of T-cells. These T-cells do not seem capable of responding normally when treated with substances known to stimulate the growth of laboratory-cultured T-cells. Neither do they produce their normal complement of immunological mediators, cytokines, through which the cells modify the behavior of other cells.

In contrast to the depression of the cellular immune response, humoral immune response of sarcoidosis patients is elevated. The humoral immune response is reflected by the production of circulating antibodies against a variety of exogenous antigens, including common viruses. This humoral component of systemic immune response is mediated by another class of lymphocytes known as B-lymphocytes, or B-cells, because they originate in the bone marrow.

In another indication of heightened humoral response, sarcoidosis patients seem prone to develop autoantibodies (antibodies against endogenous antigens) similar to rheumatoid factors.

With access to the cells and cell products in the lung tissue compartments through the bronchoalveolar technique, it also has become possible for researchers to complement the above investigations at the blood level with analysis of local inflammatory and immune events in the lungs.

In contrast to what is seen at the systemic level, the cellular immune response in the lungs seems to be heightened rather than depressed. The heightened cellular immune response in the diseased tissue is characterized by significant increases in activated T-lymphocytes with certain characteristic cell-surface antigens, as well as in activated alveolar macrophages.

This pronounced, localized cellular response is also accompanied by the appearance in the lung of an array of mediators that are thought to contribute to the disease process; these include interleukin-1, interleukin-2, B-cell growth factor, B-cell differentiation factor, fibroblast growth factor, and fibronectin.

Because a number of lung diseases follow respiratory tract infections, ascertaining whether a virus can be implicated in the events leading to sarcoidosis remains an important area of research. Some recent observations seem to provide suggestive leads on this question. In these studies, the genes of cytomegalovirus (CMV), a common disease-causing virus, were introduced into lymphocytes, and the expression of the viral genes was studied. It was found that the viral genes were expressed both during acute infection of the cells and when the virus was not replicating in the cells. However, this expression seemed to take place only when the T-cells were activated by some injurious event.

In addition, the product of a CMV gene was found capable of activating the gene in alveolar macrophage responsible for the production of interleukin-1. Since interleukin-1 levels are found to increase in alveolar macrophages from patients with sarcoidosis, this suggests that certain viral genes can enhance the production of inflammatory components associated with sarcoidosis. Whether these findings implicate viral infections in the disease process in sarcoidosis is unclear. Future research with viral models may provide clues to the molecular mechanisms that trigger alterations in lymphocyte and macrophage regulation leading to sarcoidosis.

## *Living with Sarcoidosis*

The cause of sarcoidosis still remains unknown, so there is at present no known way to prevent or cure this disease. However, doctors have had a great deal of experience in management of the illness.

If you have sarcoidosis, you can help yourself by following sensible health measures. You should not smoke. You should also avoid exposure to other substances such as dusts and chemicals that can harm your lungs.

Patients with sarcoidosis are best treated by a lung specialist or a doctor who has a special interest in sarcoidosis. Sarcoidosis specialists are usually located at major research centers.

If you have any symptoms of sarcoidosis, see your doctor regularly so that the illness can be watched and, if necessary, treated. If it heals naturally, sarcoidosis is unlikely to recur. Nevertheless, if you have had sarcoidosis, or are suspected of having the illness but have no symptoms now, be sure to have physical checkups every year, including an eye examination.

Although severe sarcoidosis can reduce the chances of becoming pregnant, particularly for older women, many young women with sarcoidosis have given birth to healthy babies while on treatment. Patients planning to have a baby should discuss the matter with their doctor. Medical checkups all through pregnancy and immediately thereafter are especially important for sarcoidosis patients. In some cases, bed rest is necessary during the last 3 months of pregnancy. In addition to family and close friends, a number of local lung organizations, other nonprofit health organizations, and self-help groups are available to help patients cope with sarcoidosis. By keeping in touch with them, you can share personal feelings and experiences. Members also share specific information on the latest scientific advances, where to find sarcoidosis specialists, and how to improve one's self-image.

## More Information

Additional information on sarcoidosis is available from a number of sources.

For information on current sarcoidosis research, write to:

**National Heart, Lung, and Blood Institute Division of Lung Diseases**
5333 Westbard Avenue
Room 6A16
Bethesda, MD 20892

If you are interested in participating in NHLBI clinical studies of sarcoidosis, have your physician write to:

**National Heart, Lung, and Blood Institute Pulmonary Branch**
9000 Rockville Pike
Building 10, Room 6D06
Bethesda, MD 20892

Information and publications for sarcoidosis patients and their families are available from:

**National Institute of Allergy and Infectious Diseases**
9000 Rockville Pike
Building 31, Room 7A32
Bethesda. MD 20892

**Sarcoidosis Family Aid and Research Foundation**
460A Central Avenue East
Orange, NJ 07018

*Sarcoidosis*

Many local chapters of the American Lung Association host support groups for sarcoidosis patients. The address and telephone number of the chapter nearest to you should be in your local telephone directory. Or you can write or call the association's national headquarters:

**American Lung Association**
1740 Broadway
New York, NY 10019-4374
(212) 315-8700

Chapter 11

# Breathing Disorders During Sleep

*"You Can Snore Your Life Away."*

This sounds more like joke than a warning. But, in fact, habitual snoring is the most common symptom of a breathing disorders that occur during sleep.

The person who snores not only sleeps restlessly, but also is at risk for serious disorders of the heart and lungs. Snoring can therefore be life-threatening because it can lead to high blood-pressure, irregular heart beats, heart attacks, and sudden death.

Normal breathing must continue at all times whether awake or asleep. The act of breathing is an automatic, highly regulated mechanical function of the body. In healthy sleeping individuals, most muscular and neural activities will slow or even shut down but respiration goes on under a neuromuscular "auto pilot." However, if something goes wrong with the auto pilot during sleep, breathing may become erratic and inefficient.

## Understanding Sleep

Sleep is a complex neurological state. Its primary function is rest and restoring the body's energy levels. Repeated interruption of sleep

---

NIH Pub. No. 93-2966; *FDA Consumer* June 1992. "Sleep Lab" excerted from "Breathless No More: Defeating Adult Sleep Apnea," by Ricki Lewis, Ph.D.

by breathing abnormalities such as cessation of breathing (apnea) or heavy snoring, leads to fragmented sleep and abnormal oxygen and carbon dioxide levels in the blood. Excessive daytime sleepiness and various disorders of the heart, lungs, and the nervous system result.

In the 1950s scientists realized that sleep is not just a quiet state of rest. In fact, two stages of sleep occur with distinct physiological patterns—rapid-eye-movement sleep (REM), and non rapid-eye-movement sleep (NREM) or deep sleep. In normal sleep, REM occurs about 90 minutes after a person falls asleep. The two sleep stages recur in cycles of about 90 minutes each, with three non-REM stages (light to deep slumber) at the beginning and REM towards the end. The amount of sleep needed by each person is usually constant although there is a wide variation among individuals.

How sleep occurs and how it restores the body are not well understood. Scientists originally believed that sleep occurs because the brain lapses into a passive resting state from lack of stimulation. Another theory proposed that sleep occurs when the body generates and accumulates sufficient amounts of a "sleep-inducing substance." However, research now suggests that sleep results when specific changes in brain function occur. By studying the brain waves, scientists can define and measure various degrees, levels, and stages of sleep.

Sleep consists of a rhythmic combination of changes in physiological, biochemical, neurophysiological and psychological processes. When the rhythm is disturbed or the individual processes are abnormal during sleep, a variety of sleep-related disorders may result.

## Sleep-Related Disorders

Sleep-related complaints appeared regularly in medical literature in the beginning of the 19th century. However, from 1900 to the mid-1960's little was published in scientific journals about the "sleepy patient" except for an occasional report on the normal or abnormal aspects of sleep physiology. Recent developments of research techniques in neurobiology, molecular biology, molecular genetics, physiology, neuropsychiatry, internal medicine, pulmonary medicine, and cardiology have allowed scientists to study the details of sleep. As a result, there has been an explosion in interest in understanding sleep and "sleep disorders."

Some sleep-related disturbances are simply temporary inconveniences while others are potentially more serious. Sleep apnea is the major respiratory disorder of sleep. Other serious sleep-related disorders are narcolepsy and clinical insomnia. "Jet lag syndrome," caused by rapid shifts in the biological sleep-wake cycle, is also an example of a temporary sleep-related disorder. So are the sleep problems experienced by shift workers.

Sleep apnea is the condition of interrupted breathing while asleep. "Apnea" is a Greek word meaning "want of breath." Clinically, sleep apnea, first described in 1965, means cessation of breathing during sleep.

Narcolepsy is a neurological disorder whose main symptom is uncontrollable, excessive sleep, regardless of the time of day or whether the person has had enough sleep during the previous night. The other features of this disorder can include brief episodes of muscle weakness or paralysis caused by laughter and anger (cataplexy), paralysis for brief periods upon awakening from sleep (sleep paralysis), and dreamlike images at sleep onset (hypnagogic hallucinations). Narcolepsy, which may affect several members of the same family, is a life-long condition. Medications help to reduce the symptoms but do not cure the disease.

Insomnia is the commonly experienced difficulty in falling asleep, remaining asleep throughout the night, and the inability to return to sleep once awakened. Its causes may be physical or psychological and it may occur regularly or only occasionally.

Even a partial list of all the disorders caused by or associated with disturbed sleep adds up to some 70 items. The costs to society due to loss of productivity, industrial accidents and medical bills are estimated to be over $60 billion. These staggering statistics led to the creation by the U.S. Congress in 1988 of a National Commission on Sleep Disorders Research. This group is charged with the task of developing a blueprint for a national effort to reduce the medical and economic consequences of sleep disorders.

## *Likely Candidates for Sleep-Related Disorders*

Some of the people most likely to have or to develop a sleep-related disorder include:

- Adults who fall asleep at inappropriate times and places (e.g., during conversation, lecturing, driving) and who exhibit night-time snoring

- Elderly men and women

- Postmenopausal women

- People who are overweight, or have some physical abnormality in the nose, throat, or other parts of the upper airway

- Night-shift workers

- People who habitually drink too much alcohol

- Blind individuals who tend to develop impaired perception of light and darkness and have disturbed circadian rhythms, the cycles of biologic activities that occur at the same time during each 24 hours

- People with depression and other psychotic disorders.

## *Sleep and Breathing Disorders*

In 1944, the important observation was made that ventilation (exchange of air between the lung and environment) normally decreases during sleep. Even in "normal" people, breathing patterns during sleep may show a few irregularities. For example, a person might experience an average of seven breathing pauses of up to 10 seconds per night without any associated symptoms or problems. However if the breathing irregularities are accompanied by reduced oxygen supply to tissue (hypoxia) and repeated loss of sleep, these people are at risk of developing more serious problems.

## *Sleep Apnea*

Sleep apnea is the most common sleep disorder in terms of mortality and morbidity, especially in middle-aged men. Perhaps the best known sleep apnea "patient" is Charles Dickens' Fat Joe in *The Posthumous Papers of the Pickwick Club*, the overweight, red-faced boy in a permanent state of sleepiness, who snored and breathed heavily. The term "Pickwickian" syndrome is now used to describe patients with the most severe form of sleep apnea that is associated with reduced levels of breathing even during the day.

Sleep apnea occurs in all age groups and both sexes, but seems to predominate in males (it may be under-diagnosed in females) and in

African Americans. The Association of Professional Sleep Societies estimates that as many as 20 million Americans have this condition. The conditions associated with sleep apnea are a cascade: apnea, arousal, sleep deprivation, and excessive daytime sleepiness. Each is related to the frequency of the prior condition.

Like obesity with which it is often associated, the clustering of sleep apnea in some families suggests a genetic abnormality. Ingestion of alcohol and sleeping pills increases the frequency and duration of breathing pauses during sleep in people with or without sleep apnea.

Because of serious disturbances in their normal sleep patterns, patients with sleep apnea feel sleepy during the day and their concentration and daytime performance suffer. The common consequences of sleep apnea range from annoying to life-threatening. They include personality changes, sexual dysfunction and falling asleep at work, on the phone, or driving.

## Symptoms of Sleep Apnea

Patients with sleep apnea have many repeated involuntary breathing pauses during sleep. The length of the breathing pause can vary within a patient, and among patients, and can last from 10 seconds to 60 seconds. Fewer than 30 such breathing pauses during a 7-hour sleep, or shorter breathing pauses, are not considered indicative of sleep apnea. Most sleep apnea patients experience 20 to 30 "apneic events" per hour, more than 200 per night. These pauses may occur in clusters.

The breathing pauses are often accompanied by choking sensations which may wake up the patient, intermittent snoring, night-time insomnia, early morning headaches, and excessive day-time sleepiness, although not all patients, for some reason, complain of day-time sleepiness. During the apneic events, a person may turn blue from low blood oxygen levels.

Other features of sleep apnea include slowing down of heart beat below 60 beats per minute (bradycardia), irregular heart beat (cardiac arrhythmias), high blood pressure (both systemic and pulmonary arterial), increase in red cells in the blood (polycythemia), and obesity. The absence of restful sleep may cause deterioration of performance, depression, irritability, sexual dysfunction, and defects in attention and concentration.

## Types of Sleep Apnea

Scientists have distinguished three types of sleep apnea: obstructive, central, and mixed. However, since all three types can have the same symptoms and signs, a sleep evaluation is needed to tell the difference among them.

**Obstructive Sleep Apnea (OSA)** is the most common type. During OSA efforts to breath continue but air cannot flow out of the patient's nose or mouth. The patient snores heavily and has frequent arousals (abrupt changes from deep sleep to light sleep) without being aware of them.

OSA occurs when the throat muscles and tongue relax during breathing and partially block the opening of the airway. When the muscles of the soft palate at the base of the tongue and the uvula (the small conical fleshy tissue hanging from the center of the soft palate) relax and sag, the airway becomes obstructed making breathing labored and noisy. Airway narrowing may also occur due to overweight, possibly because of the associated increases in the amount of tissue in the airway.

The reduction in oxygen and increase in carbon dioxide which occur during apnea cause arousals. With each arousal, a signal is sent to the upper airway muscles to open the airway; breathing is resumed with a loud snort or gasp. Although arousals serve as a rescue mechanism and are necessary for a patient with apnea, they interrupt sleep, and the patient ends up with less restorative and deep sleep than normal individuals.

**Central Apnea** occurs less frequently than obstructive apnea. There is no airflow in or out of the airways because efforts to breathe have stopped for short periods of time. In central apnea, the brain temporarily fails to send the signals to the diaphragm and the chest muscles that maintain the breathing cycle. It is present more often in the elderly than in younger people but often goes unrecognized.

In central apnea, there is periodic loss of rhythmic breathing movements. The airways remain open but air does not pass through the nose or mouth because activity of the diaphragm and the chest muscles stops. Patients with central apnea may not snore and they tend to be more aware of their frequent awakenings than those with obstructive apnea.

In **Mixed Apnea**, a period of central apnea is followed by a period of obstructive apnea before regular breathing resumes People with mixed apnea frequently snore.

## Snoring and Sleep Apnea

Snoring is a sign of abnormal breathing. It occurs when physical obstruction causes fluttering of the soft palate and the adjacent soft tissues between the mouth, external orifices of the nose (nares), the upper part of the windpipe (trachea), and the passage extending from the pharynx to the stomach (esophagus).

Snoring always occurs with obstructive sleep apnea. When diagnosing sleep disorders, obstructive sleep apnea is excluded if snoring is not a symptom. All snorers do not necessarily have sleep apnea; however, because they almost certainly have some physical obstruction in their airways, they may develop sleep apnea.

The prevalence of snoring is greater in the older population and apparently peaks in 60-year-old men and women, declining in older individuals. Men seem to snore more than women. Men also are more likely to develop sleep-disordered breathing. It is estimated that nearly half of all males over 40 snore habitually. Snoring is also more common in overweight people.

A visit to the doctor is not necessary when a person snores unless some of the other symptoms of sleep disordered breathing also occur. However, since snoring is an annoying or irritating symptom with some negative social aspects, many people have sought a "cure" for it. More than 300 devices have been patented in the U.S. which claim to control snoring. Many of these devices were developed even before medical scientists found out that heavy snoring is a potential marker of sleep apnea.

## Sleep Apnea and the Heart

Sleep apnea with snoring seems to increase the likelihood of having a variety of cardiovascular diseases. These include high blood pressure, ischemic heart disease (a condition caused by reduced blood supply to the heart muscle), cardiac arrhythmias (abnormal heartbeat rhythm), and cerebral infarction (blood clot in the brain). It is not unusual for patients with sleep apnea to be mistakenly treated for primary heart disease because cardiac arrhythmias may be more prominent than the breathing disturbances

Nearly 50 percent of sleep apnea patients have high blood pressure. Patients with the most severe sleep apnea seem to have the highest blood pressure levels and are also more likely to have trouble controlling their blood pressure than patients who do not have sleep apnea. No one knows whether a cause and effect relationship exists between high blood pressure and sleep apnea. If it does exist, the ways these conditions interact is unknown.

Snoring alone does not appear to be a risk factor for heart disease. Only when snoring occurs with sleep apnea or obesity does it seem to be associated with these conditions.

## Sleep Apnea in Infants

Before a baby is born, the mother's breathing takes care of its respiratory needs. Although the unborn baby's lungs are filled with fluid and are not ready to take in air, its respiratory muscles make breathing motions, as if "training" to take on the responsibilities of breathing after birth.

As soon as birth occurs, the normal newborn baby begins a continuous pattern of periodic breathing characterized by a succession of apneas followed by regular breathing. Apneas occasionally lasting longer than 10 to 15 seconds are common during the newborn period. Apneas are more frequent and longer in premature newborns than in full-term infants. The frequency of apnea decreases with age during the first 6 months of life.

Babies who turn blue during sleep and appear limp may be undergoing episodes of insufficient breathing. They should be checked for a sleep-related disorder.

## Sleep Apnea and Sudden Infant Death Syndrome (SIDS)

Sleep apnea is sometimes implicated in sudden infant death syndrome (SIDS), also called crib death. About 10,000 infants die every year in this country from SIDS. Scientists do not know the reasons for these deaths but sleep apnea may play a role because these babies die when they are asleep and show no evidence of trauma. On autopsy, pinpoint hemorrhages are sometimes noted in the thoracic cavity which may be caused by lack of oxygen prior to cardiac arrest and vigorous respiratory movements.

## Diagnosis of Sleep Apnea

The general physician may sometimes recognize sleep apnea, but specialists in neurology, psychiatry, pulmonary medicine and cardiology may be needed for accurate diagnosis and management. Diagnosis of sleep apnea is difficult because disturbed sleep can cause various other diseases or make them worse. Several major medical centers now have pulmonologists, neurologists, and psychiatrists with specialty training in sleep disorders on their staff. Although an evaluation for sleep apnea can sometimes be done at home, it is more reliable if it is done in a sleep laboratory.

A variety of tests can be used to diagnose sleep apnea. These include pulmonary function tests, polysomnography, and the multiple sleep latency test. Physicians continue to try to develop other simple and economical procedures for the early diagnosis of sleep apnea.

**Pulmonary function tests** taken by sleep apnea patients may show normal results unless the patient has a coexisting lung disease. To make a definitive diagnosis of sleep apnea, the physician may order an all-night evaluation of the patient's sleep stages, and of the status of breathing and gas exchange during sleep.

**Polysomnography** is a group of tests that monitors a variety of functions during sleep. These include sleep state, electrical activity of the brain (EEG), eye movement (EOG), muscle activity (EMG), heart rate, respiratory effort, airflow, blood oxygen and carbon dioxide levels. Other tests may be ordered depending on a particular patient's needs. Polysomnography sometimes helps to distinguish between different sleep disorders. These tests are used both to diagnose sleep apnea and to determine its severity.

**The Multiple Sleep Latency Test** is done during normal working hours. It consists of observations, repeated every 2 hours, of the time taken to reach various stages of sleep. In this test, people without sleep apnea take more than 10 minutes to fall asleep. On the other hand, patients with sleep apnea or narcolepsy fall asleep fairly rapidly. When it takes the patient an average of less than 5 minutes to fall asleep, it is considered pathological sleepiness. There is thus some uncertainty in the diagnosis if the sleep latency period (speed of falling asleep) is between 5 and 10 minutes. This test is important because it measures the degree of excessive day-time sleepiness and also helps to rule out narcolepsy, which is associated with the onset of REM sleep (dream sleep) in many of the naps.

## Treatment of Sleep Apnea

More than 50,000 patients are treated each year for breathing disorders of sleep. Physicians tailor therapy to the individual patient based on medical history, physical examination, and the results of laboratory tests and polysomnography.

Patients with sleep apnea can help themselves by trying to avoid doing anything that can worsen the disease. Sleeping in improper positions can increase the frequency of apnea. Use of alcohol suppresses the activity of the upper airway muscles so that the airway is more likely to collapse. Sleeping pills and sedative-hypnotic drugs suppress arousal mechanisms and prolong apneas. Moving to high altitudes may aggravate the condition because of low oxygen levels. Overweight sleep apnea patients should lose weight.

Because the exact mechanism responsible for obstructive sleep apnea is not known, there is still no treatment that directly addresses the underlying problem. In most cases, medications have not proven successful. Surgical procedures are effective only 50 percent of the time because the exact location of the airway obstruction is usually unclear.

Since patients with sleep apnea usually have significant family and work problems, the treatment should include strategies that will help them cope with these problems. Education of the patient, family, and employers is sometimes needed to help the patient return to an active normal life.

### Position Therapy

In mild cases of sleep apnea, breathing pauses occur only when the individual sleeps on the back. Thus using methods that will ensure that patients sleep on their side is often helpful.

### Nasal Continuous Positive Airway Pressure (CPAP)

CPAP is the most common effective treatment for sleep apnea. In this procedure, the patient wears a mask or a pillow over the nose during sleep and pressure from an air compressor forces air through the nasal passages. The air pressure is adjusted so that it is just enough to hold the throat open when it relaxes the most. The pressure is constant and continuous. Nasal CPAP prevents obstruction while in use but apneas return when CPAP is stopped.

The major disadvantage of CPAP is that about 40 percent of patients have difficulty using it for long periods of time. Irritation and drying in the nose occur in some patients. Facial skin irritation, abdominal bloating, mask leaks, sore eyes, and headaches are some of the other problems. Because many patients stop using nasal CPAP due to the discomfort arising from exhaling against positive pressure, the search goes on for more comfortable devices. Modifications of CPAP in the treatment of sleep apnea are currently being defined.

One device, which some patients find more comfortable, is the bilevel positive airway pressure (BiPAP). Unlike CPAP where the pressure is equal during inhalation and exhalation, BiPAP is designed to follow the patient's breathing pattern. It lowers the pressure during expiration and maintains a constant inspiratory pressure.

The ramp system, a modification of CPAP, allows the pressure to be applied only when the patient goes to sleep, increasing pressure slowly over a 30-minute period. The purpose of the ramp system is to make CPAP more comfortable.

## *Nocturnal Ventilation*

Patients can be ventilated non-invasively during sleep with positive pressure ventilation through a CPAP mask. This technique is now used in patients whose breathing is impaired to the point that their blood carbon dioxide level is elevated, as happens in patients with obesity-hypoventilation syndrome and certain neuromuscular diseases.

## *Pharmacologic Therapies*

No medications are effective in the treatment of sleep apnea. However some physicians believe that mild cases of sleep apnea respond to drugs that either stimulate breathing or suppress deep sleep. Acetazolamide has been used to treat central apnea. Tricyclic antidepressants inhibit deep sleep (REM) and are useful only in patients who have apneas in the REM state.

Oxygen administration sometimes benefits patients without any side effects. However, the role of oxygen in the treatment of sleep apnea is controversial and it is difficult to predict which patients will respond to oxygen therapy.

### Dental Appliances

Dental appliances which reposition the lower jaw and the tongue have been helpful to some patients with obstructive sleep apnea. Possible side effects include damage to teeth, soft tissues, and the jaw joint.

### Surgery

Some patients with sleep apnea may require surgical treatment. Useful procedures include removal of adenoids and tonsils, nasal polyps or other growths, or other tissue in the airway, or correction of structural deformities. Younger patients seem to benefit from surgery better than older patients.

### Tracheostomy

Tracheostomy is used only in patients with severe, life-threatening obstructive sleep apnea. In this procedure a small hole is made in the windpipe (trachea) below the Adam's apple. A T-shaped tube is inserted into the opening. This tube stays closed during waking hours and the person breathes normally. It is opened for sleep so that air flows directly into the lungs, bypassing any upper airway obstruction. Its major drawbacks are that it is a disfiguring procedure and the tracheostomy tube requires proper care to keep it clean.

### Uvulopalatopharyngoplasty (UPPP)

UPPP is a procedure used to remove excess tissue at the back of the throat (tonsils, adenoids, uvula, and part of the soft palate). This technique probably helps only half of the patients who choose it. Its negative effects include nasal speech and backflow (regurgitation) of liquids into the nose during swallowing. UPPP is not considered as universally effective as tracheostomy but does seem to be a cure for snoring. It does not appear to prevent mortality from cardiovascular complications of severe sleep apnea.

Some patients whose sleep apnea is due to deformities of the lower jaw (mandible) benefit from reconstruction or surgical advancement of the mandible. Gastric stapling procedures to treat obesity are sometimes recommended for sleep apnea patients who are morbidly obese.

## Treatment of Patients with Coexisting Lung Diseases

Asthma, chronic bronchitis, emphysema, or other lung diseases can cause breathing problems during sleep. Patients with these diseases may be frequently awakened by cough, aspiration of secretions, choking sensations, and apnea-like sleep disturbances. The treatment in these cases depends on whether the sleep disturbances are due to lung disease or sleep apnea.

## Pathophysiology of Sleep and Breathing: Highlights of the National, Heart, Lung, and Blood Institute Programs

### Sleep

The modern era of sleep research started in the mid-1950's with the discovery that sleep is not a homogeneous phenomenon. Rather, it fluctuates cyclically between two distinct sequential stages of sleep.

The first sleep stage is variously called synchronized sleep, slow sleep, slow-wave sleep, quiet sleep, or non-rapid-eye-movement (NREM) sleep. In this state the EEG is dominated by large-amplitude slow waves; body functioning generally slows; there are slow, rolling eye movements; the pupils constrict; the respiratory and heart rates decline; blood pressure decreases; and total body oxygen consumption is reduced. It is believed that NREM sleep is a recuperative state.

The second state of sleep is called synchronized sleep, fast sleep, fast-wave sleep, dream sleep, or rapid-eye-movement (REM) sleep. The EEG is synchronized, with low-voltage fast waves and there are intermittent eye movements. It is also called paradoxical sleep because of the paradox that the EEG in this sleep stage is similar to that in wakefulness or light sleep, although this is deep sleep in terms of arousability. During REM sleep, central-nervous-system (CNS) activity generally increases, and body systems are variously activated and inactivated in a complex physiological pattern. The normal adult spends some 15 to 20 percent of the sleeping hours in REM sleep; this percentage decreases with aging. In contrast, the human fetus of 30 weeks spends 80 percent of its sleep in REM sleep. This declines to 50 percent at term. The amount of quiet sleep (NREM) increases from 50 to 60 percent by 3 months and to 70 percent between 6 and 23 months.

At the biochemical level, hormone-like prostaglandins and cytokines, which are intercellular messengers found in the brain, are implicated in the mechanisms that control sleep. Some speculate that a balance between prostaglandin D2 which increases sleep, and prostaglandin E2 which increases wakefulness, may be involved in the controlling mechanism. The prostaglandins produce their effects when injected into the preoptic area of the hypothalamus, an area responsible for temperature regulation. This may explain the link between sleep and fall in temperature, and also may unify the neurophysiological and biochemical mechanisms of sleep.

Interleukin-1 is localized in the brain in areas associated with control of sleep, and is believed to play a sleep regulatory role. The amount of interleukin-1 in cerebrospinal fluid fluctuates in parallel with the normal sleep/wake cycle.

There is no clear biological answer to the fundamental question of why we sleep. A wide variety of medical and psychiatric illnesses and factors related to age and gender can interfere with falling and staying asleep, with a multitude of pathophysiological sequelae. A major goal of sleep research is the characterization of the etiology and pathophysiology of the causes and effects of disturbed sleep

*Breathing*

The two major components of breathing are inspiration and expiration. Inspiration is an active process involving contraction of the diaphragm, external intercostal, and in certain circumstances, accessory muscles. It serves to increase intrathoracic volume, decrease intrapleural pressure and allow exchange of air and carbon dioxide within the alveoli of the lungs. Oxygen is transported from the alveoli to the pulmonary blood stream by passive diffusion and is made available to tissues. Expiration, on the other hand, is a relatively passive process requiring little or no contraction of the muscles during quiet breathing. A main function of the breathing process is to bring about the exchange of oxygen and carbon dioxide and other gaseous products from biological systems.

At birth, the baby switches from dependence on placental gas exchange to air breathing. At the moment of birth there is also a switch from intermittent breathing efforts of the fetal stage to sustained breathing efforts. Since the infant's respiratory muscles are not well-equipped to sustain high workloads, respiratory muscle fatigue is a problem for premature infants, and apneic episodes requiring intervention occur in at least 50 percent of surviving infants weighing less than 1,500 grams.

## Breathing Disorders During Sleep

Breathing disorders during sleep occur either when there are deficiencies in neurally generated rhythmic respiratory efforts or when there is normal generation of rhythmic efforts but mechanically impeded airflow in upper airways. Metabolic and behavioral control systems in the brain are believed to be the control mechanisms for sleep and breathing. The metabolic system that responds to changes in carbon dioxide and oxygen seems to exert its major influence over NREM sleep. On the other hand, the behavioral control system is involved in voluntary respiratory activities and appears to influence REM sleep; many of the ventilatory changes that occur in REM sleep are similar to the behavioral ventilatory activities such as swallowing, voluntary breath holding, and hyperventilation.

Subjects without any clinical problems may exhibit obstructive or central apnea during periods of REM sleep. Although severe changes in respiratory behavior often occur during the REM sleep, sleep apnea can occur in both NREM and REM sleep. However, sleep staging in patients with severe sleep apnea syndrome is difficult because of severe sleep fragmentation. Thus it is difficult to define the relative importance of abnormal respiration detected during REM or NREM sleeps.

### Research Highlights

A recent basic research advance of potential clinical implication relates to the application of modern three dimensional medical imaging techniques to the study of pathogenesis of sleep apnea. Magnetic resonance imaging (MRI) and ultrafast X-ray computed tomography (CT) of the upper airways, combined with computer graphics and reconstructions, have begun to provide exquisite details of the geometry of the upper airway. These approaches now permit identification of the precise anatomical sites of collapse or areas of abnormal compliance to determine if the problem is in a specific area or is a more generalized multi-focal abnormality. This information will impact on the treatment options, particularly if there is more diffuse involvement since this would predict failure of localized surgical procedures.

Only 50 percent of patients with sleep apnea undergoing uvulopalatopharyngoplasty benefit from this procedure. Investigators are exploring ways to, identify those patients most likely to benefit from this procedure. A small scale clinical trial conducted to determine predictors of success for UPPP revealed that 86 percent of patients who had documented (by fiberoptic endoscopy) preoperative nasopharyngeal obstruction at the level of the soft palate, showed significant improvement in the number of apneas, arousals and in the cumulative time in apnea-hypopnea following surgery. In contrast, only 18 percent of the patients who had a collapsing segment in regions of the pharynx other than the soft palate showed any improvement following UPPP. This is the first prospective clinical study to demonstrate that closure of the passive pharynx at the level of the soft palate predicts a favorable surgical outcome.

An important opportunity for research on the pathophysiology and treatment of sleep apnea has opened up with the finding that the English bulldog seems to be a suitable animal model of sleep apnea. This model is permitting the study of the regularly occurring periodicities in neural activity of the upper airways and the inspiratory muscles, and the role of neural mechanisms in the genesis of sleep apnea. Studies with thus model revealed that the consequences of intermittent apnea (sleepiness or hypox) serve to increase the magnitude and frequency of neural inhibitory activity, thereby worsening the apnea.

Other studies exploring new treatments for obstructive sleep apnea in animals have identified buspirone, an hypnotic agent, as a potentially effective drug for sleep apnea. Buspirone seems to increase ventilation in both anesthetized and awake rats and cats without producing the traditional respiratory depressive effects. In a small-scale, controlled clinical trial, this drug decreased sleep apnea and improved respiratory status in the patients receiving the drug.

Associations between snoring, hypertension, heart disease, and stroke raise the possibility of common factors and/or causal relationships between sleep apnea and cardiovascular disorders. Such links may be related to biochemical factors such as insulin, catecholamine, or cortisol that are increased in stress. Sleep apnea may itself be a stress that produces hormonal imbalances that lead to the hypertensive state.

Alternately obesity, sleep apnea, and other cardiovascular risk factors may share common metabolic pathways and therefore may be genetically determined. These relationships are being explored by studying families with a history of sleep apnea and/or sudden infant death syndrome as well as by studying racial and genetic differences in the prevalence of sleep apnea-related illnesses.

## Research Opportunities

Since 1986, the Division of Lung Diseases, National Heart, Lung, and Blood Institute has been engaged in a concerted national program in cardiopulmonary disorders in sleep designed to fill critical gaps in the understanding of the pathogenesis, diagnosis, treatment, and prevention of sleep-disordered breathing. Some research areas of current emphasis include the following:

1. Natural history of sleep apnea with the goal of determining the magnitude of the problem and designing the most effective therapy.

2. Scientific basis for the influence of age, gender, ethnicity, smoking, obesity, and snoring on the development of sleep apnea.

3. Assessment of the severity of sleep apnea and defining the relationships of disease severity, response to treatment and prognosis.

4. Cellular and molecular basis of the role of hypoxia in excessive daytime sleepiness and sleep apnea.

5. Cardiovascular consequences of sleep apnea and the underlying neural cellular and respiratory mechanisms.

6. Improved therapeutic modalities for sleep apnea when associated with blood pressure, asthma, chronic heart failure, angina pectoris, chronic pulmonary disease and stroke.

## Sleep Lab—First Step to Treatment

Sleep apnea is often treatable. Many sufferers don't know this, however, because only 10 to 25 percent of cases are ever diagnosed. This is either because the person is unaware of the snoring or does not know that loud snoring is a symptom of apnea

Can sleep apnea really be dangerous, if you can have it and not even know it?

"I believe to some extent we have oversold [sleep apnea's] life-threatening nature. I see people in here who have had sleep apnea for

20 years. Are they dying? Only indirectly, because sleep apnea contributes to hypertension, accidents, sleepiness, and psychological problems," says John Shepard, M.D., director of the Sleep Disorders Clinic of the Mayo Clinic in Rochester, Minn.

A definitive diagnosis of sleep apnea requires a visit to one of the country's 142 sleep laboratories. Here, a variety of tests are conducted while the patient sleeps, and physiological measurements are correlated to body movements. The entire procedure is called polysomnography.

The patient arrives at the sleep lab about an hour before bedtime. If he or she normally drinks alcoholic beverages, the usual amount is consumed at the usual time, so that observations match the patient's customary experience. A technician then places dime-sized sensors on different parts of the person's body. These measure heart rate, brain wave patterns, muscle activity, leg and arm movements, and eye movements, which indicate the stage of sleep.

An elastic band holding gauges is strapped around the chest and abdomen to track movements of the muscles involved in breathing. A light mask covering the mouth and nose measures the respiratory rate, which monitors the frequency of apneic episodes. Finally, a test called oximetry measures dips in arterial oxygen saturation, the hallmark of sleep apnea.

"In oximetry, a probe is clipped onto the finger or the ear. There is a light source. The light goes through the lobe or finger, and the refraction of the light is proportional to the [amount of] oxygen in the arterioles of the blood," says Martin Scharf, Ph.D., director of the Center for Research in Sleep Disorders in Cincinnati.

The automated scanners of the sleep lab produce a readout of each measurement, and these can be displayed next to one another so that one symptom or sign is easily correlated with another. For example, cessation of breathing usually coincides with a dip in oxygen saturation, and both tend to occur when the patient is sleeping on his or her back.

A night in a sleep lab is often followed by a daytime multiple sleep latency test, which monitors a series of two-hour naps. This test distinguishes between sleep apnea and narcolepsy, in which a person falls asleep very suddenly during the day. Scharf uses the nap test to quantify a patient's report of sleepiness, and to back up polysomnography. "I see people who drive a lot, and have a history of falling asleep, like truck drivers. I won't say 'you're cured' until I repeat the multiple sleep latency test and show they're not sleepy,"he says.

Some sleep labs also study the architecture of the nose and throat, using x-rays and fiber-optic endoscopes (lights on flexible wires snaked into narrow body cavities) to picture upper airway structures. Video cameras are beginning to be used to do the work of technicians, allowing polysomnography to move from a specialized lab setting to a typical hospital ward and even to a physician's office. Physiological data are superimposed on the video of the sleeping patient.

—*Ricki Lewis, Ph D.*

## For More Information

Additional information about breathing-related sleep disorders and other disorders of sleep can be obtained from your local sleep disorders center and the following sources:

American Sleep Apnea Association
P.O. Box 3893
Charlottesville, VA 22903

The American Sleep Disorders Association
604 Second Street Southwest
Rochester, MN 55902

Association of Sleep Disorders Centers
P.O.Box 2604
Del Mar, CA 92014

AWAKE NETWORK
P.O. Box 534
Bethel Park, PA 15102

American Narcolepsy Association
P.O. Box 1187
San Carlos, CA 94070

Narcolepsy Network
155 Van Brackle Rd.
Aberdeen, NJ 07747

National Heart, Lung, and Blood Institute (NHLBI)
Communications and Public Information Branch
9000 Rockville Pike
Bethesda, MD 20892

(Other institutes at NIH that have information about sleep disorders include the National Institute of Neurological Disorders and Stroke, National Institute of Child Health and Human Development, National Institute of Mental Health, National Institute on Aging. The address for each is 9000 Rockville Pike, Bethesda, MD 20892.)

Centers for Disease Control and Prevention
600 Clifton Road, NE
Atlanta, GA 30333

Chapter 12

# Sudden Infant Death Syndrome (SIDS) and Apparent Life-Threatening Events (ALTE)

*Chapter Contents*

Section 12. 1—What is SIDS? .................................................. 470
Section 12. 2—Facts About Apnea and Other Apparent
               Life-Threatening Events ..................................... 475
Section 12. 3—Infant Positioning and SIDS ............................. 479
Section 12. 4—The Grief of Children ....................................... 480
Section 12. 5—Infant Apnea Monitors Help Parents
               Breathe Easy ....................................................... 486

## Section 12.1

# What Is SIDS?

Source: Information Sheets #1 and #4, National Sudden Infant Death Symdrome Resource Center, May 1993.

Sudden Infant Death Syndrome (SIDS) is the "sudden death of an infant under one year of age which remains unexplained after a thorough case investigation, including performance of a complete autopsy, examination of the death scene, and review of the clinical history" (Willinger et al., 1991).

### What Are the Most Common Characteristics of SIDS?

Most researchers now believe that babies who die of SIDS are born with one or more conditions that make them especially vulnerable to stresses that occur in the normal life of an infant, including both internal and external influences. SIDS occurs in all types of families and is largely indifferent to race or socioeconomic level. SIDS is unexpected, usually occurring in otherwise apparently healthy infants from 1 month to 1 year of age. Most deaths from SIDS occur by the end of the sixth month, with the greatest number taking place between 2 and 4 months of age. A SIDS death occurs quickly and is often associated with sleep, with no signs of suffering. More deaths are reported in the fall and winter (in both the Northern and Southern Hemispheres), and there is a 60-to-40-percent male-to-female ratio. A death is diagnosed as SIDS only after all other alternatives have been eliminated: SIDS is a diagnosis of exclusion.

### What Are Risk Factors for SIDS?

Risk factors are those environmental and behavioral influences that can provoke ill health. Any risk factor may be a clue to finding the cause of a disease, but risk factors in and of themselves are not causes. Researchers now know that the mother's health and behavior during her pregnancy and the baby's health before birth seem to influence the occurrence of SIDS, but these variables are not reliable in predicting how, when, why, or if SIDS will occur. Maternal risk factors include cigarette smoking during pregnancy; maternal age less than

**Data Breakdown of SIDS Deaths by Age for 1988 and 1989**

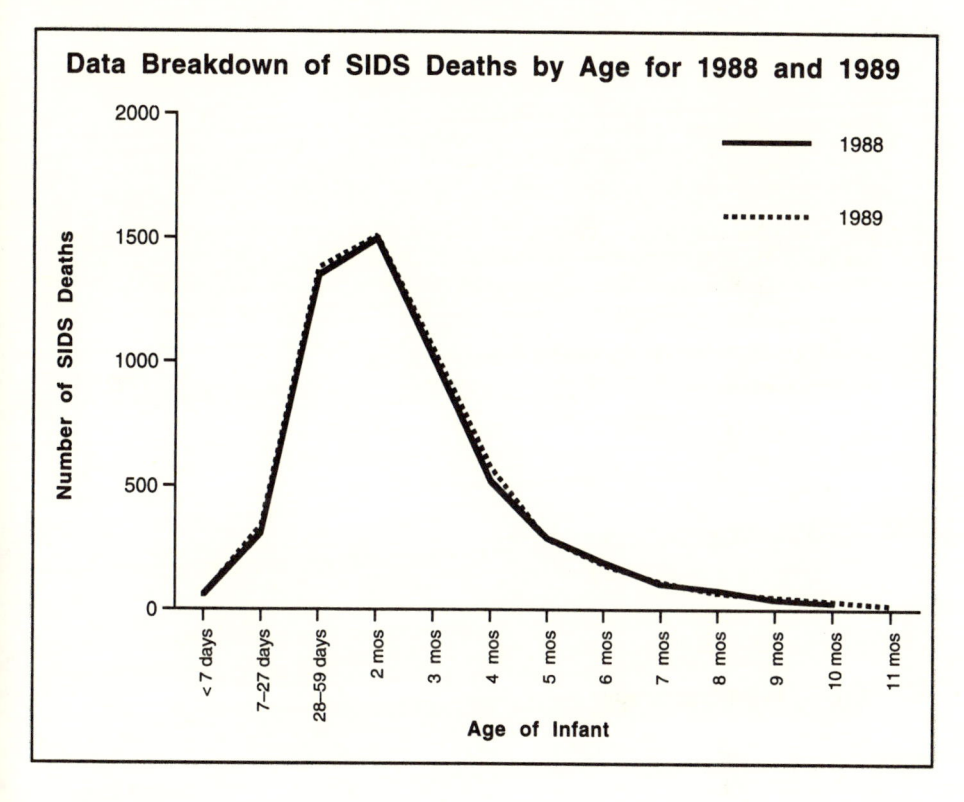

*Figure 9.1.*

20 years; poor prenatal care; low weight gain; anemia; use of illegal drugs; and history of sexually transmitted disease or urinary tract infection. These factors, which often may be subtle and undetected, suggest that SIDS is somehow associated with a harmful prenatal environment.

## How Many Babies Die From SIDS?

From year to year, the number of SIDS deaths tends to remain constant despite fluctuations in the overall number of infant deaths. The National Center for Health Statistics (NCHS) reported that, in 1988 in the United States, 5,476 infants under 1 year of age died from SIDS; in 1989, the number of SIDS deaths was 5,634 (NCHS, 1990, 1992). However, other sources estimate that the number of SIDS

The table below shows the number of SIDS deaths by age for 1988 and 1989. Data are from the National Center for Health Statistics, 6525 Belcrest Road, Hyattsville, MD 20782. For more statistical information on SIDS deaths and other infant mortality rates, call the National Center for Health Statistics at (301) 436-8500.

**Data Breakdown of SIDS Deaths by Age for 1988 and 1989**

| Under seven days | 1988 | 1989 |
|---|---|---|
| Under 1 hour | 1 | 9 |
| 1–23 hours | 6 | 5 |
| 1 day | 5 | 7 |
| 2 days | 13 | 12 |
| 3 days | 9 | 7 |
| 4 days | 7 | 5 |
| 5 days | 8 | 4 |
| 6 days | 8 | 6 |
| Total under seven days | 57 | 55 |

**Seven to twenty-seven days**

| | | |
|---|---|---|
| 7–13 days | 56 | 70 |
| 14–20 | 102 | 108 |
| 21–27 | 153 | 165 |
| Total under twenty-eight days | 368 | 398 |

**Twenty-eight days through eleven months**

| | | |
|---|---|---|
| 28–59 | 1,347 | 1,379 |
| 2 months | 1,497 | 1,508 |
| 3 months | 1,007 | 1,042 |
| 4 months | 519 | 574 |
| 5 months | 287 | 282 |
| 6 months | 191 | 178 |
| 7 months | 102 | 110 |
| 8 months | 76 | 65 |
| 9 months | 40 | 49 |
| 10 months | 25 | 33 |
| 11 months | 17 | 16 |
| Total | 5,476 | 5,634 |

*Figure 9.2.*

deaths in this country each year may actually be closer to 7,000 (Goyco and Beckerman, 1990). The larger estimate represents additional cases that are unreported or under-reported (should have been reported as SIDS cases but were not).

When considering the overall number of live births each year, SIDS remains the leading cause of death in the United States among infants between 1 month and 1 year of age and second only to congenital anomalies as the leading overall cause of death for all infants less than 1 year of age.

## How Do Professionals Diagnose SIDS?

Often the cause of an infant death can be determined only through a process of collecting information, conducting sometimes complex forensic tests and procedures, and talking with parents and physicians. When a death is sudden and unexplained, investigators, including medical examiners and coroners, use the special expertise of forensic medicine (application of medical knowledge to legal issues). SIDS is no exception.

Health professionals make use of three avenues of investigation in determining a SIDS death:

1. the autopsy,

2. death scene investigation, and,

3. review of victim and family case history.

### The Autopsy

The autopsy provides anatomical evidence through microscopic examination of tissue samples and vital organs. An autopsy is important because SIDS is a diagnosis of exclusion. A definitive diagnosis cannot be made without a thorough postmortem examination that fails to point to any other possible cause of death. Also, if a cause of SIDS is ever to be uncovered, scientists will most likely detect that cause through evidence gathered from a thorough pathological examination.

### A Thorough Death Scene Investigation

A thorough death scene investigation involves interviewing the parents, other care-givers, and family members; collecting items from the death scene; and evaluating that information. Although painful for the family, a detailed scene investigation may shed light on the cause, sometimes revealing a recognizable and possibly preventable cause of death.

### Review of the Victim and Family Case History

A comprehensive history of the infant and family is especially critical to determine a SIDS death. Often, a careful review of documented and anecdotal information about the victim's or family's history of previous illnesses, accidents, or behaviors may further corroborate what is detected in the autopsy or death scene investigation.

Investigators should be sensitive and understand that the family may view this process as an intrusion, even a violation of their grief. It should be noted that, although stressful, a careful investigation that reveals no preventable cause of death may actually be a means of giving solace to a grieving family.

## What SIDS Is and What SIDS Is Not

### SIDS Is:

- the major cause of death in infants from 1 month to 1 year of age, with most deaths occurring between 2 and 4 months
- sudden and silent—the infant was seemingly healthy
- currently, unpredictable and unpreventable
- a death that occurs quickly, often associated with sleep and with no signs of suffering
- determined only after an autopsy, an examination of the death scene, and a review of the clinical history
- designated as a diagnosis of exclusion
- a recognized medical disorder listed in the International Classification of Diseases, 9th Revision (ICD-9)
- an infant death that leaves unanswered questions, causing intense grief for parents and families

## SIDS and ALTE

**SIDS Is Not:**

- caused by vomiting and choking, or by minor illnesses such as colds or infections
- caused by the diphtheria, pertussis, tetanus (DPT) vaccines, or other immunizations
- contagious
- child abuse
- the cause of every unexpected infant death

Any sudden, unexpected death threatens one's sense of safety and security (Corr, 1991). We are forced to confront our own mortality. This is particularly true in a sudden infant death. Quite simply, babies are not supposed to die. Because the death of an infant is a disruption of the natural order, it is traumatic for parents, family, and friends. The lack of a discernible cause, the suddenness of the tragedy, and the involvement of the legal system make a SIDS death especially difficult, leaving a great sense of loss and a need for understanding.

## Section 12.2

## *Facts About Apnea and Other Apparent Life-Threatening Events*

Source: National Sudden Infant Death Syndrome Clearinghouse.

There is great concern that infants who experience frightening episodes of apnea and/or cyanosis (a bluish skin color as a result of lack of oxygen in the blood) may be at increased risk for subsequent sudden and unexpected death. The highly emotional nature of this clinical problem and the necessity to deal with these patients, despite inadequate scientific data, has led to a variety of clinical practices, and to diverse interpretations of the prognostic implications of these episodes. The purpose of this section is to summarize briefly the current state of understanding of the causes, implications, and appropriate management of infants who experience these frightening episodes, and to review recent information about the relationship of these episodes to subsequent sudden infant death syndrome.

## Apparent Life-Threatening Event (ALTE)

ALTE is an episode which is frightening to the observer. It is characterized by some combination of apnea (central or occasionally obstructive), color change (usually bluish or pallid, but occasionally reddish), marked change in muscle tone (usually limpness), or choking or gagging. In some cases the observer fears that the infant has died. Previously used terminology such as "aborted crib death" or "near-miss SIDS" should be abandoned since it implies a misleadingly close association between this type of spell and SIDS.

## What is the Relationship between ALTE and SIDS?

Recent studies indicate that no more than 5 to 7 percent of SIDS victims had experience ALTE before their death; thus it appears that most SIDS victims do not come from that population of infants. The other important way to examine the relationship between ALTE and SIDS is to ask, "what is the incidence of subsequent SIDS in infants who have experienced ALTE?" As a group, infants who have experienced ALTE are probably at approximately tenfold increased risk for SIDS when compared to the incidence of SIDS in the general population of 1.5 per 1,000 live births. However, recent studies indicate that there are certain subgroups within this overall ALTE population who may be at significantly greater risk, and in contrast most infants, whose ALTEs are relatively mild, may be at no increased risk. One study reports a subsequent mortality of 13.2 percent in 76 infants who experienced a severe, unexplained episode of apnea during sleep. If these infants required vigorous stimulation or resuscitation to terminate a subsequent episode, their mortality rose to greater than 25 percent despite the prescription of electronic home monitors. Infants with such severe spells are rare, and the great majority of ALTEs are much less serious and carry a much better prognosis.

Thus there is some overlap between SIDS and ALTE, but except for a very small, very high-risk ALTE group, that overlap is small.

The recurrent apnea which is common in prematurely born infants is not associated with an increased risk of SIDS.

## SIDS and ALTE

### How Common Is ALTE?

ALTE is observed in approximately 2 to 3 percent of the general population, making it approximately twice as frequent as SIDS.

### What Causes ALTE?

There are many different disease processes and other mechanisms which can cause ALTE, but in approximately one-half of the cases, no specific cause is identified. In some cases, evaluation indicates that the episode was caused by a specific problem such as infection, airway obstruction, heart disease, seizure, choking, or breath-holding spell. Occasional cases may actually represent a caretaker's overreaction to a normal respiratory pause (less than 20 seconds).

### How Effective are Home Monitors for ALTE?

Electronic home cardiorespiratory monitors have been prescribed for many infants with ALTE in hopes that these machines will aid the parents in knowing when an event has occurred and if intervention may be required. (See related article.) There is no proof that the use of home monitors has affected infant mortality rates, but there are many anecdotal reports of monitor alarms which alerted families to infants in serious condition. Since the ALTE population contributes such a small percentage to the total number of SIDS cases, it is not surprising that no overall effect on SIDS incidence has resulted from the use of home monitors in this population. While home monitors can be reassuring, they can also be disruptive to the family and the infant since they significantly restrict mobility. There is also a likelihood of some false alarms occurring.

### Which ALTE Infants Should be Monitored at Home?

A recent panel of experts convened by the National Institutes of Health addressed this issue and concluded that despite the lack of conclusive data base, electronic cardiorespiratory monitoring or an alternative therapy is medically indicated for infants who have experienced one of more severe ALTEs which required mouth-to-mouth resuscitation or vigorous stimulation. Home monitoring is not indicated for normal infants who are not at increased risk of sudden unexpected death, because the risks, disadvantages, and costs of monitoring outweigh the possible benefit of preventing SIDS. For infants with less severe ALTE, the panel acknowledged that the risk of death is elevated to some degree, and concluded that "the decision to monitor must be made by the family after a full discussion with the physician about the potential benefits as well as the psychosocial burdens. The decision reached will be specific to the infant, and there are no hard and fast guidelines that will apply to all cases. No family in this category should be made to feel that monitoring is necessary."

Monitors are not a cure for apnea. They are only a device which may alert parents that their infant needs immediate stimulation or resuscitation. medical and technical back-up must be continuously available to any families using monitors in the home.

There is not test which can predict which infants will subsequently die from SIDS.

*Do Infants Outgrow ALTE?*

Most of these infants do not experience severe ALTE, and the number of episodes decreases with increasing age in almost all cases. In most cases, the problem is no longer medically significant after the child is six months old.

*—John G. Brooks, M.D.,*
*Principal Investigator*
*Western New York SIDS Center.*

## Section 12.3

## Infant Positioning and SIDS

Source: Information Sheet #3, National Sudden Infant Deathy Syndrome Resource Center, May 1993.

On April 15, 1992, the American Academy of Pediatrics (AAP) released a statement on infant position and SIDS. The AAP summary statement follows, accompanied by a response from the National Institute of Child Health and Human Development (NICHHD).

*American Academy of Pediatrics Summary*

Based on careful evaluation of existing data indicating an association between Sudden Infant Death Syndrome (SIDS) and prone sleeping position for infants, the Academy recommends that normal infants, when being put down for sleep, be positioned on their side or back. The most common position currently used in the United States is prone.

This recommendation is made with the full recognition that existing studies have methodologic limitations and were conducted in countries with infant care practices and other SIDS risk factors that differ from those in the United States (e.g. maternal smoking, types of bedding, central heating, etc). However, taken as a group the studies are convincing. No reports show an advantage to the prone position with regards to SIDS incidence and there are no data proving, or even strongly suggesting, that sleeping in the lateral or supine position is harmful to normal infants. Thus, assessment of the risk/benefit balance for the prone vs non-prone positioning for such infants favors the later. It should be stressed that the actual risk of SIDS for an infant placed prone is extremely low.

*There are still good reasons for placing certain infants prone. For premature infants with respiratory distress, for infants with symptoms of gastroesophageal reflux or with certain upper airway anomalies, and perhaps for some others, prone may well be the position of choice. The proposed change in position is for healthy sleeping infants only.*

The entire article on Infant Positioning and SIDS was published in *Pediatrics* 89(6):1120-1126, June 1992.

**National Institute of Child Health and Human Development**

The National Institute of Child Health and Human Development issued a statement in response to the AAP acknowledging that, although there has been concern over whether a recommendation on sleep position should be made, the evidence for change was compelling. The United States has a lower baseline rate of SIDS than the countries studied and, due to confounding variable, it is unknown whether a nationwide change in sleeping position will change the incidence of SIDS.

Section 12.4

## *The Grief of Children*

Source: National SIDS Clearinghouse, August 1982.

One of the most difficult tasks following the death of loved one is discussing and explaining the death with children in the family. This task is even more distressing when the parents are in the midst of their own grief.

Because many adults have problems dealing with death, they assume that children cannot cope with it. They may try to protect children by leaving them out of the discussions and rituals associated with the death. Thus, children may feel anxious, bewildered, and alone. They may be left on their own to seek answers to their questions at a time when they most need the help and reassurance of those around them.

All children will be affected in some way by a death in the family. Above all, children who are too young for explanations need love from the significant people in their lives to maintain their own security. Young children may not verbalize their feelings about a death in the family. Holding back their feelings because they are so overwhelming, the children may appear to be unaffected. It is more common for them to express their feelings through behavior and play. Regardless of this ability or inability to express themselves, children do grieve, often very deeply.

## SIDS and ALTE

*Some Common Expressions of Children's Grief*

Experts have determined that those in grief pass through four major emotions: fear, anger, guilt, and sadness. It should be remembered that everyone who is touched by a death experiences these emotions to some degree—grandparents, friends, physicians, nurses, and children. Each adult and child's reactions to death are individual in nature. Some common reactions are:

- **Shock.** Children may not believe the death really happened and will act as though it did not. This is usually because the thought of death is too overwhelming.

- **Physical Symptoms.** Children may have various complaints such as headaches or stomachaches and fear that they will die too.

- **Anger.** Being mostly concerned with their own needs, children may be angry at the person who died because of the feeling of being left "all alone" or that God didn't "make the person well."

- **Guilt.** Children may think that they caused the death by having been angry with the person who died or they may feel responsible for not having been "better" in some way.

- **Anxiety and Fear.** Children may wonder who will take care of them now or fear that some other person they will die. They may cling to parents or ask other people who play important roles in their lives if they love them.

- **Regression.** Children may revert to behaviors they have previously outgrown, such as bed-wetting or thumb-sucking.

- **Sadness.** Children may show a decrease in activity—being "too quiet."

It is important to remember that all of the reactions outlined above are normal expressions of grief in children, In the grief process, time is an important factor. Experts have said that six months after a significant death in a child's life, normal routine should be resuming.

If the child's reaction seems to be prolonged, seeking professional advice of those who are familiar with the child (e.g. teachers, pediatricians, clergy) may be helpful.

## Explanations That May Not Help

Outlined below are explanations that adults may give a child hoping to explain why a person they loved has died. Unfortunately, simple but dishonest answers can only serve to increase the fear and uncertainty that the child is feeling. Children tend to be very literal—if an adult says that "Grandpa died because he was old and tired," the child may wonder when he too will be too old; he certainly gets tired—what is tired enough to die?

- "Grandma will sleep in peace forever." This explanation may result in the child's fear of going to bed or to sleep.

- "It is God' will." The child will not understand a God who takes a loved one because He needs that person Himself; or "God took him because he was so good." The child may decide to be bad so God won't take him too.

- "Daddy went on a long trip and won't be back for a long time." The child may wonder why the person left without saying goodbye. Eventually he or she will realize Daddy isn't coming back and feel that something he or she did caused Daddy to leave.

- "Jimmy was sick and went to the hospital where he died." The child will need an explanation about "little" and "big" sicknesses. Otherwise, he may be extremely fearful if he or someone he loves has to go the hospital in the future.

## Ways to Help Children

As in all situations, the best way to deal with children is honestly. Talk to the child in a language that he or she can understand. Remember to listen to the child and try to understand what the child is saying, and just as importantly, what the child is not saying. Children need to feel that the death is an open subject and that they can ex-

## SIDS and ALTE

press their thoughts or questions as they arise. Below are just a few ways adults can help children face the death of someone close to them:

*The child's first concern my be "who will take care of me now?"*

- Maintain usual routines as much as possible.
- Show affection and assure the child that he or she is still loved and protected.

*The child will probably have many questions and may need to ask them again and again.*

- Encourage the child to ask questions and give honest, simple answers that can be understood. Repeated questions require patience and continued expression of caring.
- Answers should be based on the needs the child seems to be expressing, not necessarily on the exact words used.

*The child will not know appropriate behavior for the situation.*

- Encourage the child to talk about feelings and share how you feel. You are a model for how one expresses feelings. It is helpful to cry. It is not helpful to be told how one should or should not feel.
- Allow the child to express caring for you. Loving is giving *and* taking.

*The child may fear dying or feel somehow responsible for the death.*

- Reassure the child about the cause of the death and explain that any thoughts he or she may have had about the person who died did not cause the death.
- Reassure the child that this death does not mean someone else he or she loves is likely to die soon.

*The child may wish to be a part of the family rituals.*

- Explain this to him or her and include the child in the decision on how to participate. Remember, the child should be prepared beforehand, told what to expect, and have a supporting adult to turn to. Do not force the child to do anything he or she is uncomfortable with.

*The child may show regressive behavior.*

- A common reaction to stress is to revert to an earlier stage of development. (For example, a child may begin thumb sucking, or bed-wetting; or, may need to go back into diapers or have a bottle for a time). Support the child in this and keep in mind that these regressions are temporary.

Adults can help prepare a child to deal with future losses of those who are significant by helping the child handle smaller losses through sharing their feelings when a pet dies or when death is discussed in a story or on television.

In helping children understand and cope with death, remember four key concepts: be loving, be accepting, be truthful, and be consistent.

*—Susan Woolsey, R.N. M.S.*

## For Additional Information on SIDS, Contact:

American SIDS Institute,
6065 Roswell Road, Suite 876,
Atlanta, GA 30328,
(800) 232-7437, (800) 847-7437 (within GA), (404) 843-1030, (404) 843-0577 (fax)

Association of SIDS Program Professionals (ASPP),
c/o Massachusetts Center for SIDS,
Boston City Hospital,
818 Harrison Avenue,
Boston MA 02118,
(617) 534-7437, (617) 534-5555 (fax)

National Sudden Infant Death Syndrome Resource Center (NSRC),
8201 Greensboro Drive, Suite 600,
McLean, VA 22102-3810,
(703) 821-8955, (703) 821-2098 (fax)

Southwest SIDS Research Institute, Inc.,
Brazosport Memorial Hospital,
100 Medical Drive,
Lake Jackson, TX 77566,
(409) 299-2814, (800) 245-7437, (409) 297-6905 (fax)

Sudden Infant Death Syndrome Alliance,
10500 Little Patuxent Parkway, Suite 420,
Columbia, MD 21044,
(800) 921-7437, (410) 964-8000, (410) 964-8009 (fax)

## References

Corr, C.A., Fuller, H., Barnickol, C.A., and Corr, D.M. (Eds). *Sudden Infant Death Syndrome: Who Can Help and How.* New York: Springer Publishing Co.,1991.

Goyco, P.G., and Beckerman, R.C. "Sudden Infant Death Syndrome." *Current Problems in Pediatrics* 20(6): 249-346, June 1990.

National Center for Health Statistics. "Advanced Mortality Statistics for 1989." *Monthly Vital Statistics Report*, Vol. 40, No. 8, Supp. 2, January 7, 1992, p. 44.

National Center for Health Statistics. "Advance Report of Final Mortality Statistics, 1988." *Monthly Vital Statistics Report*, Vol. 39, No. 7, Supp. 1990, p. 33.

Willinger, M., James, L.S., and Catz, C. "Defining the Sudden Infant Death Syndrome (SIDS): Deliberations of an Expert Panel Convened by the National Institute of Child Health and Human Development." *Pediatric Pathology* 11:677-684, 1991.

These articles were taken from publications produced by the National Sudden Infant Death Syndrome Resource Center, 8201 Greensboro Drive, Suite 600, McLean, VA 22102, (703) 821-8955, (operated by The Circle, Inc.). The Resource Center is an affiliate of the National Center for Education in Maternal and Child Health and is a service of the U.S. Department of Health and Human Services, Public Health Service, Health Resources and Services Administration, Maternal and Child Health Bureau.

## Section 12.5

# Infant Apnea Monitors
# Help Parents Breathe Easy

Source: *FDA Consumer.* June 1991.

It's a rare parent who hasn't tiptoed into the sleeping baby's room and listened just to make sure that tiny chest is moving in a gentle breathing rhythm.

Occasionally, though, that gentle rhythm is broken by periods of stopped breathing. As frightening as that may sound, a temporary pause from breathing, or apnea, is not always cause for alarm.

"All babies pause in their breathing," says Robert G. Meny, M.D., a pediatrician with the University of Maryland Medical School's Sudden Infant Death Syndrome Institute. "Especially after a sigh, a pause of maybe five seconds or eight seconds, depending on the baby, is completely normal."

Meny adds that "when a baby moves around a lot, you'll very often see that the child does not breathe for 10 to 15 seconds. That, too, is normal.

"The question is not if—the question is how much, how often, and how long. I begin to worry especially when I see the pauses for more than 20 seconds."

### Apparent Life-Threatening Events

**Twenty seconds.** That's the point at which apnea does become cause for alarm. When apnea lasts for more than 20 seconds, the baby may begin to turn blue or pale, choke or gag, and go limp. A pause in breathing for less than 20 seconds may also be serious if the heart rate slows significantly.

The official medical term for serious episodes of prolonged apnea that don't result in death is Apparent Life-Threatening Event or ALTE. Babies can be saved if the prolonged apnea is detected quickly enough.

"There are a whole variety of responses to apnea of 20 seconds or more," says Meny. "Very often the baby will respond to mild stimulation—a flick of the fingers on the feet or something like that. If that doesn't do the trick, then the next step is vigorous stimulation, where you give the baby a painful stimulus like a good pinch. And finally, if that doesn't work, then the parent would go to mouth and nose resuscitation."

Do not shake the baby, Meny warns. Infants do not have good head control, and vigorous shaking could cause head injury and even death.

In some cases, the episode of prolonged apnea can be traced to a specific problem such as infection, airway obstruction, heart disease, seizure, or choking, says John G. Brooks, M.D., professor of pediatrics at the University of Rochester Medical School. He adds that in approximately half the cases, however, no specific cause is identified.

When the cause isn't known, there is no known cure for infant apnea except time. The number of apnea episodes decreases as the baby gets older, and "in most cases, the problem is no longer medically significant after the child is 6 months old," says Brooks.

## Apnea Monitors

But until this time, many infants younger than 6 months who have experienced an ALTE are put on a home apnea monitor. The main function of these monitors is to sound an alarm if the baby stops breathing.

There are three types of infant apnea:

- Central or diaphragmatic—the baby makes no effort to breathe; the chest is still, and no air passes through the mouth or nose.

- Obstructive—the chest is moving but no air passes through the mouth or nose (usually due to soft tissue such as the tongue blocking the upper airway).

- Mixed—the infant has episodes of both central and obstructive all within the same event.

The variations in types of apnea complicate the function of the monitor. For example, if the apnea is obstructive, the chest will continue to move. If the monitor's only method of detecting breathing is chest movement, this type of apnea might go undetected.

For that reason, effective apnea monitors also measure a physiological function that is adversely affected within a relatively short time after the baby stops breathing. Currently, the function most monitors measure is heart rate. Normally, the monitor's alarm is set to go off if the baby stops breathing for 20 seconds or if the heart rate slows to less than 80 beats per minute.

## Government Standards

FDA is developing a mandatory performance standard for infant apnea monitors. At press time, the requirements for this standard were not final.

Many features the agency considers to be mandatory on monitors are already available on some models. Under the tentative performance standard, all monitors must be able to detect both a physiological problem that results from apnea, such as slow heart rate, as well as the absence of breathing. Some of the other requirements FDA may require include:

- battery back-up that can supply power for at least eight hours

- both audio and visual alarms

- sensors that can detect improper equipment performance, such as damaged electrodes and disconnected or improperly connected lead wires

- safeguards that prevent inadvertent or unauthorized disabling of the alarms. In some models, for example, an alarm that sounds distinctly different from the alarm that signals apnea sounds whenever the machine is turned off or unplugged without following a set procedure

- a remote alarm unit.

The remote enables parents to leave the baby's room to carry on some of their usual activities. However, parents shouldn't get too far away, warns James J. McCue Jr., director of FDA's office of standards and regulations in the agency's Center for Devices and Radiological Health.

"Once the alarm goes off, you only have a short time to get back and get that child revived before there's a possibility of permanent brain damage," says McCue. "So you don't want parents out in the garden who won't be able to run fast enough to get there in time."

## False Alarms and Missed Alarms

Apnea monitors are not perfect. "Most apnea monitors will miss some apneas," says FDA in its February 1990 safety alert letter "Important Tips for Apnea Monitor Users." The agency adds that false alarms can't be completely avoided either.

Probably the most common reason for a false alarm is shallow breathing, says Rochester's Brooks. "The baby may be doing more abdominal breathing, so the chest wall where the electrodes are isn't moving enough to register," he explains.

Another common reason is loosened wires connecting the electrodes to the monitor. This is a frequent problem because babies move around while they sleep.

FDA advises that parents be tolerant of false alarms and continue to use the monitor as instructed. "The monitor can only do its job if it is turned on and properly connected to your baby," according to the safety alert.

FDA warns, however, that while adjustments in the monitor or placement of the electrodes may help decrease the number of false alarms, parents shouldn't make those adjustments themselves; that's a job for the health professionals in charge of the baby's care.

There are also situations in which the alarms might not go off even though the baby has stopped breathing. For example, parents should not have the baby sleep in their bed because their movements might be picked up by the monitor. Other sources of interference with proper monitor function include:

- electrical appliances such as electric blankets, electric waterbed heaters, TV sets, air conditioners, and remote telephones. Keep these sources of interference at least a foot away from the monitor.

- radio signals from police stations, fire stations, or airports. In some locations such interference may keep the monitor from working properly.

Other tips from FDA's letter include:

- Keep children and pets away from the monitor and the baby to prevent the monitor from being accidentally disconnected.

- Test the monitor before each use to ensure the alarm is working.

- Make sure the monitor's breath detection indicator light flashes only once for each breath the baby takes while the baby is still. (The light may also flash when the baby moves.) If the baby is still and the light does not flash in unison with his or her breathing, contact your equipment provider immediately.

- Make sure battery and charger connections are tight. If the monitor has a light that indicates when the battery is charging, it should not flicker when the connectors are gently wiggled or twisted.

- Follow the manufacturer's recommendations and report problems to the monitor provider or, if the provider can't help you, to the manufacturer.

"It's important for parents to be as well acquainted with the monitor as they can be so they'll be able to detect problems right away," says Wally Pellerite, a consumer safety officer with FDA's Center for Devices and Radiological Health.

He says that there have been several recalls of apnea monitors over the last three years due to problems in the design or production of the devices, and while it is the distributor's and manufacturer's responsibility to notify parents about defective monitors, "it's a good idea for parents to keep the lines of communication open" with the monitor provider.

### Memory Monitors

There is no way to distinguish between false and real apnea episodes when the alarm first sounds. But even after the parents reach their baby's side, it may not be clear what happened to set off the alarm. Dorothy Bunn remembers bolting out of bed whenever her son Michael's monitor alarm sounded. "My adrenaline would really be pumping," she said. Yet, as often as the alarm sounded—"one night it went off 17 times," she said—he was always breathing when she reached his crib. "In some cases, the alarm itself will wake the baby up [and breathing will start again]," says Meny. So, while the alarm may signal a true apnea episode, parents have no way of knowing because the situation has resolved by the time they reach the crib.

Sometimes, upon hearing the alarm, parents run into the room and pick up the baby without pausing to see if the baby has truly stopped breathing. This can make it hard to determine if it was really an instance of apnea. Although it is recommended that parents turn on the light and look for signs of breathing before taking any action, it isn't easy for many parents to follow those instructions, says Brooks.

"It's hard for parents to hear an alarm, be afraid their baby's dying, run into the room, and before they touch the baby stand there and calmly assess everything," says Brooks. But whether the baby is truly not breathing or just taking shallow breaths, immediately picking the baby up frequently results in the baby taking a deep breath and waking up, and "we don't have a clue whether that was a real alarm or not."

Though parents have no way of distinguishing a false alarm from a real one if the baby is breathing when they get there, some monitors are equipped to solve the mystery after the event. Monitors with computer memories can store information, such as the length of time the monitor didn't detect any breathing and what the heart rate was. (The proposed FDA standard does not require a memory for minimum safety and effectiveness.)

Other advantages of memory monitors include:

- detecting loose lead wires: Unlike a true problem, in which the heart rate gradually drops, a loose lead wire will cause recorded heart rate to drop abruptly.

- recording how much the heart rate dropped: "Say we set the monitor to alarm if the heart rate drops below 80 beats per minute," says Teri Reid, R.N., director of the apnea clinic at Children's Hospital in Washington, D.C. "But how low did it go? Did it go to 75 or to 45? There's no way parents can know that in the home. But we know when we get the printout [from the memory]. It affects what kind of medical treatment we might give that baby."

- ensuring that parents use the machine: Memory monitors keep date and time records of when the machine is in use.

"I think memory is vital," says Meny. "I think every monitor that goes out on every baby in this country should have memory built into it, period."

Brooks disagrees. "Memory isn't essential for every baby. It is, however, an important tool when a baby has a lot of alarms that we just can't explain."

## Life with a Monitor

"I have the feeling that in the beginning several parents not only did not leave the monitor, but sat and watched it blink as well," writes Anne Barr in her booklet *At Home With a Monitor, A Guide for Parents*.

"It's very stressful," says Patricia Hughson, whose son Hassan was on a home monitor until he was 8 months old. "You're anxious about using it. You don't know what's going to happen."

According to a report from the 1986 NIH Consensus Development Conference on Infantile Apnea and Home Monitoring, the parental stress comes not only from the full-time responsibility of monitoring but also from assuming the responsibility for resuscitating a baby who stops breathing.

In addition, monitors invade every aspect of day-to-day life, says Brooks. "Because they're afraid they'll miss an alarm, many parents won't take a shower, go get the mail, or even turn on the TV in another room," says Brooks.

"There were times when it was definitely an inconvenience," Hughson says. "He slept in the room with us the first three months he was home, and if he moved the wrong way, it would go off. Of course, that would be at 2 a.m., and then just as we would doze off, he'd wake up for a 2:30 or 3 a.m. feeding."

She adds, however, that having the monitor, overall, was wonderful because on three occasions Hassan, who was born almost three months prematurely, did stop breathing.

While the stress of home monitoring is very real, it can be minimized if the parents have support. "We make sure to train our parents in CPR," says Meny. "We're also available to the parents 24 hours a day, seven days a week, and we make sure that the vendors of the home monitors are also available around the clock."

Parents of babies in the apnea clinic program at Children's Hospital in Washington, D.C., are assigned a visiting nurse. "The nurse goes to the house within 24 hours after the baby leaves the hospital," says Reid. "She reviews how to use the monitor and checks the baby's room to make sure nothing like humidifiers will interfere with the monitor's operation."

Reid has also set up a phone support program that puts parents in touch with each other. "I tried to start a support group here at the hospital, but it was too much trouble for the parents to get down here with their babies—and, of course, the monitors-in tow. It's much easier for them to call each other whenever they have a free moment."

Even the best of support programs cannot change the fact that monitor technology is still imperfect, and even when the monitor works as intended it can't save a baby's life.

"Sometimes the alarms will go off, and the parents respond appropriately, and still the baby dies," says Brooks. "It's not 100 percent effective. It seems like such a clear-cut way to prevent a baby' s death, but it's nowhere near as clear-cut and straightforward as it seems at first blush."

## Does Apnea Cause SIDS?

Talking about infant apnea without talking about sudden infant death syndrome is nearly impossible. But while apnea is of considerable interest to SIDS researchers, whether apnea causes SIDS is still unknown.

In the United States, between 5,000 and 7,000 infants die each year from SIDS, making it the leading cause of death in children between the ages of one month and one year, according to the national Centers for Disease Control in Atlanta. The incidence of SIDS has remained fairly constant since it was first recognized as a specific medical entity 20 years ago, even though infant mortality has been reduced overall.

Infants thought to be at high risk for SIDS include:

- babies born prematurely
- babies exposed before birth to drugs such as heroin or cocaine
- babies who survived an apparent life-threatening event
- twins of SIDS victims

Whether subsequent siblings of SIDS victims are at increased risk is controversial. "However, the anxiety of parents of siblings is often so intense that these babies are frequently treated as high-risk by the clinician," says pediatrician Robert G. Meny, M.D., of the University of Maryland.

—*Dori Stehlin*

Chapter 14

# Work Related Disorders

*Chapter Contents*

Section 14. 1—Lung Hazards in the Work Place .......................... 540
Section 14. 2—Farmers' Lung: Agricultural Lung Hazards ....... 545
Section 14. 3—Asbestos ................................................................ 554
Section 14. 4—Black Lung: Coal Worker's Pneumoconiosis
 and Exposure to Other Carbonaceous Dusts ..... 559
Section 14. 5—Facts About Fiberglass ........................................ 567
Section 14. 6—Irritant Gases ...................................................... 571
Section 14. 7—Silicosis ................................................................ 575

## Section 14.1

## Lung Hazards In The Workplace

Source: American Lung Association Pub. No. 0210. Used by permission.

### Lung Hazards in the Workplace

Millions of workers in hundreds of occupations are exposed to health hazards in their workplaces because of substances in the air they breathe on the job. Every year an estimated 65,000 U.S. workers develop a respiratory disease related to their jobs, and an estimated 25,000 persons die from occupational lung diseases.

### Who Is in Danger?

Lung diseases afflict workers wherever the air they breathe holds hazardous levels of dusts, sprays, fumes, gases, vapors, or radioactive materials. And the problem is becoming more complex and more dangerous to a greater number of people as industrial production of toxic substances increases in volume. New substances whose dangers are not yet fully understood expose workers to unknown hazards. Pollution in the atmosphere adds to the hazards. And workers who smoke cigarettes may significantly increase their risk of death or disability from some occupational lung diseases.

### How Do You Get an Occupational Lung Disease?

Breathing in hazardous substances can lead to a number of lung diseases as well as disease elsewhere in the body, such as nervous system disorders caused by solvent vapors. Occupational lung disease most often develops when a worker repeatedly breathes in air that contains a damaging substance. The substance may have an odor and be irritating, like formaldehyde, or it may be unnoticeable, like carbon monoxide.

Healthy lungs usually are able to withstand temporary assaults by these invaders. But disease develops when the lungs are exposed repeatedly or if the agent remains in the lung, as asbestos does, and lung tissue damage increases day after day, year after year. And because cigarette smoking also irritates the lungs and impairs their self-cleaning ability, smokers may be at greater risk of developing some lung diseases than are non-smokers.

Hazards in the air cause lung diseases in several ways. They may irritate and damage lung tissues, and eventually destroy breathing ability. They may cause diseases like bronchitis, fibrosis and lung cancer. Some may be antigens, which are substances that can cause a hypersensitive or allergic reaction and narrow the airways of susceptible persons. Occupational asthma can develop in such persons within a few years of repeated exposure to antigens. Some substances noted for causing these reactions in workers are detergent enzymes, phthalic anhydride, trimellitic anhydride, platinum salts, cereals and grains, fungi and spores, western red cedar dust, and isocyanates.

Some job hazards, such as phosgene gas, can damage the lungs instantly. These medical emergencies usually result from accidents; they are not discussed in this chapter.

### What Kinds of Substances Are Dangerous

Hazardous materials take many forms, including dusts, fumes, smoke, gases, vapors, mists, and radioactive materials. They are produced in different ways and are associated with different types of jobs.

- **DUSTS:** Many hazardous substances are in the form of dusts. They may be minerals like silica, asbestos, coal, kaolin, mica, and talc. Some dusts come from living materials like cereal grains, coffee beans, paprika, cotton, and flax. Other dusts are chemicals in powder form like enzyme powders, pesticides and dyes. Dusts cause various illnesses such as bronchitis, asthma, and cancer.

- **FUMES:** Fumes are formed when solids—usually metals—are heated to become vapors, then cool quickly and condense into fine, solid particles carried in the air. Fumes that cause lung disease may come from nickel, cadmium, chromium, and beryllium, among others. Breathed into the lungs, these particles can cause lung inflammation, bronchitis, metal fume fever, and lung cancer. Workers in industrial high heat operations like welding, smelting, furnace work, and pottery-making are most often exposed.

- **SMOKE:** Smoke is formed by burning organic materials. It contains a variety of dusts, gases, and vapors, depending upon what is burning. Severe cases of smoke inhalation are well known to cause death and injury to fire-fighters.

- **GASES:** Gases are among the most dangerous agents found in the workplace. Some can suffocate a person by displacing oxygen in the air. Others are poisonous to body systems. Many gases can damage the lungs by irritating lung tissues or causing severe hypersensitivity reactions. Gases on the job are produced by chemical reactions and high heat operations like welding, brazing, smelting, oven drying, and furnace work.

- **VAPORS:** Although some liquids do not vaporize much at working temperatures, all liquids do give off a gaseous form called a vapor. In the lungs, vapors act the same way as gases. Vapors that can damage the lungs usually irritate the nose and throat first—a valuable warning sign. Some, such as water vapors, are not harmful, but other vapors, like solvents, can cause serious illness.

- **MISTS OR SPRAYS:** Mists contain tiny droplets of liquid suspended in air or in a propellant gas. They are widely used in applying substances like paints, lacquers, hair spray, pesticides, cleaning products, acids, and solvents. Sometimes they are produced as nuisance by-products, as mists from cutting tool oil used in machine tool workshops. The amount of lung damage they can do depends on the content of the mist, its temperature and its concentration. Conditions that may be caused include irritation, asthma, bronchitis, and chemical damage to lungs.

- **RADIATION:** Radiation is a hazard threatening a growing number of workers—in the mining of radioactive ores, in industry, and in medicine. Breathing in radioactive gases or dusts can cause lung cancer.

## How to Make the Workplace Safer

Making a safer workplace is not always complicated or expensive, although it may sometimes be. The best way is to prevent hazardous conditions. New plants can be designed so problems are minimized in the structure and process before building. Where hazards are present, there are four basic approaches to controlling the hazards.

1. **CHANGE PROCEDURES:** Change ingredients, work practices, or machinery to reduce hazards in the air or separate people from them. For example,

   —Loose powders can be handled in solution or as compressed pellets or briquettes.

   —Steel shot or grit may be used instead of silica sand in abrasive blasting.

   —The filling of vats by hand can be replaced by automatic filling in which the containers remain closed to prevent dusts and vapors from escaping into the air.

2. **IMPROVE VENTILATION:** Ventilation systems can remove hazards from the air to reduce exposure and prevent build-up. General ventilation of the workplace dilutes pollutants and may be acceptable for substances of low toxicity. Local exhaust ventilation is used to extract polluted air at the point where it is generated by a hazardous process or machine and is the preferred method for substances of low toxicity.

3. **TRAIN WORKERS:** Training of workers will help minimize exposure to toxic materials. Workers should learn about the toxic effects of materials in the workplace and what the proper work procedures are.

4. **USE PERSONAL PROTECTIVE EQUIPMENT:** Respirators should be used only if hazards cannot be controlled in other ways. They should be used as temporary measures until proper engineering controls are installed in the workplace. Respirators are difficult to use but can provide protection if

they are selected according to the hazard, properly fitted, and properly maintained. It is absolutely essential for workers to be properly fitted and trained and periodically re-fitted and re-trained in their use. Management should have a program that provides for proper maintenance of personal protective equipment. For example, sand-blasters use supplied-air respirators to protect them from dust. All respirators must be carefully cleaned after each use and meticulously checked and maintained to remain in good working order.

## What Else Can Be Done?

Air in the workplace does not have to be dirty. The technology is available now to avoid most health hazards. But the actions needed to accomplish that involve everyone.

**Employers**, under federal law, have basic responsibility for workplace conditions. They need to know the hazards associated with their operations and the products they handle. Safe work practices must be observed. Just as some employers have made great gains in reducing workers' accidental injuries, it is possible to improve protection of employees from occupational diseases.

**Government Agencies** charged with the protection of public health must continue to set and enforce standards for worker health. Manufacturers must provide information about the substances used in their products. Where legislation is needed, public support is vital.

**Health Professionals** need to know how to detect occupational lung diseases; also to discover lung diseases from the use of new products and processes.

**Students** need to learn about potential hazards as they learn trades and professions.

**Engineers and Architects** need to know how to design, build and maintain safe workplaces.

**Workers** need to be alert and concerned about the possible effects of their working environment on their health. Under the law, an employee has a right to know if workplace conditions may be hazardous, to be protected from hazards, and to refuse hazardous work. The employee also has a responsibility to comply with hazard control measures such as using protective equipment.

**Smoking** adds to the health risks of people who work with hazardous substances. For example, studies of asbestos workers who

## Work Related Disorders

smoke have shown they are 50 times as likely to get lung cancer as the worker who does not smoke and does not work with asbestos.

**Hobbies** can add risk, too. Be informed about any products used at home. Many of the fumes, dusts, sprays, and chemicals used in arts and crafts can be damaging to lungs.

## Section 14.2

## *Agricultural Lung Hazards*

Source: American Lung Association Pub. No. 0213. Used by permission.

### What Are Agricultural Lung Hazards?

Agricultural lung hazards are harmful levels of chemicals or other substances in the air. These substances are in the form of dust, sprays, gases, vapors, fumes or mists, and are produced from materials found on farms and in areas where there is agricultural work.

Agricultural lung hazards may come from several sources—grain, moldy hay, animal confinement buildings, animal manure pits, grain bins, silos, farm machinery operations, and agricultural chemicals in pesticides. Exposure may result from inhaling substances that can cause lung disease ranging from mild discomfort to chronic disabling lung disease and death. Agricultural workers may contract lung diseases if they are not adequately protected while working in areas where the air contains hazardous levels of dangerous substances.

### Who Is in Danger?

Agricultural workers, their families, and veterinarians are at risk of developing agricultural lung disease. Agricultural workers who smoke tobacco face an even greater risk of disability or death from some agricultural lung diseases. Tobacco smoke together with inhalation of some airborne hazardous substances produce a risk greater than that presented by either the hazardous substance or the cigarette smoke acting alone.

## How Can Grain Handling Cause Lung Disease?

Grain dust contains dust from the grain itself, dust derived from straw, insect parts, rodent hairs, animal waste, pesticides, mold spores, grain preservatives, and field dust. Grain handling performed without adequate ventilation, equipment, and protective devices can expose the worker to harmful dust particles. Inhaling these particles may cause coughing, asthma, chronic bronchitis, and "grain fever," an acute symptom complex causing fever, coughing, breathing difficulty, and weakness. Exposure to grain dust particles can also cause eye and skin irritation.

### Protection/Prevention

A NIOSH-approved air-purifying respirator and goggles will decrease inhalation of hazardous dusts and eye irritation. The proper use of respirators requires using the right filters, frequently changing the filter cartridges, and making sure the respirator fits securely to prevent unfiltered air from leaking in around the edge of the mask. The use of vacuum cleaning equipment, rather than dry sweeping, will also decrease dust exposure. Grain handling in areas that have a continuous circulation of large volumes of fresh air will decrease the hazard of inhaling harmful levels of dusts. Good cleaning practices and elevator maintenance will help keep dust levels down. Many of the short and long-term lung diseases of grain handling can be avoided if these precautions, including not smoking, are taken.

## How Can Moldy Hay Cause Lung Disease?

Hay and grain that is stored wet will heat and foster growth of mold which releases very tiny spores. These spores remain in the hay long after mold growth has stopped. When the hay is handled later, the farm worker inhales vast numbers of microscopic spores causing a hypersensitivity reaction in some individuals. Four to twelve hours after inhaling the spores, the susceptible exposed farmer develops a flu-like illness known as Farmer's Lung with chills, fever, cough and shortness of breath. These symptoms are often mistaken for a viral illness or common cold and may last for one night or several days. The chances of developing these same symptoms whenever exposure to moldy hay occurs will be increased. Eventually, they become so severe that the victim may no longer be able to work. After repeated expo-

## Work Related Disorders

sure, chronic lung disease may develop with scarring of lung tissue, shortness of breath, and coughing. However, often the symptoms of Farmer's Lung consist only of a cough or frequent chest colds. There are other lung diseases with symptoms like those associated with Farmer's Lung that can result from the inhalation of fungal spores or dusts from organic materials.

Mycotoxicosis is another acute illness with similar symptoms. It is caused by the inhalation of mold spores that grow on the surface of moldy corn silage or grain. It is not an allergic reaction but a toxic reaction found in everyone who inhales very large amounts of the spores. There is an immediate reaction ranging from a mild cough to severe shortness of breath and is thought to be produced by the toxic effects of the "mycotoxins" found in molds. It is not known whether the respiratory symptoms result from dust, toxins, or both.

*Protection/Prevention*

Inhalation of mold spores can be avoided by the use of a NIOSH-approved air-purifying respirator for particulates and the proper handling and storage of hay. Moldy hay should be handled and stored where there is an adequate supply of fresh air circulating. Respirator masks should be appropriately selected, well fitted, and the filters changed frequently. Farm workers who find that they are ill or have a fever after pitching or handling moldy hay should seek medical attention.

### *The Dangers of Working in Animal Confinement Buildings*

Dusts and gases produced in animal confinement buildings present lung hazards.

- **DUSTS:** Dust from feed, animal hair and skin, and dried animal waste exists as very small particles that may be inhaled into the lungs. Surveys of workers who repeatedly enter animal confinement buildings and veterinarians who are frequently in and out of these buildings show that there is a high incidence of complaints such as coughing, shortness of breath, headache, and nasal irritation. Household members of these workers may also be exposed to dust carried home on work clothing.

- **GASES:** Manure pits in animal confinement buildings are designed to collect thousands of gallons of manure and urine for eventual use as fertilizer. Bacterial reaction of manure produces toxic levels of gases such as hydrogen sulfide and ammonia, as well as carbon dioxide and methane. During agitation and emptying of the pit, the release of hydrogen sulfide, a very toxic gas, may result in poisoning, causing death of the farm worker and animals.

There are other health hazards associated with exposure to gases found in and around manure pits. Toxic or poisonous gaseous reactions can occur and in high concentrations, some of the gases released by manure fermentation such as methane are explosive.

## Lung Diseases Associated with Working with Animals

Two common diseases associated with working with animals are asthma and hypersensitivity pneumonitis.

**ASTHMA** is a lung disease in which the bronchial airways overreact to dusts, vapors, gases or fumes that exist in the workplace. When these irritants are inhaled, the airway muscles tighten, the tissues swell, too much mucus is produced—all making breathing difficult. Field dust and animal hairs can cause serious episodes of breathing difficulty in allergic persons. Permanent lung damage can result if exposure continues to the substance that causes the asthma.

**HYPERSENSITIVITY PNEUMONITIS** results from the lung's alveoli (air sacs) reaction to inhaled dusts containing antigens (the offending agent). The antigens come from molds, various microorganisms, and animal proteins. Symptoms begin some hours after exposure to the offending dust and include tiredness, shortness of breath, a dry cough, fever, and chills. The symptoms may last from one to ten days. Farmer's Lung is one type of hypersensitivity disease, and perhaps, the most common. Other forms of hypersensitivity pneumonitis have been associated with raising pigeons, working with chickens and turkeys, and raising mushrooms.

*Protection/Prevention*

The appropriate NIOSH-approved air-purifying respirator mask will reduce the amount of dust inhaled into the lungs. Masks should be well-fitted and carefully cleaned after each use. They should be checked regularly to assure they are in good working condition, and replaced when they no longer perform properly. Adequate ventilation is extremely important in reducing the amount of exposure to dusts and toxic gases. However, for protection against prolonged exposure to high concentrations of toxic gases, a NIOSH-approved supplied-air mask is required. The amount of air supplied should be sufficient to avoid the dangerous risk of running out of breathing oxygen. The wearer may need a second, emergency source of breathing oxygen to enable him or her to leave the hazardous area safely. For environments with reduced oxygen content or highly toxic gases present, a supplied-air respirator should be used. Information on the proper use of supplied-air respirators should be obtained from the County Agricultural Agent, the state Occupational Health Bureau or local Fire Department. Agricultural workers should be familiar with the characteristics of toxic gases produced in confinement buildings. Some toxic gases are odorless and cannot be detected by smell. Contact your local American Lung Association for a copy of the *Agricultural Lung Hazards - Airborne Hazards Recognition Chart*.

## The Dangers of Working in Silos

When silage ferments, nitrogen dioxide known as "silo gas" is produced. Most silo gas forms during the first two weeks after corn or hay has been harvested and stored in the silo. The highest concentrations of gas are reached during the first 48 hours after filling the silo. This gas is poisonous and can injure or kill both people and livestock. Breathing low concentrations of this gas can cause coughing, choking, tightness in the chest, and nausea (Silo Filler's Disease). Symptoms can develop within a few minutes of exposure or may not appear until several hours after the exposure to silo gas. At higher concentrations it can cause pulmonary edema (fluid in the lungs) which may result in immediate death. Even after recovery from exposure, scarring of the lungs may occur after two or three weeks and can be fatal. Inhalation of the gas may also lead to chronic bronchitis or emphysema.

A related problem occurs in grain storage bins or silos where wet grain produces carbon dioxide. At high enough concentrations carbon dioxide can displace oxygen, causing unconsciousness and death when the worker enters the grain bin.

## Protection/Prevention

The silo should not be entered during the first two weeks after filling, particularly during the first 48 hours. At any time if it is necessary to enter the silo, the silo blowers or ventilation fans should be turned on. Chute doors should be kept open down to the level of the silage to prevent high concentrations of silo gas from accumulating. The air should be allowed to circulate for at least 30 minutes before anyone enters the silo, and the blower should be left on while the worker is inside the silo.

## Harmful Effects Caused by Agricultural Chemicals

Severe respiratory problems can result from unsafe handling of pesticides, fertilizers, and other agricultural chemicals. People who both smoke and work with these chemicals are at an even greater risk of developing lung diseases.

### Pesticides, Herbicides, and Fungicides

Pesticides, herbicides, and fungicides can cause serious health problems if they are not handled properly. Pesticides are used on or around livestock, field and nursery crops, as well as landscape areas. Dips, sprays, liquid pour-ons, and salves are some of the commonly used pesticide application techniques. Herbicides are applied by spraying techniques and are used for weed control and vegetation control for land clearance. Fungicides are used to control the growth of fungi on stored grain.

Some pesticides used today are related to the chemicals originally used as nerve gases during World War II. Pesticides and herbicides enter the body through breathing, swallowing, or skin and eye absorption. Breathing or skin absorption can be followed by wheezing, coughing, muscle aches, increased saliva production, stomach cramps, and diarrhea. The gradual accumulation of these poisons in the body can affect body systems including the lungs and the respiratory system. In severe cases, paralysis and death may result. Fungicides, carbon tetrachloride being the most widely used, are often applied in closed spaces, potentially resulting in unconsciousness of the worker.

# Work Related Disorders

*Protection/Prevention*

Protective gloves, clothing, and goggles will prevent chemicals from being absorbed through the skin or damaging the eyes. A chemical respirator specifically designed for workers who handle these chemicals can protect the worker from inhaling dangerous fumes, mists or vapors. Eating and drinking near chemicals should be avoided at all times, but if it must be done, extreme care should be taken to avoid food contamination. Thorough and frequent hand-washing and careful food and utensil storage and disposal is a must to protect against accidental swallowing of chemicals. It is important to read and follow the manufacturer's instructions when handling all chemicals.

*Fertilizers*

Anhydrous ammonia is an effective fertilizer. However, it is toxic and highly irritating to the eyes and mucous membranes. The chemical should be applied and handled with care. Anhydrous ammonia dissolves immediately on any moist surface to form a strong caustic that can cause skin, eye, and mouth burns. When concentrated vapor is inhaled, it will burn the lungs and may result in death. Acute symptoms such as breathing difficulty, and coughing may appear immediately after exposure.

*Protection/Prevention*

Farm workers who handle ammonia are subject to accidental exposure to the liquid or the vapor. Respirators specifically intended for use by workers who use ammonia are available but tend to saturate quickly in high concentrations. For brief ammonia exposures, eye, skin and respiratory protection is helpful. Goggles, gloves, protective clothing and NIOSH-approved respirators should be worn. To avoid exposure to high concentrations, in addition to personal protective devices, adequate ventilation is critical. For ammonia spills and for skin burns, immediate flushing with large amounts of water can save eyesight and lives. All transport and application vehicles should have a filled five gallon water container at all times. Burn victims should be seen by a doctor immediately.

## What Are the Lung Hazards of Farm Machinery Operations?

Hazards associated with industrial processes are not confined to factories. Carbon monoxide produced by gas engines and by heaters operated in poorly ventilated spaces can cause unconsciousness and sudden death. This odorless and colorless gas creates an all too frequent hazard to the unsuspecting worker.

The best protection against carbon monoxide exposure is good ventilation when gas heaters and gas engines are running. Some other potential hazards associated with farm machinery operations are inhalation of welding fumes and developing silicosis from sand-blasting. Contact your local American Lung Association for more information on these and other lung hazards.

### Selection of Respirators

Respirators must be selected according to the type of hazard to which the wearer will be exposed. The federal government's Occupational Safety and Health Administration (OSHA) requires that respirators approved by the Mine Safety & Health Administration (MSHA) or the National Institute for Occupational Safety and Health (NIOSH) be used.

A large variety of respirators are available. Air-purifying devices clean the air as it passes from the workplace into the lungs, whereas supplied-air systems insulate the wearer from the surrounding air and supply a separate, clean source of air or oxygen.

**Air-purifying Devices.** These simple respirators are useful when the airborne hazards are in low concentrations and pose no immediate threat to life or a long term danger to health and when adequate amounts of oxygen are available.

The air-purifying respirator consists of a mask that fits snugly over the nose and the mouth and allows air to enter only through a filter or other air-purifying device. However, because faces vary so greatly in shape, size and structure, unfiltered air often leaks in around the edge of the mask. Filters should never be used for hazards other than the ones they are designed to protect against. Acceptable uses will be printed on the sides of the filter cartridge.

Air-purifying devices have a limited capacity. Filters can become clogged by dust, making breathing difficult; canisters used to absorb gases and vapors can become saturated and useless. Some air-purifying canisters for gases and vapors are designed to provide some sort of signal when they are approaching capacity. The wearer should be sure he or she will recognize the signal before using the device.

**Supplied-Air Systems.** Supplied-air systems fall into two groups: demand-type respirators, which supply air as the wearer needs it, and positive-pressure respirators, which continuously pump air into the mask, and maintain a higher pressure inside than outside the mask.

Like air-purifying devices, the effectiveness of demand-type respirators is limited by their fit, which when poor, allows air to leak in around the edges. They are valuable whenever conditions are such that air-purifying devices would rapidly become saturated and when the workplace has a low concentration of oxygen.

Positive-pressure air-supplied respirators are the only ones recommended for use in air that is immediately hazardous to health. Because these respirators maintain a higher pressure inside the mask than outside, air always leaks out, rather than in, thus keeping dangerous air away from the lungs.

With either type of supplied-air system, the fact that the air supply may become depleted must be considered. The wearer may need a second, emergency source of breathing oxygen to enable him or her to leave the hazardous area safely.

### Care of Respirators

All respirators should be carefully cleaned after each use, regularly checked to assure they are in good working condition and replaced when they no longer perform properly.

### Facts on Tobacco Smoking and Agricultural Workers

Tobacco smoking increases the risk of lung disease. Quitting the smoking habit is an important step toward taking personal responsibility for protection against lung disease.

Agricultural workers who smoke are more likely to develop serious chronic lung disease than those who don't smoke.

Grain workers who smoke have twice the incidence of lung disease as those who don't.

Smoking near pesticides or grain dust is dangerous. Pesticides are mixed with petroleum-based compounds and are highly flammable. Smoking near grain dust can cause an explosion.

Contact your local American Lung Association for more information on many other lung diseases and for help with quitting the smoking habit.

*Remember! Take care of your lungs, they're only human.*

Section 4.3

# Asbestos

Source: American Lung Association Pub. No. 0206. Used by permission.

Asbestos is the general term given to a group of fluffy, fibrous minerals that resist heat and acid. Those characteristics make them valuable in many industries, but they can be harmful to workers who handle them without precautions.

Lung cancer is just one of a variety of illnesses that can be caused by asbestos particles. Your risk of developing that dreaded disease is increased many times when you combine cigarette smoking with asbestos exposure.

Breathing asbestos dust can cause lung scarring known as asbestosis. Persons who have asbestosis should seek medical advice for preventing pneumonia or influenza. Some asbestos workers develop mesothelioma, a rare form of cancer.

Asbestos-induced disease does not usually appear for 15 to 35 years after first exposure to asbestos.

## How Is Asbestos Used?

Asbestos is used to manufacture a wide variety of products. Many, including asbestos-cement pipe and sheet, roofing felt, asphalt coatings and flooring materials, are used in the construction industry.

## Work Related Disorders

Asbestos-containing brake and clutch linings, sealants, gaskets, and packings are widely used in the industrial and automotive fields. Asbestos is also used in some fireproof clothing and safety equipment.

In most modern products, the asbestos fibers are "locked-in" or encapsulated by binders such as cement, rubber or plastics so that the fibers are not easily released during normal use. Where there is a possibility of releasing dust during fabrication or removal of modern products, work practices must be established to maintain exposure well below allowable limits.

In the past, some friable (crumbly) asbestos-containing products, particularly those used for insulation, could release airborne asbestos when fabricated or handled. Most present-day insulation products no longer contain asbestos. However, workers employed in demolition, maintenance, or remodeling are likely to encounter old asbestos-containing insulation products when working on buildings or plant facilities. Both management and workers in these industries must comply with the guidelines set forth by the federal government to prevent hazardous exposures.

During World War II as many as 4.5 million Americans may have been exposed to asbestos in shipyards. Over one million persons are alive today who may have run the risk of exposure to asbestos.

### How Does Asbestos Cause Disease?

Asbestos fibers too fine to be seen can become airborne during mining and industrial processes. They are then inhaled and swallowed. Because of their size and needlelike shape, asbestos fibers can penetrate body tissues and remain for life.

As asbestos fibers build up, they produce chronic irritation. They cause scarring and thickening of your lungs' tiny air sacs or alveoli. Such scarring can interfere with the lungs' ability to get oxygen from air into blood and to remove carbon dioxide from the body. You have difficulty in breathing. The threats those asbestos fibers pose depend on amount and duration of exposure, individual susceptibility, smoking habits, and presence of other air pollutants.

Asbestos-related diseases develop slowly to undermine the health and shorten the lives of workers. Typically, the first 10 to 15 years after initial exposure to asbestos are free of signs or symptoms. After that time, early X-ray changes may appear.

## What Are the Health Warning Signals?

Asbestos can cause asbestosis, mesothelioma, and cancers of the respiratory and digestive systems.

Early *asbestosis* may be evidenced by chest X-rays before symptoms are present. In later stages, with a stethoscope, a doctor can hear a dry, crackling sound coming from your lungs during inhalation. Besides breathing difficulty, which causes a strain on the heart, the symptoms include a cough, increased sputum, and weight loss.

At the present time, over two-thirds of workers heavily exposed to asbestos for over 20 years under conditions which existed in the past have asbestosis.

*Lung cancer* is the most serious health risk to asbestos workers. It accounts for as much as 20 percent of all deaths among that occupational group. In the general population, four to five percent of deaths are caused by lung cancer. The disease is related to the amount of asbestos present in the lungs and to smoking.

Smoking greatly enhances the cancer-causing properties of asbestos. One study shows that the asbestos worker who smokes is 90 times as likely to get lung cancer as is one who has never worked with the fiber and does not smoke.

The primary symptom of lung cancer is a cough or a change in cough habit. Blood-streaked sputum and persistent chest pain unrelated to cough are also signs.

Diffuse malignant *mesothelioma* is a cancer of the chest lining and the membrane lining of the abdominal cavity. It is a rare primary tumor in the general population, constituting less than one percent of all cancers. The first symptom is usually shortness of breath or pain in the wall of your chest or abdomen. Although X-rays are of some help in diagnosing the disease, a tissue biopsy is required.

Cancers of the larynx, stomach, colon, and esophagus have been reported in heavily exposed asbestos workers. The asbestos fibers may reach the gastrointestinal tract by swallowing asbestos-contaminated mucus cleared from the lungs.

## How Can Asbestos-Related Diseases Be Prevented?

Federal regulations have been established to protect workers exposed to asbestos dust. Those Occupational Safety and Health Administration (OSHA) guidelines are designed to control exposure levels. To meet the specifications, employers must monitor dust levels, isolate dust-producing operations through engineering methods, promote good work practices, provide necessary personal safety equipment, and post caution signs in hazardous areas.

Individual health and safety precautions are essential. Wear protective clothes and follow safe work practices. Do not take work clothes home. Shower at the end of each shift. Store food, beverages, and personal belongings away from the work area. Never eat, drink, or smoke where asbestos is in use. Unrecognized exposures do occur, and unseen particles or fibers can be dangerous if breathed. If problems are recognized early, exposure levels can be reduced and complications treated. Therefore, you should have regular check-ups by your physician. If you smoke, the American Lung Association can help you quit. Even if you've smoked for years, you can decrease your disease risk by stopping the smoking habit. Practice good housekeeping while on the job to reduce dust.

If shortcomings are not corrected by employers or union representatives, you may initiate a complaint to OSHA for investigation, or request a NIOSH (National Institute for Occupational Safety and Health) Health Hazard Evaluation.

Since your family and friends may be exposed to dust carried home on work clothing, be especially sure to shower and change clothes at the job site.

Seek advice from an industrial hygienist or company health and safety director for information about your personal risk of asbestos exposure.

### Are Asbestos Substitutes Available?

Yes. One material currently being used as an alternative to asbestos insulation is fiberglass. It's a known skin irritant, but proof of it being a cancer-causing agent in humans has not been demonstrated.

### Risk Occupations

The following workers might be exposed to asbestos. Check to see if asbestos is a danger in your specific job.

Asbestos-asphalt makers
Asbestos cement makers

Asbestos insulation workers
Asbestos mill workers
Asbestos plaster makers
Asbestos rock workers
Asbestos weavers
Automobile body repairers
Automobile mechanics
Boiler makers
Brake manufacturers and repairers
Building material manufacturers
Carpenters
Caulkers
Clutch plate manufacturers
Construction workers
Demolition workers
Dock workers
Electrical appliance manufacturers
Electricians
Engineers
Filtering material manufacturers
Floor tile makers
Gasket manufacturers
Heating equipment workers
Insulation workers
Laggers
Laundry workers
Longshoremen
Machinists
Maintenance workers
Masons
Miners
Munitions manufacturers
Painters
Pipe coverers
Pipe cutters
Plumbers
Putty manufacturers
Railroad workers
Repairers
Roofers
Rubber workers

## Work Related Disorders

Sailors
Service station attendants
Ship builders
Steam fitters
Textile manufacturers
Transportation workers
Welders
Welding rod manufacturers
Wire manufacturers

## Section 14.4

# Black Lung:
# Coal Workers' Pneumoconiosis
# And Exposure To Other Carbonaceous Dusts

Source: U.S. Department of Health and Human Services Pub. No. 86-102.

## Introduction

Historical accounts of "Miners' Black Lung" date to 1831. Since that time, numerous clinical and epidemiological studies have documented the existence of Coal Workers' Pneumoconiosis (CWP) and associated lung impairment among miners. Extensive British prospective studies have established dose-response relationships between CWP and respirable coal mine dust. The Federal Coal Mine Health and Safety Act of 1969 (P.L. 91-173) established a coal mine dust standard (based upon the British data); mandated provisions for other safety and health standards; provided health surveillance, transfer rights, and rate retention for miners; provided federal compensation for "Black Lung"; and guaranteed NIOSH right of entry for further research in coal mining. In many ways, this Act served as a model for subsequent legislation and health standards from other exposures (see Table 14.1).

Because of the importance of coal as an energy source, and because of our vast coal resources, coal dust and coal products (synfuels) will continue to be produced for decades to come (see Figure 14.5 and

559

Tables 14.2 and 14.3). Graphite and carbon black represent other important carbonaceous exposures found in dozens of commercial processes in several industries; these exposures will also continue and expand in the years to come. Therefore it is essential to understand the biological effects of these exposures and how these effects may be mitigated or prevented.

## Definition

In discussing coal workers' pneumoconiosis or pneumoconiosis arising from carbon dust exposure, it is essential to define pneumoconiosis and the popular term "Black Lung." Coal Workers' Pneumoconiosis (CWP) and carbon pneumoconiosis are specific diseases resulting from the inhalation and deposition in the lung of carbonaceous dust and the lung's reaction to the dust so deposited. In CWP, the disease is manifest characteristically by the coal macule and later by coal micro-nodules and nodules resulting in simple coal workers' pneumoconiosis. In some cases large (1-3 cm) lesions, or even massive consolidated lesions, develop resulting in progressive massive fibrosis (PMF).

"Black Lung" is a legislatively defined term which encompasses the classical medical definition of coal workers' pneumoconiosis, but is defined by the Act as "a chronic dust disease of the lung arising out of employment in an underground coal mine." (Title IV—Black Lung Benefits—Part A—Federal Mine Safety and Health Act of 1977, P.L. 91-173 as amended by P.L. 95-164). This definition is used to cover disability primarily from chronic airways obstruction which is associated with coal mine dust exposure. Tuberculosis *per se* appearing in a coal miner has not qualified for benefits, nor has the development of other bacterial or viral illnesses, or lung cancer. In practice, however, miners with these and other chronic lung conditions who meet any of the qualifying criteria in the Act—if in the judgment of the examining physician and administrative law judge they have developed their condition in association with coal mine employment—may be compensated for total disability. Medical costs for these conditions have been paid by the Department of Labor. Thus the definition of "Black Lung" is broad and imprecise: it will not be discussed further in this chapter.

## Table 14.1

## COAL MINING HEALTH AND SAFETY LEGISLATION IN THE UNITED STATES

**1865:** Bill is introduced to create "Federal Mining Bureau." It is not passed.

**1910:** Bureau of Mines is established, but specifically denied right of inspection.

**1941:** Bureau of Mines is granted authority to inspect, but it is not given authority to establish or enforce safety codes (Title I Federal Coal Mine Safety Act).

**1946:** Federal Mine Safety Code for Bituminous Coal and Lignite Mines is issued by the Director, Bureau of Mines (agreement between Secretary of the Interior and the United Mine Workers of America) and included in the 1946 (Krug-Lewis) UMWA Wage Agreement.

**1947:** Congress requests coal mine operators and state agencies to report compliance with the Federal Mine Safety Code. Thirty-three percent compliance is reported.

**1952:** Title II of the Federal Coal Mine Safety Act is passed. All mines employing 15 or more persons underground must comply with the Act. Enforcement is limited to issuing orders of withdrawal for imminent danger or for failure to abate violations within a reasonable time.

**1966:** Amendments to 1952 law. Mines employing under 15 employees are included under 1952 Act; stronger regulatory powers are given to Bureau of Mines, such as the provision permitting the closing of a mine or section of a mine because of an unwarrantable failure to correct a dangerous condition.

**1969:** Federal Coal Mine Health and Safety Act is passed. In this Act the hazards of pneumoconiosis are, for the first time, given prominence, in addition to those of accidents.

**1972:** Black Lung Benefits Act of 1972 is passed. Several sections of Title IV are amended, liberalizing awarding of compensation benefits.

**1977:** Federal Mine Safety and Health Act of 1977 is passed. This Act amends Coal Mine Health and Safety Act of 1969 largely by adding health and safety standard setting, inspection, and research provisions for metal and nonmetal miners while leaving the 1969 Act largely intact. This Act also consolidated health and safety compliance activities for general industry (OSHA) and mining (MSHA) in the Department of Labor.

**1977:** Black Lung Benefits Revenue Act of 1977 was passed. This provided for an excise tax on the sale of coal by the producer to establish trust funds to pay black lung benefits.

**1977:** Black Lung Benefits Reform Act of 1977 was passed. This Act was passed to improve and further define provisions for awarding black lung benefits. Additionally, it established (a mandate) that a detailed study of occupational lung disease would be undertaken by the Department of Labor and NIOSH.

**1981:** Black Lung Benefits Revenue Act of 1981 was passed. This Act was passed to increase revenue for the Black Lung Disability Trust Fund, based on a new tax on coal with respect to sales after December 31, 1981

| Coal Type | Short Tons |
|---|---|
| Bituminous | 747,357 x $10^6$ |
| Sub-Bituminous | 485,766 x $10^6$ |
| Lignite | 478,134 x $10^6$ |
| Anthracite | 19,662 x $10^6$ |
| Total | 1,730,919,000,000 |

Source: (164)

*Table 14.2. U.S. Coal Reserves*

**Work Related Disorders**

ANTHRACITE

| Source | Short Tons |
|---|---|
| Strip Mine | 2,962,000 |
| Deep Mine | 595,000 |
| Culm Bank (Anthracite waste) | 1,480.000 |
| Total | 5,037,000 |

BITUMINOUS, SUB-BITUMINOUS AND LIGNITE

| Source | Short Tons |
|---|---|
| Strip Mine | 462,324,000 |
| Deep Mine | 306,344,000 |
| Total | 768,668,000 |

*DOE Data

Source: (81)

*Table 14.3. U.S. Coal Production for 1979 By Coal Rank And Type Of Mining*

| Work Area | Anthracite | Bituminous & Lignite |
|---|---|---|
| Underground Miners* | 483 | 141,065 |
| Surface Miners | 1,625 | 69,214 |
| Preparation Plant | 1,116 | 22,235 |
| Shop | 80 | 2,729 |
| Totals | 3,304 | 235,243 |

*Includes Mine Construction

Source: Personal Communication HSCAC, MSHA, Denver Federal Center, February 19, 1981.

*Table 14.4. Population At Risk To Exposure To U.S. Coals By Principal Work Area*

## Occupations and Industries Involved

Within coal mining, exposure is commonly divided into underground and surface operations. Coal mine construction is included legislatively, and properly so, as an underground mining exposure (see Table 14.4). Although most underground jobs result in heavier exposures to coal mine dust, certain surface jobs, particularly drillers, may have significant exposure to respirable coal dust and free silica.

Carbon black has been defined by the American Society for Testing and Materials as "a material consisting of elemental carbon in the form of near-spherical colloidal particles and coalesced particle aggregates of colloidal size, obtained from partial combustion or thermal decomposition of hydrocarbons." Carbon black is classified as furnace, thermal, or channel black depending on the manufacturing process.

As of 1976 there were eight companies operating 32 carbon black plants in the United States. Of the 2,924 million pounds sold domestically, 2,720 million were used in pigmenting and reinforcing rubber, 80 million in inks, 19 million in paints, and 3 million in the manufacture of paper. The remaining 102 million pounds were used in plastics, ceramics, foods, chemicals, and other products. The worker may be exposed during any of a number of processes including production, pelletizing, screening, packaging, loading, and unloading.

Graphite is widely used in a number of industrial applications and is the third major form of carbonaceous dust exposure. Graphite may be natural graphite, also called plumbago, or artificial or synthetic graphite. The difference is important from a respiratory disease standpoint in that natural graphite, which is mined from siliceous sediments (Sri Lanka, Madagascar, Italy, Brazil) may contain significant percentages of free silica (11% in Italian graphite). Synthetic graphite contains only traces of free silica except for pyrolitic graphite which may contain significant amounts of quartz and cristobalite.

## Estimate of Population at Risk and Disease Prevalence

Because of the extensive regulatory and health surveillance systems mandated by the Federal Coal Mine Health and Safety Act of 1969, reasonably good estimates may be made in regard to underground coal miners. Table 14.4 provides the most recent available figures on coal mining employment by type of coal mine and by type of

## Work Related Disorders

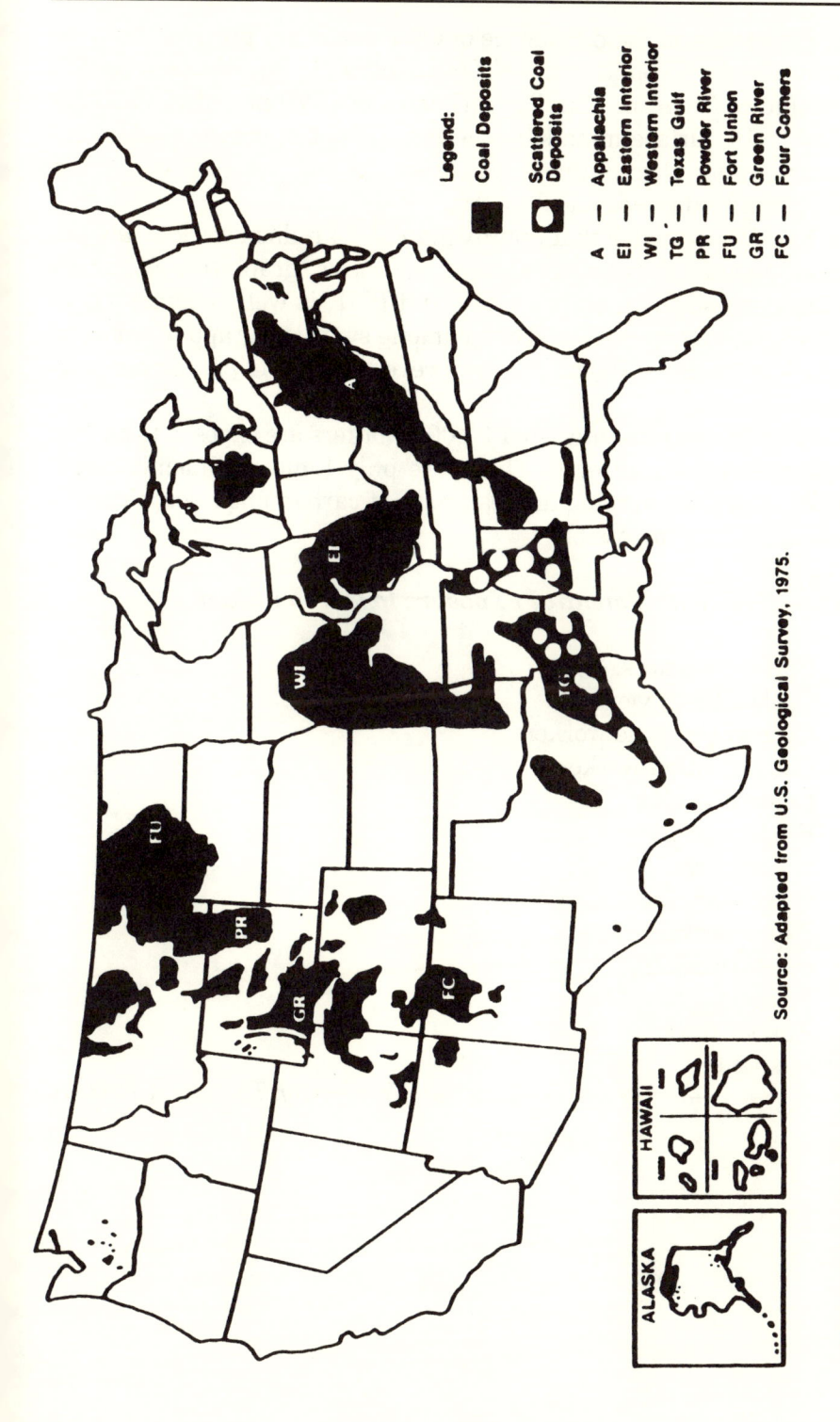

*Figure 14.5. Map Of Coal Deposits*

Source: Adapted from U.S. Geological Survey, 1975.

Legend:
- Coal Deposits
- Scattered Coal Deposits

- A — Appalachia
- EI — Eastern Interior
- WI — Western Interior
- TG — Texas Gulf
- PR — Powder River
- FU — Fort Union
- GR — Green River
- FC — Four Corners

coal. Estimates on the prevalence of CWP *per se* are provided from results of the third round of the NIOSH National Coal Workers' Health Surveillance Program. Similar estimates of CWP prevalence are not available for surface miners, as the Act did not mandate medical examinations for these miners and they are not yet covered by the health standard provision of the Act.

NIOSH estimates that approximately 2.4 million workers are potentially exposed to natural and synthetic graphites. Although pneumoconiosis, both simple CWP and PMF, is well documented in natural graphite workers and cited among synthetic graphite workers, the lack of epidemiological studies prevents making prevalence estimates.

NIOSH has estimated that 35,000 workers are exposed to carbon black directly or indirectly. There are only limited epidemiological studies available, making any estimate of carbon pneumoconiosis in these industries impossible.

*Occupations with Potential Exposure to Carbon Black*

Battery workers
Carbon black workers
Carbon electrode workers
Carburization workers
Cement workers
Food processors
Ink workers
Paint manufacture workers
Paper workers
Plastic workers
Printers
Rubber workers

—*James A. Merchant, Geoffrey Taylor, Thomas K Hodous*

Section 14.5

# Facts About Fiberglass

Source: American Lung Association   Pub. No. 0215.   Used by permission.

## What Is Fiberglass?

Fiberglass, sometimes called fibrous glass, is a man-made fiber in which the fiber-forming substance is glass. Fiberglass is used in various ways, such as reinforcing plastic materials in sports cars, boats and bathroom fixtures; as insulation in buildings, stoves, refrigerators and furnaces; and to manufacture certain textile products, such as fiberglass window drapes.

The structure and size of these glass fibers vary. The smaller fibers, which cannot be seen by the naked eye, are suspected of entering the lungs, while larger, visible fiberglass particles can be irritating to the skin, eyes, nose and throat.

## Who Is Exposed?

Workers in the building construction and maintenance industry, especially insulation workers, are at risk of exposure to fiberglass. Workers in the fiberglass manufacturing industry and automobile body repair workers may be exposed to the lung hazards of fiberglass and its associated chemicals in the work-place. According to the Federal Government, fiberglass is used in the manufacturing of about 20,000 products, and about 200,000 workers in the United States are exposed to it. "Do it yourself" homeowners who install fiberglass insulation or who disturb existing fiberglass insulation in the process of performing home repairs are also at risk.

## How Does Exposure Occur?

Workers using fiberglass may be exposed to airborne fibers from the fiberglass itself and to various chemicals associated with using it.

### Fiberglass

Direct contact with fiberglass materials or exposure to airborne fiberglass dust may irritate the skin, eyes, nose and throat. There is a possibility that these fibers cause permanent damage to the lungs or airways, or increase the likelihood of developing lung cancer. Inhaling the fibers may irritate the airways, resulting in cough and production of excess mucus, a condition known as bronchitis.

### Epoxy Resins

Epoxy resins are chemicals used in lacquers, varnishes and plastics, or in combination with other components to form plastics. They are also used to strengthen, harden, or give flexibility to fiberglass.

Breathing epoxy resins may cause chest tightness, shortness of breath or wheezing. Skin contact can cause rash.

### Styrene

Styrene is part of the polyester resin used with fiberglass. It is extremely irritating to the eyes and nose at low concentrations; at higher concentrations it causes headache, dizziness, and sometimes nausea.

### Acetone and MEK (Methyl Ethyl Ketone)

Acetone and MEK are commonly used solvents in fiberglass lay-up and spray-up. They are irritating to the eyes, nose and throat. Inhaling the vapors may cause drowsiness, breathing difficulties, and more serious damage to the lungs and nervous system.

## Prevention and Protection

There are several ways to reduce risks of exposure to fiberglass and the toxic substances often used with it.

### Laws

There are laws to protect workers from occupational hazards and risks. The Occupational Safety and Health Administration (OSHA), through the Hazard Communication Standard, requires that workers be informed about the occupational hazards they may be exposed to. Many states also have passed their own worker and/or community Right-to-Know laws.

*Work-place Environment*

- Adequate ventilation of the work area is very important.

- Employers should provide laundered work clothes or facilities in which to launder clothes.

- Washing facilities and showers should be made available to the workers to use before changing into street clothes.

- Vacuuming, wash-down procedures and wet sweeping can be helpful in reducing the dust associated with fiberglass. Dry sweeping or any other type of clean-up procedure that spreads the dust should be avoided.

Information on effective ventilation systems for dusts and solvents is available from state and federal Occupational Safety and Health Agencies, the National Safety Council, and the American Conference of Government Industrial Hygienists in its *Industrial Ventilation Manual*.

*Protective Clothing and Equipment*

- Gloves and other protective clothing can help prevent skin problems by reducing direct contact with glass fibers.

- Dust masks can help prevent or reduce the inhalation of small fiberglass particles.

- Goggles that fit properly can prevent eye irritation.

- Respirators, if properly selected, used and maintained, reduce the exposure to dusts, fibers and chemicals. Respirator selection is based on the size and concentration of the fiberglass particles.

Information on effective protective equipment is available from the state and federal Occupational Safety and Health Agencies, the National Safety Council, and the American Conference of Government Industrial Hygienists' *Industrial Ventilation Manual*.

**Work Practices and Personal Habits**

- Wash hands before eating and keep food away from the work-site.

- Eating, drinking and gum chewing at the work-site should be avoided.

- When using chemicals with fiberglass, always read and follow the manufacturer's instructions for reducing exposure.

- Be alert for possible breathing effects related to your workplace. Look out for chest tightness, wheezing, severe coughing or coughing that does not stop. If these conditions appear, see a doctor.

- Smoking cigarettes and/or marijuana may increase the risk of developing lung disease when combined with exposure to fiberglass and to chemicals used with it.

If you don't smoke, don't start. If you do smoke, your local American Lung Association can provide you with information about quitting.

Good work practices and personal habits help you to be a healthier worker.

**Work Related Disorders**

## Section 14.6

# *Irritant Gases*

Source: American Lung Association   Pub. No. 0208.   Used by permission.

Many workers are faced with dangerous gases on the job. This chapter tells about six of the gases: sulfur dioxide, chlorine, phosgene, ozone, nitrogen dioxide, and ammonia.

### Sulfur Dioxide

Sulfur dioxide is colorless and has a strong, suffocating odor. It combines easily with water vapor to become sulfurous acid or the corrosive, irritating mist sulfuric acid.

The combustion of fuels—particularly coal and oil-produces air-polluting oxides. Those sulfur oxides are also produced by chemical plants; petroleum refineries; the smelting of copper, lead, and zinc ores; and the burning of trash. Sulfur dioxide is used in the refrigeration industry and in bleaching beet sugar, manufacturing ice, and preserving fruit.

Persons exposed to sulfur dioxide show an increased susceptibility to lung infections. That is because the gas irritates the lining of your respiratory tract. Sulfur dioxide raises the risk of producing a chronic lung disease, notably bronchitis and emphysema, and aggravates existing lung conditions.

Certain people are particularly vulnerable even to relatively short-term exposures. Victims of lung ailments and cardiovascular diseases, the elderly, and children should be especially mindful of their contact with high sulfur dioxide levels. Cigarette smoking adds to the harmful effects of working with sulfur dioxide.

Whether you come in contact with sulfur dioxide at work or by breathing polluted air, you may experience a dry throat, a cough, or a burning feeling in your upper respiratory tract. Continued exposure may cause fatigue, loss of your sense of smell, increased mucus production, and shortness of breath.

Proper ventilation must be supplied by management personnel where you work. In areas where levels of sulfur dioxide gas exceeds 5 parts per million (ppm) (the government suggests an even lower level of 1 ppm to 2 ppm), you should be given supplied-air respirators. Make sure ventilation and respirator equipment are operating efficiently before beginning work.

Protective clothing, including goggles and gloves, should be worn around liquid forms of sulfur dioxide. Launder them at least twice weekly. Shower after each work shift.

### Chlorine

Chlorine is a pungent, greenish-yellow gas that is more than twice as heavy as air. Industries use chlorine in manufacturing refrigerants, pesticides, synthetic rubber, and plastics. It is an excellent bleaching agent and is used to purify drinking water, disinfect swimming pools, and treat sewage. Chlorine reacts with your body moisture to form dangerous acids. Those acids damage the delicate mucous membranes of your eyes, nose, throat, and lungs that guard those organs against disease-causing foreign particles. Initial exposure causes a burning sensation in those parts of your body. Chest pains, coughing, and sometimes vomiting result if the exposure continues. It may cause the linings of your lungs' air passages to swell and your throat muscles to cramp, and it may lead to suffocation.

Prolonged breathing of chlorine gas can corrode your teeth.

Liquid chlorine, as well as chlorine gas, can severely burn your skin and eyes. Although neither is flammable, each produces highly flammable and explosive mixtures when combined with other chemicals.

Usually, chlorine's offensive odor is sufficient warning of exposure to the health hazard. But, if you work with chlorine regularly, you may lose your ability to detect it at low concentrations.

Full-face gas masks or supplied-air respirators should be used whenever exposures in excess of 1 part per million (ppm) are encountered. In areas of high gas concentration and whenever liquid chlorine is used, wear full protective clothing and shower after each work shift. Flush your eyes with lots of water if even a little chlorine comes in contact with them.

### Phosgene

Phosgene is a noncombustible gas that has a sweet yet unpleasant odor. Eye and upper respiratory tract irritations may develop from

## Work Related Disorders

contact with the colorless gas. In liquid form it may cause severe burns.

Fire-fighters are sometimes exposed to phosgene, as are manufacturers of dyes, insecticides, and pharmaceuticals.

Symptoms of phosgene exposure include dizziness, chills, thirst, cough, and thick sputum. Unless the condition is corrected, you may develop pulmonary edema (fluid in the lungs). Chronic exposure may cause emphysema and lung scarring. Death may result from respiratory or cardiac failure.

The federally established permissible exposure limit is 0.1 ppm. Use a full-face mask or supplied-air respirator around high concentrations of gaseous phosgene. Wear protective clothing where phosgene is encountered in liquid form.

### Ozone

Known for its use as a bleach, an air purifier, and a water-sterilizing agent, ozone has also been identified as a cause of lung and heart diseases. It is an oxygen-bearing compound that occurs naturally in the atmosphere and is a part of the photochemical reaction that turns auto emissions and sunlight into smog. It is a bluish, pungent gas.

Industrial exposure to ozone also occurs. It is encountered in such processes as arc welding, aging liquor and wood, and drying varnishes and ink.

Ozone can trigger coughing, choking, headache. and severe fatigue. Its effects are strongly aggravated during periods of exercise. Although you may not feel the effects of ozone while sitting or resting, your capability and desire to perform tasks that require exercise can be greatly reduced. It can affect your life style, perhaps without your awareness.

Fluid can collect in your lungs several hours after ozone exposure has ceased. In severe cases, it may be fatal.

To protect against unnecessary ozone exposure (levels of 0.1 ppm or more), use gas masks with proper canister and full-face goggles or supplied-air respirators.

### Nitrogen Dioxide

Nitrogen dioxide enters the atmosphere as a by-product of natural gas combustion, after explosions, in industrial processes using nitric acid, and, most important, from motor vehicle emissions. It is a key element of smog. Its reddish-brown hue can significantly affect visibility.

Occupational exposures result from working with rocket fuels, fertilizers, dyes, pharmaceuticals, and chemicals. Jewelry making, food bleaching, gas and electric arc welding, lithographing, electroplating, and silo filling may also pose serious health hazards.

The high concentration of nitrogen dioxide in cigarette smoke is one reason that form of self-pollution is a major contributor to respiratory disease.

An irritant gas with a characteristic sweetish odor, nitrogen dioxide penetrates deeply into the lungs and slowly attacks the tissues. It may do extensive damage before the first symptoms occur many hours after exposure. Acute exposure to high concentrations can cause severe illness—even collapse and death.

Nitrogen dioxide levels of 5 ppm or more are dangerous. If you work in confined spaces where nitrogen dioxide may accumulate, appropriate eye and respiratory protection is a necessity. Equip yourself with a supplied-air respirator with a full face-piece or chemical goggles. Enclosed areas should be properly ventilated before you enter. It is recommended that an observer having appropriate respiratory protection be stationed outside the area and stand by to supply any aid needed.

Have regular medical examinations. Knowing your occupational exposure, your doctor can look for signs of skin, eye, pulmonary, and heart diseases. Periodic chest X-ray and pulmonary function tests are suggested.

## Ammonia

Colorless ammonia is found everywhere—in the air, water, and soil. Its characteristic pungent odor is familiar to workers in many industries. It is used in the production of fertilizers, explosives, dyes, and plastics. The refrigeration, petroleum refining, chemical, pharmaceutical, and leather tanning industries are also among those that use quantities of ammonia.

Although ammonia is not a poison and has no additive effects on the human body from repeated exposure, it is intensely irritating to your mucous membranes, eyes, and skin. Ammonia gas can produce headache, salivation, burning of the throat, perspiration, nausea, vomiting, and pain below the sternum.

## Work Related Disorders

Ventilation is the key to controlling hazards associated with gaseous ammonia. Exposure limits have been set at 50 ppm for an eight-hour period. Full-face gas masks or supplied-air respirators should be available if concentrations exceed that average. In areas where exposure to liquid ammonia occurs, goggles or face shields and protective clothing (including gloves, aprons, and boots) are required.

If you splash ammonia in your eyes, flood them with large quantities of clear water for 15 minutes or longer. Then seek medical assistance.

### Cigarette Smoking

Because cigarette smoking increases the risk of lung disease, those who work with irritant gases are advised not to smoke.

## Section 15.7

## *Silicosis*

Source: American Lung Association  Pub. No. 0204.  Used by permission.

Silicosis is a common and important dust disease. It has been known by many other names, such as miner's phthisis, stonecutter's disease, potter's asthma, and grinder's rot.

All types of mining in which the ore is extracted from quartz rock can produce silicosis. That includes the mining of gold, copper, lead, zinc, iron, anthracite coal, and some bituminous coal.

But mining is not the only industry whose workers may develop silicosis. Workers in foundries, tunneling, sandstone grinding, sandblasting, concrete breaking, granite carving, and china manufacturing also encounter silica.

### What Causes Silicosis?

Silicosis develops from breathing free crystalline silica dust on the job. It occurs in direct proportion to the percentage and the concentration of silica in the air and to the duration of exposure.

Large silica particles are stopped by the tiny hairs, mucous membranes, and other protective mechanisms of your upper respiratory tract and bronchi. But the smallest dust particles are carried to your airways and your lungs' tiny air sacs. Special defense cells engulf the dust and try to digest it. However, it often finds its way to the pulmonary lymph nodes and may block the vessels that carry lymph in and out of the nodes.

Silica may injure the special defense cells. Fibrosis—abnormal formation of wispy, fiber-like scar tissue in the lungs—may result.

If you have inhaled relatively low concentrations of dust for 10 to 20 years, you will likely have chronic or simple silicosis. That is the commonest and mildest form of the disease. The accumulated dust and tissue reaction cause small cell masses to be scattered throughout the lungs. Those cell masses have little effect. But you may experience breathlessness during exercise.

Simple silicosis has the potential of developing into a more serious condition called complicated silicosis. Some 20 to 30 percent of all simple silicosis victims progress to that advanced stage.

If you have complicated silicosis, you will likely experience breathlessness, weakness, chest pain, a cough, and increased amounts of sputum. Fibrosis—progressive massive fibrosis—spreads throughout the lungs and restricts their function. That often leads to heart disease.

Acute silicosis is a third form of the disease. It is seen in people whose occupations entail a concentrated exposure to silica dust over a relatively short period of time. If you are a sandblaster or rock driller, you may suffer acute silicosis.

A rapidly progressive disease, acute silicosis usually leads to severe disability within five years of diagnosis. Early symptoms include breathing difficulty, weight loss, fever, and coughing. Unfortunately, many victims are young and otherwise healthy people.

### Can Silicosis Cause Other Diseases?

Silicosis does not cause other diseases, but they may occur and aggravate your silicosis. Therefore, every effort should be made to shun situations that could complicate your situation. Cigarette smoking is a primary example.

Smoking damages the tiny hairlike cilia within your lungs' air passages that help move dust and other foreign materials up the airways and into the throat to be swallowed or spit out. If those cilia are not functioning properly, silica particles can be readily deposited in the air sacs. Smoking can cause emphysema or lung cancer—additional burdens for lungs already struggling to provide oxygen for your body.

Tuberculosis is a possible complication of silicosis. A person with silicosis who gets a tuberculosis infection is at high risk of developing tuberculosis disease. Chronic bronchitis occurs in a high proportion of advanced silicotics but less commonly with simple silicosis. And although pneumonia seems no more frequent in people with silicosis than in the general population, your chances for recovery are considerably decreased.

## How Can Silicosis Be Prevented?

The means of preventing silicosis must be specifically designed for each industry and each job after careful evaluation. Dust control is essential. The wetting-down of mines and improved ventilation have helped in the recent past. However, unless you have respirator protection, you should completely avoid areas where ventilation equipment is not present or is not functioning properly.

In work-places where dust concentrations cannot be reduced to safe levels, masks are a necessity. The difficulty you may have breathing through a mask and the discomfort you experience are small prices to pay when the alternative may be a crippling pulmonary disease.

See your doctor yearly for a complete physical examination, including a chest X-ray. Be sure he is aware of your occupational exposure to free silica. Take note of the slightest symptoms. Remember, silicosis is a permanent condition, irreversible by any treatment. Yet, if the disease is diagnosed in its early stages, a person with silicosis can lead a near-normal life. Only a change of job can completely eliminate silica-dust exposure. But workers showing X-ray evidence of the disease are usually only a few years from retirement and may not be able to find other employment or may lose their benefits. If you fall into that category, follow the safety recommendations proposed above, and you will likely be around to enjoy those benefits.

## How Can You Protect Yourself?

To minimize the risk of developing silicosis, you should follow several steps:

- Before starting work and periodically thereafter, make sure the ventilation system is working properly.
- Use all required and recommended protective equipment.
- Cooperate with industry management and your local union in reporting defective equipment and hazardous working conditions.
- If you experience the symptoms described above, see your doctor.
- Do not smoke! Your symptoms, discomfort, and chances of death are multiplied when you purposely inhale tobacco smoke. It's a matter of life and breath.

# Part II

# Controlling Your Breathing Environment

Chapter 15

# *Biological Agents*

## What Are They?

Biological agents include bacteria, viruses, fungi, pollen, dust mites and other insects, animal dander (tiny scales from hair, feathers, or skin) and molds. They can travel through the air and are often invisible. They are usually inhaled, either alone or by attaching themselves to particles of dust and then entering the respiratory system.

## Where Are They Found?

While the majority of biological pollutants are found indoors, some are of outdoor origin. Some of these substances are in every home. It is impossible to get rid of them all. Two conditions are essential to support biological growth—nutrients and moisture.

Bacteria, fungi and molds find nourishment and can flourish in improperly maintained air ducts, air conditioners, humidifiers, dehumidifiers, air-cleaning filters, carpets and in improperly ventilated places where moisture is likely to collect, such as bathrooms, kitchens, laundry rooms and basements. Viruses can be carried indoors by people, while plants, pets and insects are potential sources of pollen, dander, and other allergens. Dust mites and other insects can thrive in sofas, stuffed chairs, carpets and bedding.

American Lung Association Pub. No. 1186. 1990. Used by permission.

## What Are Their Health Effects?

When biological agents are allowed to flourish in poorly maintained ventilation systems, severe health problems can result that can be experienced throughout an entire building.

Infectious and non-infectious diseases can be caused by the various biological agents. They can make you sneeze, trigger allergic reactions, cause rashes, watery eyes, hoarseness, coughing, dizziness, lethargy, breathing problems, and digestive problems.

People with asthma are especially susceptible to allergic problems caused by biological agents. Their very sensitive airways can react to various allergens and irritants, making breathing difficult. The number of people with asthma has increased significantly in the last 20 years. People with breathing problems and allergies are also likely to be more sensitive to airborne biological agents.

## What Are The Problems?

Biological agents are so common that complete control over them seems hopeless. Of all indoor air pollutants, they are best described as inevitable.

## What Are The Solutions?

Give special attention to moisture control. Moisture can invade the home through many sources, including leaks and seepage and even through some appliances. Keep air-conditioner filters clean and replace them regularly. If you use a home humidifier, make sure that it is maintained and cleaned often and properly. They are excellent breeding grounds for biological agents.

Fresh air can lower the particle content of indoor air, so air your home out regularly.

Poorly maintained ventilation systems cultivate the population of biological agents. Good ventilation is important in preventing the build-up of biological particles.

Controlling dust is very important for people who are allergic to animal dander and mites. Wash bedding in hot water (at least 130° F) at least every 7 to 10 days to kill dust mites. Use synthetic bedding instead of wool blankets or feather-stuffed pillows and comforters, which do not stand up to washing.

## Biological Agents

At the office, talk to the building manager about maintenance of the ventilation system. Urge that filters be kept clean while in operation, and that there is an adequate regular exchange of air throughout the building.

A healthy dose of common sense is the best way to control the spread and multiplication of biological agents. Regular and thorough cleaning of places where biological pollutants are likely to grow will keep them at a minimum. You will never be able to get rid of them totally, but you can inhibit their growth.

Chapter 16

# Ozone Air Pollution

## What Is Ozone Air Pollution?

Ozone is a highly reactive gas that is a form of oxygen. It is the main component of the air pollution known as smog. Ozone reacts chemically ("oxidizes") with internal body tissues that it comes in contact with such as those in the lung. It also reacts with other materials such as rubber compounds, breaking them down.

## How Is It Produced?

Ozone is formed by the action of sunlight on carbon-based chemicals known as hydrocarbons, acting in combination with a group of air pollutants called oxides of nitrogen. Hydrocarbons are emitted by motor vehicles, oil and chemical storage and handling facilities, and a variety of commercial and industrial sources such as gas stations, dry cleaners and degreasing operations. Oxides of nitrogen are a by-product of burning fuel in sources such as power plants, steel mills and other heavy industry and in motor vehicles.

Ozone levels typically rise during the May through September period when higher temperatures and the increased amount of sunlight combine with the stagnant atmospheric conditions that are associated with ozone air pollution episodes. The harmful ozone in the

---

American Lung Association Pub. No. 0694. 1989. Used by permission.

lower atmosphere (troposphere) should not be confused with the protective layer of ozone in the upper atmosphere (stratosphere) which screens out harmful ultraviolet rays.

## What Are Its Health Effects?

Ozone acts as a powerful respiratory irritant at the levels frequently found in most of the nation's urban areas during summer months. Symptoms include shortness of breath, pain when inhaling deeply, wheezing and coughing. Tests carried out on healthy adults and children undergoing heavy exercise have found that exposure to ozone at a level equal to the current federal health-based air quality standard of 0.12 parts per million results in a decrease in the normal function of the lungs. A higher level of exercise results in a lower level of ozone or shorter length of exposure needed to cause these effects.

Recent research on the effects of longer exposures (6-1/2 hours) to ozone levels at or just below the health-based air quality standard have found even larger reductions in lung function, biological evidence of inflammation of the lung lining and more frequent and severe respiratory discomfort. In studies of animals, ozone exposure has been found to increase susceptibility to bacterial pneumonia infection.

Other studies of children in summer camps and adults exercising outdoors, as opposed to in a laboratory chamber, suggest that lung function decreases even at ozone levels equal to or below the current health standard. There is also evidence that the lung function changes experienced at somewhat higher ozone levels may persist for several days after the exposure.

Recently, attention has begun to focus on the effects of long-term, repeated exposures to high levels of ozone. A study of a sample of long-time residents of Los Angeles, which has the highest and most frequent ozone problem in the nation, found that the group had a higher than expected loss of lung function over time. Long-term exposures of animals to moderate ozone levels produce changes in the structure of the lung.

Based on the evidence from the studies discussed above, and from other studies, ozone air pollution represents a serious and widespread public health problem.

## Who Is at Risk?

The U.S. Environmental Protection Agency (EPA) has identified three groups of people who are at particular risk from high ozone levels:

- **People with pre-existing respiratory disease.** People with existing lung disease (e.g. chronic bronchitis, emphysema, asthma) already suffer from reduced lung function and therefore cannot tolerate an additional reduction in lung function due to ozone exposure. More than six million people with chronic bronchitis or emphysema and almost five million children and adults with asthma live in areas that exceed the federal health standard.

- **A sub-group of the general public referred to as "responders".** Studies have found that a sub-group of the general healthy population responds to ozone exposure while exercising with significantly greater losses in lung function than the average response of the overall group under study. There is currently no way to identify these "responders" prior to ozone exposure, but the EPA estimates that this sub-group represents 5 to 20 percent of the total U.S. population.

- **Individuals who exercise outdoors.** Numerous laboratory and "real world" ozone exposure studies confirm that people who exercise, or otherwise participate in activities that increase their respiratory rate, respond much more severely to ozone exposure than people at rest. Thus, adults exercising outdoors, construction workers, and children at play can all be considered at particular risk from high ozone levels.

## What are the Solutions?

The American Lung Association supports the use of stringent controls on motor vehicle and pollution emissions on the commercial and industrial sources of the hydrocarbon compounds and oxides of nitrogen that form ozone. These controls include:

- strengthening pollution control requirements for new motor vehicles,

- improving the in-use performance of existing pollution control equipment, and

- implementation of pollution controls to capture evaporating hydrocarbons in gasoline from motor vehicles and gas stations.

In addition, efforts to reduce our society's ever-increasing use of the automobile must be expanded, and controls on commercial operations and consumer products that contribute hydrocarbon compounds to the air will also be necessary.

Chapter 17

# Benefits and Concerns With the Use of Humidifiers

*Chapter Contents*

Section 17. 1—Humidifiers Increase Moisture—
and Sometimes Bacteria .................................. 590
Section 17. 2—Precautions with Certain Ventilators,
Humidifiers ....................................................... 597

## Section 17.1

# Humidifiers Increase Moisture— and Sometimes Bacteria

Source: "Humidifiers Increase Moisture—and Sometimes Bacteria." FDA *Consumer* November 1992;

If you use a humidifier in your home this winter, will your family be healthier? Whether a humidifier will make a difference in your family's health is a question still under debate in the medical community.

"It's a continuing argument," said Sam Barton, a volunteer with the American Lung Association of Northern Virginia. "If you get 10 doctors together and ask them whether they recommend using a humidifier, five would say yes and five would say no."

Barton noted, for the record, that his family does not use a humidifier. "When wintertime comes and we turn on the furnace, we just set a pan of water on the floor vent," he explained. "It puts two quarts of water in the air every day."

The term "humidifier" and "vaporizer" are often used interchangeably. Technically, however, a vaporizer is a type of humidifier that boils water before sending it into the air as steam. (See accompanying article.) The term "humidifier" will be used throughout this article to denote both humidifiers and vaporizers.

### What's Regulated, What's Not

If you opt to invest in a humidifier, keep in mind that you may be purchasing a device that is not subject to FDA regulation. Many "department store" humidifiers that consumers purchase directly off the shelf are not regulated by FDA because they make no medical claims. Some of these machines do no more than promise to increase the comfort level in your home.

Other "off-the-shelf" units promise to do more, such as produce a "warm soothing steam to help relieve congestion caused by colds and respiratory ailments." This is a medical claim, and the unit must therefore meet FDA requirements.

Some of these units have the added feature of being able to spray an over-the-counter medication (such as a nasal decongestant or cough

## Benefits and Concerns with the Use of Humidifiers

suppressant) into the air along with the soothing vapor. Such units are defined in FDA's regulations as "medicinal non-ventilatory nebulizers" or, more simply, "atomizers."

Then there are the more highly specialized devices that are used exclusively in medical settings, or that can be obtained for home use only with a physician's prescription. These FDA-regulated machines are not designed to treat the sniffles, colds, flu, or other common ailments, but serious disorders of the respiratory system such as asthma, cystic fibrosis, and other chronic pulmonary disorders. One such device, called a therapeutic humidifier, adds water vapor to breathing gases—such as oxygen—producing a vapor that pervades the area surrounding the patient, who breathes the vapor during normal respiration.

In addition to its pre-market review responsibilities, FDA also keeps an eye on respiratory medical devices after they reach the market. For example, the agency monitored the voluntary recall of 180 defective water feed sets by a manufacturer in California. The plastic tubes, used to supply distilled water from a container to a respiratory humidifier, were pulled from the market because their self-closing clamps did not work correctly. This defect could have caused the humidifier's chamber to overfill with water, possibly resulting in a decreased supply of oxygen to the patient.

### Is Wetter Better?

A number of studies suggest that relative humidity (air moisture content expressed as a percentage of its moisture-holding capacity) can, in fact, reduce the incidence of respiratory infections and allergies.

In a 1973 study, for example, 800 Army recruits were divided and placed in two barracks, only one of which was humidified. Recruits in the humidified barrack had 18 percent fewer infections between January and March than did recruits in the barrack without humidification.

Another study found a significant reduction in respiratory infections among children who attended a humidified school compared with children who attended a non-humidified school. Infections were reduced even further in children in the humidified school whose homes were also humidified.

During the study, the average weekly absentee rate due to respiratory infections was 7.1 percent for children whose schools and homes were not humidified and 1.3 percent for children with humidification at both places.

Most experts agree that some moisture in the air is a healthy thing, and that people seem to be healthiest when the relative humidity hovers in the mid-range—somewhere between 30 and 50 percent. Available data indicates that this "mid-range" of relative humidity tends to shorten the lifespan of airborne bacteria and viruses.

It's when the relative humidity gets too high or too low that certain bacteria or viruses are likely to thrive and health problems seem most likely to develop.

To keep tabs on the humidity conditions in your home, you may want to buy an instrument called a hygrometer, usually available at hardware stores.

## Wintertime Dryness

During winter, when the heat Is on, the relative humidity in your house can become very low. This is because heated air can hold much more moisture than cold air. So, as the air in your home heats up, it becomes "thirsty" and begins sucking moisture out of surrounding surfaces: plants, walls, furniture, books, paintings, human bodies, everything.

The moisture that cooking and bathing puts into the air is not likely to offset this drying effect, especially in the colder parts of the country where the furnace runs almost continuously during the winter months.

This is one reason you may find your throat getting parched more often in wintertime, your lips more chapped, and your skin more dry and itchy.

Some people are convinced that prolonged exposure to low relative humidity increases susceptibility to common colds by "drying out" the protective mucus membranes in the nose and throat. There is little evidence, however, to indicate that the mucus membranes of healthy individuals are adversely affected by low relative humidity.

"God has built a humidifier right there in your nose," said Ali Abrishami, M.D., an allergist in Greenbelt, Md. "There is moisture in your nose, and that moisture goes into the air you breathe."

Abrishami is not a strong advocate of humidifiers.

## Benefits and Concerns with the Use of Humidifiers

"If a patient asks me whether they should use a humidifier, I tell them it can't hurt, provided they aren't allergic to molds," he said. "I tell the patient that it's not harmful to add moisture to the air if it's dry.

"But too much humidity isn't good either," he added.

### The Risk Factor

If you want to keep your home's relative humidity within the "healthy," 30-50 zone during winter, you may want to take the simple approach and keep a pan of water on your floor vent or your radiator, or maybe just keep a pot of water boiling on the stove.

The other alterative is to invest in a humidifier. But there's some risk involved here. If not cleaned properly or often enough, the tanks of some models may provide an ideal breeding ground for bacteria, fungi, and other harmful microorganisms that are then sprayed into the air along with all that soothing moisture. And over-using a humidifier can cause the relative humidity to get too high, a situation that can promote the growth of dust mites and fungi (which includes molds) in your house. These organisms are capable of causing severe allergic reactions in susceptible people.

High relative humidity may also prolong the life expectancy of certain viruses that may be in your home.

### When It's Too Wet

The size of indoor populations of allergenic mites and fungi is directly dependent on the relative humidity.

Mites are the culprits behind house dust allergies, and laboratory studies show that these microscopic creatures like life on the moist side; they begin multiplying rapidly as the humidity climbs above 50 percent.

In a two-year study involving 98 houses, fewer than 10 live mites per gram of house dust were found when the relative humidity fell below 40 to 50 percent.

In another two-year study involving two houses, no mites at all were found when the relative humidity fell below 50 percent. Both studies found that mite density was not affected by the age of the house, or by how clean the house was kept.

Mites aren't the only house guests that enjoy humidity. Fungi, which include molds, usually need relative humidities in excess of 75 percent to grow. They are known to cause allergic reactions such as asthma attacks or rhinitis (an inflammation of the mucous membranes of the nose).

Because they like it wet, most fungi populations stay in areas such as the kitchen and bathroom, unless, of course, you own a humidifier and run it too much in some other room.

For someone allergic to certain molds, running a humidifier (especially in the bedroom at night) can be double trouble: Fungi may grow in the humidifier's tank and be sprayed into the air for the person to breathe; and the excessively humid environment may cause fungi to begin forming on furniture, walls, carpets, clothes, and other surfaces in the person's room.

## White Dust

If you use tap water in your humidifier, the minerals in the water will be dispersed into the air and coat your floors, walls and furniture with a fine white dust, sometimes called humidifier dust. According to Ken Giles of the U.S. Consumer Product Safety Commission, this white dust may contain particles small enough to enter the lungs.

"The health effects from inhaling humidifier dust are not clear," said Giles. "Any impact on human health will depend upon the types and amounts of the minerals found in the water."

Since the medical community remains unsure about the effects of white dust, play it safe and use distilled water in your machine.

## The Whole-House Approach

If you live in a house with forced-air heat, you can add a humidifier to your heating system. It's an efficient way to go. But some of these systems—if not properly maintained—can breed microorganisms just as easily as stand-alone units. And they have the added feature of being able to spread allergens and pathogens throughout your entire home, not just one room.

If you or someone in your family is sensitive to molds or dust mites, you may want to talk to your family doctor, or even a respira-

## Benefits and Concerns with the Use of Humidifiers

tory specialist, before deciding whether you want to install one of these units.

A humidifier of any kind won't accomplish much if your house isn't insulated, or if it doesn't have a vapor barrier, because the moisture will be lost. (Most houses built before 1950 don't have a vapor barrier—a layer of plastic, foil, or treated paper on the room side of the insulation.) A humidifier won't moisturize the air sufficiently in a house that lacks insulation or vapor barrier. The moisture will simply escape to the outside.

If your house isn't insulated, you probably don't need a humidifier. The air exchange rate in a leaky house is usually so great that indoor air doesn't have time to get too dry or thirsty. Your heating bills may be outrageous, but you at least have the satisfaction of knowing that your relative humidity is probably well within the healthy zone.

### How Humidifiers Work

Humidifiers come in all shapes and sizes, from hatbox-sized portable units to furniture-sized consoles. But they all do the same thing: They put moisture in the air. And they do it in one of five ways.

*Evaporation*

Evaporative units have a fan inside them that blows air through a wet pad, and this moisture-laden air then continues on into the room. ("Wicking" humidifiers do the same thing, only the air is blown through a moisturized filter instead of a pad.) Evaporative units don't produce a spray and are therefore less likely to spread germs than are units that throw a cool mist into the air. The wet pads, however, can become a breeding ground for bacteria if not cleaned regularly.

*Steam*

These units, sometimes called vaporizers, boil water and send it into the air as steam. They tend not to put microorganisms into the air; after all, it would take an extraordinarily tough germ to survive the boiling process. Unlike other kinds of humidifiers, they produce little or no "white dust." Steam units leave the minerals behind when they boil water in their tanks.

### Warm mist

These units boil water just like steam vaporizers, only the steam is cooled slightly before exiting the unit, resulting in a "mist" of warm water droplets instead of real steam.

### Cool mist

These units break up water into tiny droplets and spray a cool mist into the air. Because the water isn't boiled, the cool vapor may contain potentially harmful organisms if the tank is not properly cleaned and sanitized.

### Ultrasonic

These units use high-frequency vibrations to break up water droplets into an extremely fine mist. The mist produced by these machines contains no molds and comparatively few live bacteria. It is thought that the ultrasonic vibrations may "break up" and shatter living organisms along with the water droplets. However, while these bits of dead microbes may not cause respiratory infections, they may still trigger allergic reactions in sensitive people.

## Keep It Clean

To reduce the possibility of health hazards from dirty humidifiers, the Consumer Product Safety Commission recommends the following precautions:

- Clean your humidifier every day.

- Empty any left-over water, wipe all surfaces dry with a soft towel, and refill with clean water. Some units may require special maintenance steps, so carefully follow the manufacturer's instructions.

- Sanitize your humidifier every seven days (or every 14 days if your humidifier has a capacity of five or more gallons). Empty left-over water and fill with a weak bleach solution (one teaspoon of bleach per gallon of water). Let the solution soak for 20 minutes, swishing it around the sides every few minutes.

## Benefits and Concerns with the Use of Humidifiers

Rinse the tank with water until you can no longer smell bleach. Remove any scale or mineral deposits using a soft brush or towel and a vinegar solution (half vinegar, half water).

- Use distilled or demineralized water to reduce the build-up of scale (which is composed of minerals that have settled out of the water) and the release of humidifier dust (minerals that are released in the mist and settle as a fine, white dust). Don't use tap water because it contains more minerals. Use demineralization cartridges or filters if they are supplied or recommended.

- Clean or replace sponge filters or belts as needed.

- Sanitize and thoroughly dry the appliance before storing it. Clean it after summer storage, and remove dust on the outside of the unit, too.

*—Tom Cramer*

## Section 17.2

## Precautions with Certain Ventilators, Humidifiers

Source: "Precautions with Certain Ventilators, Humidifiers." FDA *Consumer* March 1994.

After receiving several reports of death and injuries from malfunctioning volume ventilators and heated humidifiers, FDA last September alerted physicians to use precautions with these devices. Though most commonly used in health-care facilities, these medical devices are sometimes used at home when prescribed by a physician.

FDA recommends the following precautions with prescription volume ventilators and heated humidifiers:

- Immediately stop using the device if it shows signs of overheating, smoking, or electrical malfunction such as sparking or causing shocks. Have the unit evaluated and repaired by a factory-authorized representative before using it again.

- Use an audible alarm that senses gas temperature in the line to the patient with any humidifier used together with a volume ventilator. Test the alarm periodically.

- Make sure the device is serviced and maintained according to all the manufacturer's recommendations. Keep appropriate records of service and maintenance work. This is especially important for used or remanufactured equipment.

- Check power cords regularly for damage inside or outside the unit. Ensure that power cords are fitted with strain relief devices.

Chapter 18

# Environmental Tobacco Smoke (ETS)

## What is ETS?

Environmental tobacco smoke (ETS) is the combination of two forms of smoke from burning tobacco products:

- Sidestream smoke, or smoke that comes from a burning cigarette, pipe, or cigar between puffs, and

- Mainstream smoke, or the smoke that is exhaled by the smoker.

When a cigarette is smoked, about one-half of the smoke generated is sidestream smoke emitted from the burning cigarette between puffs. This sidestream smoke contains essentially all of the same carcinogenic (cancer-causing) and toxic agents that have been identified in the mainstream smoke inhaled by the smoker, but at greater levels.

More than 4,000 individual compounds have been identified in tobacco and tobacco smoke. Among these are about 60 compounds that are carcinogens, tumor initiators (substances that can result in irreversible changes in normal cells), and tumor promoters (substances that can lead to tumor growth once cell changes begin). Some of these

---

National Cancer Institute. Pub. No. 3.9. May 31, 1994.

compounds are tar, carbon monoxide, hydrogen cyanide, phenols, ammonia, formaldehyde benzene, nitrosamine, and nicotine.

The exposure of nonsmokers to ETS is referred to as involuntary smoking, passive smoking, and secondhand smoke. Nonsmokers who are exposed to ETS absorb nicotine and other compounds just as smokers do, and the greater the exposure to ETS, the greater the level of these harmful compounds in the body.

Although the smoke to which an involuntary smoker is exposed is less concentrated than that inhaled by smokers, research has demonstrated that the health risk from inhaling smoke is significant. For example, scientists estimate that ETS causes about 3,000 lung cancer deaths each year.

## How Strong Is the Evidence Linking ETS With Lung Cancer and Respiratory Disease?

In 1986, two reports were published on the association between ETS exposure and adverse health effects in nonsmokers: one by the U.S. Surgeon General and the other by the Expert Committee on Passive Smoking, National Academy of Sciences' National Research Council (NAS/NRC). Both of these reports concluded that:

- ETS can cause lung cancer in healthy adult nonsmokers;

- Children of parents who smoke have more respiratory symptoms and acute lower respiratory tract infections, as well as evidence of reduced lung function, than do children of nonsmoking parents; and

- Separating smokers and nonsmokers within the same air space may reduce but does not eliminate a nonsmoker's exposure to ETS.

More recent epidemiologic studies support and reinforce these earlier reports. The firmly established causal relationship between lung cancer and mainstream smoke, coupled with the chemical similarities between ETS and the smoke inhaled by smokers, led researchers to conclude that involuntary smoking is likely to have similar effects on the lung.

In light of the widespread presence of ETS in both the home and work-place and its absorption by the body, the U.S. Environmental Protection Agency (EPA) released a report in 1992 in which ETS was classified as a Group A carcinogen—a category reserved only for the most dangerous cancer-causing agents in humans.

The overall results of 30 epidemiologic studies of lung cancer and involuntary smoking further justify a Group A classification. In these studies, female never-smokers who are married to smokers are compared with female never-smokers who are married to nonsmokers. Higher exposures cause higher risks, and people whose spouses smoke in the home face a higher risk than that of people whose spouses do not smoke at home. In studies of ETS in the work-place, exposures are often even greater than exposure at home from spousal smoking.

While the EPA report focuses only on the respiratory health effects of involuntary smoking, there may be other health effects of concern as well. Recent studies suggest that ETS exposure also may be a risk factor for cardiovascular disease. In addition, a few studies link ETS exposure to cancers of sites other than the lung.

## ETS Exposure in Infants and Children

Studies dating from the early 1970s have consistently shown that children and infants exposed to ETS in the home have significantly elevated rates of respiratory symptoms and respiratory tract infections. More than 50 recently published studies confirm these previous conclusions:

- ETS exposure due to parental smoking, especially the mother's, contributes to 150,000 to 300,000 cases annually of lower respiratory tract infection (pneumonia, bronchitis, and other infections) in infants and children under 18 months of age; 7,500 to 15,000 of these cases require hospitalization.

- ETS exposure is associated with increased respiratory irritation (cough, phlegm production, and wheezing) and middle ear infections, as well as upper respiratory tract symptoms (sore throats and colds) in infants and children.

- ETS exposure increases the number of episodes and the severity of asthma in children who already have the disease. The

EPA report estimates that ETS worsens the condition in 200,000 to 1 million asthmatic children. Moreover, ETS exposure increases the number of new cases of asthma in children who have not previously exhibited symptoms.

- ETS exposure in utero and in infancy can alter lung function and structure and create other changes that are known to predispose children to long-term pulmonary risks.

- In the United States, sudden infant death syndrome (SIDS) is the major cause of death in infants between the ages of 1 month and 1 year, and the linkage with maternal smoking is well established. Current evidence strongly suggests that infants whose mothers smoke are at an increased risk of dying of SIDS, independent of other known risk factors for SIDS, including low birth weight and low gestational age, both of which are specifically associated with active smoking during pregnancy. Additional studies are needed to determine whether the increased risk is related to in utero or postnatal exposure to tobacco smoke, or to both.

These findings prompted recommendations that ETS be eliminated from the environment of small children. Thus, smoking should not be allowed in day care centers, nurseries, or other settings where infants and young children are cared for.

### ETS Exposure in Nonsmokers with Existing Health Problems

ETS can worsen existing pulmonary symptoms in people with asthma and chronic bronchitis, as well as for people with allergic conditions. Even individuals who are not allergic can suffer eye irritation, sore throat, nausea, and hoarseness. Contact lens wearers can find tobacco smoke very irritating.

### Public Policies Restricting Smoking

Following the release of the Surgeon General's report and the NAS/NRC review, many new laws, regulations, and ordinances were enacted that severely restrict or ban public smoking. With the release of the EPA report, many more such laws can be expected:

## Environmental Tobacco Smoke

- On the Federal level, the General Services Administration issued regulations restricting smoking to designated areas only in Federal office buildings. Many agencies within the Public Health Service, which includes the National Institutes of Health, have banned smoking completely.

- By law, all airline flights of 6 hours or less within the United States and all interstate bus travel are smoke free.

- ETS meets the criteria of the Occupational Safety and Health Administration (OSHA) for classification as a potential occupational carcinogen. (OSHA is the Federal agency responsible for health and safety regulations in the work-place.)

- The National Institute for Occupational Safety and Health (NIOSH) is another Federal agency that is concerned with ETS exposure in the work-place. NIOSH conducts ETS-related research, evaluates work-sites for possible health hazards, and makes safety recommendations. NIOSH recommends that ETS be regarded as a potential occupational carcinogen, in conformance with the OSHA carcinogen policy, and that exposures to ETS be reduced to the lowest possible levels.

- Currently, nearly every state has some form of legislation to protect nonsmokers; some states require private employers to enact policies that protect employees who do not smoke. In addition to state legislation, more than 560 local jurisdictions have enacted ordinances addressing nonsmokers' rights, and most are more restrictive than their state counterparts.

### *Additional Resources About the Effects of ETS*

The NAS/NRC report *Environmental Tobacco Smoke: Measuring Exposures and Assessing Health Effects* (POD #318) is published by the National Academy Press. It may be ordered from the National Academy Press, Box 285, 2101 Constitution Avenue NW, Washington, DC 20055; the telephone number is 202-334-3313, and the toll-free number is 1-800-624-6242. The price is $58.25 plus $4.00 for shipping and handling per order. Orders must be prepaid by check or charged to VISA, MasterCard, or American Express.

*The Health Consequences of Involuntary Smoking: A Report of the Surgeon General* (stock number 017-001-00458-8) is available for $11.00 from the U.S. Government Printing Office, Post Office Box 371954, Pittsburgh, PA 15250-7954; the telephone number is 202-783-3238.

The EPA report *Respiratory Health Effects of Passive Smoking: Lung Cancer and Other Disorders* (stock number 055-000-00407-2) is available for $29.00 from the U.S. Government Printing Office, Post Office Box 371954, Pittsburgh, PA 15250-7954; the telephone number is 202-783-3238. The summary of this report and additional information on ETS are available free of charge from the U.S. Environmental Protection Agency, Indoor Air Quality, Post Office Box 37133, Washington. DC 20013-7133; the toll-free telephone number is 1-800-438-4318.

The NIOSH report *Current Intelligence Bulletin 54, Environmental Tobacco Smoke in the Work-place* is available from NIOSH's Office of Information, 4676 Columbia Parkway/ Mailstop C-19, Cincinnati, OH 45226. The toll-free telephone number is 1-800-35-NIOSH (1-800-356-4674).

In cooperation with Americans for Nonsmokers' Rights, the National Cancer Institute (NCI) completed an inventory of all existing local laws in 1989. A revised version of this publication is being prepared. Single copies of Major Local Smoking Control Ordinances in the United States can be ordered free from NCI through the Cancer Information Service (1-800 4-CANCER). A related NCI publication, *Smoking Policies: Questions and Answers*, provides answers to the 10 questions most often asked about smoking control policies at worksites.

The Office of Smoking and Health, Centers for Disease Control and Prevention, distributes materials on ETS. The Office can be contacted at 1600 Clifton Road, Rhodes Building/NE Mail Stop K-50, Atlanta, GA 30341-3724; the telephone number is 404-488-5705.

Additional information on lung disease, cancer, and smoking is provided by the American Lung Association and the American Cancer Society. Local chapters of these organizations are listed in telephone directories.

The Cancer Information Service (CIS), a program of the National Cancer Institute, provides a nationwide telephone service for cancer patients and their families, the public, and health care professionals. CIS information specialists have extensive training in providing up-to-date and understandable information about cancer and cancer research. They can answer questions in English and Spanish and can send free printed material. In addition, CIS offices serve specific geographic areas and have information about cancer-related services and resources in their region. The toll-free number of the CIS is 1-800-4-CANCER, (1-800 422-6237).

Chapter 19

# The Health Benefits of Smoking Cessation: A Report of the Surgeon General, 1990

## Preface to the Executive Summary

This Report of the Surgeon General is the twenty-first report of the U.S. Public Health Service on the health consequences of smoking and the first issued during my tenure as Surgeon General. Whereas previous reports have focused on the health effects of smoking, this Report is devoted to the benefits of smoking cessation.

The public health impact of smoking is enormous. As documented in the 1989 Surgeon General's Report, an estimated 390,000 Americans die each year from diseases caused by smoking. This toll includes 115,000 deaths from heart disease; 106,000 from lung cancer; 31,600 from other cancers; 57,000 from chronic obstructive pulmonary disease; 27,500 from stroke; and 52,900 from other conditions related to smoking. More than one of every six deaths in the United States are caused by smoking. For more than a decade the Public Health Service has identified cigarette smoking as the most important preventable cause of death in our society.

It is clear, then, that the elimination of smoking would yield substantial benefits for public health. What are the benefits, however, for the individual smoker who quits? A large body of evidence has accumulated to address that question and derives from cohort and case-control studies, cross-sectional surveys, and clinical trials. In studies of

---

U.S. DHHS Pub. No. 90-8416, 1990.

the health effects of smoking cessation, persons classified as former smokers may include some current smokers; this misclassification is likely to cause an underestimation of the health benefits of quitting. Taken together, the evidence clearly indicates that smoking cessation has major and immediate health benefits for men and women of all ages.

## *Overall Benefits of Smoking Cessation*

People who quit smoking live longer than those who continue to smoke. To what extent is a smoker's risk of premature death reduced after quitting smoking? The answer depends on several factors, including the number of years of smoking, the number of cigarettes smoked per day, and the presence or absence of disease at the time of quitting. Data from the American Cancer Society's Cancer Prevention Study II (CPS-II) were analyzed in this Report to estimate the risk of premature death in ex-smokers versus current smokers. These data show, for example, that persons who quit smoking before age 50 have one-half the risk of dying in the next 15 years compared with continuing smokers.

Smoking cessation increases life expectancy because it reduces the risk of dying from specific smoking-related diseases. One such disease is lung cancer, the most common cause of cancer death in both men and women. The risk of dying from lung cancer is 22 times higher among male smokers and 12 times higher among female smokers compared with people who have never smoked. The risk of lung cancer declines steadily in people who quit smoking; after 10 years of abstinence, the risk of lung cancer is about 30 to 50 percent of the risk for continuing smokers. Smoking cessation also reduces the risk of cancers of the larynx, oral cavity, esophagus, pancreas, and urinary bladder.

Coronary heart disease (CHD) is the leading cause of death in the United States. Smokers have about twice the risk of dying from ChD compared with lifetime nonsmokers. This excess risk is reduced by about half among ex-smokers after only 1 year of smoking abstinence and declines gradually thereafter. After 15 years of abstinence the risk of CHD is similar to that of persons who have never smoked.

Compared with lifetime nonsmokers, smokers have about twice the risk of dying from stroke, the third leading cause of death in the United States. After quitting smoking, the risk of stroke returns to the level of people who have never smoked; in some studies this reduction

## Health Benefits of Smoking Cessation

in risk has occurred within 5 years, but in others as long as 15 years of abstinence were required.

Cigarette smoking is the major cause of chronic obstructive pulmonary disease (COPD), the fifth leading cause of death in the United States. Smoking increases the risk of COPD by accelerating the age-related decline in lung function. With sustained abstinence from smoking, the rate of decline of lung function among former smokers returns to that of never smokers, thus reducing the risk of developing COPD.

Influenza and pneumonia represent the sixth leading cause of death in the United States. Cigarette smoking increases the risk of respiratory infections such as influenza, pneumonia, and bronchitis, and smoking cessation reduces the risk.

Cigarette smoking is a major cause of peripheral artery occlusive disease. This condition causes substantial mortality and morbidity; complications may include intermittent claudication, tissue ischemia and gangrene, and ultimately, loss of limb. Smoking cessation substantially reduces the risk of peripheral artery occlusive disease compared with continued smoking.

The mortality rate from abdominal aortic aneurysm is two to five times higher in current smokers than in never smokers. Former smokers have half the excess risk of dying from this condition relative to current smokers.

About 90 million Americans currently have, or have had, an ulcer of the stomach or duodenum. Smokers have an increased risk of developing gastric or duodenal ulcers, and this increased risk is reduced by quitting smoking.

### Benefits at All Ages

According to a 1989 Gallup survey, the proportion of smokers who say they would like to give up smoking is lower for smokers aged 50 and older (57 percent) than for smokers aged 18-29 (68 percent) and 30-49 (67 percent). Older smokers may be less motivated to quit smoking because the highly motivated may have quit already at younger ages, leaving a relatively "hard-core" group of older smokers. But many long-term smokers may lack motivation to quit for other reasons. Some may believe they are no longer at risk of smoking-related diseases because they have already survived smoking for many years. Others may believe that any damage that may have been caused by smoking is irreversible after decades of smoking. For similar reasons, many physicians may be less likely to counsel their older patients to quit.

CPS-II data were used to estimate the effects of quitting smoking at various ages on the cumulative risk of death during a fixed interval after cessation. The results show the benefits of cessation extend to quitting at older ages. For example, a healthy man aged 60-64 who smokes 1 pack of cigarettes or more per day reduces his risk of dying during the next 15 years by 10 percent if he quits smoking.

These findings support the recommendations of the Surgeon General's 1988 Workshop on Health Promotion and Aging for the development and dissemination of smoking cessation messages and interventions to older persons. I am pleased that a coalition of organizations and agencies is now working toward implementation of those recommendations, including the Centers for Disease Control; the National Cancer Institute; the National Heart, Lung, and Blood Institute; the Administration on Aging; the Department of Veterans Affairs; the Office of Disease Prevention and Health Promotion; the American Association of Retired Persons; and the Fox Chase Cancer Center. The major message of this campaign will be that it is never too late to quit smoking.

Two Pacts point to the urgent need for a strong smoking cessation campaign targeting older Americans:

1. Seven million smokers are aged 60 or older; and

2. Smoking is a major risk factor for 6 of the 14 leading causes of death among those aged 60 and older, and is a complicating factor for 3 others.

### Benefits for Smokers with Existing Disease

Many smokers who have already developed smoking-related disease or symptoms may be less motivated to quit because of a belief that the damage is already done. For the same reason, physicians may be less motivated to advise these patients to quit. However, the evidence reviewed in this report shows that smoking cessation yields important health benefits to those who already suffer from smoking-related illness.

Among persons with diagnosed CHD, smoking cessation markedly reduces the risk of recurrent heart attack and cardiovascular

## Health Benefits of Smoking Cessation

death. In many studies, this reduction in risk has been 50 percent or more. Smoking cessation is the most important intervention in the management of peripheral artery occlusive disease; for patients with this condition, quitting smoking improves exercise tolerance, reduces the risk of amputation after peripheral artery surgery, and increases overall survival. Patients with gastric and duodenal ulcers who stop smoking improve their clinical course relative to smokers who continue to smoke. Although the benefits of smoking cessation among stroke patients have not been studied, it is reasonable to assume that quitting smoking reduces the risk of recurrent stroke just as it reduces the risk of recurrence of other cardiovascular events.

Even smokers who have already developed cancer may benefit from smoking cessation. A few studies have shown that persons who stopped smoking after diagnosis of cancer had a reduced risk of acquiring a second primary cancer compared with persons who continued to smoke. Although relevant data are sparse, longer survival might be expected among smokers with cancer or other serious illnesses if they stop smoking. Smoking cessation reduces the risk of respiratory infections such as pneumonia, which are often the immediate causes of death in patients with an underlying chronic disease.

The important role of health care providers in counseling patients to quit smoking is well recognized. Health care providers should give smoking cessation advice and assistance to all patients who smoke, including those with existing illness.

### Benefits for the Fetus

Maternal smoking is associated with several complications of pregnancy including abruptio placentae, placenta previa, bleeding during pregnancy, premature and prolonged rupture of the membranes, and preterm delivery. Maternal smoking retards fetal growth, causes an average reduction in birth-weight of 200 g, and doubles the risk of having a low birth-weight baby. Studies have shown a 25- to 50-percent higher rate of fetal and infant deaths among women who smoke during pregnancy compared with those who do not.

Women who stop smoking before becoming pregnant have infants of the same birth-weight as those born to women who have never smoked. The same benefit accrues to women who quit smoking in the first 3 to 4 months of pregnancy and who remain abstinent throughout the remainder of pregnancy. Women who quit smoking at later stages of pregnancy, up to the 30th week of gestation, have infants with higher birth-weight than do women who smoke throughout pregnancy.

Smoking is probably the most important modifiable cause of poor pregnancy outcome among women in the United States. Recent estimates suggest that the elimination of smoking during pregnancy could prevent about 5 percent of perinatal deaths, about 20 percent of low birth-weight births, and about 8 percent of preterm deliveries in the United States. In groups with a high prevalence of smoking (e.g., women who have not completed high school), the elimination of smoking during pregnancy could prevent about 10 percent of perinatal deaths, about 35 percent of low birth-weight births, and about 15 percent of preterm deliveries.

The prevalence of smoking during pregnancy has declined over time but remains unacceptably high. Approximately 30 percent of U.S. women who are cigarette smokers quit after recognition of pregnancy, and others quit later in pregnancy. However, about 25 percent of pregnant women in the United States smoke throughout pregnancy. A shocking statistic is that half of pregnant women who have not completed high school smoke throughout pregnancy. Many women who do not quit smoking during pregnancy reduce their daily cigarette consumption; however, reduced consumption without quitting may have little or no benefit for birth-weight. Of the women who quit smoking during pregnancy, 70 percent resume smoking within 1 year of delivery.

Initiatives have been launched in the public and private sectors to reduce smoking during pregnancy. These programs should be expanded, and less educated pregnant women should be a special target of these efforts. Strategies need to be developed to address the problem of relapse after delivery.

### Benefits for Infants and Children

As a pediatrician, I am particularly concerned about the effects of parental smoking on infants and children. Evidence reviewed in the 1986 Surgeon General's Report, *The Health Consequences of Involuntary Smoking*, indicates that the children of parents who smoke, compared with the children of non-smoking parents, have an increased frequency of respiratory infections such as pneumonia and bronchitis. Many studies have found a dose-response relationship between respiratory illness in children and their level of tobacco smoke exposure.

Several studies have shown that children exposed to tobacco smoke in the home are more likely to develop acute otitis media and persistent middle ear effusions. Middle ear disease imposes a substantial burden on the health care system. Otitis media is the most frequent diagnosis made by physicians who care for children. The myringotomy-and-tube procedure, used to treat otitis media in more than 1 million American children each year, is the most common minor surgical operation performed under general anesthesia.

The impact of smoking cessation during or after pregnancy on these associations has not been studied. However, the dose-response relationship between parental smoking and frequency of childhood respiratory infections suggests that smoking cessation during pregnancy and abstinence after delivery would eliminate most or all of the excess risk by eliminating most or all of the exposure.

If parents are unwilling to quit smoking for their own sake, I would urge them to quit for the sake of their children.

Passive-smoking-induced infections in infants and young children can cause serious and even fatal illness. Moreover, children whose parents smoke are much more likely to become smokers themselves.

## Smoking Cessation and Weight Gain

The fear of post-cessation weight gain may discourage many smokers from trying to quit. The fear or occurrence of weight gain may precipitate relapse among many of those who already have quit. In the 1986 Adult Use of Tobacco Survey, current smokers who had tried to quit were asked to judge the importance of several possible reasons for their return to smoking. Twenty-seven percent responded that "actual weight gain" was a "very important" or "somewhat important" reason why they resumed smoking; 22 percent said that "the possibility of gaining weight" was an important reason for their relapse. Forty-seven percent of current smokers and 48 percent of former smokers agreed with the statement that "smoking helps control weight."

Fifteen studies involving a total of 20,000 persons were reviewed in this report to determine the likelihood of gaining weight and the average weight gain after quitting. Although four-fifths of smokers who quit gained weight alter cessation, the average weight gain was only 5 pounds (2.3 kg). The average weight gain among subjects who continued to smoke was 1 pound. Thus, smoking cessation produces a 4-pound greater weight gain than that associated with continued smoking. This weight gain poses a minimal health risk. Moreover, evidence suggests that this small weight gain is accompanied by favorable changes in lipid profiles and in body fat distribution. Smoking cessation programs and messages should emphasize that weight gain after quitting is small on average.

Not only is the average post-cessation weight gain small, but the risk of large weight gain after quitting is extremely low. Less than 4 percent of those who quit smoking gain more than 20 pounds. Nevertheless, special advice and assistance should be available to the rare person who does gain considerable weight after quitting. For these individuals, the health benefits of cessation still occur, and weight control programs rather than smoking relapse should be implemented.

Increase in food intake and decreases in resting energy expenditure are largely responsible for post-cessation weight gain. Thus, dietary advice and exercise should be helpful in preventing or reducing post-cessation weight gain. Unfortunately, minor weight control modification to smoking cessation programs do not generally yield beneficial effects in terms of reducing weight gain or increasing cessation rates. A few studies have investigated pharmacologic approaches to post-cessation weight control; preliminary results are encouraging but more research is needed. High priority should be given to the development and evaluation of effective weight control programs that can be targeted in a cost-effective manner to those at greatest need of assistance.

## Psychological and Behavioral Consequences of Smoking Cessation

Nicotine withdrawal symptoms include anxiety, irritability, frustration, anger, difficulty concentrating, increased appetite, and urges to smoke. With the possible exception of urges to smoke and increased appetite, these effects soon disappear. Nicotine withdrawal peaks in first 1 to 2 days following cessation and subsides rapidly during the following weeks. With long-term abstinence, former smokers are likely to enjoy favorable psychological changes such as enhanced self-esteem and increased sense of self-control.

Although most nicotine withdrawal symptoms are short-lived, they often exert a strong influence on smokers' ability to quit and maintain abstinence. Nicotine withdrawal may discourage many smokers from trying to quit and may precipitate relapse among those who have recently quit. In the 1986 Adult Use of Tobacco Survey, 39 percent of current smokers reported that irritability was a "very important" or "somewhat important" reason why they resumed smoking after a previous quit attempt.

Smokers and ex-smokers should be counseled that adverse psychological effects of smoking subside rapidly over time. Smoking cessation materials and programs, nicotine replacement, exercise, stress management, and dietary counseling can help smokers cope with these symptoms until they abate, after which favorable psychological changes are likely to occur.

## Support for a Causal Association Between Smoking and Disease

Tens of thousands of studies have documented the associations between cigarette smoking and a large number of serious diseases. It is safe to say that smoking represents the most extensively documented cause of disease ever investigated in the history of biomedical research. Previous Surgeon General's reports, in particular the landmark 1964 Report of the Surgeon General's Advisory Committee on Smoking and Health and the 1982 Surgeon General's Report on smoking and cancer, examined these associations with respect to epidemiologic criteria for causality. These criteria include the consistency, strength, specificity, coherence, and temporal relationship of the association. Based on these criteria, previous reports have recognized a causal association between smoking and cancers of the lung, larynx, esophagus, and oral cavity; heart disease; stroke; peripheral artery occlusive disease; chronic obstructive pulmonary disease; and intrauterine growth retardation. This Surgeon General's Report is the first to conclude that the evidence is now sufficient to identify cigarette smoking as a cause of cancer of the urinary bladder; the 1982 report concluded that cigarette smoking is a contributing factor in the development of bladder cancer.

The causal nature of most of these associations was well established long before publication of this report. Nevertheless, it is worth noting that the findings of this report add even more weight to the evidence that these associations are causal. The criterion of coherence requires that descriptive epidemiologic findings on disease occurrence correlate with measures of exposure to the suspected agent. Coherence would predict that the increased risk of disease associated with an exposure would diminish or disappear after cessation of exposure.

As this report shows in great detail, the risks of most smoking-related diseases decrease after cessation and with increasing duration or abstinence.

Evidence on the risk of disease after smoking cessation is especially important for the understanding of smoking-and-disease associations of unclear causality. For example cigarette smoking is associated with cancer of the uterine cervix, but this association is potentially confounded by unidentified factors (in particular by a sexually transmitted etiologic agent). The evidence reviewed in this report indicates that former smokers experience a lower risk of cervical cancer than current smokers even after adjusting for the social correlates of smoking and risk of sexually acquired infections. This diminution of risk after smoking cessation supports the hypothesis that smoking is a contributing cause of cervical cancer.

## Conclusion

The Comprehensive Smoking Education Act of 1984 (Public Law 98-474) requires the rotation of four health warnings on cigarette packages and advertisements. One of those warnings reads "SURGEON GENERAL'S WARNING: Quitting Smoking Now Greatly Reduces Serious Risks to Your Health." The evidence reviewed in this report confirms and expands that advice.

The health benefits of quitting smoking are immediate and substantial. They far exceed any risks from the average 5-pound weight gain or any adverse psychological affects that may follow quitting. The benefits extend to men and women to the young and the old, to those who are sick and to those who are well. Smoking cessation represents the single most important step that smokers can take to enhance the length and quality of their lives.

Public opinion polls tell us that most smokers want to quit. This report provides smokers with new and more powerful motivation to give up this self-destructive behavior.

## Summary of Chapter 7: Smoking Cessation and Non-malignant Respiratory Diseases

1. Smoking cessation reduces rates of respiratory symptoms such as cough, sputum production, and wheezing, and respi-

## Health Benefits of Smoking Cessation

ratory infections such as bronchitis and pneumonia, compared with continued smoking.

2. For persons without overt chronic obstructive pulmonary disease (COPD), smoking cessation improves pulmonary function about 5 percent within a few months after cessation.

3. Cigarette smoking accelerates the age-related decline in lung function that occurs among never smokers. With sustained abstinence from smoking, the rate of decline in pulmonary function among former smokers returns to that of never smokers.

4. With sustained abstinence, the COPD mortality rates among former smokers decline in comparison with continuing smokers.

*—Antonia C. Novello, M.D.. M.P.H.,*
*Surgeon General*

Chapter 20

# Clearing the Air:
# How to Quit Smoking...
# and Quit for Keeps

This chapter guides you from thinking about stopping smoking through actually doing it—from the day you quit to quitting for keeps. It gives tips on fighting temptation—and what to do if you give in— and on avoiding weight gain (a handy Snack Calorie Chart is included). By telling you what to expect, it can help you through the day-by-day process of becoming a nonsmoker.

In this chapter, you'll find a variety of tips and helpful hints on kicking your smoking habit. Take a few moments to look at each suggestion carefully. Pick those you feel comfortable with and decide today that you're going to use them to quit. It may take a while to find the combination that's right for you, but you can quit for good, even if you've tried to quit before.

Many smokers have successfully given up cigarettes by replacing them with new habits without quitting "cold turkey," planning a special program, or seeking professional help.

The following approaches include many of those most popular with ex-smokers. Remember that successful methods are as different as the people who use them. What may seem silly to others may be just what you need to quit. So don't be embarrassed to try something new. These methods can make your own personal efforts a little easier.

Pick the ideas that make sense to you. And then follow through. You'll have a much better chance of success.

---

National Institutes of Health   Pub. No. 94-1647.

## Preparing Yourself for Quitting

- Decide positively that you want to quit. Try to avoid negative thoughts about how difficult it might be.

- List all the reasons you want to quit. Every night before going to bed, repeat one of those reasons 10 times.

- Develop strong personal reasons in addition to your health and obligations to others. For example, think of all the time you waste taking cigarette breaks, rushing out to buy a pack, hunting for a light, etc.

- Begin to condition yourself physically: Start a modest exercise program; drink more fluids; get plenty of rest; and avoid fatigue.

- Set a target date for quitting—perhaps a special day such as your birthday, your anniversary, or the Great American Smokeout. If you smoke heavily at work, quit during your vacation so that you're already committed to quitting when you return. Make the date sacred and don't let anything change it. This will make it easy for you to keep track of the day you became a nonsmoker and to celebrate that date every year

## Knowing What to Expect

- Have realistic expectations—quitting isn't easy, but it's not impossible either. More than 3 million Americans quit every year.

- Understand that withdrawal symptoms are temporary. They usually last only 1-2 weeks.

- Know that most relapses occur in the first week after quitting, when withdrawal symptoms are strongest, and your body is still dependent on nicotine. Be aware that this will be your hardest time and use all your personal resources, willpower, family, friends, and the tips in this booklet—to get you through this critical period successfully.

- Know that most other relapses occur in the first 3 months after quitting, when situational triggers, such as a particularly stressful event, occur unexpectedly. These are the times when people reach for cigarettes automatically, because they associate smoking with relaxing. This is the kind of situation that's hard to prepare yourself for until it happens, so it's especially important to recognize it if it does happen. Remember that smoking is a habit, but a habit you can break.

- Realize that most successful ex-smokers quit for good only after several attempts. You may be one of those who can quit on your first try. But if you're not, don't give up. Try again.

## Involving Someone Else

- Bet a friend you can quit on your target date. Put your cigarette money aside for every day you don't smoke and forfeit it if you smoke. (But if you do smoke, don't give up. Simply strengthen your resolve and try again.)

- Ask your friend or spouse to quit with you.

- Tell your family and friends that you're quitting and when. They can be an important source of support both before and after you quit.

## Ways of Quitting

### Switch Brands

- Switch to a brand you find distasteful.

- Change to a brand that is low in tar and nicotine a couple of weeks before your target date. This will help change your smoking behavior. However, do not smoke more cigarettes, inhale them more often or more deeply, or place your fingertips over the holes in the filters. These actions will increase your nicotine intake, and the idea is to get your body used to functioning without nicotine.

*Cut Down the Number of Cigarettes You Smoke*

- Smoke only half of each cigarette.

- Each day, postpone the lighting of your first cigarette 1 hour.

- Decide you'll only smoke during odd or even hours of the day.

- Decide beforehand how many cigarettes you'll smoke during the day. For each additional cigarette, give a dollar to your favorite charity.

- Change your eating habits to help you cut down. For example, drink milk, which many people consider incompatible with smoking. End meals or snacks with something that won't lead to a cigarette.

- Reach for a glass of juice instead of a cigarette for a "pick-me-up."

- Remember: Cutting down can help you quit, but it's not a substitute for quitting. If you're down to about seven cigarettes a day, it's time to set your target date to quit and get ready to stick to it.

*Don't Smoke "Automatically"*

- Smoke only those cigarettes you really want. Catch yourself before you light up a cigarette out of pure habit.

- Don't empty your ashtrays. This will remind you of how many cigarettes you've smoked each day, and the sight and the smell of stale cigarettes butts will be very unpleasant.

- Make yourself aware of each cigarette by using the opposite hand or putting cigarettes in an unfamiliar location or a different pocket to break the automatic reach.

- If you light up many times during the day without even thinking about it, try to look into a mirror each time you put a match to your cigarette—you may decide you don't need it.

## Clearing the Air: How to Quit Smoking and Quit for Keeps

### Make Smoking Inconvenient

- Stop buying cigarettes by the carton. Wait until one pack is empty before you buy another.

- Stop carrying cigarettes with you at home or at work. Make them difficult to get.

### Make Smoking Unpleasant

- Smoke only under circumstances that aren't especially pleasurable for you. If you like to smoke with others, smoke alone. Turn your chair to an empty corner and focus only on the cigarette you are smoking and all its many negative effects.

- Collect all your cigarette butts in one large glass container as a visual reminder of the filth made by smoking.

### Just Before Quitting

- Practice going without cigarettes.

- Don't think of *never* smoking again. Think of quitting in terms of *1 day at a time*.

- Tell yourself you won't smoke today and then, don't.

- Clean your clothes to rid them of the cigarette smell, which can linger for a long time.

### On the Day You Quit

- Throw away all your cigarettes and matches. Hide your lighters and ashtrays.

- Visit the dentist and have your teeth cleaned to get rid of tobacco stains. Notice how nice they look and resolve to keep them that way.

- Make a list of things you'd like to buy for yourself or someone else. Estimate the cost in terms of packs of cigarettes and put the money aside to buy these presents.

- Keep very busy on the big day. Go to the movies, exercise, take long walks, go bike riding.

- Remind your family and friends that this is your quit date and ask them to help you over the rough spots of the first couple of days and weeks.

- Buy yourself a treat or do something special to celebrate.

## *Immediately After Quitting*

- Develop a clean, fresh, non-smoking environment around yourself, at work and at home. Buy yourself flowers. You may be surprised how much you can enjoy their scent now.

- The first few days after you quit, spend as much free time as possible in places where smoking isn't allowed, such as libraries, museums, theaters, department stores, and churches.

- Drink large quantities of water and fruit juice (but avoid sodas that contain caffeine).

- Try to avoid alcohol, coffee, and other beverages that you associate with cigarette smoking.

- Strike up conversation instead of a match for a cigarette.

- If you miss the sensation of having a cigarette in your hand, play with something else, such as a pencil, a paper clip, a marble.

- If you miss having something in your mouth, try toothpicks or a fake cigarette.

## Avoid Temptation

- Instead of smoking after meals, get up from the table and brush your teeth or go for a walk.

- If you always smoke while driving, listen to a particularly interesting radio program or your favorite music, or take public transportation for a while, if you can.

- For the first 1-3 weeks, avoid situations you strongly associate with the pleasurable aspects of smoking, such as watching your favorite TV program, sitting in your favorite chair, or having a cocktail before dinner.

- Until you are confident of your ability to stay off cigarettes, limit your socializing to healthful, outdoor activities or situations where smoking is not allowed.

- If you must be in a situation where you'll be tempted to smoke, such as a cocktail or dinner party, try to associate with the nonsmokers there.

- Try to analyze cigarette ads to understand how they attempt to "sell" you on individual brands.

## When You Get the Crazies

- Keep oral substitutes handy. Try carrots, pickles, sunflower seeds, apples, celery, raisins, or sugarless gum instead of a cigarette.

- Take 10 deep breaths and hold the last one while lighting a match. Exhale slowly and blow out the match. Pretend it's a cigarette and crush it out in an ashtray.

- Take a shower or bath if possible.

- Learn to relax quickly and deeply. Make yourself limp, visualize a soothing, pleasing situation and get away from it all for a moment. Concentrate on that peaceful image and nothing else.

- Light incense or a candle instead of a cigarette.

- Never allow yourself to think that "one won't hurt" —it will.

**Find New Habits**

- Change your habits to make smoking difficult, impossible, or unnecessary. For example, it's hard to smoke while you're swimming, jogging, or playing tennis or handball. When your desire for a cigarette is intense, wash your hands or the dishes, or try new recipes.

- Do things that require you to use your hands. Try crossword puzzles, needlework, gardening, or household chores. Go bike riding or take the dog for a walk; give yourself a manicure; write letters.

- Enjoy having a clean-mouth taste and maintain it by brushing your teeth frequently and using a mouthwash.

- Stretch a lot.

- Get plenty of rest.

- Pay attention to your appearance. Look and feel sharp.

- Try to find time for the activities that are the most meaningful, satisfying, and important to you.

**About Gaining Weight**

Many people who are considering quitting are very concerned about gaining weight. If you are concerned about weight gain, keep these points in mind:

- Quitting doesn't mean you'll automatically gain weight. When people gain, it's because they often eat more once they quit.

- The benefits of giving up cigarettes far outweigh the drawbacks of adding a few pounds. You'd have to gain a very large amount of weight to offset the many substantial health ben-

# Clearing the Air: How to Quit Smoking and Quit for Keeps

efits that a normal smoker gains by quitting. Watch what you eat, and if you are concerned about gaining weight, consider the tips that follow.

## *Tips To Help You Avoid Weight Gain*

- Make sure you have a well balanced diet, with the proper amounts of protein, carbohydrates, and fat.

- Don't set a target date for a holiday, when the temptation of high-calorie food and drinks may be too hard to resist.

- Drink a glass of water before your meals.

- Weigh yourself weekly.

- Chew sugarless gum when you want sweet foods.

- Plan menus carefully and count calories. Don't try to lose weight; just try to maintain your pre-quitting weight.

|  | *Snacks* | *Calories\** |
|---|---|---|
| BEVERAGES | **Carbonated** (per 8-ounce glass) | |
| | Cola-type | 95 |
| | Fruit flavors (10-13% sugar) | 115 |
| | Ginger ale | 75 |
| | **Fruit drinks** (per 1/2 cup) | |
| | Apricot nectar | 70 |
| | Cranberry juice | 80 |
| | Grape drink | 70 |
| | Lemonade (frozen) | 55 |
| | **Fruit juices** (per 1/2 cup) | |
| | Apple juice, canned | 60 |
| | Grape juice, bottled | 80 |
| | Grapefruit juice, canned, unsweetened | 50 |
| | Orange juice, canned, unsweetened | 55 |
| | Pineapple juice, canned, unsweetened | 70 |
| | Prune juice, canned | 100 |
| | **Vegetable juices** (per 1/2 cup) | |
| | Tomato juice | 25 |
| | Vegetable juice cocktail | 20 |
| | **Coffee and tea** | |
| \* Data from published sources. References are available upon request. | Coffee, black | 3-5 |
| | with 1 tsp. sugar | 18-20 |
| | with 1 tsp. cream | 13-15 |
| | Tea, plain | 0-1 |
| | with 1 tsp. sugar | 15-16 |

*Figure 20.1.* Snack Calorie Chart, continued on next page

| | | |
|---|---|---|
| CANDY, CHIPS, AND PRETZELS | **Candy** (per ounce) | |
| | Hard candy | 110 |
| | Jelly beans | 105 |
| | Marshmallows | 90 |
| | Gumdrops | 100 |
| | **Chips** (per cup) | |
| | Corn chips | 230 |
| | Potato chips | 115 |
| | **Popcorn** (air-popped, without butter) | 25 |
| | **Pretzels** | |
| | Dutch, 1 twisted | 60 |
| | Stick, 5 regular | 10 |
| CHEESE (per ounce) | American, processed | 105 |
| | Cottage, creamed | 30 |
| | Cottage, low-fat (2%) | 25 |
| | Swiss, natural | 105 |
| CRACKERS | Butter, 2-inch diameter | 15 |
| | Graham, 2 1/2 inches square, 2 | 55 |
| | Matzoh, 6-inch diameter | 80 |
| | Rye | 45 |
| | Saltine | 50 |
| FRUITS (raw) | Apple, 1 medium | 80 |
| | Apricots, fresh, 3 medium | 50 |
| | Apricots, dried, 5 halves | 40 |
| | Banana, 1 medium | 105 |
| | Blackberries, 1/2 cup | 35 |
| | Blueberries, 1/2 cup | 40 |
| | Cantaloupe, 1/4 melon | 50 |
| | Cherries, 10 | 50 |
| | Dates, dried, 3 | 70 |
| | Fig, dried, 1 medium | 50 |
| | Grapefruit, 1/2 | 40 |
| | Grapes, 20 | 30 |
| | Orange, 1 medium | 60 |
| | Peach, 1 medium | 35 |
| | Pear, 1 medium | 100 |
| | Pineapple, 1/2 cup | 40 |
| | Prunes, dried, 3 | 60 |
| | Raisins, 1/4 cup | 110 |
| | Strawberries, 1 cup | 45 |
| | Watermelon, 1 cup | 50 |
| NUTS (per 2 tablespoons) | Almonds | 105 |
| | Brazil nuts | 115 |
| | Cashews | 100 |
| | Peanuts | 105 |
| | Pecans, halves | 95 |
| VEGETABLES (raw) | Carrots, 1/2 cup grated | 35 |
| | Celery, 5-inch stalks, 3 | 10 |
| | Pickle, 1 | 15-20 |

- Have low-calorie foods on hand for nibbling. Use the Snack Calorie Chart to choose foods that are both nutritious and low in calories. Some good choices are fresh fruits and vegetables, fruit and vegetable juices, low-fat cottage cheese, and air-popped popcorn without butter.

- Take time for daily exercise or join an organized exercise group.

## What Happens After You Quit Smoking

### *Immediate Rewards*

Within 12 hours after you have your last cigarette, your body will begin to heal itself. The levels of carbon monoxide and nicotine in your system will decline rapidly, and your heart and lungs will begin to repair the damage caused by cigarette smoke.

Within a few days you will probably begin to notice some remarkable changes in your body. Your sense of smell and taste may improve. You will breathe easier, and your smoker's hack will begin to disappear, although you may notice that you will continue to cough for a while. And you will be free of the mess, smell, inconvenience, expense, and dependence of cigarette smoking.

### *Immediate Effects*

As your body begins to repair itself, instead of feeling better right away, you may feel worse for a while. It's important to understand that healing is a process—it begins immediately, but it continues over time. These "withdrawal pangs" are really symptoms of the recovery process (See "Withdrawal Symptoms and Activities That Might Help")

Immediately after quitting, many ex-smokers experience "symptoms of recovery" such as temporary weight gain caused by fluid retention, irregularity and dry, sore gums or tongue. You may feel edgy, hungry, more tired, or more short-tempered than usual; you may have trouble sleeping or notice that you are coughing a lot. These symptoms are the result of your body clearing itself of nicotine, a powerful addictive chemical. Most nicotine is gone from the body in 2—3 days.

*Long-Range Benefits*

It is important to understand that the after-effects of quitting are only temporary and signal the beginning of a healthier life. Now that you've quit, you've added a number of healthy, productive days to each year of your life. Most important, you've greatly improved your chances for a longer life. You have significantly reduced your risk of death from heart disease, stroke, chronic bronchitis, emphysema, and several kinds of cancer—not just lung cancer. More than 400,000 deaths in the United States each year are from smoking-related illnesses.

## Withdrawal Symptoms and Activities That Might Help

Adapted from Quitting Times: A Magazine for Women Who Smoke, funded by the Pennsylvania Department of Health; prepared by Fox Chase Cancer Center, Philadelphia.

**Dry mouth; sore throat, gums or tongue:** Sip ice-cold water or fruit juice, or chew gum.

**Headaches:** Take a warm bath or shower. Try relaxation or meditation techniques.

**Trouble sleeping:** Don't drink coffee, tea, or soda with caffeine after 6:00 p.m. Again, try relaxation or meditation techniques.

**Irregularity:** Add roughage to your diet, such as raw fruit, vegetables, and whole-grain cereals. Drink 6-8 glasses of water a day.

**Fatigue:** Take a nap. Try not to push yourself during this time; don't expect too much of your body until it's had a chance to begin to heal itself over a couple of weeks.

**Hunger:** Drink water or low-calorie liquids. Eat low-fat, low calorie snacks. (See "Snack Calorie Chart")

**Tenseness, irritability:** Take a walk, soak in a hot bath, try relaxation or meditation techniques.

## Clearing the Air: How to Quit Smoking and Quit for Keeps

**Coughing:** Sip warm herbal tea. Suck on cough drops or sugarless hard candy.

## Quitting for Keeps

Congratulations! Now you are ready to develop a new habit-not smoking. Like any other habit, it takes time to become a part of you; unlike most other habits, though, not smoking will take some conscious effort and practice. This section of the booklet can be a big help. You will find many techniques to use for developing the non-smoking habit and holding on to it.

By reading this section of the chapter carefully and reviewing it often, you'll become more aware of the places and situations that prompt the desire for a cigarette. You will also learn about many non-smoking ways to deal with the urge to smoke. These are called coping skills. Finally, you will learn what to do in case you do slip and give in to the smoking urge.

### Keep Your Guard Up

The key to living as a nonsmoker is to avoid letting your urges or cravings for a cigarette lead you to smoke. Don't kid yourself—even though you have made a commitment not to smoke, you will sometimes be tempted. But instead of giving in to the urge, you can use it as a learning experience.

First, remind yourself that you have quit and you are a nonsmoker. Then look closely at your urge to smoke and ask yourself:

- Where was I when I got the urge?
- What was I doing at the time?
- Who was with me?
- What was I thinking?

The urge to smoke after you've quit often hits at predictable times. The trick is to anticipate those times and find ways to cope with them—without smoking. Naturally, it won't be easy at first. In fact, you may continue to want a cigarette at times. But remember, even if you slip, it doesn't mean an end to the non-smoking you. It does mean that you should try to identify what triggered your slip, strengthen your commitment to quitting, and try again.

Look at the following list of typical triggers. Do many of them ring a bell with you? Check off those that might trigger an urge to smoke, and add any others you can think of:

- Working under pressure
- Feeling blue
- Talking on the telephone
- Having a drink
- Watching television
- Driving your car
- Finishing a meal
- Playing cards
- Drinking coffee
- Watching someone else smoke

If you are like many new nonsmokers, the most difficult place to resist the urge to smoke is the most familiar—home. The activities most closely associated with smoking urges are eating, partying, and drinking. And, not surprisingly, most urges occur when a smoker is present.

### *How to Dampen That Urge*

There are seven major coping skills to help you fight the urge to smoke. These tips are designed for you, the new nonsmoker, to help you nurture the non-smoking habit.

1. Think about why you quit. Go back to your list of reasons for quitting. Look at this list several times a day, especially when you are hit with the urge to smoke. The best reasons you could have for quitting are very personally yours, and these are also the best reasons to stay a nonsmoker.

2. Know when you are rationalizing. It is easy to rationalize yourself back into smoking. (See "Common Rationalizations") Don't talk yourself into smoking again. A new nonsmoker in a tense situation may think, "I'll just have one cigarette to calm myself down." If thoughts like this pop into your head, stop and think again! You know better ways to relax, nonsmokers' ways, such as taking a walk or doing breathing exercises.

## Clearing the Air: How to Quit Smoking and Quit for Keeps

Concern about gaining weight may also lead to rationalizations. Learn to counter thoughts, such as "I'd rather be thin, even if it means smoking." Remember that a slight weight gain is not likely to endanger your health as much as smoking would. (Cigarette smokers have about a 70-percent higher rate of premature death than nonsmokers.) And review the list of healthy, low-calorie snacks that you used when quitting.

3. Anticipate triggers and prepare to avoid them. By now you know which situations, people, and feelings are likely to tempt you to smoke. Be prepared to meet these triggers head-on and counteract them. Keep using the skills that helped you cope in cutting down and quitting:

—Keep your hands busy—doodle, knit, type a letter.

—Avoid people who smoke; spend more time with nonsmoking friends.

—Find activities that make smoking difficult (gardening, washing the car, taking a shower). Exercise to help knock out the smoking urge; it will help you to feel and look good as well.

—Put something other than a cigarette in your mouth. Chew sugarless gum or nibble on a carrot or celery stick.

—Avoid places where smoking is permitted. Sit in the non-smoking section of restaurants, trains, and planes.

—Reduce your consumption of alcohol, which often stimulates the desire to smoke. Try to have no more than one or two drinks at a party. Better yet, have a glass of juice, soda, or mineral water.

4. Reward yourself for not smoking. Congratulations are in order each time you get through a day without smoking. After a week, give yourself a pat on the back and a reward of some kind. Buy a new tape or compact disc. Treat yourself to a movie or concert. No matter how you do it, make sure you

reward yourself in some way. It helps to remind yourself that what you are doing is important.

5. Use positive thoughts. If self-defeating thoughts start to creep in, remind yourself again that you are a nonsmoker, that you do not want to smoke, and that you have good reasons for quitting. Putting yourself down and trying to hold out using willpower alone are not effective coping techniques. Mobilize the power of positive thinking!

6. Use relaxation techniques. Breathing exercises help to reduce tension. Instead of having a cigarette, take a long deep breath, count to 10, and release it. Repeat this five times. See how much more relaxed you feel?

7. Get social support. The commitment to remain a nonsmoker can be made easier by talking about it with friends and relatives. They can congratulate you as you check off another day, week, and month as a nonsmoker. Tell the people close to you that you might be tense for a while, so they know what to expect. They'll be sympathetic when you have an urge to smoke and can be counted on to help you resist it. Remember to call on your friends when you are lonely, or you feel an urge to smoke. A buddy system is a great technique.

### Not Smoking Is Habit-Forming

Good for you! You have made a commitment not to smoke, and by using this chapter, you know what to do if you are tempted to forget that commitment. It is difficult to stay a nonsmoker once you have had a cigarette so do everything possible to avoid it.

If you follow the advice in this chapter and use at least one coping skill whenever you have an urge to smoke, you will have quit for keeps!

### Relapse: If You Do Smoke Again

If you slip and smoke, don't be discouraged. Many former smokers tried to stop several times before they finally succeeded. Here's what you should do:

# Clearing the Air: How to Quit Smoking and Quit for Keeps

- Recognize that you have had a slip. A slip means that you have had a small setback and smoked a cigarette or two. But your first cigarette did not make you a smoker to start with, and a small setback does not make you a smoker again.

- Don't be too hard on yourself. One slip doesn't mean you're a failure or that you can't be a nonsmoker, but it is important to get yourself back on the non-smoking track immediately.

- Identify the trigger: Exactly what was it that prompted you to smoke? Be aware of the trigger and decide now how you will cope with it when it comes up again.

- Know and use the coping skills described above. People who know at least one coping skill are more likely to remain non-smokers than those who do not know any.

- Sign a contract with yourself to remain a nonsmoker.

- If you think you need professional help, see your doctor. He or she can provide extra motivation for you to stop smoking. Your doctor may also prescribe nicotine gum or a nicotine patch as an alternative source of nicotine while you break the habit of smoking.

## *Marking Progress*

- Each month, on the anniversary of your quit date, plan a special celebration.

- Periodically, write down new reasons you are glad you quit and post these reasons where you will be sure to see them.

- Make up a calendar for the first 90 days. Cross off each day and indicate the money you saved by not smoking.

- Set other intermediate target dates and do something special with the money you have saved.

## Common Rationalizations

Adapted from Clinical Opportunities for Smoking Intervention-A Guide for the Busy Physician. National Heart, Lung, and Blood Institute. NIH Pub. No. 86-2178. August 1986.

*I'm under a lot of stress, and smoking relaxes me.*

Your body is used to nicotine, so you naturally feel more relaxed when you give your body a substance upon which it has grown dependent. But nicotine really is a stimulant; it raises your heart rate, blood pressure, and adrenaline level. Most ex-smokers feel much less nervous just a few weeks after quitting.

*Smoking makes me more effective in my work.*

Trouble concentrating can be a short-term symptom of quitting, but smoking actually deprives your brain of oxygen

*I've already cut down to a safe level.*

Cutting down is a good first step, but there's a big difference in the benefits to you between smoking a little and not smoking at all. Besides, smokers who cut back often inhale more often and more deeply, negating many of the benefits of cutting back. After you've cut back to about seven cigarettes a day, it's time to set a quit date.

*I smoke only safe low-tar/low-nicotine cigarettes.*

These cigarettes still contain harmful substances, and many smokers who use them inhale more often and more deeply to maintain their nicotine intake. Also, carbon monoxide intake often increases with a switch to low-tar cigarettes.

*It's too hard to quit. I don't have the willpower.*

Quitting and staying away from cigarettes is hard, but it's not impossible. More than 3 million Americans quit every year It's important for you to remember that many people have had to try more than once, and try more than one method, before they became ex-smokers, but they have done it and so can you.

## Clearing the Air: How to Quit Smoking and Quit for Keeps

*I'm worried about gaining weight.*

Most smokers who gain more than 5—10 pounds are eating more. Gaining weight isn't inevitable. There are certain things you can do to help keep your weight stable (See "Tips To Help You Avoid Weight Gain")

*I don't know what to do with my hands.*

That's a common complaint among ex-smokers. You can keep your hands busy in other ways; it's just a matter of getting used to the change of not holding a cigarette. Try holding something else, such as a pencil, paper clip, or marble. Practice simply keeping your hands clasped together. If you're at home, think of all the things you wish you had time to do, make a list, and consult the list for alternatives to smoking whenever your hands feel restless.

*Sometimes I have an almost irresistible urge to have a cigarette.*

This is a common feeling, especially within the first 1—3 weeks. The longer you're off cigarettes, the more your urges probably will come at times when you smoked before, such as when you're drinking coffee or alcohol or are at a cocktail party where other people are smoking. These are high-risk situations, and you can help yourself by avoiding them whenever possible. If you can't avoid them, you can try to visualize in advance how you'll handle the desire for a cigarette if it arises in those situations.

*I blew it I smoked a cigarette.*

Smoking one or a few cigarettes doesn't mean you've "blown it." It does mean that you have to strengthen your determination to quit and try again—harder. Don't forget that you got through several days, perhaps even weeks or months, without a cigarette. This shows that you don't need cigarettes and that you can be a successful quitter.

### For Further Information

The Cancer Information Service, a program of the National Cancer Institute, is a nationwide telephone service for cancer patients and their families and friends, the public, and health care professionals.

The staff can answer questions (in English or Spanish) and can send free National Cancer Institute materials about cancer. They also know about support groups and other resources and services. One toll-free number, 1-800-4-CANCER (1-800-422-6237), connects callers with the office that serves their area.

The following organizations also can help you. Contact them to learn more about quitting for keeps.

American Cancer Society
1599 Clifton Road, NE
Atlanta, GA 30329
(404) 320-3333

The American Cancer Society (ACS) is a voluntary organization composed of 58 divisions and 3,100 local units. Through "The Great American Smokeout" in November, the annual Cancer Crusade in April, and the numerous educational materials, ACS helps people learn about the health hazards of smoking and become successful ex-smokers.

American Heart Association
7272 Greenville Avenue
Dallas, TX 75231
(214) 373-6300

The American Heart Association (AHA) is a voluntary organization with 130,000 members (physicians, scientists, and lay persons) in 55 state and regional groups. AHA produces a variety of publications and audiovisual materials about the effects of smoking on the heart. AHA also has developed a guidebook for incorporating a weight-control component into smoking cessation programs.

American Lung Association
1740 Broadway
New York, NY 10019-4374
(212) 315-8700

The oldest voluntary health agency with 57 state associations and 60 affiliates throughout the United States, the American Lung Association (ALA) provides help for smokers who wish to quit through their "Freedom From Smoking" self-help smoking cessation program. The organization actively supports legislation and information campaigns for nonsmokers' rights and conducts public information programs about the health effects of smoking. Consult your local telephone directory for listings of local chapters.

Office on Smoking and Health
Centers for Disease Control
Mail Stop K-50
4770 Buford Highway, NE
Atlanta, GA 30341-3724
(404) 488-5705

The Office on Smoking and Health (OSH) is the Department of Health and Human Services' lead agency in smoking control. OSH sponsors distribution of publications on smoking-related topics, such as free flyers on relapse after initial quitting, helping a friend or family member quit smoking, the health hazards of smoking, and the effects of parental smoking on teenagers.

Chapter 21

# I Mind Very Much If You Smoke

## Other People's Smoke

Every year, 434,000 people die of illnesses related to their smoking. But smokers are not the only ones whose health can suffer. Their tobacco smoke in the air is called environmental tobacco smoke (ETS) or secondhand smoke. Breathing it can be a hazard to your health and to the health of your child.

Secondhand smoke contains smaller amounts of the same chemicals that harm smokers. ETS is so harmful that the U.S. Environmental Protection Agency (EPA) has classified it as a "Group A" carcinogen. "Group A" carcinogens are the most toxic substances known to cause cancer in humans, also including benzene, radon, and asbestos.

The more often you're around secondhand smoke, the greater your risk for health problems. Each year it causes about 3,000 lung cancer deaths in U.S. adults who don't smoke. Secondhand smoke increases the nonsmoker's risk for heart disease and makes worse the symptoms of adults already suffering from asthma, allergies, or bronchitis.

Children are usually innocent victims—unable to choose whether or not to be in a smoke-filled environment. Among infants to 18 months of age, secondhand smoke is associated with as many as 300,000 cases of bronchitis and pneumonia each year. It also increases

---

NIH Pub. No. 93-3544. June 1993.

the chances for middle ear problems, causes coughing and wheezing, and worsens asthma conditions.

Facts like these show that other people's smoke is more than an annoyance. Secondhand smoke is a serious threat to your good health.

## Saying No to Secondhand Smoke

As long as people continue to smoke tobacco, secondhand smoke will threaten the health of nonsmokers. Still, you can take steps to protect yourself and your children from other people's smoke-at home, at work, and in public places.

## Saying No at Home

Your husband or wife smokes and you don't. Every time your mother visits and smokes, your son has an asthma attack. Your babysitter smokes.

How can you and your children share air space at home with smokers without risking your health? Here are some ideas to help you clear the air.

### *If You Live With a Smoker*

- Ask him or her not to smoke inside your home. Look at this booklet together and discuss how his or her habit puts you and your children at risk.

- If he/she is unwilling to go outside, suggest ways to limit the exposure to smoke for you and your children. Maybe a room could be set aside for smoking-one that is seldom used by other members of the household. Some smokers protect others at home by smoking near an open window or when no one is around.

- Keep rooms well-ventilated. Open windows.

- Support smokers who decide to quit.

## When Visitors Come to Call

- Ask all smokers who visit not to smoke in your house or apartment. It's your right to keep your home free of this health risk.

- Don't keep ashtrays around.

## In Others' Homes

- Tell friends and relatives politely that you'd appreciate it if they do not smoke while you're there.

- Let people know when their smoke is causing immediate problems. If it is making your allergies worse, making you cough or wheeze, or making your eyes sting—say so. Some smokers may put their cigarettes away when they see the discomfort it causes.

## If You Have Children

- Insist that babysitters, grandparents, or other care-givers not smoke around your children. Be firm if necessary; your child's health is worth it.

- Help children avoid secondhand smoke if smokers do use tobacco around them. Have them leave the room or play outside while an adult is smoking. Air rooms out after smoking occurs. Keep smokers away from places children sleep.

## *Saying No at Work*

The person next to you smokes all day long, and you go home with itchy, watery eyes. You cough and sneeze after your regular office meetings because a few of your co-workers smoked.

When smoking is allowed at the work-place, nonsmokers cannot avoid secondhand smoke. Often, the ventilation system brings other people's smoke into your breathing space.

A report from the National Institute for Occupational Safety and Health (NIOSH) recommends that employee exposure to ETS be reduced to the lowest possible amount.

If your company still allows smoking, you can help limit your exposure by taking steps like these:

- Give your employer copies of the EPA and NIOSH reports on the harmful health effects of environmental tobacco smoke. (See ORGANIZATIONS, at the end of this chapter.)

- Ask to work near other nonsmokers and as far away from smokers as possible.

- Ask smokers if they would not smoke around you. Thank those who care enough to stop.

- Use a fan and open windows to keep the air moving.

- Hang a "Thank You For Not Smoking" sign in your work area.

- Talk to your employer about the company's smoking policy. Be sure your management knows that medical leaders think secondhand smoke is a serious problem that can make the workplace unsafe for nonsmokers. Give them a copy of this article or the EPA report.

- Volunteer to help develop a fair company policy that protects nonsmokers.

## Saying No in Public Places

Your hotel room smells like stale smoke and you wake up coughing and sneezing. The sign says "NO Smoking." Still, smoke is so thick inside the sports arena that you cannot enjoy the game. Cigarette smoke from other tables makes it hard to relish-or even taste-your restaurant meal.

In some cities and towns, smoking is forbidden in most public places, and many restaurants are completely smoke-free. Yet in other localities, restaurants, bars, sports centers, bowling alleys, theater lobbies, waiting rooms, and other public places, remain smoke-filled. Of course, enforcement of smoking bans is often lax.

How can you avoid other people's smoke in public areas? Take full advantage of non-smoking spaces and limit the time you spend in places that don't protect nonsmokers.

## I Mind Very Much If You Smoke

*Here are some ideas:*

- Always take the "non-smoking" options that are available. Today, many restaurants have non-smoking sections and hotels offer non-smoking rooms and floors. You can even get a non-smoking rental car. If one place doesn't offer non-smoking, choose another that does. The strongest statement against smoking in public places is made by taking your business elsewhere.

- Don't accept what you can change. If a restaurant puts you at a table near smokers (even if you're in a non-smoking section), ask to move. If smokers don't obey non-smoking rules, ask those in charge to enforce the rules. When people near you are smoking, ask them politely to either stop, move the ashtray, or hold their cigarette away from you.

- Keep children out of smoking areas. Choose "non-smoking" even if people in your group smoke. They can smoke outside or go into the smoking section if they need a cigarette. If there are no non-smoking sections, go someplace else.

### If You Want to Do More

Most Americans believe that smokers should never smoke around nonsmokers. Yet many work-places and public buildings still allow smoking. To protect themselves and their children, some nonsmokers are trying to change the rules. They are working to convince lawmakers and businesses to protect nonsmokers from cancer-causing tobacco smoke.

Some steps for nonsmokers include:

- Find out about laws that may require your employer to ban or limit smoking. The organizations listed at the end of this booklet can give you more information.

- Urge your child's school, including preschool, to ban all indoor smoking. When smoking is allowed in some places (such as the teacher's lounge, storage areas, or private offices), second-hand smoke may reach your child through the ventilation system.

- Write to public officials, newspapers, and businesses to promote policies protecting nonsmokers.

- Attend public meetings and express your views.

- Know the law. When laws exist to protect you, insist that those in charge enforce them.

- Support organizations in your area that are working to protect nonsmokers. These include local or state offices of the the American Cancer Society, American Lung Association, or the American Heart Association.

## Organizations

The following organizations may provide more information about the health effects of secondhand smoke or how to deal with it.

Action on Smoking and Health (ASH)
2013 H Street, NW
Washington, DC 20006
(202) 659-4310

American Cancer Society
1599 Clifton Road, NE
Atlanta, GA 30329
1-800-ACS-2345

Americans for Nonsmokers' Rights
2530 San Pablo Avenue, Suite J
Berkeley, CA 94702
(510) 841-3032

National Cancer Institute
Building 31, Room 10A24
Bethesda, MD 20892
1-800-4-CANCER

National Institute for Occupational Safety and Health
4676 Columbia Parkway
Cincinnati, OH 42226-1998
1-800-35-NIOSH

Office on Smoking and Health
Centers for Disease Control
Mail Stop K-50
4770 Buford Highway, NE
Atlanta, GA 30341-3724
1-800-CDC-1311

U.S. Environmental Protection Agency (EPA)/Indoor Air Quality Information Clearinghouse
(IAQ INFO)
P.O. Box 37133
Washington, D.C. 20013-7133
1-800-438-4318

The National Heart, Lung, and Blood Institute
Information Center
PO. Box 30105
Bethesda, MD 20824-0105

## Referenced Reports

EPA Report—*Respiratory Health Effects of Passive Smoking: Lung Cancer and Other Disorders.*

NIOSH Report—*Environmental Tobacco Smoke in the Workplace: Lung Cancer and Other Health Effects.*

# Part III

# Current Research into Respiratory Illness, Treatment, and Prevention

Chapter 22

# Respiratory Problems in Minorities

*Chapter Contents*

Section 22. 1—Asthma in Minorities ............................................. 652
Section 22. 2—African Americans and Smoking at a Glance ..... 660
Section 22. 3—Alaska Natives Fight TB ...................................... 674
Section 22. 4—Minorities Over-Represented in Lung
          Diseases ................................................................... 676
Section 22. 5—Smoking Education Program Sends Out
          Stop Smoking Message .......................................... 678
Section 22. 6—Link Between Respiratory Disease and
          Poverty Needs Study ............................................. 680

## Section 22.1

## Asthma In Minorities

Source: Excerpted from Proceedings of the 4th National Forum on Cardiovascular Health, Pulmonary Disorders, and Blood Resources, June 1992.

### Poor Assessment Causes Increased Death Among Asthma Patients of All Races

In recent years, physicians have been faced with a troubling and confusing statistic regarding asthma. Despite the wide range of treatments available for asthma and a fairly extensive understanding of its characteristics among health care providers, the number of hospital admissions for asthma has begun to increase.

"We don't really understand this," said Elena Reece, Chief of the Department of Allergy and Immunology at Howard University. "If we look at emergency department visits, they have been increasing as well, and the mortality trend is upward."

To stop this trend from getting worse, Reece believes that the health care community has to become more aware of the problems that are causing the trend.

Reece outlined some of those problems as follows:

- **The need for more diagnosis of asthma.** "The first problem we have is convincing patients that they indeed have asthma," she said. "And we have problems in terms of defining asthma, because even our trainees are often ill-informed as to its nature."

- **Convincing patients of asthma's seriousness.** "This is a diagnosis that indicates a really chronic condition. There is some indication that some children—maybe 30 percent—will outgrow their asthma. But we have to take into account that many of these people will present with the condition later in life."

- **Recognizing the inflammatory nature of asthma.** "We don't see any drops in asthma mortality until you have anti-inflammatory medications being used," she noted.

- **Realizing the danger of under-treatment.** "Why do patients die? Because they have been inadequately assessed by the physician, or they have inadequately assessed themselves. They have over-relied on the medications that give them a quick fix and under-relied on the medications that reverse the inflammatory components of their asthma."

- **Recognizing the symptoms of asthma.** "Constant complaint of coughing after exertion or at night. Wheezing. Breathlessness."

- **Grading the severity of asthma.** Mild—"An intermittently symptomatic type of condition." Moderate—"Patients tend to have symptoms on a continuous basis." Severe—"Patients have constant symptoms and require multiple drug treatment modalities."

- **Determining response to medications.** "We have a way of classifying patients based on their reactivity to medications that induce bronchospasm. It takes a lot of methacholine to change pulmonary function data in normal people, a little less for people with mild asthma, and even less for severe cases.

- **Understanding asthma inflammation.** "We can think of it pathologically as being very much like a burn of the airways. Burns tend to ooze, so these patients basically drown in secretions."

In addition to changing the general understanding of asthma, Reece urged health care providers to change their method of treatment:

- **Emphasize anti-inflammatory treatment.** "When the patient walks in to the emergency department, you have got to start anti-inflammatory treatment immediately. If you can reverse the episode, maybe the patient won't have to come back to the emergency department a few hours later."

- **Be comprehensive.** "This involves patient education. It involves control of the environment. It involves drug treatment and may involve immunotherapy and behavior modification."

- **Teach patients to avoid allergens.** "House dust, molds, house-dust mites, cockroach allergens—these are all important."

Another area of concern is drug intervention. Reece believes that drug regimens are often inadequate or used improperly by the patient; and she suggested a few guidelines:

- **Mild patients.** May require the occasional use of a beta$_2$-antagonist.

- **Moderate patients.** Require the use of both anti-inflammatories and bronchodilators.

- **Severe patients.** Require anti-inflammatories, bronchodilators, and the addition of steroids, either orally or by injection.

- **Proper administration.** "The vast majority of patients are using inhaled medications in an inappropriate way. You have to emphasize the proper use."

- **Proper education.** "The patient does not have to call you to find out the first thing they should do about an attack," she said. "Watch your patients, make sure they are getting better, and use the medications according to the severity of the condition."

*—Elena Reece, M.D.*

## *Asthma in Hispanic Community Impairs Child Health, Family Functioning*

Although current data on asthma among Hispanics are not extensive, the information that exists seems to be nothing but bad news. In attempting to address the asthma problem in this minority population, Humberto Hidalgo, Assistant Professor, Department of Pediatrics for the University of Texas Health Sciences Center, quoted from a study of one group of poor, urban Hispanic children with moderate asthma living in San Antonio, Texas.

According to the findings of this study, asthma is currently having a highly negative impact on Hispanic children and families and is not receiving adequate attention.

"The burden of asthma for these patients and their families is considerable," Hidalgo noted. "Some of the reasons relate to cultural beliefs and attitudes, but there are more important reasons, such as poverty and inadequate access to health care."

Hidalgo went on to outline the parameters of the San Antonio findings and summarized what was learned from the study:

- **Demographics.** In the study, 90 percent were Mexican Americans ages 6 to 16 years; four out of five had both parents living at home.

- **Objective.** Collect information on asthma morbidity in three main areas: child functioning, family functioning, use of health care services.

- **Impaired child functioning.** An assessment of school absenteeism showed an average 7.4 percent, or 2.5 weeks, of school missed. Parents reported that children were impaired by their asthma 20 percent of the time, or about 1 day a week.

- **Moderate impairment of family functioning.** From 84 to 92 percent of parents believed that their children were somewhat or seriously ill; 33 percent thought the child's health was worse than their peers.

- **Persistence of asthma impairment.** "If you look at these measures over time, there is absolutely no change," he reported. "There was no improvement."

Hidalgo found these results alarming, but he was even more disturbed by the lack of knowledge about their causes. "We need to find out why and how asthma poses such a burden on these children and their families," he said. "We need to look at the major barriers to providing better care for these children."

Among the most critical barriers, Hidalgo listed the following:

- Lack of access to good health care, including lack of transportation, lack of money to pay for prescriptions and doctors' visits, and lack of preventive care.

- Lack of appropriate medication. "Despite the severity of the disease, less than half the children took any anti-inflammatory drugs regularly," he noted. "Almost none were monitored for peak expiratory flow rate."

- Smoking in the home. "Forty-four percent of the children were exposed to cigarette smoke in the home," he said.

- Shortage of culturally compatible providers.

- Shortage of research data pertinent to the problem; shortage of educational materials pertinent to the patients.

For health care providers, addressing this problem will mean making changes and "thinking small." "Whatever your role or interest in delivering care to minorities, all I want to remind you is to think small," Hidalgo said. "Forget the big picture for a while and focus on the details."

—*Humberto Hidalgo, M.D.*

## Asthma Researchers Need Objective, Quantitative Measure of the Disease

Before the minority community can make progress toward treating asthma, the first task is to define asthma clearly so that it will be recognized when it's encountered. Floyd Malveaux, Professor of Microbiology for the Howard University School of Medicine, underscored this problem with a quote from a senior pulmonologist at Johns Hopkins: " 'Asthma is like love. Everybody knows what it is, but nobody can define it.'"

Despite the difficulty in defining asthma, Malveaux believes that important strides can be made with this disease by developing objective measures of its effects on the body.

"One major thing in the definition of asthma is that airway inflammation is really very important in making the diagnosis of asthma and also in managing asthma," he reported. "Something else that is very characteristic of asthma is the nocturnal variation. In virtually every person with asthma, there is usually higher lung function or better lung function in the evenings, and it tends to decline as it gets later into the night; in the early morning it is really at its lowest point."

In addition to these two measures, Malveaux emphasized the value of peak flow measures (measures of air flow out of the lungs). "This is very important in determining the severity of the disease in the individual at any point in time," he said.

Malveaux offered a rough scale of peak flow levels that help in determining asthma severity:

- **Mild.** "They tend to have greater than 80 percent of predicted or personal best peak flow."

- **Moderate.** "In addition to increased symptoms, less tolerance of activity, more days missed from school or work, individuals tend toward 60 to 80 percent of predicted capacity."

- **Severe.** "Less than 60 percent of the predicted or personal best peak flow."

Peak flow measures are helpful not only in checking for air flow obstruction but also for testing reversibility, according to Malveaux. "After the use of a bronchodilator, you can then demonstrate reversibility. That reversibility may be very small, but in any case most individuals will show reversibility."

Peak flow can also help monitor progress and check for changes in the patient's condition. These measures can be used in conjunction with spirometers, which can measure flow volume loops.

In addition, peak flow measurement has other advantages such as simplicity, reproducibility, portability, and the fact that it is a quantitative measure.

Malveaux's desire for change in asthma control doesn't stop with peak flow measures. He also wants more investigation of asthma triggers in the work-place and in schools.

Communication between patient and provider could also be improved, in his view, and more could be done to create action plans for patients and providers to follow after a diagnosis of asthma has been confirmed. "You can't monitor peak flow levels in isolation. You have to have an action plan. That action plan enables the patient and provider to actually communicate."

When a patient takes a peak flow measure, that patient should know what to do if the reading isn't in a good (green) range, Malveaux said. "If they get into the yellow zone, indicating lower air flow, their asthma may not be under control. They may need to increase medication or adjust their maintenance therapy. And of course the red zone is a medical alert and immediate bronchodilation should occur."

Malveaux favors a peak flow measure system with which the patient determines the level of air flow according to a color-coded system, rather than a numerical one. "It's a means by which patients can actually see that they are getting into trouble," he said.

—*Floyd Malveaux, M.D., Ph.D.*

## Asthma Education Needed That Will Empower the Patient

To make the other components of asthma care work, Virginia Taggart, health program specialist, NHLBI, wants to see more education for asthma patients. But not the kind of education in which clinicians tell patients what to do and how to do it. In Taggart's view, that style of education doesn't work anyway.

"Our studies show that less than 30 to 40 percent of patients understand or follow our instructions," she said. "Giving information is necessary, but it isn't enough to effect the kind of behavior change needed for adequate asthma management."

Taggart wants to see clinicians go beyond information giving to building a partnership with the patient, a partnership in which both sides have rights and responsibilities.

"The clinician has to provide the medical expertise to select the right treatment. The clinician needs to teach the management skills," she explained. "The patient has to learn the management skills, adhere to the treatment plan, report difficulties, and communicate concerns. Both the clinician and the patient negotiate together to develop a plan that is medically sound and practically acceptable."

To make this partnership work, Taggart believes that it's best to go back to basics, with an education program made up of "four R's": reaching agreement on goals, rehearsing, repeating, and reinforcing.

- **Reaching agreement on goals.** "One of the first goals or jobs of the clinician is to convince patients that the goals for asthma therapy can be high. That has to be balanced with what the patients want and what their needs and concerns are."

  Under this R, Taggart feels it is critical that clinicians address the patients' fears, including fear of the toxicity of the medicines, of side effects, of steroids and confusion about their purpose, of addiction, of becoming immune to the benefits of the medicine, and of physical activity.

  This is also where clinicians must help patients face and dispel myths about asthma—that it is largely a psychosomatic illness, that it is a permanent handicap, and that they will become invalids because of it.

  Clinicians must then help patients set priorities in the management of their illness. "We need to help patients set this up in a priority step-wise plan that gives them a chance to succeed. A written action plan tells patients what they need to be doing on a daily basis and what to do when their asthma starts to worsen," Taggart said.

  Patients also need assistance in overcoming barriers to treatment, such as cost, convenience, side effects, a lack of perceived benefit, a lack of skill in using medications, and basic confusion over the plan itself.

- **Rehearsal.** "We have specific skills that we are emphasizing in asthma management. We have to demonstrate these skills with the patient and go back to the old adage, 'If I hear something I know it, if I see it I understand it, if I practice it I can do it.'"

- **Repetition.** "We've found in studies that 5 minutes after a visit, 50 percent of the people remembered what the doctor said. But when the message was repeated three times, 100 percent recalled it."

- **Reinforcement.** Taggart listed several possible reinforcement tools and techniques, including keeping a diary, a reward system for compliance, making the treatment part of the patient's daily habits, involving the family and calling the patient with reminders.

The last component of an effective education system, according to Taggart, is delivery. Many patients can't afford the time or money to attend special education programs, so the program has to be incorporated into the provision of medical care. It has to come to them.

"An education effort for a partnership in asthma care is really important, not only for making quality care available to the patient but also in giving the patient and clinician some real satisfaction that quality care is possible," she said.

—*Virginia Taggart, M.P.H.*

Section 22.2

## African Americans and Smoking at a Glance

Source: Centers For Disease Control

"At a time when our people desperately need the message of health promotion, the [Tobacco Industry's] message is more disease, more suffering, and more death for a group already bearing more than its share of smoking-related illnesses and mortality," according to Louis W. Sullivan, M.D., Secretary U.S. Department of Health and Human Services

Smoking is responsible for one of every five deaths in the United States. Moreover, it is the single most important preventable cause of death in our society.

More black Americans smoke cigarettes, over other tobacco products, than their white counterparts. Although the smoking rate for blacks is higher than for white smokers, black smokers smoke fewer cigarettes per day. Black smokers suffer from a higher incidence of smoking-related illnesses than white smokers.

The following summarizes the most recent smoking information for African Americans in the United States.

## Respiratory Problems in Minorities

| Disease | Men Black | Men White | Women Black | Women White |
|---|---|---|---|---|
| Lung and bronchus | 125.1 | 82.0 | 40.4 | 38.1 |
| Esophagus | 19.4 | 5.3 | 5.0 | 1.7 |
| Oral cavity/pharynx | 25.1 | 16.4 | 6.0 | 6.3 |
| Cancer (all sites) | 519.2 | 435.7 | 325.2 | 340.4 |

*age-adjusted to 1970 U.S. Population

Source: NIH, SEER Program Data 1986-87, National Cancer Institute, Bethesda, Maryland: Public Health Service.

**Table 22.1.** *Cancer Incidence Rates\* for Selected Smoking-Related Cancers (new cases per 100,000 persons, 1986-87)*

| Disease | Men Black | Men White | Women Black | Women White |
|---|---|---|---|---|
| Respiratory system cancers | 84.2 | 58.6 | 24.3 | 23.8 |
| Heart disease | 287.1 | 225.9 | 180.8 | 116.3 |
| Stroke | 57.1 | 30.3 | 46.7 | 26.3 |
| Chronic obstructive pulmonary disease | 24.0 | 27.4 | 9.5 | 13.7 |
| All causes | 1,023.2 | 668.2 | 586.2 | 384.1 |

*age-adusted

Source: National Center for Health Statistics: Vital Statistics of the United States, Vol. II, Mortality, Part A, for data years 1950-87. Public Health Service.

**Table 22.2.** *Death Rates\* from Smoking Related Disease (deaths per 100,000 persons, 1987)*

## Respiratory Diseases and Disorders Sourcebook

| Race | Men° | Women° | Total† |
|---|---|---|---|
| Black | 33,288 | 14,405 | 47,692 |
| White | 249,214 | 129,442 | 378,657 |
| Total Population*† | 286,820 | 147,352 | 434,175 |

*(includes whites, blacks, and racial category "other" and deaths among nonsmokers from lung cancer attributable to passive smoking)
†(sum may not equal total because of rounding)
°(includes pediatric deaths)

Source: Centers for Disease Control. Smoking-attributable mortality and years of potential life lost—United States, 1988. *Morbidity and Mortality Weekly Report,* 1990; 40:62-71.

**Table 22.3.** *Smoking-Attributable Mortality, 1988*


| Race | Men | Women | Both Sexes |
|---|---|---|---|
| Black | 702.9 | 231.5 | 437.3 |
| White | 555.8 | 244.2 | 389.3 |
| Total Population† | 558.6 | 240.7 | 387.8 |

*per 100,000 persons ≥ 35 years old adjusted to the 1980 U.S. population
†includes racial category "other" and passive smoking-related deaths

Source: Centers for Disease Control. Smoking-attributable mortality and years of potential life lost—United States, 1988. *Morbidity and Mortality Weekly Report,* 1990; 40: 62-71.

**Table 22.4.** *Smoking-Attributable Death Rate*, 1988*


| Men | 18-24 | 25-44 | 45-64 | 65+ |
|---|---|---|---|---|
| White | 19.9 | 39.9 | 56.2 | 77.5 |
| Black | 11.8 | 25.5 | 39.6 | 55.5 |

| Women | 18-24 | 25-44 | 44-54 | 65+ |
|---|---|---|---|---|
| White | 26.9 | 37.7 | 42.5 | 59.1 |
| Black | 16.7 | 21.9 | 38.9 | 58.0 |

Quit ratio = proportion of persons who have ever smoked cigarettes and who have stopped smoking cigarettes [(number of former smokers)/(number of current + number of former smokers)].

Source: National Health Interview Survey, 1987, OSH unpublished data

**Table 22.5.** *Quit Ratios by Race, Sex, and Age, United States, 1987*

## Cigarette Smoking Prevalence

- Smoking rates among black adults are higher than those for whites, even though the pattern of decline in smoking rates is similar for both groups.

- In 1988, more than 50 million Americans smoked cigarettes. Of those 50 million current smokers, about 6 million are black.

- In 1987, 34.0% of black adults (aged 20+) smoked, compared with 29.0% of white adults (aged 20+); in 1966, 43.0% of black adults and 40.0% of white adults smoked.

- Both black men and black women are more likely to smoke cigarettes, rather than other forms of tobacco, than their white counterparts. In 1987, 39.0% of black men (aged 18+) (30.5% of white men) and 28.0% of black women (aged 18+) (26.7% of white women) smoked cigarettes.

## Cigarette Smoking Behavior

Recent studies demonstrate that cigarette smoking behaviors vary by race and by sex.

- Black smokers (aged 17+ years) report smoking an average of 15 cigarettes per day; white men smoke nearly 24 cigarettes per day; and white women smoke an estimated 20 cigarettes per day.

- Heavy smoking (25+ cigarettes per day) is much less common among blacks than among whites.

- Black smokers are more likely to smoke higher tar and nicotine brands than are white smokers; and smoking higher tar brands is associated with higher lung cancer incidence and mortality rates.

- Blacks also are more likely to smoke mentholated cigarettes. Of blacks who smoke, 75% of those aged 17 and over smoke mentholated cigarettes but only 23% of whites who smoke use mentholated brands.

- Three mentholated brands represent 55% of the market among black smokers.

    1. Newport (Lorrilard, Inc.)

    2. Kool (Brown & Williamson)

    3. Salem (R.J. Reynolds)

## Prevalence of Other Forms of Tobacco Use

- A 1987 study of smokers 18 years of age and over indicated that cigarettes are the most popular tobacco product among blacks, as they are among the general population. However, blacks do use other forms of tobacco.

- The prevalence for pipe smoking is the same for black and white men (3.4%).

- More white men (5.6%) smoke cigars than do black men (4.0%).

- Use of chewing tobacco and snuff varies significantly by race and sex.

- Black men (3.4%) use chewing tobacco less than white men (4.2%).

- More black women (1.7%) chew tobacco than white women (0.1 %).

- White men use snuff at a rate of 3.3%, compared with a 1.1 % rate for black men.

- Among black women, 2.2% use snuff whereas only 0.3% of white women use this product.

## Smoking and Occupational Status

In examining smoking and the work-place, researchers have found a link between smoking behavior and occupations.

- Smoking prevalence varies by occupational category. Smoking rates are generally higher in male and female blue-collar workers than in their white-collar counterparts. In 1987, 26.1% of white-collar men and 26.6% of white-collar women smoked cigarettes. Among blue-collar workers, 42.1 % of men and 36.6% of women smoked during that year. (Note: blacks of both sexes are more concentrated in blue-collar occupations.)

- The National Health Interview Survey 1978-1980 revealed a relationship between smoking behavior and occupations. Among men, blue-collar workers had considerably higher smoking rates than white-collar workers within each racial group, and black male blue-collar workers exhibited the highest smoking rate (52.1%). Among black women, there was little difference in smoking prevalence between occupations. However, among white women, the expected white-collar, blue-collar, service worker differences prevailed; blue-collar and service workers were more likely to smoke (39.6% and 38.7%, respectively) than white-collar workers (32.0%).

- Black workers are considerably less likely than their white counterparts to be heavy smokers (smoke 20 or more cigarettes daily). This trend holds true for all categories of workers and for men and women.

## Health Consequences

Black Americans suffer from smoking-related diseases at a higher rate than whites.

- Black men and women have a higher incidence of respiratory system cancers than do white men and women (Table 1).

- This trend also is present for incidences of esophagus and oral cavity cancer.

Blacks experience excessive mortality for many tobacco-related cancers.

- The average (annual age-adjusted) mortality is higher among black men than among white men for cancers of the respiratory system, heart disease, and stroke (Table 2).

- The death rates for black women are higher than for white women for cancers of the respiratory system, heart disease, and stroke.

In 1988, nearly 48,000 black Americans died from smoking-attributable causes—these are deaths that could have been prevented (Table 3).

- Smoking-attributable deaths among black men are double those among black women. This ratio is not as high among white men and women.

The rate of smoking-attributable deaths is higher among blacks than among whites (Table 4).

- The death rate due to smoking for black men is triple that for black women; and 1.3 times higher than the death rate for white men. The death rate from smoking for white men is double that for white women.

- The death rates for white women are higher relative to those of black women.

## Years of Potential Life Lost Smoking and Pregnancy (YPLL)

Studies conducted by the Centers for Disease Control report that black Americans have not only a higher death rate from cigarette smoking than do whites, but have a greater loss of productive years of life.

- Blacks tend to become ill from smoking at younger ages than do whites.

## Respiratory Problems in Minorities

- In 1988, blacks lost an estimated 268,437 years of potential life to age 65 due to smoking. Whites lost an estimated 913,943 years. (Note: The U.S. Census reported that black Americans comprised 12% of the total population in 1990).

- Although whites lost more years in total, the rate of smoking attributable YPLL (before age 65 per 100,000 persons 35 years of age) for blacks (2,472) was twice that for whites (1,225). NOTE: Smoking-attributable YPLL is the sum of years of life lost for deaths attributed to smoking for all diagnoses related to smoking.

### Smoking and Pregnancy

In general, women in the lowest age and socioeconomic categories are most likely to smoke during pregnancy.

- Among pregnant teenagers, smoking rates between 1967-1980 remained constant at about 38% among whites and 27% among blacks.

- Among all pregnant women over age 20, decreases in smoking prevalence between 1967-1980 varied considerably by race. Smoking prevalence among pregnant white women over age 20 declined from 40% in 1967 to 25% in 1980; among pregnant black women (aged 20+ years), it declined from 33% to 23%.

- Older black women (25 to 44 years of age) are less likely to smoke during pregnancy than white women (43% versus 53%). Among pregnant women who smoke, blacks smoke fewer cigarettes per day than whites.

- Among white women over age 20, the proportion who quit smoking during pregnancy increased from 11% to 16%; among blacks (aged 20+ years) the proportion who quit decreased from 17% to 11%.

## Smoking and Youth

Every day more than 3,000 American teenagers become regular smokers—that's more than 1 million annually. Most regular smokers start in their teens. However, this trend is more dominant among white teenagers.

- According to the National Institute on Drug Abuse (NIDA) National High School Senior Survey, the prevalence of daily smoking has fallen substantially among black high school seniors, from 26% in 1976 to 6% in 1989. During the same period, prevalence among white high school seniors declined from 29% to 22%.

- Another indirect measure of smoking initiation is the prevalence of smoking among persons aged 20 to 24 years. Ninety percent of persons who will become regular smokers have begun smoking by age 20. Among blacks, the prevalence among 20- to 24-year-olds declined by one-third between 1983 and 1987 (from 38.7% to 25.6%).

- Among whites, the prevalence of smoking for persons in this age group declined by only 17% (from 36.8% to 30.5%) (Note: the age of initiation for blacks is somewhat older than that for whites).

## Black Americans and Quitting

Black Americans quit more often than whites; however, whites are more likely to continue not to smoke.

- Overall, the proportion of quitters is lower for blacks than for whites. In 1987, the quit ratio (proportion of persons who have ever smoked cigarettes and who have stopped smoking) was 31.5% for blacks and 46.4% for whites.

- Since 1974, the rate of increase in the quit ratio has been the same for blacks and whites.

## Respiratory Problems in Minorities

- Among men, the quit ratio for blacks is lower in every age category than for whites (Table 5).

- The quit ratio is lower for black women under age 65 than for white women in this age group. Among women age 65 or older, the quit ratio is similar for blacks and whites (Table 5).

- Black smokers are more likely than white smokers to have quit for at least one day during the previous year. Blacks, however, are less likely than whites to remain abstinent for one year or more.

### Black Americans and Advertising

- Cigarette companies heavily target mentholated cigarette advertising to blacks. For example, mentholated brands are more commonly advertised in black-oriented than in white-oriented magazines.

- Cigarette companies advertise heavily in popular black magazines, but they also successfully target the African American community by sponsoring entertainment, sporting, and cultural events and political and literacy campaigns.

- Billboards advertising tobacco products are placed in African American communities four to five times more often than in white communities. In 1985, tobacco companies spent $5.8 million for advertisements on eight-sheet billboards in African American communities, accounting for 37% of total advertising in this medium.

- Data from the six major U.S. cigarette manufacturers revealed that in 1988, United States cigarette advertising and promotional expenditures reached an all-time high of $3.3 billion—a 26.9% increase over 1987 expenditures of $2.6 billion.

- Black magazines receive proportionately more revenues from cigarette advertising than do other consumer magazines. In 1987, tobacco and smoking accessories accounted for only

6.1% of advertising in 166 consumer magazines; the percentages of cigarette advertising were higher in black magazines:

Jet-10.2%
Essence-9.2%
Ebony-7.5%

## Policy Issues Related to Tobacco

- According to a 1990 survey of blacks in California:

  About 28% of black smokers reported that they would support a future tax increase on cigarettes; the majority would not.

- Black smokers supported an overall ban on tobacco advertisements: banning sponsorships (about 58%), banning print ads (about 60%), and banning billboard ads (about 62%).

- Black community leaders have acted to restrict tobacco and alcohol advertising in several African American communities, including those in New York, Michigan, the District of Columbia, and Pennsylvania. This is one part of a growing battle against alcohol and tobacco ads in black inner-city neighborhoods.

## References

1. Office On Smoking and Health. *Reducing the health consequences of smoking: 25 years of progress. A report of the Surgeon General.* Washington, D.C.: U.S. Department of Health and Human Services, Public Health Service, Office on Smoking and Health, 1989. DHHS publication no. (CDC)89-8411.

2. Alcohol, Drug Abuse, and Mental Health Administration. *National Institute on Drug Abuse, National household survey on drug abuse: population estimates 1988.* Washington, D.C.: U.S. Department Of Health and Human Services, Public Health Service, Alcohol, Drug Abuse, and Mental Health Administration, 1989. DHHS publication no. (ADM)89-1636.

3. Schoenborn CA, Boyd G. *Smoking and other tobacco use: United States, 1987.* Washington, D.C.: U.S. Department of Health and Human Services, Public Health Service, National Center for Health Statistics, 1987. DHHS publication no. (PHS)89-1591. (Vital and health statistics, series 10, no. 169).

4. Office On Smoking and Health. *Adult use of tobacco, 1986.* Washington, D.C.: U.S. Department of Health and Human Services, Public Health Service, Office on Smoking and Health, 1989. DHHS publication no. (OM)90-2004.

5. Centers for Disease Control. "Cigarette brand use among adult smokers—United States, 1986." *Morbidity and Mortality Weekly Report 1990*; 39:665, 671-673.

6. National Health Interview Survey, 1987, Office on Smoking and Health, unpublished data.

7. Office On Smoking and Health. *The health consequences of smoking: cancer and chronic lung disease in the work-place. A report of the Surgeon General.* Washington, D.C.: U.S. Department of Health and Human Services, Public Health Service, Office on Smoking and Health, 1985. DHHS publication no. (PHS)8550207

8. National Center for Health Statistics. *Health, United States, prevention profile 1989.* Hyattsville, Maryland: U.S. Department of Health and Human Services, Public Health Service, 1990. DHHS publication no. (PHS)90-1232.

9. National Institutes of Health. *Cancer statistics review 1973-87, surveillance, epidemiology, and end results report (SEER), 1978-81.* Washington, D.C.: U. S. Department of Health and Human Services, Public Health Service, National Cancer Institute, 1990. NIH publication no. (NIH)90-2789.

10. Centers for Disease Control. "Smoking-attributable mortality and years of potential life lost—United States, 1988." *Morbidity and Mortality Weekly Report 1990*; 40:62-71.

11. Centers for Disease Control. "Smoking-attributable mortality and years of potential life lost—United States, 1984." *Morbidity and Mortality Weekly Report 1987*; 36:693-697.

12. Niswander KR, Gordon M. *The women and their pregnancies. The collaborative perinatal study of the National Institute of Neurological Diseases and Stroke.* Washington, D.C.: U.S. Department of Health, Education, and Welfare, Public Health Service, National Institutes of Health, 1972. DHEW publication no. (NIH)73379.

13. Mosher WD, Pratt, WF. *Fecundity, infertility, and reproductive health in the United States, 1982.* Washington, D.C.: Public Health Service, Government Printing Office, 1988. National Center for Health Statistics, 1988. DHHS publication no. (PHS)88-1591. (Vital and Health Statistics, series 2, no.106).

14. National Institute on Drug Abuse. Monitoring the Future Project, 1989, Office On Smoking and Health, unpublished data.

15. Office On Smoking and Health. *The health benefits of smoking cessation.* Washington, D.C.: U.S. Department of Health and Human Services, Public Health Service, Office on Smoking and Health, 1990. DHHS publication no.(CDC)90-8416.

16. Fiore MC, Novotny TE, Pierce JP, Hatziandrea EJ, Patel KM, Davis RM. "Trends in cigarette smoking in the United States: the changing influence of gender and race." *Journal of the American Medical Association* 1989; 261 :49-55.

17. Davis, RM. "Current trends in cigarette advertising and marketing." *New England Journal of Medicine* 1987; 316:725-732.

18. Cummings KM, Giovino G, Mendicino AJ. *Cigarette advertising and racial differences in cigarette brand preference.* Public Health Reports 1987; 102:698-701.

19. Federal Trade Commission. *Report to Congress for 1987 pursuant to the Federal Cigarette Labeling and Advertising Act.* Washington, D.C.: U.S. Federal Trade Commission, 1989.

20. McMahon ET, Taylor PA. *Citizens' action handbook on alcohol and tobacco billboard advertising.* Washington, D.C.: Center for Science in the Public Interest, 1990.

21. Ramirez A. "A cigarette campaign under fire." *New York Times* .1990 Jan 12: D1, D4.

22. California Department of Health Services. *Tobacco use in California 1990: preliminary report documenting the decline of tobacco use.* San Diego: University of California, 1990.

23. Marcus M, Glick D, Lewis SD. "Fighting ads in the inner city: a grassroots battle against 'minority marketing.'" *Newsweek.* 1990 Feb 5: 46.

*For more information, write to:*

Office on Smoking and Health Centers for Disease Control
Mail Stop K-50 1600 Clifton Road, NE
Atlanta, GA 30333

## Section 22.3

## Fight Against Tuberculosis Continues for Alaska Natives

Source: Proceedings of the 4th National Forum on Cardiovascular Health, Pulmonary Disorders, and Blood Resources, June 1992.

Alaska Natives face a number of unique problems that usually aren't encountered by other minority groups . They live in a region with few roads, unpredictable weather, and unreliable communications technology and they often treat their health problems alone, with the help of a "radio sick call" to a physician.

In addition to these challenges, Alaskans are still fighting an outbreak of tuberculosis (TB) that started in the 18th and 19th centuries.

"We still see Alaska Natives bearing the significant burden of TB infection and disease," said Theodore Mala. "Although we comprise only 16 percent of the State's population, we have 50 to 90 percent of all TB cases."

Mala attributes this problem to many factors, beginning with what he calls "the remarkably intense transmission of microbacterium TB during the first half of this century."

He offered some statistics to give a sense of the scope of the problem and to show how much progress has been made against the disease:

- Between 1926 and 1930, 36 percent of the 2,767 deaths that occurred among Alaska Natives were related to TB.

- In 1946, TB was listed as the cause of death on 43 percent of all death certificates for Alaska Natives.

- In 1950, the death rate for Alaska Natives from TB was 673.3 per 100,000, compared to 17.9 for whites.

- In a 1952 study of TB skin tests, the proportion of children in the 5- to 8-year-old age group with positive results ranged from 89 percent for Alaska Natives to 22 percent for southeast Indians.

- In 1990, race-specific TB cases were 1.4 per 100,000 for whites, 5.3 for blacks, and 60.7 for Alaska Natives.

"We certainly have outbreaks of TB still on the small islands," Mala noted. "Potentially, all of these cases are preventable."

Another problem that is reaching epidemic levels in Alaska is death from tobacco-caused lung cancer, Mala said. In 1950, the death rate from lung cancer was 5.6 per 100,000. It is now 89 per 100,000. The Alaska Native population is also struggling with a high death rate due to injuries and a high rate of illness and injury related to alcohol.

However, progress is being made against other health problems in Alaska. Mala offered several statistics that indicate improvement overall:

- In 1950, infant mortality was 101 per 1,000. Now it is 22.3.

- In 1950, the death rate among Alaska Natives was 1,742 per 100,000. Now it is 726 per 100,000.

- In 1950, life expectancy among Alaska Natives was age 47. Now it is age 67 and continues to increase.

- In 1950, numerous deaths were caused by measles, whooping cough, rheumatic fever, syphilis, typhoid, and polio. There have been no recently reported deaths from these illnesses.

For the future, Mala hopes for continued improvement. "There are quite a few things we know we can prevent, and certainly social factors are a major contributor to that."

*—Theodore Mala, M.D., M.P.H.,*
*Commissioner, State of Alaska*
*Department of Health and Social Services,*
*Juneau, Alaska*

## Section 22.4
# Minorities Over-Represented in Lung Diseases

Source: Proceedings of the 4th National Forum on Cardiovascular Health, Pulmonary Disorders, and Blood Resources, June 1992.

Given the higher prevalence of poverty, overcrowding, smoking, AIDS, and environmental and occupational risks among minority communities, Alvin Thomas sees a clear relationship between these risk factors and a higher incidence of respiratory disease and lung problems among minority groups.

In recent years, an increasing number of minorities have suffered from a respiratory disease that was thought to be under control in the United States: tuberculosis (TB).

Thomas places much of the blame for this increase at poverty's door. "It's certainly a problem in TB," he said. "There are some recent data from CDC where they looked at median income and TB incidence per 100,000. As you go from less poor to more poor, the incidence rate increases substantially."

The sudden increase in TB cases took many researchers by surprise, according to Thomas. In 1984, after many years of steady decreases in TB rates, the rate suddenly jumped 15.5 percent.

"If you look at recent data, you see that 70 percent of the total cases in 1990 were in a minority group," he reported. However, TB is only one disease on the increase among minority groups. Minorities suffer from other lung and respiratory conditions at a disproportionate rate compared to the general population. Thomas outlined some of the most serious trends, including:

- **Lung cancer.** Black males have a 45 percent higher incidence than non-blacks. Southeast Asian males have an 18 percent higher incidence. In both black and white women, lung cancer incidence is increasing 5 percent per year.

- **Pneumonia.** African Americans are nearly three times more likely to die from pneumonia than is the general population.

- **Bronchial asthma.** Prevalence among blacks is now 12.2 cases per 100 population and growing. Mortality among blacks is three times greater than among whites.

- **Sickle cell anemia.** A trait which is found in 8 to 12 percent of the black population may develop respiratory complications.

- **Sarcoidosis.** Among blacks, this disease is 10 to 17 times more prevalent than in whites.

*Risk Factors for Respiratory Diseases*

In terms of risk factors leading to higher rates of respiratory disease, Thomas puts occupation near the top of the list. "One thing is clear. If you start collecting data [on minority lung disease], you'll find that **occupational lung problems** are over-represented in minorities."

Pointing out that people below poverty level have death rates twice that of people above it, Thomas' list of risk factors includes poverty, plus many others:

- **Heredity.** "It' s an important problem in sickle cell anemia and in some forms of lung cancer. In chronic obstructive pulmonary disease (COPD), asthma, and sarcoidosis there are some hints at it," he reported.

- **Smoking.** The decline of the prevalence of smoking among whites (0.5 percent per year) is higher than among blacks (0.4 percent per year).

- **AIDS.** "It is an important risk factor associated with the increase of TB, especially among the 25- to 45-age group which represents almost 70 percent of all cases," Thomas noted.

- **Passive tobacco smoke.** "A substantial cause of disease in nonsmokers," he reported.

Despite these serious problems, Thomas had good news about respiratory research and bronchial asthma. Studies of alpha$_1$ protease inhibitors have turned up some exciting findings. "Data developed over the last 3 to 5 years suggest that problems with this inhibitor may be a substantial problem in people with asthma."

In other areas of respiratory disease, much more needs to be done. Research initiatives are needed in the areas of environmental tobacco smoke, TB, alpha$_1$-protease inhibitors, sarcoidosis, and COPD. "We need much better data bases than we have now," Thomas said. "And we certainly need better elucidation of natural history in these diseases."

—*Alvin Thomas, M.D.,*
*Associate Professor of Medicine,*
*Chief,*
*Division of Pulmonary and Critical Care Medicine,*
*Howard University, Washington, D.C.*

Section 22.5

## Stop Smoking Education Program Sends Out the Stop Smoking Message

Source: Proceedings of the 4th National Forum on Cardiovascular Health, Pulmonary Disorders, and Blood Resources, June 1992.

According to newly released data on smoking in the United States, the stop-smoking message is apparently getting through to many groups. Glen Bennett, coordinator of the NHLBI's Smoking Educational Program (SEP), outlined some of the good news:

- A significant drop in smoking rates among black women has brought them below the rate for white women.

- Significant decreases in smoking rates among black men have reduced the gap between black and white men.

- Over the past 15 years, smoking rates have come down for all population groups.

- Younger blacks are not smoking at the same rates as in the past, suggesting that they are not starting to smoke at the same rate.

However, problems still exist:

- People who are continuing to smoke have the least amount of education.

- A substantial portion of children of all races, and a considerably higher portion among blacks, live in households with smokers.

- About half of smokers who see a physician are not advised to quit smoking.

With much work still left to do in this area, Bennett reported that the NHLBI SEP is focusing on "preparing physicians, nurses, respiratory therapists, and other health care providers to intervene with smokers when they enter health care settings." This approach is called Clinical Opportunities for Smoking Intervention. Bennett outlined some of its components:

- Training package. The centerpiece is a 25-minute video with four segments that allows viewers to stop between segments and discuss key elements. It also contains guides for counseling patients to quit smoking.

- The training package was validated with medical residents at Interfaith Medical Center in Brooklyn, N.Y. "About 70 percent of the resident physicians were born outside the United States, and roughly 90 percent of the patients were inner-city blacks and Hispanics. We trained about 35 of their residents in this activity, and we saw a substantial increase in the amount of counseling by these residents."

- Clinical Opportunities Guide for Respiratory Care Providers: "When you target a specific group like respiratory therapists, they like the recognition and are more likely to adopt the strategy. This is very important because respiratory therapists are key professionals in organizing hospital-based smoking intervention efforts."

- Clinical Opportunities Guide for Nurses: "Our most successful product to date. Due primarily to concerns about costs, we often face pressure to develop a generic guide for use by all health care professionals. However, it was not until this product came out that we saw nurses excited about smoking intervention in clinical practice."

The program's latest effort in the stop-smoking campaign is to put together a package dealing with infant exposure to passive smoke.

*—Glen Bennett, M.P.H.,
Coordinator, NHLBI Smoking Education Program,
National Heart, Lung, and Blood Institute,
National Institutes of Health,
Bethesda, Maryland.*

Section 22.6

# Link Between Respiratory Disease and Poverty Needs Further Study

Source: Proceedings of the 4th National Forum on Cardiovascular Health, Pulmonary Disorders, and Blood Resources, June 1992.

In his discussion of the higher prevalence of respiratory diseases among minority populations, Kevin Gibson called for more study of the relationship between disease and socioeconomic status.

"In examining the true impact of disease on prevalence, morbidity, and mortality, we should look at the relationship of poverty and disease in this manner: Namely, that poverty acts through ethnicity and race in a manner that is perhaps influenced by factors such as environment, information and knowledge on the part of the patient, genetic factors, risk promotion, and lifestyle behaviors to increase prevalence, morbidity, and mortality."

To call attention to the need for research initiatives in this area, Gibson reported on the current status of four respiratory diseases as they relate to minority populations: chronic obstructive pulmonary disease, lung cancer, sarcoidosis, and tuberculosis

- Chronic obstructive pulmonary disease (chronic bronchitis, emphysema, and asthma). Data suggest that COPD is actually much less prevalent in minority populations than in the general population. Gibson partly attributes this to higher CVD mortality rates among minorities. "However, the data are just not that good. We need more epidemiological data to really characterize chronic obstructive pulmonary disease in this population."
Death rates from asthma for Puerto Ricans and Mexican Americans show a huge disparity. "I think what this points out is that we still have a great deal of difficulty in doing epidemiological studies in minority population subgroups because it's hard to believe that this is the case."

- Lung cancer. Death rates among black males are much higher than the general population. "An argument might be made that maybe black males die from lung cancer sooner because they present much later in their disease," Gibson said. "We really need much better studies to determine exactly why this occurs."

- Sarcoidosis. "The risk factors for this disease are totally unknown. We know nothing about why people get it. But those who practice medicine in minority communities and black communities in particular will attest to the fact that this is a very, very common disease associated with a significant morbidity among blacks."

- Tuberculosis. "In minorities, the disease appears to be affecting a younger population of patients," Gibson said. "The disease in minority patients is not only more prevalent and has a higher incidence, but it is more likely to be contagious and will spread to other segments of the population."

Gibson concluded by emphasizing the need for more studies of the link between disease and social factors. "It is very important in our studies that we look at this in the context of race and ethnicity and the impact of environmental factors, education, genetic factors, risk behavior, and access to health care."

—*Kevin Gibson, M.D., Chair, Working Group on Respiratory Health in Minorities for the National Heart, Lung, and Blood Institute, Division of Lung Diseases, Assistant Professor of Medicine, University of Pittsburgh, Pittsburgh, Pennsylvania.*

Chapter 23

# Research Highlights

*Chapter Contents*

Section 23. 1—Asthma Allergens: Examining the Role of
    Eosinophils ............................................................ 684
Section 23. 2—A Trigger for Asthma at the Tip of Your Toes .... 688
Section 23. 3—Respiratory Illness Associated with Inhalation
    of Mushroom Spores ............................................. 689

Section 23.1

## Asthma Allergens: Examining the Role of Eosinophils

Source: *Research Resources Reporter,* March/April 1993.

A protein component of white blood cells known as eosinophils may play a direct role in constricting lung airways and in provoking increased airway sensitivity to allergens. These are reactions typically seen in patients with asthma and other allergic lung reactions, according to scientists at the Mayo Medical School in Rochester, Minnesota, and Boehringer Ingelheim Pharmaceuticals in Ridgefield, Connecticut. Their studies suggest that eosinophils are not beneficial in allergic reactions, as had been hypothesized, but rather are part of the problem, says Dr. Robert H. Gundel, principal scientist at the pulmonary inflammation laboratory, Boehringer Ingelheim Pharmaceuticals.

### The Research

Dr. Gundel and Dr. Gerald J. Gleich, professor of immunology and medicine at the Mayo Medical School, Mayo Clinic and Foundation, collaborated to examine the effects of injecting purified proteins produced by human eosinophils directly into the tracheas, or windpipes, of anesthetized monkeys. The proteins are known as granule proteins because they combine to form microscopic dark-staining granules in the cell. The granule protein known as major basic protein (MBP) produced an immediate temporary constriction of the monkeys' bronchi, the tubes leading to the lungs, as well as a dose-related airway hyperresponsiveness to inhaled methacholine, a chemical to which the airways of asthmatics are extremely reactive.

"This in vivo study shows for the first time that one of the granule proteins from the eosinophil has this biological effect. This is important because, until recently, the role of the eosinophil in asthma was unclear," says Dr. Gundel. Eosinophils are known to congregate in the air passages of asthmatics and release enzymes that reverse some aspects of allergic reactions; however, only in the past few years have

## Research Highlights

the cells also been implicated as contributors to the symptoms of asthma.

Recent studies have shown a correlation between bronchial hyperactivity and increased numbers of airway eosinophils and increased levels of MBP in the lung fluid of primate models for asthma; similar findings were noted in patients with the disease, Dr. Gleich says. All these studies suggested that "some component of the eosinophil must play a role in asthma," he says.

To test this hypothesis Dr. Gundel and his colleagues studied the ways human eosinophil proteins affected the respiratory tracts of five anesthetized cynomolgus monkeys. The scientists first monitored the animals' baseline airway function and then observed the effects when the monkeys inhaled increasing concentrations of aerosolized methacholine. Each animal subsequently received an intratracheal injection of an inert salt solution or one of the following diluted eosinophil granule proteins: MBP, eosinophil cationic protein, eosinophil peroxidase, or eosinophil-derived neurotoxin. Respiratory responsiveness to inhaled methacholine was monitored at 1, 2, and 4 hours after protein injection. In separate experiments extending over several months each animal received intratracheal injections of each of the four purified granule proteins.

Both MBP and eosinophil peroxidase produced an immediate constriction of the airways that was resolved after 60 minutes, the scientists say, but only MBP induced hyper-responsiveness to inhaled methacholine. The increased airway sensitivity to methacholine developed 2 hours after MBP was injected and returned to baseline values by 4 hours. The other eosinophil granule proteins tested had no effect on airway sensitivity or function. The investigators suggest that MBP may induce the release of chemical mediators that alter the responsiveness of the muscles of the airway and contribute to asthma and other inflammatory airway diseases.

"It is also interesting to note that MBP can cause hyper-responsiveness at subcytotoxic doses," Dr. Gundel says. Until recently, he says, these biological effects were believed to be related to the destruction of the cells lining the airway. However, in the primate study hyper-responsiveness began 2 hours after the animals were exposed to the irritant and returned to normal after 4 hours, which suggests that no such cell deaths occurred.

## Preventing or Reversing the Toxic Effects of MBP

The scientists recently completed a follow-up study that demonstrates how the toxic effects of MBP might be prevented or at least reversed. The investigators successfully blocked MBP toxicity in monkeys by pretreating the animals with polyglutamic acid aerosol inhalations. Because MBP has a very basic pH, the scientists speculated that a specific inhibitor of MBP—one that is as acidic as MBP is basic—might play a role in counteracting the toxicity of MBP. According to Dr. Gundel, an acidic subsection of newly synthesized MBP may initially neutralize the protein's toxicity, but this subsection and the protection it affords may be lost when MBP is incorporated into the eosinophil granule. Although the acidic subsection has not yet been isolated, Dr. Gundel and his colleagues were able to use polyglutamic acid to mimic its neutralizing action.

The researchers are now pursuing another approach that may lead to a new drug therapy for asthma. Knowing that MBP initially has a neutral pH, Dr. Gleich and his coworkers are looking for the enzyme responsible for cleaving off the acidic section of MBP. Once this enzyme has been identified, the scientists hope to find an inhibitor to block the enzyme's action, and the inhibitor may be used to treat patients who have asthma.

"To cure asthma one must deal not only with the broncho-constricting effects associated with the disease but also with the inflammation that is produced," says Dr. Gundel, whose area of expertise is inflammation. Some of his current research addresses the questions of how and why eosinophils enter the bronchi, release their toxic proteins, and alter airway function.

Several investigators are now studying the role played by T-cells, a type of white blood cell that produces several substances that affect the activation of eosinophils. Dr. Gundel likens the T-cell to a general who gives eosinophils their marching orders. "There are two possible approaches to therapy: We could look for inhibitors that will block the harmful effects of eosinophils once they are already in the bronchi, or we could try to modulate T-cell function to block the release of substances that call for the release of eosinophils. The latter may be a better approach to therapy," he says.

Dr. Gundel and his colleagues are now examining substances called cytokines that are released by T-cells and act as chemical messengers between cells. According to Dr. Gundel, cytokines promote

## Research Highlights

growth and differentiation of eosinophils in bone marrow and activate those cells already present in the circulation and tissues. In patients with asthma certain cytokines are found in elevated numbers.

"Asthma has not been an easy disease to understand," says Dr. Gleich. In more than two decades of studying asthma, it took 10 years to realize that the eosinophil is not beneficial, he says, and another decade to show how the eosinophil causes harm. "This work is a landmark in a long odyssey of work dealing with eosinophilia," he says.

Dr. Gleich speculates that the results of this study may have implications for understanding other inflammatory diseases. He hypothesizes that the MBP manufactured by eosinophils may produce similar effects in other organs, including the eye, the nose, the gastrointestinal tract, and possibly the bladder. "The mechanisms we observed in the lungs may also occur in other parts of the body. This granule protein may prove to be quite important," he says.

### Additional Reading

1. Barker, R. L., Gundel, R. H., Gleich, G. J., et al., Acid polyamino acids inhibit human eosinophil granule major protein toxicity. *Journal of Clinical Investigation* 88:798-805, 1991.

2. Gundel, R. H., Letts, L. G., and Gleich, G. J., Human eosinophil major basic protein induces airway constriction and airway hyper-responsiveness in primates. *Journal of Clinical Investigation* 87:1470-1473, 1991.

3. Gundel, R. H., Gerritsen, M. E., Gleich, G. J., and Wegner, C. D., Repeated antigen inhalation results in a prolonged airway eosinophilia and airway hyper-responsiveness in primates. *Journal of Applied Physiology* 68:779-786, 1990.

4. Gundel, R. H., Gerritsen, M. E., and Wegner, C. D., Antigen-coated sepharose beads induce airway eosinophilia and airway hyper-responsiveness in cynomolgus monkeys. *American Review of Respiratory Disease* 140:629-633, 1989.

The research described in this chapter was supported by the General Clinical Research Centers Program of the National Center for Research Resources, the National Institute of Allergy and Infectious Diseases, and the Mayo Foundation.

—L. Anne Hirschel, D.D.S

## Section 23.2

## A Trigger for Asthma at the Tip of Your Toes

Source: NCRR *Reporter*; July 29, 1994.

Researchers at the University of Virginia GCRC are studying the role that a fungus known as *Trichophyton*—commonly found on human skin, hair, and toenails—might play in the development of severe asthma. Although most asthma causes can be traced to household allergens like dust mites, cockroaches, or cat or dog dander, some causes of asthma are more difficult to pinpoint.

Dr. Thomas Platts-Mills and his colleagues report that *Trichophyton* and other fungi that colonize the body may be the culprit behind some cases of so-called intrinsic asthma, which does not improve when a patient is removed from household allergens. "In these cases the allergen may be already within the body, or intrinsic to the person," says Dr. Platts-Mills. He and his associates are working to detail their patients' immune responses to *Trichophyton* and to determine potential implications for treatment.

In one study now under way, Dr. Platts-Mills and his colleagues are studying whether the antifungal drug fluconazole can reduce bronchial obstruction and ease breathing. Ten patients who are allergic to *Trichophyton* take oral doses of fluconazole (100 mg per day) for either 22 or 44 weeks. Preliminary results suggest that the antifungal therapy leads to reduced lung sensitivity to *Trichophyton*, dramatic increases in the patients' sense of well-being, and progressive reduction in the doses of steroids needed to control asthma.

The patients who received this experimental therapy have a severe form of asthma that did not respond well to conventional treatments. "Fluconazole not only proved to be effective in treating these patients, but also turned out to be a very benign drug for long-term use," says Dr. Platts-Mills. Other investigational drugs for severe asthma—including methotrexate, gold, and cyclosporine-A—are more toxic than fluconazole, he says.

The Virginia researchers are now in the midst of conducting a double-blind control trial to study the effects of fluconazole and another antifungal drug, itraconazole, on asthma. Other common fungi, such as *Aspergillus* and *Candida*, are also being investigated as possible triggers for intrinsic asthma.

Section 23.3

# Respiratory Illness Associated with Inhalation of Mushroom Spores—Wisconsin, 1994

Source: *Morbidity and Mortality Weekly Report,* July 29, 1994.

During April 8-14, 1994, eight persons aged 16-19 years from southeastern Wisconsin visited physicians for respiratory illness associated with inhalation of *Lycoperdon perlatum* (i.e., puffball mushrooms). On April 19, the Bureau of Public Health, Wisconsin Division of Health, was notified of these cases. This report summarizes the case investigations.

On April 3, the adolescents attended a party during which they inhaled and chewed puffball mushrooms. It was unknown whether other persons at the party participated in this activity. No illicit drugs were reportedly used at the party. Three persons reported nausea and vomiting within 6-12 hours after exposure. Within 3-7 days after exposure, all patients developed cough, fever (temperature up to 103 F [39.4 C]), shortness of breath, myalgia, and fatigue.

Five persons required hospitalization; two were intubated. Two patients had a history of asthma and were using steroid inhalers. Chest radiographs on all hospitalized patients indicated bilateral reticulonodular infiltrates. Two patients underwent transbronchial lung biopsy, and one had an open lung biopsy. Histopathologic examination of the lung biopsy specimens revealed an inflammatory process and the presence of yeast-like structures consistent with Lycoperdon spores. Fungal cultures of the lung biopsy tissue were negative.

All hospitalized patients received corticosteroids, and four received antifungal therapy with either amphotericin B or azole drugs. All patients recovered within 1-4 weeks with no apparent sequelae.

Lycoperdonosis is a rare respiratory illness caused by inhalation of spores of the mushroom Lycoperdon. Puffballs, which are found worldwide, grow in the autumn and can be edible then. In the spring, they desiccate and form spores can be easily released by agitating the mushroom (1). One puffball species (*L. marginatum*) can produce psychoactive effects (2).

Only three cases of lycoperdonosis have been reported previously (1,3)—two in children and one in an adolescent. These three patients had inhaled large quantities of puffball spores, one unintentionally and two deliberately (as a folk remedy to control nosebleed). All patients had evidence of bilateral infiltrates on chest radiographs. Whether the pulmonary process results from a hypersensitivity reaction, an actual infection by the spores, or both is unknown.

The efficacy of using antifungal agents to treat lycoperdonosis is unknown. Physicians should be aware of this illness, especially in children and young adults presenting with a compatible clinical history and progressive respiratory symptoms.

*References*

1. Strand RD, Neuhauser EBD, Sornberger CF. Lycoperdonosis. N Engl J Med 1967; 277:89-91.

2. Lincoff G, Mitchel DH. Toxic and hallucinogenic mushroom poisoning. Williams WK, ed. New York: Van Nostrand Reinhold Company, 1977.

3. Henriksen NT. Lycoperdonosis Acta Paediatr Scand 1976; 65:643-5.

Reported by: *TA Taft, MD, RC Cardillo, MD, D Letzer, DO, CT Kaufman, DO, Milwaukee; JJ Kazmierczak, DVM, JP Davis, MD, Communicable Disease Epidemiologist, Bureau of Public Health, Wisconsin Div of Health. Div of Respiratory Disease Studies, National Institute for Occupational Safety and Health; Div of Bacterial and Mycotic Diseases, National Center for Infectious Diseases, CDC.*

Chapter 24

# New Drugs, Treatments, and Problems

*Chapter Contents*

Section 24. 1—Specialists Recommend Changes in Asthma
            Treatment............................................................. 692
Section 24. 2—FDA Licenses Cystic Fibrosis Treatment .......... 693
Section 24. 3—Prevalence of Penicillin-Resistant
            Streptococcus ...................................................... 694
Section 24. 4—Pneumococcal Polysaccharide Vaccine
            Recommendations of the Immunization
            Practices Advisory Committee ........................... 697
Section 24. 5—Combination TB Drug Approved ....................... 705

## Section 24.1

## *Specialists Recommend Change in Asthma Treatment*

Source: FDA *Consumer* July/August 1992.

The form of asthma medication most commonly prescribed in the United States should no longer be considered the first line of defense against the lung disease, according to an international panel of asthma experts.

Beta-agonist bronchodilators should be abandoned as first-line therapy for anything more than occasional mild asthma, according to a report by the International Asthma Management Project, a team of 18 asthma specialists from 11 countries. The report, issued in March 1992, says physicians should instead prescribe regular use of anti-inflammatory drugs, preferably inhaled corticosteroids. The beta-agonist bronchodilators should be reserved for pretreatment of exercise-induced asthma and to relieve symptoms of asthma attacks when anti-inflammatory therapy is insufficient.

The report advises physicians to stop focusing treatment on episodic asthma attacks and instead manage the chronic, persistent inflammation that exists in the airways of asthma sufferers.

"Since inflammation is the predominant feature in asthma, medications to reverse and prevent inflammation are key to effective asthma management," says Stephen T. Holgate, M.D., clinical professor of immunopharmacology at Southampton General Hospital, Southampton, England, and a panel member.

In addition to drug therapy, the report recommends a six-part asthma management program that includes:

- patient education
- frequent measurements of lung function to assess asthma severity
- avoidance and control of asthma triggers
- written medication plans for chronic management
- action plans for handling asthma attacks
- regular follow-up care.

The International Asthma Management Project was convened by the National Heart, Lung, and Blood Institute. The countries represented on the panel were Australia, Belgium, Canada, Denmark, France, Germany, Italy, Poland, Spain, the United Kingdom, and the United States.

## Section 24.2

## FDA Licenses Cystic Fibrosis Treatment

Source: FDA *Consumer* March 1994;

Licensing of the first product in 30 years specifically developed to treat cystic fibrosis was announce in December 1993. The biologic product was licensed nine months after it was submitted for review by FDA. It was jointly reviewed with the Canadian Health Protection Branch and licensed simultaneously in both countries.

Dornase alfa, commonly called DNase, a product of recombinant DNA technology, reduces the frequency of respiratory infections and improves lung function in cystic fibrosis patients.

Cystic fibrosis, an inherited disorder that affects about 30,000 Americans, is characterized by thick mucous secretions in the lungs. The retention of this mucous in the airways contributes to reduced lung function and chronic lung infections. Respiratory complications are the major cause of death among patients.

In providing an expedited review, FDA followed procedures established to implement the Prescription Drug User Fee Act of 1992, which provides additional resources to FDA to speed up review of drugs and biologics submitted to the agency for approval.

Due to the relatively low incidence of cystic fibrosis, FDA has designated DNase an "orphan" product. This designation provides financial incentives for companies developing products for rare diseases—those affecting fewer than 200,000 people in the United States.

DNase was evaluated in a six-month, multi-center, placebo-controlled clinical trial of 968 cystic fibrosis patients 5 years and older. Daily doses of DNase, used in conjunction with standard therapies, reduced the risk of severe respiratory tract infections by 27 percent and increased patients' lung function.

No clinical trials were conducted to demonstrate safety and effectiveness of DNase in children younger than 5, in patients with breathing function measured at less than 40 percent, or in patients for longer than 12 months.

Side effects include inflammation of throat, chest pain, voice alteration, and laryngitis.

DNase is manufactured by Genentech Inc. of San Francisco, and is marketed under the trade name Pulmozyme.

## Section 24.3

## *Prevalence of Penicillin-Resistant* Streptococcus Pneumoniae—*Connecticut, 1992—1993*

Source: *Morbidity and Mortality Weekly Report*, April 1994.

Streptococcus pneumoniae is an important cause of community-acquired bacterial pneumonia, meningitis, acute otitis media, and other infections. Infants, young children, and the elderly are most severely affected by pneumococcal disease. although *S. pneumoniae* was once considered to be routinely susceptible to penicillin, since the mid-1980s the incidence of resistance of this organism to penicillin and other antimicrobial agents has been increasing in the United States. National surveillance for drug-resistant *S. pneumoniae* (DRSP) is limited to testing invasive isolates from sentinel hospitals in 13 states. To determine the extent of antimicrobial susceptibility testing of *S. pneumoniae* and the prevalence of penicillin resistance among pneumococcal isolates from July 1992 through June 1993, in August 1993 the Connecticut Department of Public Health and Addiction Services (DPHAS) surveyed all 44 hospitals with clinical microbiology laboratories in Connecticut. This chapter summarizes the results of that survey.

Hospital laboratories were asked whether pneumococcal isolates were tested for resistance to penicillin, which isolates were tested, which tests were used, the number of isolates tested from different

## New Drugs, Treatments, and Problems

body sites from July 1992 through June 1993, and the minimal inhibitory concentrations (MICs) for any resistant isolates. Forty-three (98 percent) of 44 hospital laboratories responded.

Of the 43 hospital laboratories, 33 reported performing antimicrobial susceptibility tests on pneumococcal isolates, nine sent pneumococcal isolates to other laboratories for testing, and one neither performed such tests on pneumococcal isolates nor sent isolates to other laboratories for testing.

In 15 of the 33 laboratories, penicillin susceptibility testing was limited to qualitative disk diffusion (using an oxacillin disk). Nine laboratories screened pneumococcal isolates by disk diffusion, then confirmed penicillin resistance by determination of a quantitative MIC. Nine laboratories determined the penicillin MIC for all pneumococcal isolates.

MIC data were provided by 14 of the 18 laboratories that performed such tests for pneumococcal isolates. MICs were reported for 846 isolates collected during July 1992—June 1993. Penicillin resistance was defined as MIC 0.1 $\mu$g/mL, and high-level resistance was defined as MIC 2.0 $\mu$g/mL. Penicillin-resistant isolates were reported from four of 14 hospitals. Eighteen isolates (2.1 percent) from any body site were penicillin resistant, including five (1.3 percent) of 400 isolates from usually sterile sites. Overall, three isolates (one each from blood, sputum, and nasal fluid) were highly resistant. Two of these isolates had penicillin MICs 4.0 $\mu$g/mL.

The spread of DRSP strains may increase the public health impact of *S. pneumoniae* infections because of increased morbidity and reductions in the effectiveness of antimicrobial treatment for pneumococcal disease. Of special concern is resistance to extended-spectrum cephalosporins, which are often used as empiric therapy for meningitis.

Durinq 1979—1987, only one (0.02 percent) of 4585 pneumococcal sterile-site isolates submitted to CDC's sentinel hospital surveillance system was highly resistant to penicillin; in comparison, during 1992, seven (1.3 percent) of 544 such isolates were highly resistant. In some pediatric populations, up to 30 percent of pneumococcal isolates are penicillin resistant at some level, with a substantial proportion of strains resistant to multiple drugs. Although information regarding resistance to other antimicrobial drugs was unavailable in the Connecticut survey, the overall prevalence of penicillin-resistant strains in Connecticut was low through June 1993. However, resistant pneumococcal strains can spread rapidly in communities, and DPHAS is conducting surveillance for antimicrobial resistance.

Because penicillin susceptibility cannot be assumed, pneumococcal isolates associated with disease should be screened routinely for penicillin resistance by disk diffusion using a 1-$\mu$g oxacillin disk, which is highly sensitive—although not 100 percent specific—for penicillin resistance. Screening cannot reliably quantify the degree of penicillin resistance; therefore, pneumococcal isolates with oxacillin zone sizes less than or equal to 19 mm should be further tested by determination of MICs for penicillin, as well as for other drugs likely to be used in treatment. Some pneumococci with either intermediate or high-level penicillin resistance also may be resistant to extended-spectrum cephalosporins; therefore, penicillin-resistant isolates should be tested by MIC for susceptibility to either ceftriaxone or cefotaxime.

To optimize empiric regimens and initial therapy for pneumococcal infections, clinical health-care providers must be informed about the prevalence and patterns of drug resistance among isolates in their communities. Statewide surveillance for DRSP as a notifiable condition has been initiated in Colorado, Connecticut, and New Jersey. CDC in collaboration with the Council of State and Territorial Epidemiologists and the Association of State and Territorial Public Health Laboratory Directors, is developing strategies for collecting information on pneumococcal drug resistance in other states and for preventing morbidity and death associated with infection with resistant strains. Because antimicrobial susceptibility testing should be conducted routinely on invasive pneumococcal isolates, emphasis must be placed on developing methods to compile and analyze results, alerting health-care providers in communities in which resistant pneumococcal strains are prevalent, and identifying areas requiring more intensive epidemiologic assessment.

In areas where pneumococci resistant to extended-spectrum cephalosporins are prevalent, empiric therapy with vancomycin and an extended-spectrum cephalosporin should be considered for cases of life-threatening infection (e.g., meningitis) potentially caused by *S. pneumoniae* until results of culture and susceptibility testing are known. The emergence of drug-resistant pneumococcal infections underscores the need for adherence to recommendations of the Advisory Committee on Immunization Practices that persons aged 2 years with medical conditions placing them at increased risk for serious pneumococcal infection and all persons aged 65 years should receive 23-valent pneumococcal capsular polysaccharide vaccine; no pneumococcal vaccine is licensed for children less than 2 years old.

## Section 24.4

# Pneumococcal Polysaccharide Vaccine: Recommendations of the Immunization Practices Advisory Committee

Source: *Morbidity and Mortality Weekly Report*, February 1989.

Disease caused by *Streptococcus pneumoniae* (pneumococcus) remains an important cause of morbidity and mortality in the United States, particularly in the very young, the elderly, and persons with certain high-risk conditions. Pneumococcal pneumonia accounts for 10—25 percent of all pneumonias and an estimated 40,000 deaths annually. Although no recent data from the United States exist, in the United Kingdom pneumococcal infections may account for 34 percent of pneumonias in adults who require hospitalization. The best estimates of the incidence of serious pneumococcal disease in the United States are based on surveys and community-based studies of pneumococcal bacteremia. Recent studies suggest annual rates of bacteremia of 15—19/100,000 for all persons, 50/100,000 for persons 65 years old or older, and 160/100,000 for children 2 years old or younger. These rates are 2—3 times those previously documented in the United States. The overall rate for pneumococcal bacteremia in some Native American popuiations can be six times the rate of the general population. The incidence of pneumococcal pneumonia can be 3—5 times that of the detected rates of bacteremia. The estimated incidence of pneumococcal meningitis is 1—2/100,000 persons.

Mortality from pneumococcal disease is highest in patients with bacteremia or meningitis, patients with underlying medical conditions, and older persons. In some high-risk patients, mortality has been reported to be >40 percent for bacteremic disease and 55 percent for meningitis, despite appropriate antimicrobial therapy. Over 90 percent of pneumococci remain very sensitive to penicillin.

In addition to the very young and persons ≥65 years old, patients with certain chronic conditions are at increased risk of developing pneumococcal infection and severe pneumococcal illness. Patients with chronic cardiovascular diseases, chronic pulmonary disease, diabetes mellitus, alcoholism, and cirrhosis are generally immunocompetent but have increased risk. Other patients at greater risk because of decreased responsiveness to polysaccharide antigens or more rapid decline in serum antibody include those with functional or anatomic asplenia (e.g., sickle cell disease or splenectomy), Hodgkin's disease, lymphoma, multiple myeloma, chronic renal failure, nephrotic syndrome, and organ transplantation. In a recent population-based study, all persons 55-64 years old with pneumococcal bacteremia had at least one of these chronic conditions. Studies indicate that patients with acquired immunodeficiency syndrome (AIDS) are also at increased risk of pneumococcal disease, with an annual attack rate of pneumococcal pneumonia as high as 17.9/1000. This observation is consistent with the B-cell dysfunction noted in patients with AIDS. Recurrent pneumococcal meningitis may occur in patients with cerebrospinal fluid leakage complicating skull fractures or neurologic procedures.

## Pneumococcal Polysaccharide Vaccine

The current pneumococcal vaccine (Pneumovax® 23, Merck Sharp & Dohme, and Pnu-lmune® 23, Lederle Laboratories) is composed of purified capsular polysaccharide antigens of 23 types of *S. pneumoniae* (Danish types 1, 2, 3, 4, 5, 6B, 7F, 8, 9N, 9V, 10A, 11A, 12F, 14, 15B, 17F, 18C, 19F, 19A, 20, 22F, 23F, 33F). It was licensed in the United States in 1983, replacing a 14-valent vaccine licensed in 1977. Each vaccine dose (0.5 mL) contains 25µg of each polysaccharide antigen. The 23 capsular types in the vaccine cause 88 percent of the bacteremic pneumococcal disease in the United States. In addition, studies of the human antibody response indicate that cross-reactivity occurs for several types (e.g., 6A and 6B) that cause an additional 8 percent of bacteremic disease.

Most healthy adults, including the elderly, show a twofold or greater rise in type-specific antibody, as measured by radioimmunoassay, within 2—3 weeks of vaccination. Similar antibody responses have been reported in patients with alcoholic cirrhosis and diabetes mellitus requiring insulin. In immunocompromised patients, the response to vaccination may be less. In children <2 years old, antibody response to most capsular types is generally poor. In addition, re-

## New Drugs, Treatments, and Problems

sponse to some important pediatric pneumococcal types (e.g., 6A and 14) is decreased in children <5 years old.

Following vaccination of healthy adults with polyvalent pneumococcal vaccine, antibody levels for most pneumococcal vaccine types remain elevated at least 5 years; in some persons, they fall to prevaccination levels within 10 years. A more rapid decline in antibody levels may occur in children. In children who have undergone splenectomy following trauma and in those with sickle cell disease, antibody titers for some types can fall to prevaccination levels 3—5 years after vaccination. Similar rates of decline can occur in children with nephrotic syndrome.

Patients with AIDS have been shown to have an impaired antibody response to pneumococcal vaccine. However, asymptomatic HIV-infected men or those with persistent generalized lymphadenopathy respond to the 23-valent pneumococcal vaccine.

### Vaccine Efficacy

In the 1970s, pneumococcal vaccine was shown to reduce significantly the occurrence of pneumonia in young, healthy populations in South Africa and Papua New Guinea, where incidence of pneumonia is high. It was also demonstrated to protect against systemic pneumococcal infection in hyposplenic patients in the United States. Since then, studies have attempted to assess vaccine efficacy in other U.S. populations (see Table 24.1). A prospective, ongoing case-control study in Connecticut has shown an overall protective efficacy of 61 percent against pneumococcal bacteremia caused by vaccine—and vaccine-related serotypes. The protective efficacy was 60 percent for patients with alcoholism or chronic pulmonary, cardiac, or renal disease and 64 percent for patients 55 years old without other high-risk chronic conditions. In another multicenter case-control study, vaccine efficacy in immunocompetent persons 55 years old was 70 percent. A smaller case-control study of veterans failed to show efficacy in preventing pneumococcal bacteremia, but determination of the vaccination status was judged to be inadequate and the selection of controls was considered to be potentially biased.

Studies based on CDC's pneumococcal surveillance system suggest an efficacy of 60-64 percent for vaccine-type strains in patients with bacteremic disease. For all persons ≥65 years of age (including persons with chronic heart disease, pulmonary disease, or diabetes mellitus), vaccine efficacy was 44—61 percent (CDC unpublished

## Respiratory Diseases and Disorders Sourcebook

| Location | Method | No. persons | Type infection | Vaccine efficacy (%) | 95% C.I. |
|---|---|---|---|---|---|
| Connecticut (25,26) | Case-control* | 543 cases 543 controls | VT[†], VT-related | 61 | 42, 73 |
| Philadelphia (27) | Case-control* | 122 cases 244 controls | All serotypes | 70 | 37, 86 |
| Denver (28) | Case-control* | 89 cases 89 controls | All serotypes | –21 | –221, 55 |
| CDC-1 (29) | Epidemiologic* | 249 vaccinated 1638 unvaccinated | VT | 64 | 47, 76 |
| CDC-2 (unpublished) | Epidemiologic* | 240 vaccinated 1527 unvaccinated | VT | 60 | 45, 70 |
| VA cooperative study (30) | Randomized controlled trial[§] | 1145 vaccinated 1150 controls | All serotypes VT | –34[¶] –19[¶] | –119, 18[¶] –164, 47[¶] |

*Only patients with isolates from normally sterile body sites were included.
[†]Vaccine-type pneumococcal infection.
[§]Pneumococcal pneumonia and bronchitis were diagnosed primarily by culture of respiratory secretions.
[¶]Values calculated from the published data.

*Table 24.1. Clinical Effectiveness of Pneumococcal Vaccination in U.S. Populations*

data). In addition, estimates of vaccine efficacy for serologically related types were 29—66 percent. Limited data suggest that clinical efficacy may decline ≥6 years after vaccination (CDC, unpublished data).

A randomized, double-blind, placebo-controlled trial among high-risk veterans showed no vaccine efficacy against pneumococcal pneumonia or bronchitis; however, case definitions used were judged to have uncertain specificity. In addition, this study had only a 6 percent ability to detect a vaccine efficacy of 65 percent for pneumococcal bacteremia. In contrast, a French clinical trial found pneumococcal vaccine to be 77 percent effective in reducing the incidence of pneumonia in nursing home residents.

Despite conflicting findings, the data continue to support the use of the pneumococcal vaccine for certain well-defined groups at risk.

### Recommendations for Vaccine Use

#### Adults

1. Immunocompetent adults who are at increased risk of pneumococcal disease or its complications because of chronic ill-

## New Drugs, Treatments, and Problems

nesses (e.g., cardiovascular disease, pulmonary disease, diabetes meliitus, alcoholism, cirrhosis, or cerebrospinal fluid leaks) or who are ≥65 years old.

2. Immunocompromised adults at increased risk of pneumococcal disease or its complications (e.g., persons with splenic dysfunction or anatomic asplenia, Hodgkin's disease, lymphoma, multiple myeloma, chronic renal failure, nephrotic syndrome, or conditions such as organ transplantation associated with immunosuppression).

3. Adults with asymptomatic or symptomatic HIV infection.

### Children

1. Children ≥ 2 years old with chronic illnesses specifically associated with increased risk of pneumococcal disease or its complications (e.g., anatomic or functional asplenia [including sickle cell disease], nephrotic syndrome, cerebrospinal fluid leaks, and conditions associated with immunosuppression).

2. Children ≥2 years old with asymptomatic or symptomatic HIV infection.

3. The currently available 23-valent vaccine is not indicated for patients having only recurrent upper respiratory tract disease, including otitis media and sinusitis.

### Special Groups

Persons living in special environments or social settings with an identified increased risk of pneumococcal disease or its complications (e.g., certain Native American populations).

## ADVERSE REACTIONS

Approximately 50 percent of persons given pneumococcal vaccine develop mild side effects, such as erythema and pain at the injection site. Fever, myalgia, and severe local reactions have been reported in <1 percent of those vaccinated. Severe systemic reactions, such as anaphylaxis, rarely have been reported.

## PRECAUTIONS

The safety of pneumococcal vaccine for pregnant women has not been evaluated. Ideally, women at high risk of pneumococcal disease should be vaccinated before pregnancy.

## TIMING OF VACCINATION

When elective splenectomy is being considered, pneumococcal vaccine should be given at least 2 weeks before the operation, if possible. Similarly, for planning cancer chemotherapy or immunosuppressive therapy, as in patients who undergo organ transplantation, the interval between vaccination and initiation of chemotherapy or immunosuppression should also be at least 2 weeks.

## REVACCINATION

In one study, local reactions after revaccination in adults were more severe than after initial vaccination when the interval between vaccinations was 13 months (see Table 24.2). Reports of revaccination after longer intervals in children and adults, including a large group of elderly persons revaccinated at least 4 years after primary vaccination, suggest a similar incidence of such reactions after primary vaccination and revaccination (unpublished data).

Without more information, persons who received the 14-valent pneumococcal vaccine should not be routinely revaccinated with the 23-valent vaccine, as increased coverage is modest and duration of protection is not well defined. However, revaccination with the 23-valent vaccine should be strongly considered for persons who received the 14-valent vaccine if they are at highest risk of fatal pneumococcal infection (e.g., asplenic patients). Revaccination should also be considered for adults at highest risk who received the 23-valent vaccine 6 years before and for those shown to have rapid decline in pneumococcal antibody levels (e.g., patients with nephrotic syndrome, renal failure, or transplant recipients). Revaccination after 3—5 years should be considered for children with nephrotic syndrome, asplenia, or sickle cell anemia who would be 10 years old at revaccination.

## New Drugs, Treatments, and Problems

| Study | Vaccinees Condition | Age | No. | Revaccination period | Reactions |
|---|---|---|---|---|---|
| Borgono, et al. 1978 (33) | Normal | Adults | 7 | 13 mos | Increase in local reactions |
| Carlson, et al. 1979 (34) | Normal | 21–62 yrs | 23 | 12–18 mos | Increase in local reactions |
| Rigau-Perez, et al. 1983 (35) | Sickle cell disease | ≥3 yrs | 28 | 28–35 mos | No increase in reactions compared with primary vaccination |
| Lawrence, et al. 1983 (36) | Normal | 2–5 yrs | 52 | 35 mos (mean) | Increase in local reactions |
| Mufson, et al. 1984 (37) | Normal | 23–40 yrs | 12 | 24–48 mos | No increase in reactions compared with primary vaccination |
| Weintrub, et al. 1984 (17) | Sickle cell disease | 10–27 yrs | 17 | 8–9 yrs | No "serious" local reactions |
| Kaplan, et al. 1986 (38) | Sickle cell disease | 4–23 yrs | 86 | 37–53 mos | Four "severe" reactions* |

*Severe reaction was defined as presence of local pain, redness, swelling, and axillary temperature >100 F (37.8 C); two patients aged 21 and 23 years had temperatures of 102 F (38.9 C).

*Table 24.2. Reactions to Revaccination with Pneumococcal Vaccine*

## Strategies for Vaccine Delivery

Recommendations for pneumococcal vaccination have been made by the ACIP, the American Academy of Pediatrics, the American College of Physicians, and the American Academy of Family Physicians. Recent analysis indicates that pneumococcal vaccination of elderly persons is cost-effective. The vaccine is targeted for approximately 27 million persons aged ≥ 65 years and 21 million persons aged <65 years with high-risk conditions. Despite Medicare reimbursement for costs of the vaccine and its administration, which began in 1981, annual use of pneumococcal vaccine has not increased above levels observed in earlier years (see Figure 24.3). In 1985, <10 percent of the 48 million persons considered to be at increased risk of serious pneumococcal infection were estimated to have ever received pneumococcal vaccine.

Opportunities to vaccinate high-risk persons are missed both at time of hospital discharge and during visits to clinicians' offices. Two thirds or more of patients with serious pneumococcal disease had been hospitalized at least once within 5 years before their pneumococcal illness, yet few had received pneumococcal vaccine. More effective programs for vaccine delivery are needed, including offering pneumococcal vaccine in hospitals (at the time of discharge), clinicians' offices, nursing homes, and other chronic-care facilities. Many patients who receive pneumococcal vaccine should also be immunized with influenza vaccine, which can be given simultaneously at a different site. In contrast to pneumococcal vaccine, influenza vaccine is given annually.

## Vaccine Development

A more immunogenic pneumococcal vaccine preparation is needed, particularly for children <2 years old. The development of a protein-polysaccharide conjugate vaccine for selected capsular types holds promise.

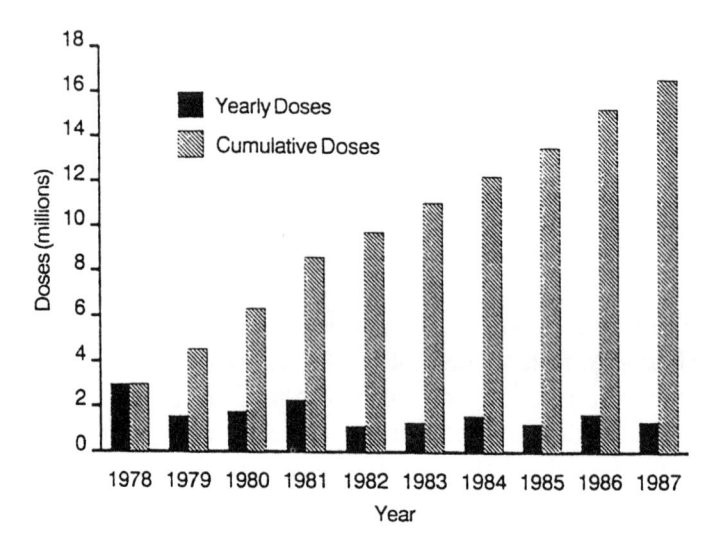

*Figure 24.3* Pneumococcal Vaccine Distribution—United States, 1978—1987.

**New Drugs, Treatments, and Problems**

Section 24.5

## Combination TB Drug Approved

Source: FDA *Consumer* September 1994.

Rifater, a product that combines three existing tuberculosis drugs into a single tablet, was approved by FDA last May 31. The fixed-dose product was developed to make it easier for patients to comply with the standard long-term, multi-drug regimen of isoniazid, rifampin and pyrazinamide.

Patients may fail to take the full amount of the three drugs individually—as many as 13 pills a day—and this has been a public health concern in the control of the disease. The single-tablet dosage form reduces the number of pills to six a day.

Use of the combination drug should also slow emergence of multi-drug-resistant tuberculosis, a problem partly attributable to not following the dosing regimen.

Rifater's use will also prevent inadvertent under- or overdosing with any of the three component drugs, and will safeguard against patients deciding to stop taking any of the drugs.

Rifater has been used in Europe, Africa and Hong Kong since the mid-1980s. Nearly two years ago, FDA encouraged Marion Merrell Dow, the drug's manufacturer, to seek U.S. marketing approval.

Chapter 25

# Single and Double Lung Transplantation

## Introduction

Allogeneic lung transplantation (LT) involves the grafting of one or both lungs from a brain-dead or cadaveric donor to a selected patient with end-stage pulmonary vascular or parenchymal disease who has failed standard therapies and for whom no other treatment option exists. The first use of a living related donor for LT using a lobe rather than a whole lung has already been reported (JAMA 1990;264:2724), and the use of live donors, related or unrelated will probably evolve as a common clinical option.

The transplant is used in three clinical procedures:

- combined heart-lung transplantation (HLT)
- single lung transplantation (SLT) and
- double lung transplantation (DLT), either performed en bloc with the bronchial tree or including transplant of each lung separately with bilateral bronchial anastomoses.

End-stage pulmonary disease is a term defining irreversibility of severe anatomic changes in the lungs leading to incapacitating clinical manifestations and eventual respiratory failure (often associated

---

U.S. Department of Health and Human Services, Health Technology Assessment Report Number 5, 1991.

with right ventricular failure). The lungs have exhausted all reserves for gas exchange, and patients frequently require oxygen or assisted ventilation therapy to sustain life. Examples of such life-threatening diseases are severe emphysema, pulmonary fibrosis, cystic fibrosis, and pulmonary hypertension resulting from arterial or venous vascular disease or congenital heart defects. Lung transplantation can potentially be applied to thousands of patients yearly who might otherwise die from these acute or chronically progressive end-stage pulmonary diseases.

Chronic obstructive pulmonary disease (COPD) affects approximately 10 million people in the United States, the majority of whom have emphysema. For those patients having severe progressive disease relatively early in life, LT offers the only possibility of preventing a premature demise. Emphysema may also be secondary to an inherited deficiency of a $alpha_1$-antitrypsin (AAT), which affects an estimated 40,000 Americans.

Primary pulmonary hypertension affects relatively young persons (mean age at diagnosis is 34), but the prognosis of these patients is poor, and only 20 percent survive five years.

The prevalence of pulmonary fibrosis is estimated to be 3—5 cases per 100,000 population, and the disease in these patients generally runs an aggressive and usually fatal course.

Cystic fibrosis is a common multivisceral recessive genetic disease having an incidence of one case per 2,000 in white and one case per 17,000 in black births. There are an estimated 20,000 cases in the United States (including 2,000 adults) and approximately 1,000 new cases annually. There is no medical treatment for these patients other than supportive care, and pulmonary disease as a consequence of exocrine gland obstruction by viscous secretions commonly results in bronchiectasis, peribronchial fibrosis, and airway obstruction. Survival in patients with CF has dramatically increased in the past two decades secondary to improvement in antibiotics, nutrition management, physiotherapy, and specialized centers for treatment. However, 50 percent of patients die of respiratory failure by the age of 16, and the others rarely survive longer than 30 years.

Despite the limited availability of suitable donor lungs, which restricts the application of this technology, there has been a dramatic increase in the number of lung tranplants performed in the United States in recent years: 32 in 1988, 84 in 1989, approximately 200 in 1990, and an extimated 500 to be completed in 1991. The estimated cost of an LT is $150,000 in the first year and $20,000 annually thereafter.

In addition to the relatively standardized surgical technique, successful LT involves a large team of professionals attending to patient and donor selection, pre-operative and post-operative rehabilitation, lifelong immunosuppression, and long-term follow-up.

## Background

Progress in LT has lagged behind that of other solid organ transplantation in part because of a lack of a suitable experimental model (the transplantation of normal lungs into nondiseased experimental animals is dramatically different from the transplantation of lungs into chronically ill humans). The initial poor results of LT (survival period of less than one month) accounted, in part, for the hiatus in clinical interest in LT between 1963 and 1982, when the first "long-term" success was reported.

The lung is a very fragile organ. During transplantation, it is at increased risk for infection because of exposure to organisms in the atmosphere. Lung allografts are unique among solid organ transplants in that they do not have their systemic arterial blood supply reconstructed at the time of surgery. The fine network of bronchial vessels is interrupted and are not amenable to reattachment. In the absence of positive intervention, the airway is at risk for ischemic complications until local adequate revascularization (usually requiring 2-3 weeks) can occur across the healing bronchial anastomosis. The experience with primates at Stanford University suggested that reconstruction of the bronchial arteries is probably required to ensure a slough-free donor bronchus, decreasing the risk of dehiscence. However, the technique of LT has rarely included direct microsurgical methods of reestablishing bronchial circulation and these have been almost universally unsuccessful because of the caliber of the vessels.

Early concerns about LT included the uncertainty of recurrent disease, especially in patients with CF or interstitial fibrosis. Poor results in some of the early clinical experiences were associated with a ventilation/perfusion (V/P) imbalance. In addition, there were fears that SLT would not provide sufficient pulmonary function and adaptation to the normal cardiac output without abnormal elevation of pulmonary artery pressure. To date, it appears that these concerns were exaggerated. Recurrent disease has not been reported, the ability of

SLT to provide total respiratory function has been abundantly demonstrated in preclinical studies and confirmed in humans, and it has been shown that significant V/P imbalance does not occur in the absence of other adverse conditions, e.g. infection or rejection, which may themselves be prevented or respond to treatment.

The surgical feasibility of LT has been based largely on experiments in normal animals. The operative techniques of LT were derived from canine models, and the first successes were reported in 1950 by Metras in France and in 1954 by Hardin and Kittle in the United States.

After extensive transplantation experience in more than 400 dogs, Hardy and associates performed the first human SLT in 1963. Although the patient survived only 18 days, adequate lung function was established, and LT was thus demonstrated to be feasible in humans.

Two 1970 reviews of LT noted no long-term survivors in the 25 transplants performed to that time. In subsequent reviews of more than 40 cases of LT through 1985 (including three HLT and four lobe transplants) reported by 26 teams worldwide, the median survival time was 8.5 days, and only two patients survived longer than two months. The longest survivors (six and ten months) obtained significant palliation. Most patients died within days or weeks from respiratory failure, pulmonary sepsis, rejection, or bronchial anastomotic complications.

Prior to 1980, there were important technical advances including extracorporeal bypass, improved positive end-expiratory pressure techniques, fiberoptic oximetry and bronchoscopy, and the introduction of cyclosporine immunosuppression. Short-term data had accumulated from both animal and human LT experience demonstrating that adequate (but not normal) respiratory function could be maintained despite pulmonary deservation. However, the major limiting factor in LT still appeared to be bronchial anastomic complications.

Although ischemia is the primary source of such airway complications, immunosuppressant effects on bronchial anastomotic healing also play a significant role. These airway complications include necrosis, strictures, dehiscence, and the development of retrotracheal airspace.

Bronchial anastomotic complications secondary to ischemia following LT are in sharp contrast to the situation following HLT, wherein consistent satisfactory tracheal anastomotic healing is almost assured. This is attributed to preservation of mediastinal collateral arterial circulation from the coronary arteries through the pericardium and directly into the bronchial circulation of the lower trachea and carina.

An early major technical advance in LT, introduced by Metras, was related to the high incidence of thrombosis of the pulmonary venous anastomosis. This surgical innovation involved transecting a cuff of donor left atrium including the ostia of the pulmonary veins, thereby avoiding the need for anastomosis of these vessels.

The majority of early LT recipients who lived more than two weeks died in the third week from disruption of the bronchial anatomosis. The recognition that a significant proportion of the major complications contributing to the realtively poor success of LT was related to immunosuppressant steroid inhibition of bronchial anastomotic collagen synthesis and wound healing, in addition to the local ischemic problem, prompted additional canine experiments. This led to the reduction or elimination of routine early use of steroids in the immunosuppressive regimens and the use of omental pedicle flaps (bronchial omentopexy) to promote bronchial revascularization and physically support the anastomotic site to prevent bronchovascular or bronchopleural fistulae.

The use of omentum as a vascularized pedicle to wrap the bronchial anastomosis is now commonly performed as a highly successful technique to promote bronchial integrity. Collateral circulation between the omental and bronchial vessels is often rapidly accomplished within a few days rather than 2-3 weeks, and problems of bronchial anastomotic healing have been dramatically reduced.

The first long-term survivor with an allografted lung was a patient subjected to HLT who remained alive and well 10 months after surgery (reported by the Stanford University group in 1982). The first long-term successes with SLT were reported by the Toronto Lung Transplant Group in 1986. Two patients were alive and well at 26 months and 14 months after the procedure.

Single lung transplantation was initially introduced and, on the basis of early clincal experience, recommended as a treatment for restrictive interstitial lung disease. The ideal candidates for SLT, i.e. those with end-stage pulmonary fibrosis, generally do not have chronic pulmonary infections. The reduced compliance and increased vascular resistance of the remaining fibrotic lung facilitate preferential ventilation and perfusion of the transplanted lung, which in turn increase pulmonary artery to bronchial artery blood flow and decrease the likelihood of airway ischemia. Patients with emphysema were thought to be poor candidates for SLT because of the belief that hyperexpansion of the native lung and mediastinal shift would result in restricted ventilation of the transplant. However, in practice this did not present a significant problem. Therefore, end-stage emphysema patients (especially those with AAT deficiency) as well as patients with pulmonary hypertension or COPD are currently regarded as candidates for SLT.

Single lung transplantation is almost universally regarded as unsuitable for patients with chronically infected lungs (e.g., those with CF or bronchiectasis), which remain a focus for continuous for sepsis, especially in the environment of immunosuppression.

Although transplantation of both lungs without the heart is technically more complex than HLT, the value of preservation of the recipient's heart has become apparent. Experience from investigations of DLT has evolved a technique to avoid the problems and need for replaced the heart in patents having only end-stage parenchymal pulmonary disease for whom HLT was the only other treatment option available.

In 1971, Veith and associates described a dog model for bilateral simultaneous lung allotransplantation. An en bloc DLT in dogs was first described by Vanderhoeft et al in Belgium in 1972. This experimental technique was further developed by Dark and the Toronto Lung Group in 1986, and it was introduced clinically by Patterson and associates in 1988.

Double lung transplantation was initially performed in patients with obstructive lung disease, based on the belief that such patients were not suitable for SLT because of V/P imbalance and crowding of the transplant by hyperinflation of the native lung. More recent experience indicates that SLT achieves very satisfactory results in such patients. Double lung transplantation is now applied to patients with end-stage pulmonary disease and adequate cardiac function who are not candidates for SLT. These patients commonly have bilateral pulmonary sepsis, COPD, CF, or pulmonary hypertension. While the technical feasibility of DLT has been established, the incidence of airway complications is higher than that associated with SLT as a consequence of a greater bronchial area subject to ischemia. In addition, after DLT the pulmonary artery flow is equally distributed to each lung; therefore, collateral flow to each lung is reduced, in contrast to the situation described for SLT.

Recent modifications in the technique of DLT have included bilateral sequential transplantation of the lungs, which reduces the requirement for cardiopulmonary bypass during en bloc procedures and substitutes bilateral bronchial anastomosis (without omentopexy) for the tracheal anastomosis, which itself was associated with significant airway problems.

## Summary

Lung transplantation currently involves the allografting of one or both lungs from a cadaver or brain-dead donor to selected patients with progressive end-stage pulmonary disease for whom there are no other viable treatment options.

Expanding experience since 1986 in Canada, the United States, and Europe has demonstrated that both SLT and DLT can provide adequate pulmonary function and palliation for extended periods in some patients with otherwise fatal lung disease. A more rapid expansion of this technology has been constrained by the scarcity of suitable donors and the current limits of organ preservation time. Lung transplantation has evolved as a clinical prodedure achieving a favorable risk-benefit ratio and acceptable one-to-two year survival rates.

Lung transplantation is applied as a therapeutic option for patients with end-stage pulmonary disease. However, the transplant community has not yet reached consensus regarding patient selection criteria or absolute contra-indications to LT. Specific selection criteria for the optimal treatment of all LT candidates do not exist as yet and are currently evolving. The majority of candidates have had pulmonay fibrosis, bronchiectasis, emphysema, pulmonary hypertension, or CF.

Additional clinical information and experience will be useful in refining evaluation of risk-benefit ratios of SLT and DLT, which may vary for specific subsets of patients.

# Part IV

# Glossary

Chapter 26

# Glossary of Medical Terms

This glossary contains many of the terms used throughout this and other volumes of the *Health Reference Series*. The definitions given are not dictionary definitions but are those most applicable to usage relating to respiratory diseases and disorders.

## A

**Abscess.** A collection of pus formed by dead and dying cells and tissues, which can result from infections.

**Absorption.** In physiology, the passage or uptake of substances into or across tissues, such as the uptake of digested food and water from the intestines to the bloodstream. Because of a lack of digestive enzymes, some foods eaten by patients with CF may not be adequately absorbed.

**ACE.** Angiotensin-inverting enzyme.

**Acid-fast bacilli (AFB).** Bacteria that retain certain dyes after being washed in an acid solution. Most acid-fast organisms are mycobacteria. When AFB are seen on a stained smear of sputum or other clini-

---

Excerpted from CDC Pub No. 1094; NIH Pub No. 91-3093, 93-2020, and 93-2391; DHHS Pub Questions and Answers About Tuberculosis; Morbidity and Mortality Weekly Report October 28, 1994 Vol 43 No RR-13.

cal specimen, a diagnosis of TB should be suspected; however, the diagnosis of TB is not confirmed until a culture is grown and identified as M. tuberculosis.

**Acute Respiratory Failure Sudden.** Severe condition in which a sufficient supply of oxygen does not reach the bloodstream, and carbon dioxide is not adequately removed from the blood and lungs. Requires emergency care.

**Acute.** A term used to denote a disease or condition which is sudden, severe, and of short duration. Not chronic. Although CF is a chronic disease, it is often marked by acute episodes of infection or other clinical complications.

**Adenoids.** Gland-like tissue growths in the nose above the throat which obstruct breathing when swollen.

**Adherence.** Refers to the behavior of patients when they follow all aspects of the treatment regimen as prescribed by the medical provider, and also refers to the behavior of health care workers and employers when they follow all guidelines pertaining to infection control.

**Aerosol.** A solution of a drug which is made into a fine mist for use in inhalation therapy. Some drugs for treating respiratory complications of CF are used in this form.
The droplet nuclei that are expelled by an infectious person (e.g., by coughing or sneezing); these droplet nuclei can remain suspended in the air and can transmit M. tuberculosis to other persons.

**AIA.** The American Institute of Architects, a professional body that develops standards for building ventilation.

**Air mixing.** The degree to which air supplied to a room mixes with the air already in the room, usually expressed as a mixing factor. This factor varies from 1 (for perfect mixing) to 10 (for poor mixing), and it is used as a multiplier to determine the actual airflow required (i.e., the recommended ACH multiplied by the mixing factor equals the actual ACH required).

**Air changes.** The ratio of the volume of air flowing through a space in a certain period of time (i.e., the airflow rate) to the volume of that

## Glossary of Medical Terms

space (i.e., the room volume); this ratio is usually expressed as the number of air changes per hour (ACH).

**Airway obstruction.** A narrowing, clogging, or blocking of the passages that carry air to the lungs.

**Airways.** Tubes conducting air from the outside into the lungs. The lungs contain many airways of different sizes. The largest airway is the central airway called the trachea. This branches into other airways called the bronchi, which then divide into even smaller branches called bronchioles. (Also see Bronchus, Bronchioles, Respiratory System.)

**Allergy.** The body's reaction to a specific substance (allergen) to which the individual is sensitive.

**Alpha$_1$.** A substance in blood transported to the protease lungs that inhibits the digestive activity of inhibitor trypsin and other proteases which digest proteins. Deficiency of this substance is associated with emphysema. (See alpha$_1$ protease inhibitor.)

**Alpha$_1$ antitrypsin Deficiency.** Inherited condition in which the lung tissue is destroyed through an abnormality of the body's immune system. Caused by a lack of alpha$_1$ antitrypsin, a protein in the blood which controls the action of the enzyme trypsin, involved in the digestion. When alpha$_1$ antitrypsin is not present, the enzyme will attack and destroy the lung tissue as well as the liver.

**Alveoli.** The millions of tiny air sacs in the lungs that lie at the end of the bronchial tree, where oxygen and carbon dioxide are exchanged with the bloodstream. In CF, a patient's alveoli may become clogged with mucus, thereby interfering with the oxygen/carbon dioxide exchange. They are the site where TB infection usually begins. (Also see Respiratory System.)

**Alveolitis.** Inflammation of the alveoli.

**Amino Acids.** Building blocks of proteins, which are essential in development and maintenance of body functions.

**Aminoglycoside.** Any of a group of antibiotics that are used to combat bacterial infections. Tobramycin and gentamicin are examples of these antibiotics and are often used by CF patients.

**Amniocentesis.** A technique used to identify or "screen" genetic defects in the unborn child. A hollow needle is inserted through the mother's abdominal wall into the womb and a small sample of amniotic fluid surrounding the fetus is withdrawn and analyzed.

**Amniotic Fluid.** The liquid surrounding the fetus in the womb.

**Anergy.** Absence of immune response to particular substances. The inability of a person to react to skin-test antigens (even if the person is infected with the organisms tested) because of immunosuppression.

**Angina.** Chest pain that originates in the heart.

**Anoxia.** The absence or lack of oxygen supply in the body.

**Antenatal.** Refers to the period before birth. (Also see Prenatal.)

**Anterior-posterior A-P Diameter.** (front to back) Measurement of the chest. This measurement is usually increased in children with CF. It is related to long-term mucous obstruction of the lungs and its effects on breathing patterns.

**Anteroom.** A small room leading from a corridor into an isolation room; this room can act as an airlock, preventing the escape of contaminants from the isolation room into the corridor.

**Antibiotic.** A drug which can destroy or inhibit growth of infectious organisms, such as bacteria. Antibiotics are frequently administered to individuals with CF to combat respiratory infections. Among the antibiotics used in CF treatment are penicillin, tetracycline, gentamicin, and carbenicillin.

**Antibody.** Part of the body's immune defense system. Antibodies are proteins produced in the blood in response to foreign organisms in the body.

## Glossary of Medical Terms

**Antielastases or Elastase Inhibitors.** Substances in the blood transported to the lungs and other organs which prevent the digestive action of elastases.

**Antigen.** Substances, such as bacteria or toxins, which stimulate formation of antibody.

**Aorta.** Blood vessel that delivers oxygen-rich blood from the left ventricle to the body; it is the largest blood vessel in the body.

**A-P Diameter Anterior-posterior (front to back).** Measurement of the chest. This measurement is usually increased in children with CF. It is related to long-term mucous obstruction of the lungs and its effects on breathing patterns.

**Apnea.** Cessation of breathing.

**Applied Research.** Investigations which focus on "applying" findings from basic research to practical problems (such as disease, symptoms, etc.). Development of new respiratory equipment or studies of cell defects in the sweat glands of CF patients can be considered examples of applied research.

**Area.** A structural unit (e.g., a hospital ward or laboratory) or functional unit (e.g., an internal medicine service) in which health care workers provide services to and share air with a specific patient population or work with clinical specimens that may contain viable M. tuberculosis organisms. The risk for exposure to M. tuberculosis in a given area depends on the prevalence of TB in the population served and the characteristics of the environment.

**Arousal.** An abrupt change from deep sleep to a lighter stage of sleep which may or may not lead to awakening.

**Arrhythmia.** Any variation from the normal rhythm of the heart beat. It is sometimes seen in advance cases of CF in which pulmonary complications begin to interfere with heart and lung function. (Also see Cor Pulmonale.)

**ASHRAE.** The American Society of Heating, Refrigerating and Air-Conditioning Engineers, Inc., a professional body that develops standards for building ventilation.

**Aspirate.** The process of mechanical suctioning of liquids or gases from the lungs. This method is often used to remove excess mucus from the lungs of patients with CF. Also means to inhale food or other material.

**Asymptomatic.** Without symptoms, or producing no symptoms.

**Atelectasis.** Collapsed portion of the lung which does not contain air. This can be caused by excessive accumulations of mucous secretions which interfere with complete inhalation.

**Atrium.** One of the two receiving chambers of the heart. The right atrium receives oxygen-poor blood from the body. The left atrium receives oxygen-rich blood from the lungs. The plural of atrium is atria.

**Autosomal Recessive.** A genetic trait or disorder which appears only when an individual inherits a pair of chromosomes, each containing the gene for the trait. One chromosome of the pair comes from the father and the other from the mother. Autosomal recessive disorders can occur only if both parents are carriers of the trait. CF is inherited in this manner. (Also see Carrier, Chromosome, Gene.)

# B

**Bacillus of Calmette and Guerin (BCG) vaccine.** A TB vaccine used in many parts of the world.

**BACTEC.** One of the most often used radiometric methods for detecting the early growth of mycobacteria in culture. It provides rapid growth (in 7-14 days) and rapid drug-susceptibility testing (in 5 6 days). When BACTEC is used with rapid species identification methods, M. tuberculosis can be identified within 1>14 days of specimen collection.

**Bacteria.** Microscopic one-celled organisms frequently responsible for many infections. Patients with CF are particularly susceptible to bac-

## Glossary of Medical Terms

terial infections in the lungs (Staphylococcus aureus and Pseudomonas aeruginosa). However, some bacteria normally found in the body perform useful functions. (E. coli lives in the intestines and helps with digestion.)

**Barrel Chest.** Enlarged rib cage caused by some lung diseases, including CF

**Base Pairs.** Small building blocks that make up genetic material.

**Basic Science Research.** Investigations aimed at increasing understanding of the fundamental aspects of life processes. To obtain data on the causes underlying CF, scientists conduct basic science investigations, ranging from genetic studies to research on the cell and how the cell membrane is involved in the movement of substances from the cell's interior to the surrounding environment.

**BCG.** A vaccine for TB named after the French scientists Calmette and Guerin. BCG is not widely used in the United States, but it is often given to infants and small children in other countries where TB is common.

**Berylliosis.** A lung disease resulting from exposure to beryllium metal.

**Biopsy.** Surgical removal of tissue from a living body for microscopic examination to aid in diagnosis.

**Birth Defect.** Any defect present when a child is born. Birth defects are disorders of body structure, function, or chemistry which may be inherited or may result from environmental interference during embryonic or fetal life.

**Blood Pressure.** Force exerted by the heart in pumping blood from its chambers. The pressure of blood against the walls of a blood vessel or heart chamber. Unless there is reference to another location, such as the pulmonary artery or one of the heart chambers, it refers to the pressure in the systemic arteries, as measured, for example, in the forearm.

**Booster phenomenon.** A phenomenon in which some persons (especially older adults) who are skin tested many years after infection with M. tuberculosis have a negative reaction to an initial skin test, followed by a positive reaction to a subsequent skin test. The second (i.e., positive) reaction is caused by a boosted immune response. Two-step testing is used to distinguish new infections from boosted reactions (see Two-step testing).

**Bronchi.** Larger air passages of the lungs.

**Bronchial Lavage.** A procedure in which large volumes of saline are rinsed through the lungs, followed by suction. It may be used in the treatment of CF to aspirate mucus secretions which cannot be removed through postural drainage. (Also see Aspirate.)

**Bronchial Drainage.** A form of physical therapy used for CF patients in which the chest is pounded from several different angles and positions to help loosen mucus in the lungs. CF patients undergo bronchial drainage up to several times per day. (Also see Physical Therapy, Postural Drainage.)

**Bronchiectasis.** Long-term condition in which the bronchi of the lungs are stretched or dilated beyond their normal dimensions. This condition leads to abnormal breathing patterns, coughing, and coughing up of mucus from the lungs. This condition can occur in CF patients. (Also see Respiratory System.)

**Bronchiole.** Finer air passages of the lungs.

**Bronchioles.** The smallest of the air tubes (airways) leading to the lung. (Also see Respiratory System, Bronchus, Airways.)

**Bronchitis.** An inflammation of the bronchi caused by infection, exposure to cold, or irritants. Symptoms include fever and cough. Many individuals with CF have frequent attacks of bronchitis.

**Broncho-constriction.** Tightening of the muscles surrounding bronchi, the tubes that branch from the windpipe.

**Bronchodilator.** A drug that relaxes the smooth muscles and opens the constricted airway. Medication which dilates or opens bronchial

## Glossary of Medical Terms

tubes to allow freer breathing. Often prescribed to relieve bronchospasm.

**Bronchoscope.** A long, narrow tube with a light at the end that is used by the doctor for direct observation of the airways, as well as for suction of tissue and other materials.

**Bronchoscopy.** Internal examination of the lungs by using an illuminated tube-like instrument (bronchoscope) which is inserted into the lungs through the throat, pharynx and trachea (windpipe). Allows direct examination of the interior of the bronchial tubes. (Also see Respiratory System.)

**Bronchospasm.** Tightening or contracting of muscles surrounding and supporting bronchial tubes interfering with normal breathing and causing respiratory distress. Occurs in asthma attacks and in CF.

**Bronchus (plural: Bronchi).** The large tubes which transport air from the trachea toward the lungs. The bronchi subdivide into smaller tubes (bronchioles) which lead to the alveoli of the lungs. In CF, the bronchi are often clogged by mucus, thereby interfering with breathing. (Also see Respiratory System.)

## C

**Calipers.** Forceps-like instruments used to measure the thickness of objects, such as the A-P diameter of the chest of children with CF and other lung diseases.

**Capillaries.** The smallest blood vessels in the body through which most of the oxygen, carbon dioxide, and nutrient exchanges take place.

**Capreomycin.** An injectable, second-line anti-TB drug used primarily for the treatment of drug-resistant TB.

**Cardiac output.** Total amount of blood being pumped by the heart over a particular period of time.

**Cardiac arrest.** Sudden cessation of cardiac function.

**Cardiac arrhythmia.** Variation in the nomlal rhythm of the heartbeat.

**Carrier.** A person possessing a single gene for a genetic trait or disorder, such as CF. Carriers show no signs of the trait. In CF, every parent of a CF child is a carrier of a single CF gene.

**Catheter.** Thin, flexible medical tube; one use is to insert it into a blood vessel to measure blood pressure.

**Cavity.** A hole in the lung where TB bacteria have eaten away the surrounding tissue. If a cavity shows up on your chest x-ray, you are more likely to cough up bacteria and be infectious. A hole in the lung resulting from the destruction of pulmonary tissue by TB or other pulmonary infections or conditions. TB patients who have cavities in their lungs are referred to as having **cavitary disease**, and they are often more infectious than TB patients without cavitary disease.

**Celiac Disease.** Intestinal disorder with symptoms (diarrhea, with bulky foul-smelling stools; failure to thrive; and protruding abdomen) similar to the digestive complications of CF. Celiac disease is a disorder of intestinal absorption caused by an intolerance to gluten, the protein found in wheat, barley, and rye, and is apparently inherited. If foods containing gluten are avoided, symptoms usually disappear, and the child will grow normally and have a normal life expectancy. Many children with celiac disease eventually are able to tolerate small amounts of gluten.

**Cell.** The basic unit of living organisms.

**Cephalosporins.** Any of a group of antibiotics used to combat bacterial infections of the lungs. (Also see Antibiotics, Bacteria.)

**Chemotherapy.** Treatment of an infection or disease by means of oral or injectable drugs.

**Chest x-ray.** A picture of the inside of your chest. A chest x-ray is made by exposing a film to x-rays that pass through your chest. A doctor can look at this film to see whether TB bacteria have damaged your lungs.

## Glossary of Medical Terms

**Chorionic Villus Biopsy.** Biopsy of a very small portion of the placenta. This is done during the early stages of pregnancy to obtain tissue for genetic diagnosis. Prenatal diagnosis of cystic fibrosis can be made on examination of this tissue if there is a child with cystic fibrosis already in the family. The tissue is obtained by inserting a hollow needle into the womb and taking a very small piece of the placenta. (Also see Amniocentesis, Prenatal.)

**Chromosome.** The thread-like material which carries genes, the units of heredity. Chromosomes are located in the nucleus of every living cell. Normally, every person has 23 pairs of chromosomes.

**Chronic.** Term applied to any disease or condition of long duration. Persistent, not acute. CF is a chronic disease.

**Cilia.** Hair-like structures found on the surface of a variety of tissues. In the respiratory system, cilia line the airways. The regular waving motions of the cilia help sweep inhaled particles, dust, and other foreign material from the lungs and toward the trachea (windpipe) where they can be coughed out or eventually swallowed. Thick mucous secretions, infection, cigarette smoke, and other irritants can slow the cilia and thus hinder this natural cleaning mechanism.

**Circadian rhythm.** Natural daily fluctuation of physiological and behavioral functions.

**Cirrhosis.** Fibrosis and scarring of the liver which can be caused by a number of diseases. A unique form of cirrhosis occurs in approximately one percent of cystic fibrosis patients. This is caused by obstruction of the bile ducts in the liver by thick secretions.

**Clinical Research.** Investigations aimed at improving methods of diagnosis and treatment. Studies on antibiotics, respiratory function testing, nutrition, and various methods of "sweat testing" are examples of clinical research on CF.

**Clinical trials.** Medical studies of patients that evaluate the effectiveness of treatment.

**Clubbing.** Rounded, enlarged tips of the fingers and toes. Clubbing usually indicates a chronic deficiency of oxygen in the bloodstream.

Occurs in CF and congenital heart disease, as well as in some other heart, lung, and gastrointestinal diseases.

**Cluster.** Two or more PPD skin-test conversions occurring within a 3-month period among health care workers in a specific area or occupational group, and epidemiologic evidence suggests occupational (nosocomial) transmission.

**Congenital.** Refers to a condition existing at or dating from birth.

**Constrict** Tighten; narrow.

**Contact.** A person who has shared the same air with a person who has infectious TB for a sufficient amount of time to allow possible transmission of M. tuberculosis.

**Continuous positive airway pressure (CPAP).** A mechanical ventilation technique used to deliver continuous positive airway pressure.

**Contraindicated.** Not indicated; used to describe situations in which certain medications and therapies should not be prescribed.

**Conversion, PPD.** See PPD test conversion.

**Cor pulmonale.** Heart disease due to lung problems. Enlargement of the right ventricle of the heart due to resistance of the passage of blood through the lungs. Can often lead to right heart failure. This can be a major complication of chronic pulmonary diseases such as CF.

**Corticosteroids.** A group of hormones produced by adrenal glands.

**Cough.** A natural body mechanism for ridding the respiratory tract of irritating and harmful substances such as smoke, gases, dust, and excessive accumulations of mucus.

**CPAP.** A mechanical ventilator used to deliver continuous positive airway pressure.

**Crackle.** Another name for rale. Clicking sounds in the chest caused by excessive mucus or fluid in the lungs. Usually heard by using a stethoscope.

## Glossary of Medical Terms

**Culture.** A test to see whether there are TB bacteria in your phlegm or other body fluids. This test can take 2 to 4 weeks in most laboratories. The process of growing bacteria in the laboratory so that organisms can be identified.

**Cyanosis.** Bluish coloration of skin due to insufficient oxygen in the bloodstream. May occur in a CF patient during acute respiratory failure.

**Cycloserine.** A second-line, oral anti-TB drug used primarily for treating drug-resistant TB. Directly observed therapy {DOT}: An adherence-enhancing strategy in which an health care worker or other designated person watches the patient swallow each dose of medication.

## D

**Decongestant.** A drug that reduces swelling and congestion in the nose, sinuses and respiratory system. Decongestants often are used to reduce the symptoms of colds and infections.

**Diabetes (Diabetes mellitus).** A pancreatic disorder which causes abnormal insulin production. This affects the body's ability to utilize sugar and other food substances and usually is treated by diet modification (restricted sugar intake) and use of insulin. In cystic fibrosis, disruption of pancreatic function sometimes leads to diabetes.

**Diaphragm.** The wide dome-shaped sheath of muscle which separates organs of the chest from the stomach, intestines, and other abdominal organs. The most important breathing muscle. The major respiratory muscle that participates in the act of breathing. The diaphragm separates the chest and abdominal areas.

**Diastolic pressure.** The lowest pressure to which blood pressure falls between contractions of the ventricles.

**Digestive System.** The group of organs involved in ingestion, digestion, and elimination of food. Includes the mouth, salivary glands, pharynx, esophagus, stomach, intestines, liver, pancreas, colon, rectum, and anus. In CF, thick mucous secretions can block the passages in some parts of the digestive system, particularly between the pancreas and intestines.

**Dilate.** Relax: expand.

**Directly observed therapy (DOT).** A way of helping patients take their medicine for TB. If you get DOT, you will meet with a health care worker every day or several times a week. You will meet at a place you both agree on. This can be the TB clinic, your home or work, or any other convenient location. You will take your medicine at this place.

**DNA probe.** A technique that allows rapid and precise identification of mycobacteria (e.g., M. tuberculosis and M. bovis) that are grown in culture. The identification can often be completed in 2 hours.

**DNA Deoxyribonucleic acid.** The chemical coding for a gene. DNA determines the "genetic message" within each cell, organ, and organism. (Also see Chromosomes, Genes.)

**Droplet nuclei.** Microscopic particles produced when a person coughs, sneezes, shouts, or sings. The droplets produced by an infectious TB patient can carry tubercle bacilli and can remain suspended in the air for prolonged periods of time and be carried on normal air currents in the room.

**Drug-susceptibility pattern.** The anti-TB drugs to which the tubercle bacilli cultured from a TB patient are susceptible or resistant based on drug-susceptibility tests.

**Drug-susceptibility tests.** Laboratory tests that determine whether the tubercle bacilli cultured from a patient are susceptible or resistant to various anti-TB drugs.

**Drug resistance, acquired.** A resistance to one or more anti-TB drugs that develops while a patient is receiving therapy and which usually results from the patient's non-adherence to therapy or the prescription of an inadequate regimen by a health-care provider.

**Drug resistance, primary.** A resistance to one or more anti-TB drugs that exists before a patient is treated with the drug(s). Primary resistance occurs in persons exposed to and infected with a drug-resistant strain of M. tuberculosis.

**Duct.** A tube or passageway for secretions. Ducts are found in many organs, organ systems, and in exocrine glands. In CF, thick mucus can block ducts and prevent the passage of secretions.

**Dysfunction Malfunction.** Irregular function.

**Dyspnea.** Shortness of breath; difficult or labored breathing.

**E**

**Edema.** Abnormal amount of fluid in body tissues. Swelling due to the buildup of fluid.

**Elastase Inhibitors or Antielastases.** Substances in the blood transported to the lungs and other organs which prevent the digestive action of elastases.

**Elastin degrading enzymes (elastases).** Substances in the blood transported to the lungs and other organs which digest or breakdown elastin.

**Elastin.** An elastic substance in the lungs (and some other body organs) that support their structural framework.

**Endocrine Glands.** Ductless glands which secrete substances (hormones) into the blood stream. Includes pituitary, adrenal, and thyroid glands. (Not directly affected in CF.)

**Endothelial cells.** The delicate lining, only one cell thick, of the organs of circulation.

**Enzyme.** Substance, made by living cells, that causes specific chemical changes. Substance which helps produce and/or accelerate certain chemical processes in the body, such as breaking down of foods during digestion. In CF, mucus often blocks the passageways through which digestive enzymes from the pancreas flow. Consequently, individuals with cystic fibrosis may need enzyme replacements to help with proper digestion of food. (Also see Digestive System, Pancreas.)

**Epithelial.** Tissue Cells which form a lining on the outside of the body and on the inside of the respiratory and digestive tracts.

**Erythema nodosum.** Red bumps that tend to appear on the face, arms, and shins.

**Erythrocytes.** Red blood cells containing hemoglobin, the substance which carries oxygen in the bloodstream.

**Ethambutol.** A first-line, oral anti-TB drug sometimes used concomitantly with INH. rifampin, and pyrazinamide.

**Ethionamide.** A second-line, oral anti-TB drug used primarily for treating drug resistant TB.

**Exocrine Glands.** Glands which secrete substances through ducts to surrounding surfaces. Includes sweat, salivary and tear glands, as well as the mucous glands in the digestive, respiratory, and genitourinary systems. These glands are greatly affected in CF. Their ducts may be obstructed by mucus.

**Expectorant.** Medication which loosens the mucus in the lungs, so that it can be removed through coughing. Used often to treat pulmonary complications of CF.

**Expectorate.** Process of expelling substances~ such as mucus, from the lungs.

**Expiration.** Exhalation, breathing out.

**Exposure.** The condition of being subjected to something (e.g., infectious agents) that could have a harmful effect. A person exposed to M. tuberculosis does not necessarily become infected (see Transmission).

**Extra-pulmonary TB.** TB disease in any part of the body other than the lungs (for example, the kidney or lymph nodes).

**F**

**False Negative.** Test reaction which incorrectly indicates the absence or lack of a disease or condition. A false negative "sweat test" incor-

## Glossary of Medical Terms

rectly indicates that the patient does not have CF when, in fact, he/she does have CF. (Also see Sweat Test.) False Positive Test reaction which incorrectly indicates the presence of a disease or condition. A false positive "sweat test" indicates that the patient has CF, when, in fact, he/she does not. False positive tests for CF do not occur frequently.

**Fibrosis.** Formation of fiber or scar tissue as a result of structural change or other damage. Occurs in the pancreas and lungs of many children with CF, as a result of abnormal mucous accumulations. Process by which inflamed tissue becomes scarred.

**Fibrotic tissue.** Inflamed tissue that has become scarred.

**First-line drugs.** The most often used anti-TB drugs (i.e., INH, rifampin, pyrazinamide, ethambutol, and streptomycin).

**Fixed room-air HEPA recirculation systems.** Non-mobile devices or systems that remove airborne contaminants by recirculating air through a HEPA filter. These may be built into the room and permanently ducted or may be mounted to the wall or ceiling within the room. In either situation, they are fixed in place and are not easily movable.

**Flatulence.** Gas passed through the rectum or belched through the mouth. Because of the digestive problems of the disease, flatulence may occur in patients with CF.

**Fluorochrome stain.** A technique for staining a clinical specimen with fluorescent dyes to perform a microscopic examination (smear) for mycobacteria. This technique is preferable to other staining techniques because the mycobacteria can be seen easily and the slides can be read quickly.

**Fomites.** Linens, books, dishes, or other objects used or touched by a patient. These objects are not involved in the transmission of M. tuberculosis. Gastric aspirate: A procedure sometimes used to obtain a specimen for culture when a patient cannot cough up adequate sputum. A tube is inserted through the mouth or nose and into the stomach to recover sputum that was coughed into the throat and then swallowed. This procedure is particularly useful for diagnosis in children, who are often unable to cough up sputum.

## G

**Gamma Globulin.** Antibody-like proteins found in blood plasma which function to help the body fight disease.

**Gas Exchange.** A primary function of the lungs involving transfer of oxygen from inhaled air into blood and of carbon dioxide from blood into lungs.

**Gastroenterology.** The study of the digestive system, particularly the stomach and intestines; and diseases of these organs. Gastroenterology is relevant to study and treatment of the digestive complications of CF. (Also see Digestive System.)

**Gene.** Basic, functional unit of heredity (hundreds of genes are carried on each chromosome). Genes determine or influence a large portion of an individual's physical and chemical characteristics (eye color, facial features, stature, and many health conditions). CF is caused by a defect or abnormality of a gene. However, the specific gene has not yet been identified. A child inherits CF at conception, when he or she receives two genes for the disease, one from each parent. (Also see Autosomal Recessive. Chromosome.)

**Genetic Hereditary.** inherited.

**Genetics.** Study of heredity.

**Granulomas.** Small lumps in tissues caused by inflammation.

## H

**Heartbeat.** One complete contraction of the heart.

**Hemoptysis.** Coughing up blood, often with sputum. Results from broken small blood vessels in the lungs. This condition may occur in CF due to pulmonary complications.

**Hemorrhage.** Escape of blood from blood carrying tissue.

**Hemothorax.** Accumulation of blood in the cavity around the lungs. This can be an advanced complication of CF.

## Glossary of Medical Terms

**Hereditary Traits.** or conditions that are genetically passed on from parents to children. (Also see Gene, Genetic.)

**Heterozygote.** A person who has inherited a single gene for a particular trait. A person who is heterozygous for cystic fibrosis has inherited one gene for CF and one "normal" gene. Therefore, the person does not have CF; he or she is a carrier without symptoms. A parent of a child with CF is a heterozygote. (Also see Autosomal Recessive, Chromosome, Gene.) Homozygote A person who has inherited two genes for a particular trait. A person with CF is a CF gene homozygote, having inherited a gene for CF from each parent.

**High-efficiency particulate air (HEPA) filter.** A specialized filter that is capable of removing 99.97% of particles 0.3 $\mu$m in diameter and that may assist in controlling the transmission of M. tuberculosis. Filters may be used in ventilation systems to remove particles from the air or in personal respirators to filter air before it is inhaled by the person wearing the respirator. The use of HEPA filters in ventilation systems requires expertise in installation and maintenance.

**HIV infection.** Infection with the human immunodeficiency virus, the virus that causes AIDS (acquired immunodeficiency syndrome). A person with both TB infection and HIV infection is at very high risk for TB disease.

**Hormone.** Secretion of the endocrine glands. Involved in regulating many body functions (growth, maturation, heart rate). Hormones are not known to be affected by CF.

**Human immunodeficiency virus (HIV) infection.** Infection with the virus that causes acquired immunodeficiency syndrome (AIDS). HIV infection is the most important risk factor for the progression of latent TB infection to active TB.

**Hyper-reactive.** Describes a situation in which a body tissue is especially likely to have an exaggerated reaction to a particular situation.

**Hyperglycemia.** High blood sugar. Can occur in CF patients as a result of lesions in the pancreas. This condition is easily controlled through use of insulin. (Also see Diabetes, Digestive System.)

**Hypertension.** Abnormally high blood pressure.

**Hyperventilation.** A state in which abnormally fast and deep respiration results in the intake of excessive amount of oxygen into the lung and reduced carbon dioxide levels in the blood.

**Hypotension.** Abnormally low blood pressure.

**Hypoventilation.** A state in which there is an insufficient amount of air entering and leaving the lungs to bring oxygen into tissues and eliminate carbon dioxide

**Hypoxemia.** Deficient oxygenation of the blood.

**Hypoxia.** Low blood oxygen. May occur in lung diseases such as CF. A state in which there is oxygen deficiency.

# I

**Immunology.** A branch of biomedical science concerned with the body's (immune) defenses against infection.

**Immunosuppressed.** A condition in which the immune system is not functioning normally (e.g., severe cellular immunosuppression resulting from HIV infection or immunosuppressive therapy). Immunosuppressed persons are at greatly increased risk for developing active TB after they have been infected with M. tuberculosis. No data are available regarding whether these persons are also at increased risk for infection with M. tuberculosis after they have been exposed to the organism.

**In Vitro.** Latin term literally meaning "in glass." Usually used to refer to research conducted under laboratory conditions, and outside the body.

**In Vivo.** In a living body or organism. Usually refers to research done in the body.

**Incidence.** The number of new cases of a condition occurring in a given population during a specified time, such as a year.

## Glossary of Medical Terms

**Induration.** An area of swelling produced by an immune response to an antigen. In tuberculin skin testing or anergy testing, the diameter of the indurated area is measured 48-72 hours after the injection, and the result is recorded in millimeters.

**Infection.** The condition in which organisms capable of causing disease (e.g., M. tuberculosis) enter the body and elicit a response from the host's immune defenses. TB infection may or may not lead to clinical disease.

**Infectious TB.** TB disease of the lungs or throat, which can be spread to other people

**Infectious person.** A person who can spread TB to others because he or she is coughing TB bacteria into the air. INH or isoniazid - a drug used to prevent TB disease in people who have TB infection. INH is also one of the five drugs often used to treat TB disease.

**Infectious.** Capable of transmitting infection. When persons who have clinically active pulmonary or laryngeal TB disease cough or sneeze, they can expel droplets containing M. tuberculosis into the air. Persons whose sputum smears are positive for AFB are probably infectious.

**Inflammation.** A basic response of the body to injury, usually showing up in skin redness, warmth, swelling, and pain.

**Injectable.** A medication that is usually administered by injection into the muscle (intramuscular [IM]) or the bloodstream (intravenous [IV]).

**Inpatient.** Hospitalized patient

**Intermittent therapy.** Therapy administered either two or three times per week, rather than daily. Intermittent therapy should be administered only under the direct supervision of an health care worker or other designated person (see Directly observed therapy [DOT]).

**Intermittent positive pressure breathing machine (IPPB).** A device that assists intermittent positive pressure inhalation of therapeutic breathing aerosols without hand coordination required in the use of hand nebulizers or metered dose inhalers.

**Intradermal.** Within the layers of the skin.

**Ischemic heart.** Heart disease from restricted blood disease supply due to obstruction in blood vessels.

**Isoniazid (INH).** A first-line, oral drug used either alone as preventive therapy or in combination with several other drugs to treat TB disease. Kanamycin: An injectable, second-line anti-TB drug used primarily for treatment of drug-resistant TB.

**L**

**Laser.** In the context of a therapeutic tool, it is a device that produces a high-intensity light that can generate extreme heat instantaneously when it hits a target

**Latent TB infection.** Infection with M. tuberculosis, usually detected by a positive PPD skin-test result, in a person who has no symptoms of active TB and who is not infectious.

**Lavage.** To wash a body organ.

**Lesion.** An abnormal structural change in body tissues or organs. For example, the scar tissue in the lungs of a child with CF.

**Leukocyte.** White blood cell, involved in body defense systems.

**Lipids.** Fatty molecules which are used by the body for energy. They are an important part of cell structure. CF interferes with the digestive breakdown of fats into lipids.

**Lung volume.** The amount of air the lungs hold.

**Lung-damaging Diseases.** Diseases characterized by destruction of lung tissue. Includes tuberculosis, lung abscess, lung cancer, immune deficiency disorders, cystic fibrosis, chronic bronchitis, bronchiectasis, asthma, "childhood emphysema," disorders of lung development and recurrent pneumonia.

## Glossary of Medical Terms

**Lymph nodes.** Small, bean-shaped organs of the immune system distributed throughout the body tissue.

**Lymphoma.** Cancer of the lymph nodes.

## M

**M. tuberculosis.** Bacteria that cause TB infection and TB disease.

**M. tuberculosis complex.** A group of closely related mycobacterial species that can cause active TB (e.g., M. tuberculosis, M. bovis, and M. africanum); most TB in the United States is caused by M. tuberculosis.

**Malabsorption.** Inadequate uptake of nutrients from food for use by the body. In CF, mucous plugs in ducts of digestive organs may block the secretion of enzymes and hormones needed for digestion. As a result, many nutrients are not available for use in body maintenance and growth. This is associated with a common symptom of CF: failure to thrive. (Also see Absorption, Digestive System.) Meconium The first stool of a newborn infant, usually passed within a few hours after birth. Contains mucus and other secretions of intestinal glands. (Also see Meconium Ileus.)

**Mantoux test.** A method of skin testing that is performed by injecting 0.1 ml of PPD tuberculin containing S tuberculin units into the dermis {i.e., the second layer of skin) of the forearm with a needle and syringe. This test is the most reliable and standardized technique for tuberculin testing (see Tuberculin skin test and Purified protein derivative [PPD]-tuberculin test).

**Mean blood pressure.** The average blood pressure, taking account of the rise and fall that occurs with each heartbeat. It is often estimated by multiplying the diastolic pressure by two, adding the systolic pressure, and then dividing this sum by three.

**Meconium Ileus Equivalent.** Obstruction of the intestines by abnormal stool in an older infant, child, or adult with CF. Obstruction may be partial or complete.

**Meconium Ileus.** Obstruction of the intestines of a newborn infant with abnormally thick meconium. Earliest symptom of cystic fibrosis. Occurs in seven to 10 percent of patients with CF.

**Metabolism.** The chemical and physical process by which food is transformed into basic elements and used by the body for energy and growth.

**Miliary TB.** TB disease that has spread to the whole body through the bloodstream.

**Morbidity.** Refers to illness.

**Mortality.** Refers to death.

**Mucolytic Agents.** Drugs which are used to loosen mucus so that it can be coughed up.

**Mucopurulent.** Secretion containing mucus and pus.

**Mucous Plugs.** Very thick mucus in a duct or airway that partially or completely blocks the flow of secretions or air. Occurs in CF. (Also see Ducts.)

**Mucous Membrane.** Tissue which contains mucous-producing glands. Found in the nose, mouth, lungs, esophagus, stomach, and intestines. (Also see Epithelial Tissue.)

**Mucoviscidosis.** Term once used for cystic fibrosis, still generally used in Europe. Mucoviscidosis was coined in 1944 to describe the abnormally viscid (thick and sticky) mucous secretions characteristic of CF.

**Mucus.** A fluid secreted by mucous membranes and glands. Generally thin and slippery. In people with CF, mucus is usually thick and sticky.

**Multi-drug-resistant tuberculosis (MDR-TB).** Active TB caused by M. tuberculosis organisms that are resistant to more than one anti-TB drug; in practice, often refers to organisms that are resistant to both INH and rifampin with or without resistance to other drugs (see Drug resistance, acquired and Drug resistance, primary).

## Glossary of Medical Terms

**Mutation.** A permanent change in genetic material that usually involves a single gene. This may be in the form of a loss (deletion), a gain (translocation), or an exchange (transduction) of base pairs.

## N

**Nares.** Openings in the nasal cavities-nostrils.

**Nasal Polyps.** Small growths of swollen mucous membrane which project into the nasal passages. Common in children with CF, they are usually multiple or recurrent and can be surgically removed.

**Nebulizer.** A device used for delivering a mist. In the treatment of CF, nebulizers may be used for inhaling aerosol antibiotics or mucolytic drugs. (Also see Aerosol, Antibiotics, Mucolytic Agents.)

**Negative.** Usually refers to a test result. If you have a negative TB skin test reaction, you probably do not have TB infection.

**Negative pressure.** The relative air pressure difference between two areas in a health-care facility. A room that is at negative pressure has a lower pressure than adjacent areas, which keeps air from flowing out of the room and into adjacent rooms or areas.

**Neonatal.** Refers to the period directly after birth. Period up to the first 4 weeks after birth.

**Neonate.** The newborn child.

**NonREM sleep (NREM).** A nonuniforn series of four stages of sleep which occur early in the night and are characterized by the absence of movement and slow wave brain activity. NREM generally preceded the first REM period.

**Nosocomial.** An occurrence, usually an infection, that is acquired in a hospital or as a result of medical care.

## O

**Outpatient.** A patient who is not hospitalized, but who receives treatment at a doctor's office or a medical clinic (such as a CFF care center).

## P

**Palliative.** Anything used to lessen the pain or severity of symptoms, but not for providing a cure.

**Palpitation.** The sensation of rapid heartbeats.

**Pancreas.** Elongated glandular organ located behind the stomach. The duct portion of the pancreas secretes digestive enzymes into the intestine to help break down food. In CF, the pancreatic ducts may be obstructed by mucous secretions, thereby hampering the digestion of food. Another portion of the pancreas contains endocrine tissue which produces the hormone insulin, con trolling storage and oxidation of sugar. Also see Digestive System, Duct.)

**Para-aminosalicylic acid.** A second-line, oral anti-TB drug used for treating drug-resistant TB.

**Pathogenesis.** The changes and mechanisms which affect the development and course of a disease. In CF, the pathogenesis begins with a genetic defect which causes changes in cellular and organ functions. These events, in turn, affect development of other complications, such as susceptibility to respiratory infections. (Also see Cor Pulmonale, Digestive System, Respiratory System.) The pathologic, physiologic, or biochemical process by which a disease develops.

**Pathogenicity.** The quality of producing or the ability to produce pathologic changes or disease. Some non-tuberculous mycobacteria are pathogenic (e.g., Mycobacterium kansasii ), and others are not (e.g., Mycobacterium phlei ).

**Pathology.** The study of the nature of disease, and the structural and functional changes caused by disease.

**Percussor.** A device which delivers short, sharp blows. In the management of CF, percussors may be used to perform chest physical therapy to help loosen mucus in the lungs. (Also see Physical Therapy).

## Glossary of Medical Terms

**Perfusion.** Flow.

**Pertussis.** Whooping cough.

**PFT.** Pulmonary function test.

**Phlegm.** Mucus secreted from glands lining the lungs and bronchial tubes. Sputum.

**Physical Therapy.** Treatment of disease by physical means, employing heat, cold, water, light, electricity, manipulation, massage, exercise, and mechanical devices. A physical therapy used in CF is bronchial drainage, used to help loosen mucus in the lungs.

**Pilocarpine iontophoresis.** A technique in which sweating is stimulated by applying the chemical pilocarpine onto a small area of the skin, which then receives a small electrical current. Quantitative pilocarpine iontophoresis is the most generally recommended procedure for sweat testing.

**Plasma.** The fluid portion of the blood containing clotting factors. (Also see Serum.)

**Pleura.** The thin, two-layered membrane surrounding and protecting the lungs. (Pleurisy is the inflammation of the pleura.) Pneumonia An inflammation of the lungs often caused by bacterial infection. Pneumonia is a major problem in individuals with cystic fibrosis.

**Pneumonia.** Inflammation of the lungs.

**Pneumonitis.** A disease caused by inhaling a wide variety of substances such as dusts and molds. Also called "farmer's disease."

**Pneumothorax.** A sudden, partial or complete collapse of the lung. Results from the rupture of lung tissue, which allows air to escape from the lung and become trapped between lung and chest wall. Can be an advanced complication of CF.

**Polysomnography.** The continuous recording of a number of physiological functions and events during sleep.

**Portable room-air HEPA recirculation units.** Free-standing portable devices that remove airborne contaminants by recirculating air through a HEPA filter.

**Positive.** Usually refers to a test result. If you have a positive TB skin test reaction, you probably have TB infection.

**Positive PPD reaction.** A reaction to the purified protein derivative (PPD)-tuberculin skin test that suggests the person tested is infected with M. tuberculosis. The person interpreting the skin-test reaction determines whether it is positive on the basis of the size of the induration and the medical history and risk factors of the person being tested.

**Postural bronchial drainage (Also called bronchial drainage).** A form of physical therapy, during which the chest of the patient is "pounded" or gently clapped to dislodge mucus in the lungs. Careful attention is given to body position (e.g., head drainage below chest) during the therapy to make removal of mucus easier. (Also see Bronchial Drainage, Physical Therapy.)

**Prenatal.** Refers to the period before birth.

**Preventive therapy.** Treatment for people with TB infection that prevents them from developing TB disease.

**Preventive therapy.** Treatment of latent TB infection used to prevent the progression of latent infection to clinically active disease.

**Productive Cough.** Cough resulting in removal of phlegm from the lungs.

**Prognosis.** The prospect for the course of an illness or disease.

**Prophylactic.** Referring to prevention, such as drugs used to prevent or ward off infections.

**Prostaglandins.** A group of fat-derived chemicals involved in the regulation of a number of body functions.

**Pseudomonas Aeruginosa.** Bacteria which frequently colonize the

## Glossary of Medical Terms

lungs of patients with CF and are a major cause of respiratory infections. Infections caused by these bacteria are often difficult to treat.

**Pulmonary.** The medical discipline which studies normal function and diseases of the lungs and other parts of the respiratory system. (Also see Respiratory System.)

**Pulmonary hypertension.** Abnormally high blood pressure in the arteries of the lungs.

**Pulmonary artery.** Blood vessel delivering oxygen-poor blood from the right ventricle to the lungs.

**Pulmonary Function Tests (PFTs).** Test procedures used to evaluate lung function. Along with patient history and physical examination, pulmonary function tests are used to make the diagnosis, plan therapy, and determine prognosis. Can be used with adults and with children at least five to six years of age. Pulmonary function tests are used to measure: flows (of air) and timed volumes; tidal volume (amount of air entering and leaving the lungs during natural respiration); maximum voluntary ventilation (amount of air forcefully expired during one minute); residual volume of air remaining in the lungs after maximum voluntary expiration); total lung capacity (total amount of air in the lungs after maximum inspiration); and vital capacity (maximum amount of air expired after a full inspiration.)

**Pulmonary TB.** TB disease that occurs in the lungs, usually producing a cough that lasts longer than 2 weeks. Most TB disease is pulmonary.

**Purified protein derivative (PPD)-tuberculin.** A purified tuberculin preparation that was developed in the 1930s and that was derived from old tuberculin. The standard Mantoux test uses 0.1 ml of PPD standardized to 5 tuberculin units.

**Purified protein derivative (PPD). Tuberculin test conversion.** A change in PPD test results from negative to positive. A conversion within a 2-year period is usually interpreted as new M. tuberculosis infection, which carries an increased risk for progression to active disease. A booster reaction may be misinterpreted as a new infection (see Booster phenomenon and Two-step testing).

**Purified protein derivative (PPD)-tuberculin test.** A method used to evaluate the likelihood that a person is infected with M. tuberculosis. A small dose of tuberculin (PPD) is injected just beneath the surface of the skin, and the area is examined 48-72 hours after the injection. A reaction is measured according to the size of the induration. The classification of a reaction as positive or negative depends on the patient's medical history and various risk factors (see Mantoux test).

**Pyrazinamide.** A first-line, oral anti-TB drug used in treatment regimens.

# R

**Radiography.** A method of viewing the respiratory system by using radiation to transmit an image of the respiratory system to film. A chest radiograph is taken to view the respiratory system of a person who is being evaluated for pulmonary TB. Abnormalities (e.g., lesions or cavities in the lungs and enlarged lymph nodes) may indicate the presence of TB.

**Radiometric method.** A method for culturing a specimen that allows for rapid detection of bacterial growth by measuring production of $CO_2$ by viable organisms; also a method of rapidly performing susceptibility testing of M. tuberculosis.

**Rale.** Clicking sounds in the chest caused by excessive mucus or fluid in the lungs. Often called "crackle." Usually heard by using a stethoscope.

**Rapid eye movement (REM).** A stage of sleep in which dreaming is associated with mild involuntary muscle movements. Adults cycle in and out of REM at about 90 minute intervals. REM occupies 20 percent of total sleep.

**Recirculation.** Ventilation in which all or most of the air that is exhausted from an area is returned to the same area or other areas of the facility.

**Rectal Prolapse.** Protrusion of rectum. May occur in children with CF as a result of digestive complications. CF is the most common cause of rectal prolapse in American infants and children.

## Glossary of Medical Terms

**Regimen.** Any particular TB treatment plan that specifies which drugs are used, in what doses, according to what schedule, and for how long.

**Registry.** A record-keeping method for collecting clinical, laboratory, and radiographic data concerning TB patients so that the data can be organized and made available for epidemiologic study.

**Resistance.** The ability of some strains of bacteria, including M. tuberculosis, to grow and multiply in the presence of certain drugs that ordinarily kill them; such strains are referred to as drug-resistant strains.

**Resistant bacteria.** Bacteria that can no longer be killed by a certain drug.

**Respiratory System.** That portion of body including all organs through which air passes during breathing. Also includes the structures (pleura, ribs, and intercostal muscles) which support these organs. The upper respiratory tract includes the nose, sinuses, pharynx (throat), and larynx (voice box). The lower respiratory tract includes the trachea (windpipe), bronchial tubes (two branches from the windpipe), bronchioles (smaller bronchial tubes), and alveoli (sacs where the exchange of oxygen and carbon dioxide occurs). The thick mucous secretions in CF obstruct components of the respiratory system.

**Respiratory Diseases.** Diseases affecting the respiratory tract. Includes asthma, influenza, sinusitis, hay fever, common cold, sore throat, pneumonia and tuberculosis, and frequently, CF.

**Respiratory Rate.** Number of breaths per minute.

**Rifampin.** A first-line, oral anti-TB drug that, when used concomitantly with INH and pyrazinamide, provides the basis for short-course therapy.

**RNA (Ribonucleic acid).** Molecules of nucleic acid which are formed in the cell's nucleus (as directed by DNA). RNA is responsible for assembling proteins.

## Respiratory Diseases and Disorders Sourcebook

**Room-air HEPA recirculation systems and units.** Devices (either fixed or portable) that remove airborne contaminants by recirculating air through a HEPA filter.

## S

**Saline.** A mixture of salt and water.

**Sclera.** Outer coat of the eyeball.

**Second-line drugs.** Anti-TB drugs used when the first-line drugs cannot be used (e.g., for drug-resistant TB or because of adverse reactions to the first-line drugs). Examples are cycloserine, ethionamide, and capreomycin. Single-pass ventilation: Ventilation in which 100% of the air supplied to an area is exhausted to the outside.

**Serum.** The clear, liquid portion of blood which separates in the clotting of blood. (Also see Plasma.)

**Sign.** Objective indication of disease. (Also see Symptom.)

**Sinusitis.** An infection of the lining of the air spaces (sinuses) in the bones of the skull which drain into the nasal cavity. Some patients with CF also seem susceptible to this type of infection. Spirometer Instrument used to measure lung air volumes and flow rates. (Also see Pulmonary Function Test.)

**Sleep hygiene.** Conditions and practices that promote effective and continuous sleep, e.g., regular bedtime and arise time; restriction of alcohol, coffee etc.

**Sleep fragmentation.** Interruption of a sleep stage by awakening or appearance of another sleep stage.

**Sleep latency.** Time measured from "lights out" or bedtime to actually falling asleep.

**Smear (AFB smear).** A laboratory technique for visualizing mycobacteria. The specimen is smeared onto a slide and stained, then examined using a microscope. Smear results should be available within 24 hours. In TB, a large number of mycobacteria seen on an AFB

## Glossary of Medical Terms

smear usually indicates infectiousness. However, a positive result is not diagnostic of TB because organisms other than M. tuberculosis may be seen on an AFB smear (e.g., non-tuberculous mycobacteria).

**Smooth muscle.** Muscle that performs automatic tasks, such as constricting blood vessels.

**Source control.** Controlling a contaminant at the source of its generation, which prevents the spread of the contaminant to the general work space.

**Source case.** A case of TB in an infectious person who has transmitted M. tuberculosis to another person or persons.

**Specimen.** Any body fluid, secretion, or tissue sent to a laboratory where smears and cultures for M. tuberculosis will be performed (e.g., sputum, urine, spinal fluid, and material obtained at biopsy}.

**Spirogram.** A record of the amounts of air being moved in and out of the lungs.

**Sputum smear, positive.** AFB are visible on the sputum smear when viewed under a microscope. Persons with a sputum smear positive for AFB are considered more infectious than those with smear-negative sputum.

**Sputum.** Mucus and other materials coughed up from lungs. Phlegm coughed up from deep inside the lungs. Sputum is examined for TB bacteria using a smear; part of the sputum can also be used to do a culture. If a patient has pulmonary disease, an examination of the sputum by smear and culture can be helpful in evaluating the organism responsible for the infection. Sputum should not be confused with saliva or nasal secretions.

**Sputum induction.** A method used to obtain sputum from a patient who is unable to cough up a specimen spontaneously. The patient inhales a saline mist, which stimulates a cough from deep within the lungs.

**Staphylococcus Aureus.** Bacteria which can cause generalized infections. In CF, "staph" commonly causes respiratory infections. Can often be effectively treated with antibiotics. (Also see Antibiotics, Bacteria.)

**Steatorrhea.** An excessive amount of fats in the stool. In cystic fibrosis, this is caused by blockage of pancreatic ducts. Fats are not properly broken down and absorbed and are therefore excreted in the stools. (Also see Digestion, Enzymes, Pancreas.)

**Streptomycin.** A first-line, injectable anti-TB drug.

**Sweat Test.** The diagnostic test for CF. Measures the concentration of salt (sodium and chloride) in sweat. (Also see Pilocarpine iontophoresis.)

**Sweat Electrolytes.** Chemical ions contained in sweat Some electrolytes (sodium and chloride) are elevated in CF.

**Symptom.** Subjective evidence of a disease or a patient's condition. Symptoms of CF include: persistent cough; wheezing; frequent, bulky, foul-smelling stools; failure to thrive; nasal polyps; rectal prolapse. (Also see Bacteria, Nasal Polyps, Rectal Prolapse.)

**Symptomatic.** Having symptoms that may indicate the presence of TB or another disease (see Asymptomatic).

**Syncope.** Fainting; temporary loss of consciousness.

**Systemic.** Relating to a process that affects the body generally; in this instance, the way in which blood is supplied through the aorta to all body organs except the lungs.

**Systolic pressure.** The highest pressure to which blood pressure rises with the contraction of the ventricles.

**T**

**TB infection.** A condition in which TB bacteria are alive but inactive in the body. People with TB infection have no symptoms, don't feel sick, can't spread TB to others, and usually have a positive skin test reaction. But they develop TB disease later in life if they do not receive preventive therapy.

## Glossary of Medical Terms

**TB disease.** An illness in which TB bacteria are multiplying and attacking different parts of the body. The symptoms of TB disease include weakness, weight loss, fever, no appetite, chills, and sweating at night. Other symptoms of TB disease depend on where in the body the bacteria are growing. If TB disease is in the lungs (pulmonary TB), the symptoms may include a bad cough, pain in the chest, and coughing up blood.

**TB skin test.** A test that is often used to detect TB infection. A liquid called tuberculin is injected under the skin on the lower part of your arm. If you have a positive reaction to this test, you probably have TB infection.

**TB case.** A particular episode of clinically active TB. This term should be used only to refer to the disease itself, not the patient with the disease. By law, cases of TB must be reported to the local health department.

**Thoracic Cage.** The bony structure formed by 12 pairs of ribs, the breast bone and back bone.

**Tissue.** A group of cells of a similar type, having a similar function.

**Tissue Culture.** Individual cells grown in the laboratory for use in research studies. (Also see In Vitro.)

**Tracheostomy.** Surgical insertion of a tube into the airway through the neck to maintain an opening for the outside air to enter the lungs.

**Transmission.** The spread of an infectious agent from one person to another. The likelihood of transmission is directly related to the duration and intensity of exposure to M. tuberculosis (see Exposure). Treatment failures: TB disease in patients who do not respond to chemotherapy and in patients whose disease worsens after having improved initially.

**Tubercle bacilli.** M. tuberculosis organisms.

**Tuberculin.** A liquid that is injected under the skin on the lower part of your arm during a TB skin test. If you have TB infection, you will probably have a positive reaction to the tuberculin.

**Tuberculin skin test.** A method used to evaluate the likelihood that a person is infected with M. tuberculosis. A small dose of PPD-tuberculin is injected just beneath the surface of the skin, and the area is examined 4>72 hours after the injection. A reaction is measured according to the size of the induration. The classification of a reaction as positive or negative depends on the patient's medical history and various risk factors (see Mantoux test, PPD test).

**Tuberculosis (TB).** A clinically activej symptomatic disease caused by an organism in the M. tuberculosis complex (usually M. tuberculosis or, rarely, M. bovis or M. africanum).

**Two-step testing.** A procedure used for the baseline testing of persons who will periodically receive tuberculin skin tests (e.g., HCWs) to reduce the likelihood of mistaking a boosted reaction for a new infection. If the initial tubercuiin-test result is classified as negative, a second test is repeated 1-3 weeks later. If the reaction to the second test is positive, it probably represents a boosted reaction. If the second test result is also negative, the person is classified as not infected. A positive reaction to a subsequent test would indicate new infection (i.e., a skin-test conversion) in such a person.

# U

**Ultraviolet germicidal irradiation (UVGI) lamps.** Lamps that kill or inactivate microorganisms by emitting ultraviolet germicidal radiation, predominantly at a wavelength of 254 nm (intermediate light waves between visible light and X-rays). UVGI lamps can be used in ceiling or wall fixtures or within air ducts of ventilation systems.

**Ultraviolet germicidal irradiation (UVGI).** The use of ultraviolet radiation to kill or inactivate microorganisms.

# V

**Vaccination.** Administration of weakened or killed bacteria or virus to stimulate immunity and protection against further exposure to that agent.

**Vas Deferens.** A duct in the reproductive system of the male. Carries

## Glossary of Medical Terms

sperm from the testes to the prostate gland. In males with CF, this duct is usually obstructed, resulting in sterility.

**Vasodilator** An agent that widens blood vessels.

**Ventilation.** The process of exchange of air between the lungs and the atmospheric air leading to exchange of gases with blood.

**Ventilation, local exhaust.** Ventilation used to capture and remove airborne contaminants by enclosing the contaminant source (i.e., the patient) or by placing an exhaust hood close to the contaminant source.

**Ventilation, dilution.** An engineering control technique to dilute and remove airborne contaminants by the flow of air into and out of an area. Air that contains droplet nuclei is removed and replaced by contaminant-free air. If the flow is sufficient, droplet nuclei become dispersed, and their concentration in the air is diminished.

**Ventricle.** One of the two pumping chambers of the heart. The right ventricle receives oxygen-poor blood from the right atrium and pumps it to the lungs through the pulmonary artery. The left ventricle receives oxygen-rich blood from the left atrium and pumps it to the body through the aorta.

**Virulence.** The degree of pathogenicity of a microorganism as indicated by the severity of the disease produced and its ability to invade the tissues of a host. M. tuberculosis is a virulent organism.

**Virus.** An organism smaller than bacteria, capable of causing various infections and contagious diseases, such as influenza, viral pneumonia, and hepatitis.

**Viscid.** Thick and sticky.

**Vital Signs.** Temperature, pulse, respiration and blood pressure. These vital signs indicate a patient's condition.

**Vitamins.** Substances that occur in foods in small amounts and are necessary for the normal functioning of the body. In cystic fibrosis, when digestive enzymes are blocked, vitamins from foods may not be sufficiently absorbed by the body, and vitamin supplements are needed. (Also see Digestion, Pancreas.)

# *Index*

# Index

## A

23-valent pneumococcal capsular polysaccharide vaccine 697
AAT deficiency 161, 162, 175, 176, 185-187
absenteeism 19, 36, 48, 75, 212, 655
acetaminophen 217
acetylcholine 29
acquired immunodeficiency syndrome (AIDS)
  AIDS 698, 735
action on Smoking and Health (ASH) *see* associations
African American *see* ethnic groups
adenoviruses 213
adolescent *see* age groups
adult *see* age groups
adrenergic bronchodilators 132, 133, 152
aerobid 51
aged *see* age groups
age groups
  adolescent 15, 19, 30, 36, 39, 52, 53, 379, 438, 452, 491, 636
  adult 15, 19, 379, 438, 452
  aged 545
  child 23, 32, 35, 37, 142, 143, 154
  infant 486, 487, 493

age groups, continued
  middle age 15, 19, 379, 438, 452
  teenagers 42, 45, 53, 59, 142, 217, 229, 230, 233, 262, 263, 286, 336, 639, 667, 668
agricultural chemicals 550
air-purifying devices 552, 553
  air conditioning systems 552, 553
  air-purifying respirator 133, 169
  HEPA filters high-efficiency particulate activating filters 100, 401, 402
  humidifier 444
  humidity conditions 444
Alaska Natives *see* ethnic groups
Allerest 227
allergen 22, 27, 28, 42, 87, 688, 719
allergies 5, 19, 21-23, 29, 32, 33, 37, 42, 47, 59, 62, 64, 68, 69, 79, 81, 117, 143, 144, 150, 151, 154, 174, 209, 219, 222, 224, 226, 227, 433, 531, 582, 591, 593, 641, 643
Allergy and Asthma Network/Mothers of Asthmatics *see* associations
allergy shots 31, 42, 59, 117, 174
allogeneic lung transplantation (LT 707)
allografting 713
alpha$_1$ antitrypsin (AAT) 161, 182, 183, 185, 186, 708
alpha$_1$ protease inhibitor 161, 162, 678

757

Alupent 52, 133
alveoli 4, 5, 19, 161, 163, 164, 182, 183, 186, 251, 415-417, 423, 432, 433, 439, 462, 515, 516, 548, 555, 719, 725, 747
AMERICA 2000 74
American Academy of Allergy & Immunology *see* associations
American Academy of Pediatrics Committee on Drugs *see* associations
American SIDS Institute *see* associations
amiloride 265, 326, 327
Aminophylline 53, 96, 99, 100
aminorex fumarate 405
ammonia 200, 548, 551, 571, 574, 575, 600
amniocentesis 244, 323, 341, 364, 720, 727
amphotericin B 372, 690
ampicillin 99, 100, 169
anabolic steroids 40
analgesics 89, 227
anaphylaxis 113, 702
anesthetic 6, 89
angiotensin-converting enzyme (ACE) 441
anorexia 509
anti-inflammatory drugs 42, 265, 692
antibiotics 49, 53, 112, 169, 179, 184, 214, 217, 231, 254-256, 258, 265, 292, 293, 295, 320, 326, 376, 380, 381, 384, 510, 518, 529, 708, 720, 726, 727, 741, 750
antibodies 21, 22, 33, 216, 218, 232, 234, 389, 391, 444, 720
anticholinergic drug 29
anticoagulant 218, 401, 403
antihistamines 122, 217, 221-224, 226-229, 258
antimicrobial susceptibility testing 694, 696
antitussives 226, 228, 229
antiviral drugs 218, 219
apneic events 453
asbestos 7, 540, 541, 544, 545, 554-558, 641
asbestosis 554, 556
Asian *see* ethnic groups
Asian flu 235
aspirin 23, 42, 66, 216, 217, 229-231, 233
asplenia 698, 701, 702

associations
 Action on Smoking and Health (ASH) 576
 Allergy and Asthma Network/Mothers of Asthmatics 28
 American Academy of Allergy & Immunology 138, 142, 143, 150, 151, 153, 154
 American Academy of Pediatrics Committee on Drugs 138, 142, 143, 150, 151, 153, 154
 American SIDS Institute 138, 142, 143, 150, 151, 153, 154
 Association of SIDS Program Professionals (ASPP) 221, 222
 Asthma and Allergy Foundation of America 133, 135
 Asthma Foundation of Southern Arizona 133, 135
 College of American Pathologists (CAP) 212-219, 226, 228, 367, 546, 747
 Mothers of Asthmatics 255
 National Jewish Center for Immunology and Respiratory Medicine 39, 40, 53, 146, 175, 196, 292, 741
 Sudden Infant Death Syndrome Alliance 23, 24, 33, 42
Asthma and Allergy Foundation of America *see* associations
asthma attack 31, 36, 40, 44, 69, 71, 73, 144, 642
asthma education programs 137, 140, 141
asthma episode 38, 44-46, 48, 50-56, 58-60, 75, 80-83, 117, 127, 129, 130, 147
Asthma Foundation of Southern Arizona *see* associations
asthma management program 75, 77, 78, 692
asthma medications 26, 49, 53, 81, 85, 88, 94, 149
Asthma Symptom and Peak Flow Diary 128, 130, 131
atropine 29, 89, 169
autosomal recessive 243, 722, 734, 735
azatadine 221
Azathioprine 387, 418, 443
Azmacort 51

# Index

## B

B-cell growth factor 444
B-cells 444
B-lymphocytes 444
bacillus Calmette-Guerin (BCG) 216, 218, 231-237, 377, 380-384, 500, 520, 522, 524, 528, 529, 697-704, 722, 723
bacteremia 383, 384, 697-700
bacterial pneumonia 235, 377, 378, 380, 383, 384, 586, 694
barbiturates 170
barrel chest 35, 723
basic defect 246, 247, 265
beclomethasone 88, 111, 169
Beclovent 51
Bennett, Glen 678, 680
berylliosis 438, 723
beta adrenergic antagonist 24, 29, 30, 34
beta blockers 24, 136
beta-agonists 39, 115
beta2-agonist 88, 89, 120, 122, 129, 130
bilateral sequential transplantation 712
bilevel positive airway pressure (BiPAP) 459
biopsy 244, 417, 441, 524, 556, 689, 723, 727, 749
birth defects 97, 226, 274, 723
bitolterol 133
blood clot 396, 398, 415, 455
blood tests 162, 372, 416, 440, 441
Boeck's disease 435
bradycardia 91, 453
breast-feed 32, 33
Brethaire 133
Brethine 52
Bricanyl 52
brompheniramine maleat 221, 228
bronchial airways 19, 69, 227, 548
bronchial asthma 18, 19, 676, 677
bronchial disease 37
bronchial drainage 171, 254, 268, 297, 300, 302, 303, 724, 743, 744
bronchial pneumonia 377
bronchiectasis 181, 258, 708, 712, 713, 724, 738
bronchiolitis 22, 37, 428, 430
bronchoalveolar lavage 416, 441, 443, 444
bronchodilator 30, 39, 61, 72, 73, 88, 128,

bronchodilator, continued 135, 175, 179, 184, 425, 657, 724
bronchoscopy 5, 6, 536, 710, 725
bronchospasm 37, 42, 57, 69, 89, 133, 136, 150, 653, 725
Bronkaid Mist 133
Bronkolixir 227
bronkometer 133
Bronkotabs 227
brothers *see* family

## C

calf surfactant 431, 433, 434
camphor 228
Canadian Health Protection Branch *see* government agencies
Cancer Information Service (CIS) *see* government agencies
cardiac arrhythmias 453, 455
cardiorespiratory monitors 477
carrier screening 333-341, 344-350, 352, 354, 355, 357, 360-364
carrier status 324, 332, 337, 338, 342, 350-352, 356, 362, 364, 451
caucasians *see* ethnic groups
Centers for Disease Control and Prevention *see* government agencies
central apnea 454, 455, 459, 463
CF Research Trust 336
CFF care center 263, 264, 267, 300
CFF Home Health Service 270
cheekbrush test 324
chest physical therapy 252, 254, 255, 258, 259, 268, 292, 294
chickenpox 217, 229, 230, 233
child *see* age groups
chlorambucil 418, 443
chlorine 571, 572
chloroquine 443
ChlorTrimeton Decongestant Tablets 227
cholesterol 273, 280, 327, 366
chorionic villus biopsy 244
chronic asthmatic 35
chronic cough 8, 146, 166, 180, 181, 535
chronic hypertensive disease 93
chronic obstructive pulmonary disease 7, 8, 133, 160, 161, 168, 177-179, 407, 461, 546, 549, 577, 587, 602, 617, 630,

759

chronic obstructive pulmonary disease, continued 681, 708, 738
Churg-Strauss syndrome 25
cigarette smoking 7, 8, 59, 94, 160, 166, 168, 175, 177, 181, 184, 188, 273, 412, 470, 541, 554, 575, 576, 609, 615, 617, 624, 663, 672
ciliated cell 5
cimetidine 113
circadian rhythms 452
Civilian Health and Medical Program of the Uniformed Services 346
clemastine 221
climate 257, 280, 335
clinical insomnia 451
clubbing 248, 258, 415, 727
Co-Tylenol Cold Medication 227
coaches 73
coal miners' lungs 7
cockroach allergy 120
codeine 170, 228
colchicine 418
College of American Pathologists (CAP) see associations
Collins, Francis 315, 324, 328
compliance 463, 511, 512, 514, 519, 523, 530, 561, 562, 659, 711
complicated silicosis 576
complications 21, 30, 85, 97, 113, 217, 231-233, 235, 236, 258, 330, 381, 401, 411, 412, 460, 557, 609, 611, 677, 693, 700, 701, 709-712, 718, 721, 726, 732, 734, 742, 746
Comprehensive Smoking Education Act of 1984 616
computed tomography 416
Comtrex 227
continuous positive airway pressure 728
Cooley's Anemia 334
cooling towers 387, 390
coronaviruses 213
corpulmonale 165, 169, 259, 608
corticosteroids 30, 31, 38, 40, 41, 51, 52, 71-73, 88, 89, 110, 152, 169, 418, 442, 443, 690, 692, 728
cortisone 40, 52
cough suppressants 170, 226-228, 257, 293
coughing 8, 38, 40, 44, 45, 55, 68, 69, 71, 75, 76, 83, 85, 114, 120, 127, 128, 133,

coughing, continued 135, 160, 166, 172, 174, 179-181, 192, 227, 231, 240, 255, 257, 261, 292-294, 297, 299, 301, 302, 400, 438, 439, 498, 520, 532, 533, 536, 546, 547, 549-551, 570, 572, 573, 576, 582, 586, 629, 631, 642, 644, 653, 718, 724, 732, 734, 737, 751
coxsackieviruses 213
cromolyn sodium 29, 71, 88, 165, 407, 475, 729
cyclophosphamide 418, 443
cyclosporine-A 689
cyproheptadine 221
Cystic Fibrosis 240, 241, 243-245, 247, 248, 251, 254, 258, 260, 264, 266, 267, 269-272, 276, 277, 284, 286, 291, 292, 294, 295, 315, 320-322, 326-328, 330, 331, 333, 335, 361, 362, 364, 366, 591, 693, 708, 727, 729, 731, 738, 740, 743, 750
cytokines 444, 461, 686, 687

# D

D-penicillamine 443
day-time sleepiness 453
Decadron 52
decongestants 217, 225, 227, 229, 235, 255, 258, 729
deep sleep 450, 454, 459, 461, 721
delivery 88, 92, 96, 109, 114, 117, 163, 208, 268, 283, 338, 345, 346, 367, 429, 431, 432, 611-613, 660, 703, 704
delta F508 324, 328, 329
dental appliances 460
depression 42, 58, 418, 443, 444, 452, 453
desoxyephedrine 229
dexamethasone 169
dexbrompheniramine 228
dextromethorphan 228
diabetes 30, 56, 65, 72, 110, 136, 226, 233, 315, 352, 355, 381-383, 387, 400, 498, 519, 532, 698, 699, 701, 729, 735
diet 42, 49, 53, 174, 180, 200, 214, 267, 272-276, 279-281, 284, 286, 293, 326, 380, 381, 413, 419, 509, 627, 630, 729
dietary supplements 283
diffusing capacity 168
digestive problems 247, 291, 292, 733
digitalis 170

760

## Index

digoxin 170
dimenhydrinate 221, 222
diphenhydramine hydrochlorid 113, 221, 222, 228
diphenylpyraline 221
directly observed therapy (DOT) program 504
discrimination 333, 335, 338, 349, 355, 356
diuretics 53, 170, 259, 410
DNA 316-319, 323, 327, 330-333, 338, 339, 341, 357-360, 362, 364, 366, 367, 510, 693, 730, 747
DNase 265, 330, 331, 693, 694
Dornase alfa 330, 693
double lung transplantation 410, 707, 712
doxylamine 221, 226, 228
Dristan 227
drugs 19, 21, 23, 24, 29, 30, 33, 34, 38-42, 49, 53, 66, 67, 71, 97, 99-101, 115, 132, 133, 136, 143, 152, 154, 170, 175, 179, 184, 215, 217-219, 221, 222, 224-227, 230, 234, 256, 265, 319, 320, 326, 330, 361, 366, 380, 387, 399, 401, 403, 410, 412, 417, 423-425, 432, 443, 458, 459, 471, 493, 496, 499, 500, 502-504, 507, 511-515, 517-519, 522, 525-529, 532, 534, 656, 689, 690, 692, 693, 695, 696, 705, 718, 726, 730, 733, 737, 738, 740, 741, 744, 747, 748
dust 7, 21, 22, 28, 29, 35, 41, 42, 46, 47, 62, 64, 68, 76, 79, 81, 86, 90, 111, 116, 118, 119, 151, 166, 171, 178-180, 199, 215, 246, 251, 369-371, 373, 379, 407, 409, 415, 436, 438, 439, 541, 544-548, 552, 554-557, 559, 560, 564, 568-570, 575-577, 581, 582, 593-595, 597, 654, 688, 727, 728, 731

## E

early onset emphysema 183
echocardiogram 408
echoviruses 213
eczema 22
education 14, 73, 74, 78, 80-83, 117, 123, 126, 129, 137-142, 144-147, 156, 161, 162, 172, 262, 263, 269, 270, 334-336, 338, 343-346, 350, 362, 458, 485, 518,

education, continued 530, 616, 653, 654, 658, 660, 672, 678-681, 692, 731
electrocardiogram 401, 407
ELISA test 234
Elixophyllin 53
embolus 398, 400, 401
emphysema 7, 8, 33, 45, 63, 133, 160-162, 175-178, 181-188, 226, 227, 400, 407, 461, 549, 571, 573, 577, 587, 630, 681, 708, 711-713, 719, 738
endocrine glands 240, 731, 735
enteroviruses 213
environmental tobacco smoke (ETS) 599
enzyme replacement therapy 5, 23, 162, 247, 268, 272, 277, 278, 280, 284-286, 293, 316-320, 322, 323, 326, 514, 517, 541, 684, 717, 731, 739, 742, 750, 753
eosinophils 20, 22, 684-687
ephedrine 170, 229
epidemiology 94, 236, 522, 523, 671
epinephrine 39, 113, 133, 135
Equal Employment Opportunity Commission (EEOC) Regulations 356
erythema nodosum 436, 440, 732
erythromycin 53, 112, 113, 169, 387
ethambutol 502, 518, 732, 733
ethnic groups 255, 268
  African American 255, 268
  Alaska Natives 133, 169
  Asian 320
  caucasians 94, 139, 236, 385, 388, 468, 493, 537, 604, 652, 666, 671, 672
  European 6, 20-22, 25, 29, 32, 40-43, 45, 51, 54-58, 63, 68-72, 77, 81, 85, 112, 116, 122, 144, 147, 149, 150, 169, 171, 180, 183-185, 187, 214, 252, 254, 255, 261, 265, 293, 294, 340, 381, 392, 398, 404, 407, 408, 412, 413, 419, 573, 576, 586, 587, 611, 614, 615, 620, 624, 629, 633, 692, 743
  French Canadian 20, 23, 38, 41, 45, 46, 79, 172, 178, 179, 183, 540, 541, 545, 548, 551, 552
  Hispanics 21, 22, 40, 69, 89, 217, 222
  Italians 689
  Japanese 451
  Jews 324, 329, 334
  Native Americans 39, 40, 53, 146, 175, 196, 292, 741

## Respiratory Diseases and Disorders Sourcebook

ethnic groups, continued
   Northern European 174, 185, 265, 267, 268, 271, 272, 274, 276, 277, 279, 281, 284, 286, 371, 513, 514, 708, 727
   Orientals 241
ETS exposure 600-602
European *see* ethnic groups
exocrine glands 240, 246, 249, 731, 732
expectorants 170
eye disease 439

## F

familial emphysema 162, 175, 176, 185
family 42, 45-48, 64, 80, 121, 137, 138, 140, 141, 143, 147, 148, 155, 161, 172, 187, 234, 243, 244, 247, 248, 250, 260, 262-264, 266, 268, 269, 271-276, 280, 281, 285, 286, 301, 323, 333, 337-341, 345, 347-349, 351, 353, 354, 356, 361, 380, 406, 413, 419, 437, 446, 451, 458, 473-475, 477, 478, 480, 483, 497, 500, 504-507, 510, 557, 590, 594, 620, 621, 624, 639, 654, 655, 659, 703, 727
   brothers 171
   mothers 22, 64, 88, 93, 113, 241-243, 354, 424, 427, 432, 642, 722
   parents 22, 58, 60, 76, 77, 80, 81, 140, 222, 243, 246, 285, 291, 301, 329, 332, 343, 486, 487, 726, 734, 735
   sisters 224, 372, 674, 752
Fanconi, Dr. Guido 241
farmer's lung disease 438
female 92, 241, 243, 436, 470, 601, 608, 665
fentanyl 89
fetal complications 85, 113
fetus 50, 85, 88, 89, 93, 113, 244, 323, 334, 348, 354, 362, 364, 423, 461, 611, 720
fiberglass 557, 567-570
fibroblast growth factor 444
fibronectin 444
financial services 90, 111, 264
flu 41, 77, 117, 122, 173, 212, 220, 224, 225, 227, 229-237, 257, 261, 369, 371, 372, 380, 384, 546, 591
fluconazole 688, 689

Flumadine 234, 235
flunisolide 169
food 6, 21, 24, 33, 45, 55, 68, 122, 147, 150, 187, 194, 195, 222, 225, 231, 247, 262, 272, 274-279, 281-286, 293, 294, 320, 359, 366, 379, 388, 433, 442, 443, 551, 557, 570, 574, 614, 627, 717, 722, 729, 731, 739, 740, 742
Food and Drug Administration *see* government agencies
forced expiratory volume 86, 91, 167
forced vital capacity 167
Foundation for Asthma/Tucson Medical Center 139
French Canadian *see* ethnic groups
fungal infections 438
fungus 369-372, 379, 688

## G

gallium scanning 441
gases 3, 167, 379, 440, 540-542, 545, 547-550, 553, 571, 575, 591, 722, 728, 753
gastric stapling 460
gastroesophageal reflux 25, 26, 479
gene jumping technique 318
Genentech Inc. 331, 694
genes 175, 242, 243, 245, 246, 250, 291, 294, 316, 317, 319, 323, 324, 326, 327, 332, 366, 367, 433, 444, 445, 727, 730, 734, 735
genetic 161, 162, 175, 244, 250, 265, 291, 316, 317, 320, 321, 323, 324, 327, 329-335, 337-339, 341-356, 358-362, 366-368, 412, 427, 453, 464, 680, 681, 708, 720, 722, 723, 726, 727, 730, 734, 735, 741, 742
Genzyme Corp. 324
Georgetown University Hospital 230
germ line gene therapy 367
gestational hypertension 85, 94
Gibson, Kevin 680, 682
glucose intolerance 278
glycopyrrolate 89
gold 575, 689
government agencies 139, 544
   Canadian Health Protection Branch 7, 8, 45, 181, 273, 274, 317, 355, 366, 387, 399, 400, 403, 437, 438, 498,

# Index

government agencies, continued
  Canadian Health Protection Branch, continued 510, 541, 542, 545, 554, 556, 557, 560, 568, 577, 599-601, 604, 605, 607, 608, 610, 611, 615, 616, 630, 637, 638, 641, 645-647, 661, 663, 665, 671, 675-677, 680, 681, 702, 738, 739
  Cancer Information Service (CIS) 221
  Centers for Disease Control and Prevention 94, 139, 236, 385, 388, 468, 493, 537, 604, 652, 666, 671, 672
  Food and Drug Administration 53
  Mine Safety & Health Administration (MSHA) 575
  National Center for Human Genome Research 39, 40, 53, 146, 175, 196, 292, 741
  National Center for Nursing Research 14, 73, 74, 83, 117, 123, 126, 129, 137, 140-142, 145-147, 156
  National Center for Research Resources (NCRR) 39, 40, 53, 146, 175, 196, 292, 741
  National Heart Lung and Blood Institute (NHLBI) 566
  National Institute for Occupational Safety and Health (NIOSH) 14, 73, 74, 83, 117, 123, 126, 129, 137, 140-142, 145-147, 156
  National Institute of Diabetes and Digestive and Kidney Disease (NIDDKD) 14, 73, 74, 83, 117, 123, 126, 129, 137, 140-142, 145-147, 156
  National Institutes of Health (NIH) 14, 73, 74, 83, 117, 123, 126, 129, 137, 140-142, 145-147, 156
  Occupational Safety and Health Administration (OSHA) 540, 557, 564, 566, 576, 665
  Office of Educational Research and Improvement 711
  Office of Technology Assessment 711
  Office on Smoking and Health (OSH) 711
  Pharmacopoeia 463
  Public Health Service's Advisory Committee on Immunization 689
  Surgeon General 463

government agencies, continued
  U.S. Department of Education 463
  U.S. Department of Energy (DOE) 463
  U.S. Department of Health and Human Services 463
granulomas 435, 438-441, 443, 516, 517, 734
granulomatous diseases 438
Greenfield filter 402
grief 470, 474, 480, 481
grinder's rot 575

# H

hay fever 22, 35, 144, 222, 747
HEPA filters high-efficiency particulate activating filters *see* air purifying devices
heart 3, 4, 6, 7, 14, 24, 30, 39, 53, 57, 63, 65-67, 70, 71, 73, 74, 86, 87, 91, 136, 137, 139, 148, 160, 164, 165, 169, 170, 174, 176, 178, 184, 226, 255, 258, 259, 266, 273, 327, 378, 381-383, 387, 398-402, 404-413, 415, 419, 420, 425, 427, 429, 430, 434, 437-440, 442, 443, 446, 449, 450, 453, 455-457, 461, 464-466, 468, 477, 486-488, 491, 556, 573, 574, 576, 607, 608, 610, 615, 629, 630, 636, 638, 641, 646, 647, 666, 680, 682, 693, 699, 707, 708, 712, 720-723, 725, 728, 734, 735, 738, 753
hemoptysis 259, 734
heredity 37, 160, 242, 243, 272, 317, 414, 437, 677, 727, 734
Hidalgo, Humberto 654, 656
high blood pressure 39, 67, 72, 127, 136, 226, 273, 274, 327, 408, 415, 443, 453, 456, 736, 745
high-frequency ventilator 424-426
Hispanics *see* ethnic groups
histoplasma capsulatum 369
histoplasmosis 369-373
HIV 233, 234, 382, 383, 498-502, 507, 511-517, 519, 521-523, 525-528, 530-536, 699, 701, 735, 736
home care 270
home oxygen therapy 168
Hong Kong flu 235
Hospital for Sick Children in Toronto 315, 328

763

humidifier *see* air purifying devices
humidity conditions *see* air purifying devices
Hutchinson's disease 435
hyaline membrane disease 422, 424, 431, 432
hygiene 381, 508, 748
hygrometer 592
hyper-coagulable 399
hyperemesis gravidarum 85, 93
hypersensitivity 7, 37, 438, 444, 516, 542, 546, 548, 690
hypertension 85, 93, 94, 110, 404, 405, 407-413, 415, 418, 464, 466, 708, 712, 713, 736, 745
hyperthyroidism 25, 27
hyperventilation 25, 38, 90, 463, 736
hypnagogic hallucinations 451
hypotension 88, 91, 113, 410, 736
hypoxia 85, 88, 91, 93, 452, 465, 736

# I

ibuprofen 23, 42, 326
idiopathic 21, 25, 414, 415, 417-419
IgE 21-23, 30, 111
illegal drugs 49, 53, 471
immunological inertness 443
immunoreactive trypsinogen test 250
immunotherapy 31, 87, 653
Indiana University Medical Center 424
indomethacin 23
indoor air pollutants 582
infant *see* age groups
infection 5, 9, 22, 23, 25, 26, 33, 37, 41, 52, 72, 111, 112, 165, 169, 179, 180, 184, 185, 212, 214-216, 218, 219, 233, 234, 251-253, 255-257, 262, 276, 320, 326, 327, 370, 372, 373, 376, 378-380, 382, 383, 386, 393, 414, 415, 428-431, 440, 445, 471, 477, 487, 496-502, 507, 511, 515-517, 519-522, 524, 525, 527-530, 535, 536, 577, 586, 601, 674, 690, 696, 698, 699, 701-703, 709, 710, 718, 719, 724, 726, 727, 735-739, 741, 743-745, 748-752
influenza 112, 173, 180, 185, 213, 216, 217, 231-237, 257, 376, 378, 380, 554, 609, 704, 747, 753

inhalation therapy 174, 718
inhaled steroids 34, 41, 52, 123, 169
inhaler 39-42, 48, 49, 51-53, 56, 60, 61, 64, 66, 72, 114, 123-126, 134-136, 189, 227
injections 36, 224, 685
insulin 110, 278, 464, 698, 729, 735, 742
insurance 274, 300, 301, 333, 346-349, 351-354, 356, 357
interferon 218, 528
interleukin-1 462
interleukin-2 444
intermittent positive pressure breathing 737
International Asthma Management Project 692, 693
intracellular adhesion molecule-1 219
ipratropium 52, 169
irritant gases 571, 575
ischemia 609, 710-712
isoetharine 133
isoniazid (INH) 502, 518, 523, 738
isoproterenol 133, 169
Isuprel 133
Italians *see* ethnic groups

# J

Japanese *see* ethnic groups
Jews *see* ethnic groups

# K

ketamine 89
Kendig, James W. 431
kinins 215, 219
Kveim test 441, 442

# L

labor 87-89, 91, 96, 97, 108, 114, 117, 360, 560, 562
lactation 97
lamina propria 20
latency test 457, 466, 467
Latin America 499, 500, 507
legionella 386-391, 393
Legionnaires' disease 386-390

# Index

life expectancy 264, 361, 593, 608, 675, 726
lobar pneumonia 376
Lp-1 antigen 392
lung cancer 7, 8, 45, 181, 400, 541, 542, 545, 554, 556, 560, 568, 600, 601, 604, 607, 608, 630, 647, 663, 675-677, 680, 681, 738
lung hazards in the workplace 540
lycoperdonosis 690
lymph glands 440
lymphoma 438, 698, 701, 739

# M

macrophages 5, 444, 445, 514-516
magnesium sulfate 89
major basic protein (MBP) 684
Mala, Theodore 674, 675
male 92, 241, 243, 436, 470, 608, 665, 752
Malveaux, Floyd 656, 658
Mantoux test 517, 739, 745, 746, 752
mast cells 21, 22
Maternal and Child Health (MCH) Block Grant (Public Law 97-35) 346
maternal hypoxemia 87, 113
maternal serum alpha-fetoprotein (MSAFP) screening 337
maternal smoking 479, 602, 611
Maxair 133
mechanical aids 254
Medicaid 346, 349
medical equipment 196, 300
medical expenses 361
medical records 50, 144, 353
Medicare 232, 346, 382-384, 703
medications 25-27, 29, 31, 32, 38, 41, 42, 49-53, 58, 59, 64-67, 76, 77, 79, 81, 85-88, 94, 100, 111, 142, 144, 145, 147, 149, 151, 152, 169, 194, 213, 217, 224, 226, 228, 258, 261-263, 265, 270, 286, 293, 451, 458, 459, 652-654, 659, 692, 728
Medihaler 133
meningitis 383, 516, 694-698
menthol 228
menus 276, 286, 627
meperidine 170

mesothelioma 554, 556
metaprel 52
metaproterenol 133, 169
metered-dose inhaler 114, 123, 126, 134
methacholine sensitivity 96
methotrexate 443, 689
methylprednisolone 89
methylprednisone 52
methylxanthines 29, 30, 169, 170
middle age *see* age groups
Mine Safety & Health Administration (MSHA) *see* government agencies
minorities 512, 530, 652, 656, 676, 677, 681, 682
mists 541, 542, 545, 551
mixed apnea 455
monitoring 29, 31, 70, 76, 86-88, 100, 110, 153, 263, 431, 477, 478, 492, 672
monoclonal antibody subtype (MAS) 391
morbidity 93, 94, 161, 386, 390, 393, 428, 452, 609, 655, 671, 672, 680, 681, 684, 692, 695-697, 717, 740
morphine 170
mortality 7, 17, 18, 85, 93, 94, 146, 161, 386, 390, 393, 426, 428, 430, 432, 452, 460, 475-477, 485, 493, 609, 617, 652, 660, 662, 663, 666, 671, 672, 675, 676, 680, 681, 684, 692, 697, 717, 740
mothers *see* family
Mothers of Asthmatics 255
mucosal membranes 28
mucous glands 20, 246, 732
mucus 5, 19, 20, 25, 26, 29, 30, 37, 38, 40, 44, 52, 53, 59, 63, 69, 117, 146, 161, 163, 170, 177, 179, 181, 214, 215, 227, 240, 246-248, 251-255, 257-259, 261, 265, 277, 291-295, 297, 299, 315, 320, 322, 326, 548, 556, 568, 571, 592, 719, 722, 724, 725, 728, 731, 732, 739, 740, 742-744, 746, 749
multi-drug-resistant TB (MDR TB) 507
multiple sleep latency test 457, 467
mycobacterium tuberculosis 496, 510, 512, 523
mycoplasma pneumonia 379, 380
mycotoxicosis 547

# N

naproxen 42, 326
narcolepsy 451, 457, 466-468
nasal polyposis 23
National Asthma Education Program 74, 83
National Center for Human Genome Research *see* government agencies
National Center for Nursing Research *see* government agencies
National Center for Research Resources (NCRR) *see* government agencies
National Heart Lung and Blood Institute (NHLBI) *see* government agencies
National Institute for Occupational Safety and Health (NIOSH) *see* government agencies
National Institute of Diabetes and Digestive and Kidney Disease (NIDDKD) *see* government agencies
National Institutes of Health (NIH) *see* government agencies
National Jewish Center for Immunology and Respiratory Medicine *see* associations
Native Americans *see* ethnic groups
nephrotic syndrome 698, 699, 701
neutrophils 20
newborns 97, 161, 250, 331, 424, 427, 432, 456
nitrogen dioxide 549, 571, 573, 574
non-familial emphysema 162
non-REM stages 450
nonprescription drug 217, 224, 225, 227
Northern European *see* ethnic groups
Nyquil 227

# O

obesity 273, 453, 456, 459, 460, 464, 465
obstructive sleep apnea 454
Occupational Safety and Health Administration (OSHA) *see* government agencies
occupational lung problems 677
Office of Educational Research and Improvement *see* government agencies
Office of Technology Assessment *see* government agencies
Office on Smoking and Health (OSH) *see* government agencies
Open Airways for Schools 144
open lung biopsy 417, 689
oral corticosteroids 41, 52
oral steroids 52
Orenstein, Jan M. 400
Orientals *see* ethnic groups
orthomyxoviruses 213
osmolar agents 230
osteoporosis 30
Otulana, Tunde 71
oximetry 466, 710
oxtriphylline 30
Oxygen therapy 168, 169, 174, 259, 459
oxytocin 89
ozone 28, 185, 571, 573, 585-587

# P

Packard Children's Hospital at Stanford 429
pain 9, 23, 40, 44, 66, 69, 112, 136, 170, 181, 214, 224, 320, 331, 372, 378, 380, 383, 384, 386, 396, 399, 400, 407, 409, 439, 443, 498, 501, 503, 510, 517, 532, 556, 574, 576, 586, 694, 701, 720, 737, 742, 751
pancreas 241, 247, 277, 278, 320, 322, 328, 332, 608, 729-731, 733, 735, 742, 750, 754
parainfluenza 22, 213, 230, 402, 440, 451, 550
paramyxoviruses 213
paraoxonase (PON) 317
parasympathomimetics 169
parents *see* family
peak expiratory flow rat 31, 86
peak flow meter 31, 48, 50, 66, 76, 80, 115, 126-128, 142, 149, 153, 154
penicillamine 418, 443
percussion 172, 297-299, 302
perfusion lung scan 408
perinatal 85, 93, 94, 612, 672
peripartum 91, 92
personal protective equipment 544
pets 28, 42, 47, 120, 484

# Index

phagocytes 371
pharmacist 61, 64, 152, 221
pharmacokinetics 97, 99, 528
Pharmacopoeia *see* government agencies
phenindamine 221, 228
phenylbutazone 23
phenylephrine hydrochloride 229
phosgene 541, 571-573
pirbuterol 133
pneumococcal bacteremia 697-700
pneumococcal pneumonia 180, 184, 185, 379-384, 697, 698
pneumococcal vaccine 382-384, 698-700, 702-704
pneumococcusis 377
pneumocystis carinii pneumonia (PCP) 379
pneumonia 37, 173, 180, 184, 185, 231, 235, 248, 252, 292, 320, 326, 376-384, 386, 388-393, 400, 517, 521, 554, 577, 586, 601, 609, 611, 612, 617, 641, 676, 694, 697-700, 738, 743, 747, 753
pneumothorax 259, 425, 433, 508, 743
pollen 21, 22, 28, 35, 42, 45, 48, 62, 64, 68-70, 72, 76, 111, 118, 215, 581
pollution 37, 41, 45, 48, 62, 160, 173, 177, 183, 185, 202, 540, 574, 585-588
polymerase chain reaction 362, 518, 525
polysaccharide antigens 698
polysomnography 457, 458, 466, 467, 743
portable oxygen unit 196, 413
positive-pressure air-supplied respirators 553
postnatal 602
postural bronchial drainage 171, 744
potter's asthma 575
PPD-skin test reactivity 523
PPH-patient registry 411
prednisone 52, 326, 387, 418, 442
preeclampsia 85, 93
pregnancy 25, 26, 85-87, 89-94, 96, 97, 99-107, 110-116, 126, 147, 153, 154, 233, 241, 246, 274, 276, 323, 337, 342, 343, 347, 349, 354, 364, 412, 413, 419, 445, 446, 470, 602, 611-613, 666, 667, 702, 727
prenatal 92, 244, 247, 265, 334, 337, 345, 348, 354, 362-365, 471, 720, 727, 744
Prescription Drug User Fee Act 330, 693
preterm labor 89, 97

preventive therapy 497, 501, 502, 507, 519, 520, 738, 744, 750
primary atypical pneumonia 379
primary pulmonary hypertension 405, 410-412, 708
Primatene Mist 133
professional education 345
promethazine hydrochloride 227
propoxyphene 170
propylhexedrine 229
prostacycline 410, 411
prostaglandins 23, 461, 744
protective equipment 544, 570, 578
Proventil 52, 133
pseudoephedrine hydrochlorid 111-113, 229
psittacosis 379
Public Health Service's Advisory Committee on Immunization *see* government agencies
pulmonary artery 4, 401, 404, 405, 409, 412, 709, 711, 712, 723, 745, 753
pulmonary edema 93, 549, 573
pulmonary embolism 396, 398-403
pulmonary function tests 5, 86, 252, 253, 268, 408, 416, 440, 457, 745
Pulmozyme 331, 694
purified protein derivative (PPD) 532, 744-746
pyrazinamide 502, 518, 528, 705, 732, 733, 746, 747
pyrilamine 221, 228

## Q

Q fever 379
Quibron 53

## R

radioactive materials 540, 541
radioimmunoassay 389, 391, 698
ragweed 21, 22, 42
rapid-eye-movement sleep (REM) 450
Raynaud's disease 406
recipes 195, 283, 626
recreation 207
regulation 227, 228, 278, 347, 357, 359, 360, 445, 461, 590, 744

relaxation techniques 55, 171, 634
REM 450, 457, 459, 461, 463, 741, 746
research 7, 34, 73, 74, 97, 139, 141, 142, 168, 174, 176, 182, 184, 187, 214, 215, 218, 219, 242, 246, 265, 266, 269, 270, 291, 294, 315-317, 319, 320, 323, 327, 333, 336, 350, 382, 398, 412, 413, 417, 419, 423, 427, 428, 431, 434, 437, 443-446, 450, 451, 461-466, 485, 508-510, 514, 521, 522, 524-527, 529-531, 559, 562, 586, 600, 603, 605, 614, 615, 656, 677, 680, 684, 686-688, 721, 723, 727, 736, 751
residual volume 91, 167, 745
respirator 424, 546-549, 551, 552, 570, 572-574, 577, 735
Respiratory Club at Gaylord Hospital 188
respiratory distress syndrome 422, 424
respiratory syncytial virus (RSV) 428
respiratory therapy 140, 195
restriction fragment length polymorphism (RFLP) 316
retin-A 53
Reye's syndrome 217, 229, 230, 233
rheumatic fever 438, 675
rhinitis 22, 29, 110-112, 147, 150, 594
rhinoviruses 213, 215, 216, 218, 219
ribavirin 428-431
rickettsia 379, 380
rifampin 502-504, 518, 519, 528, 534, 705, 732, 733, 740, 747
rifater 705
right-heart cardiac catheterization 409
risk factors 86, 87, 160, 174, 398, 470, 602, 676, 677, 681, 744, 746, 752
Rocky Mountain spotted fever 379

# S

di Sant-Agnese, Dr. Paul 316
salicylates 233
Sander, Nancy 36
sarcoidosis 435-447, 677, 678, 680, 681
sedatives 170, 224
serum antibody titer 391, 393
sex 15, 128, 147, 189, 243, 275, 276, 278, 279, 321, 327, 391, 392, 662-664
sexual dysfunction 453
short-course chemotherapy 518

sickle cell anemia 334, 335, 381, 677, 702
side effects 30, 31, 40, 41, 49, 52, 53, 71, 72, 74, 76, 81, 123, 135, 143, 152, 170, 183, 217, 218, 222-224, 226, 233, 235, 331, 372, 383, 384, 418, 433, 443, 459, 460, 503-505, 507, 512, 518, 659, 694, 701
SIDS 456, 470-480, 484, 485, 493, 494, 602
silicosis 498, 552, 575-577
Silo Filler's Disease 549
silo gas 549, 550
simple silicosis 576, 577
single lung transplantation 707, 711, 712
sinusitis 25, 26, 110, 112, 113, 217, 258, 701, 747, 748
skin rashes 135, 436
skin sarcoidosis 438, 439
skin tests 449, 465, 466
sisters *see* family
sleep apnea 449, 451-461, 463-467
apnea 449-461, 463-467, 470, 475, 476, 478, 486-493, 721
sleep paralysis 451
sleep-inducing substance 450
sleeping pills 66, 170, 224, 453, 458
sleeping position 479, 480
sleepy patient 450
slit-lamp examination 442
Slo-Phyllin 53
Slobid 53
smoke 9, 20, 33, 41, 45, 46, 48, 53, 58, 59, 62-64, 67, 68, 77, 87, 116, 121, 160-162, 173, 178, 180, 181, 183, 184, 186, 187, 206, 387, 399, 403, 419, 445, 540-542, 545, 550, 553, 556, 557, 570, 574, 575, 578, 599-604, 608, 611-614, 620-623, 625, 626, 629-636, 641-647, 656, 660, 663-665, 667, 668, 677-680, 727, 728
smoker's emphysema 162
Smith, David W. 428
snoring 449-451, 453, 455, 456, 460, 464, 465
somatic cell therapy 366, 367
Somophyllin 53
Southeast Asia 507
spinhaler 40
spirometer 86, 167, 440, 748
spores 46, 111, 370-373, 541, 546, 547, 689, 690

# Index

sports 42, 43, 49, 57, 68, 81, 82, 149, 255, 567, 644
sputum 8, 9, 22, 160, 161, 165, 166, 169, 174, 252, 253, 259, 299, 378, 379, 386, 389, 498, 510, 515, 517, 521, 523, 524, 533, 536, 556, 573, 576, 616, 695, 717, 733, 734, 737, 743, 749
staphylococcus aureus 252, 723, 749
statistics 14, 36, 37, 139, 146, 156, 212, 422, 451, 471, 472, 485, 671, 672, 674, 675
steroids 31, 34, 40, 41, 52, 110, 115, 123, 151, 169, 265, 654, 659, 688, 711
stonecutter's disease 575
stopping smoking 7, 8, 33, 48, 53, 59, 64, 67, 94, 116, 121, 160-162, 164, 166, 168, 172, 174, 175, 177-181, 183, 184, 186-188, 204, 206, 227, 273, 403, 412, 413, 465, 470, 479, 541, 544, 546, 553-557, 570, 571, 575-577, 598, 600-604, 607-617, 619, 621-626, 629-639, 641-647, 652, 656, 660-673, 676-680
streptococcus pneumoniae 694, 697
streptokinase 401
streptomycin 502, 509, 733, 750
stress 26, 32, 45, 58, 64, 147, 192, 201, 214, 269, 364, 407, 412, 464, 484, 492, 615, 636
students 56, 73-82, 154, 233, 267, 270, 286, 291, 544
submucous glands 20
substance abuse 498
Sudafed Plus 227
sudden infant death syndrome (SIDS) 602
Sudden Infant Death Syndrome Alliance *see* associations
sulfur dioxide 178, 571, 572
supplied-air respirators 544, 549, 572, 573
support groups 140, 413, 638
surfactant 422-425, 427, 431-434
Surgeon General *see* government agencies
surgery 6, 259, 373, 396, 399, 402, 403, 417, 460, 464, 508, 611, 709, 711
Sutter Memorial Hospital 428, 430
sweat glands 240, 246, 249, 250, 316, 328, 721
sweat test 247, 249, 250, 316, 321, 322,

sweat test, continued 732, 733, 750
Symmetrel 234, 235
sympathomimetics 169, 170
symptoms 6, 8, 9, 22, 25-28, 31, 32, 34, 38, 40-42, 44-46, 48, 49, 51, 54, 55, 59, 60, 63-65, 69-71, 73, 75, 76, 82, 85-88, 90, 96, 110, 111, 113-118, 129, 130, 132, 133, 135, 142, 147, 149, 151, 160, 162, 164, 166, 168, 172, 178, 182-188, 194, 212-215, 217-219, 222-226, 228-231, 233, 234, 242, 243, 247-250, 252, 253, 272, 273, 292, 294, 315, 320-323, 326-328, 351, 354, 361, 370-372, 378, 379, 381, 386, 396, 399, 400, 402, 406, 407, 409, 412, 414, 415, 435, 436, 438-440, 442, 445, 451-455, 479, 481, 496-498, 501, 503, 504, 516, 517, 521, 524, 528, 532, 533, 535, 537, 546-549, 551, 555, 556, 573, 574, 576-578, 586, 600-602, 610, 614-616, 620, 629, 630, 641, 653, 657, 685, 690, 692, 721, 722, 724, 726, 729, 735, 738, 742, 750, 751
synthetic human surfactant 427
Szefler, Stanley 70

# T

T-cells 443-445, 686
T-lymphocytes 443, 444
tachypnea 90
Taggart, Virginia 660
Tay-Sachs disease 334, 509
TB control strategies 511
TB research 514, 522, 527, 529, 530
TB transmission 513, 514, 522, 534
TB-related clinical trials 527
teenagers *see* age groups
teens 43, 45, 46, 56, 62, 229, 668
terbutaline 133, 169
terfenadine 221
tetracycline 169, 720
theophylline 30, 39, 41, 52, 53, 99, 100, 152, 169, 227
therapy 30, 39, 76, 85-89, 99, 111-113, 140, 154, 168-170, 174, 176, 195, 252-256, 258, 259, 261, 265, 268, 277, 279, 285, 292-294, 301, 320, 327, 328, 361, 366-368, 396, 401, 428, 431-434, 442, 458, 459, 465, 477, 497, 501, 502, 504, 505, 507, 512, 518-521, 527, 528, 532,

therapy, continued 534, 658, 659, 686, 688, 690, 692, 695-697, 702, 708, 718, 724, 729, 730, 736-738, 742-745, 747, 750
third trimester 86, 90-92, 337
Thomas, Alvin 676, 678
thorax 3, 5
thrombus 398
thrush 41, 52, 72
tissue plasminogen activator 401
tocolytic therapy 89
Tornalate 133
total lung capacity 91, 167, 745
toxemia 85, 93
trachea 4-6, 19, 37, 315, 432, 455, 460, 711, 719, 725, 727, 747
tracheobronchial tree 4, 6
tracheostomy 460, 751
tranquilizers 49, 53, 66, 170, 224
transmission 215, 216, 390, 392, 393, 510, 511, 513-515, 522, 531, 534, 674, 728, 732, 733, 735, 751
travel 6, 43, 48, 50, 60, 64-67, 81, 90, 114, 173, 198, 204, 205, 222, 254, 400, 402, 581, 603, 658, 747
treatment centers 139, 143
triamcinolone 169
trichophyton 688
trigger 21-23, 25-27, 32, 37, 40-42, 45-48, 50, 57-59, 69, 72, 81, 82, 117, 118, 414, 437, 445, 573, 582, 596, 632, 635, 688
trimethoprim-sulfamethoxazole 169
tripelennamine 111, 221
triprolidine 221, 228
trypsin 322, 719
trypsinogen 250, 322
Tsui, Lap-Chee 317, 328
tubercle bacillus 514
tuberculin 499, 516, 517, 519, 521, 532, 737, 739, 744-746, 751, 752
tuberculosis 45, 181, 219, 369, 371, 372, 379, 438, 496, 508, 510-517, 520, 521, 523-525, 529, 531, 532, 537, 560, 577, 674, 676, 680, 681, 705, 717, 718, 721, 722, 724, 728, 730-733, 735-740, 744-747, 749, 751-753
typhus 379

## U

University of Alabama Hospital 146
University of California 673
University of Iowa Hospitals and Clinics 70
University of Michigan 315, 318, 328
University of Utah 317, 323
uridine triphosphate (UTP) 327
urokinase 401
U.S. Department of Education *see* government agencies
U.S. Department of Energy (DOE) *see* government agencies
U.S. Department of Health and Human Services *see* government agencies

## V

vaccines 232, 233, 235, 265, 475, 520, 522, 524, 529
vaginal hemorrhage 85, 93
Vanceril 51
vaporizer 226, 590
vapors 540-543, 545, 548, 551, 553, 568
vasculitis 21, 25
vasoconstrictor 111
vasodilator 410, 753
vasomotor rhinitis 110-112
venogram 399
ventilation systems 543, 570, 582, 735, 752
ventilator 423-426, 429, 432, 598, 728
Ventolin 52, 133
vibration 297, 298, 302
Vicks Vaporub 227
vincristine sulfate 418
viokase 326
viral pneumonia 378, 380, 383, 384, 753
viral upper respiratory infection 37, 111, 112
Virchow, Rudolf 396
Virchow's triad 398
virus 22, 213, 215-219, 231-235, 327, 367, 378, 414, 428, 437, 444, 445, 498, 511, 512, 531, 735, 752, 753
vitamin C 217, 218
vitamins 262, 268, 274, 281, 283, 293, 753

volunteers 523, 528, 536

# W

warfarin 401
weight loss 252, 273, 436, 498, 532, 556, 576, 751
Western Blot test 234
wheezing 35, 38, 45, 50, 55, 59, 63, 68, 69, 75, 76, 83, 85, 113, 114, 120, 127, 128, 133, 135, 166, 187, 248, 252, 292, 400, 550, 568, 570, 586, 601, 616, 642, 653, 750
Weiler, John 70
World Health Organization (WHO) 521
wrongful birth 342
wrongful life 342, 343

# X

x-ray crystallography 218
x-rays 5, 6, 176, 326, 372, 416, 440, 467, 517, 521, 524, 533, 556, 726, 752